PAEDIATRIC ORTHOPAEDIC TRAUMA

Protocols and Techniques

PAEDIATRIC ORTHOPAEDIC TRAUMA
Protocols and Techniques

Binoti Sheth

M.S. Othopaedics, D.N.B., F.C.P.S., D. Ortho

Fellowship
Paediatric Orthopaedics
UK

Associate Professor and Head of Unit
Department of Orthopaedics
Lokmanya Tilak Municipal Medical College
Sion
Mumbai

Sandeep Vaidya

M.S. Othopaedics, D.N.B., D. Ortho
MRCSEd (UK)

Fellowship
Paediatric Orthopaedics
Korea, Singapore

Consultant Paediatric Orthopaedic Surgeon
Pinnacle Orthocentre Hospital
Thane

Bai Jerbai Wadia Hospital for Children
Mumbai

Jupiter Hospital
Thane

Mandar Agashe

M.S. Othopaedics

Fellowship
Paediatric Orthopaedics
India, Korea, USA

Consultant Paediatric Orthopaedic Surgeon
AGASHE Hospital
Kurla, Mumbai

SRCC children's Hospital
Haji Ali, Mumbai

Assistant Honorary Consultant
BJ Wadia Hospital
Mumbai

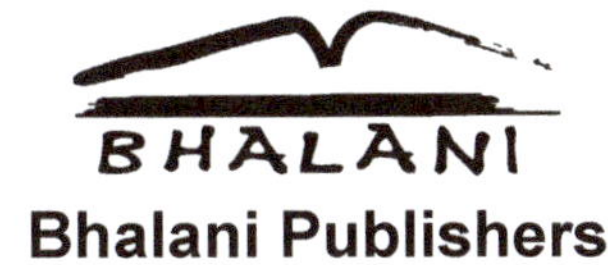

Bhalani Publishers

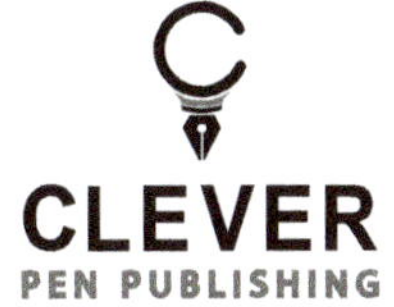

First Edition: 2021

Published by:

BHALANI PUBLISHERS and
Clever Pen Publishing
(A joint venture between Bhalani Publishers and National Medical Book House)
D-2 Neelkanth Business Park Co-op. Premises Society Lt.
Nathani Road
Vidyavihar (West)
Mumbai 400086
Mob.: 09867214519

Email:
bhalanipublishers@gmail.com
cleverpen9@gmail.com

ISBN 978-93-83794-11-9

Printed & Bound in India

PREFACE

Orthopaedic trauma in children is an immensely fulfilling experience to the clinician with the tremendous remodelling potential of the child leading to magical healing and correction of many post-traumatic deformities. However, it is a difficult and challenging field, as well. The often-used adage "A child is NOT a miniature adult" is especially true in this aspect with many ill-chosen, unindicated and poorly performed surgeries with "adult" orthopaedic principles doing more harm than good. The child with limb trauma presents with certain unique problems which require a different protocol for management, which is many a time not given in standard orthopaedic textbooks.

With this as a backdrop, we, the authors of this book have attempted to make a concise textbook for all orthopaedic surgeons who are interested in, and routinely perform Paediatric trauma as a part of their day-to-day practice. This textbook takes the clinician right from the diagnosis of a particular fracture or injury, its classification, diagnosis and the various modalities of management in a precise protocolised manner. The text is well-illustrated with surgical diagrams including positioning, key steps and method of fixation, making it ideal for the busy practitioner who wants a quick refresher before starting the surgery. It also contains adequate number of pre-operative and post-operative radiographs showing standard methods of treatment.

We, the authors are uniquely qualified in attempting this task. All three of us are attached to major teaching hospitals with busy paediatric trauma work along with our private practice with an almost equal number of patients but with slightly different expectations and demands. We have made this textbook with a lot of care and research trying to encompass standard teaching and steps with the authors' own unique tips and tricks, finally summing up with a flowchart to help the surgeon manage the patient in a systematic manner. We hope that this textbook becomes a standard text for all orthopaedic surgeons, junior or senior, when dealing with a child with limb trauma.

Thank you all and Happy reading!!

Dr. Binoti Sheth
Dr. Sandeep Vaidya
Dr. Mandar Agashe

FOREWORD

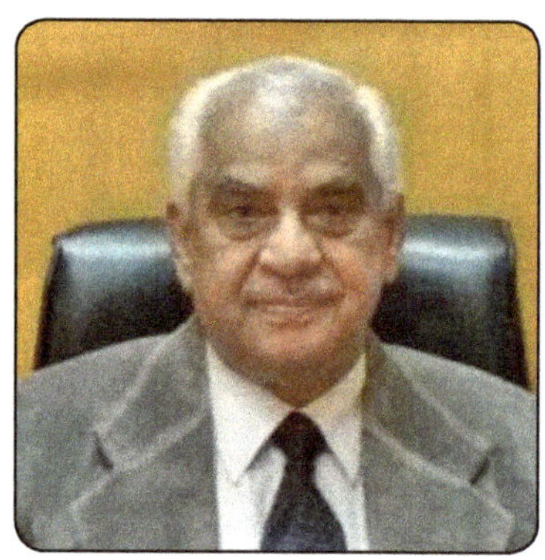

Dr. Nandkishore S. Laud Awarded Padma Bhushan by President
M.S. (Orth.), F.R.C.S (ENG), D.Sc (Hon)

Ex- Professor and Head
Department of Orthopaedics
LTMG Hospital and LTMM College, Sion

Ex- President
Indian Orthopaedic Association
Maharashtra Orthopaedic Association
Indian Society for Surgery of Hand
Bombay Orthopaedic Society

It was a pleasant surprise when Mandar met me on behalf of Binoti and Sandeep and asked me to write a few words for their book on "Pediatric Orthopedic Trauma - Protocols and Techniques".

I looked at this as an opportunity to revisit the challenges facing orthopedic surgeons in managing Pediatric Orthopedic trauma. Going through the pages of the book, I noticed the rapid changes happening in the past few decades. The old dictum was - "reduce the fracture, immobilize it, relieve pain and the fracture will heal. In case of loss of alignment, the remodeling will correct it." Now, this no longer holds true.

Few things are worth mentioning in this book; There is a sea-change in presentations of Pediatric trauma, mainly due to increased level of sporting activity in children, desire to compete and attain perfection in sports like gymnastics and athletics.

Today, Pediatric trauma forms more than 50% of cases presenting to orthopaedic surgeons. Need to arrive at a correct diagnosis, initiate specific therapy and aim to achieve excellent results is mandatory. The squeal of improper diagnosis and inadequate treatment may lead to life-long disability, altered function and it may even affect the child's personality.

The book illustrates the role of proper history taking, clinical assessment and adequate radiological examination. In injuries involving growth plates, the role of CT scan and MRI cannot be overstressed. The chapter on the role of arthrography in epiphyseal injuries explains its importance in diagnosis and planning specific treatment. I was impressed by the sketches which bring clarity to the clinical case presentations and convince one the role of proper protocol to follow. The often quoted phrase, " A child is not a half man" is true ! However, in injuries to pelvis, spine and hip and their etiology, presentation and management is almost the same as in adult trauma.

The design and availability of elastic nails, especially titanium, low profile implants and well-designed instrumentation make the surgeon's life comfortable. The book makes easy reading, has clarity in understanding and gives us ability to solve a problem because of its content. Even after many years in active orthopaedic practice, I learnt a lot and got over confusion and misconceptions about paediatric trauma issues from this book.

In my opinion, this book is a must in every institutional library and a ready reference book for an orthopedic surgeon. I am convinced that the orthopaedic surgeons referring to this book will be able to prevent post-trauma deformities or shortening, give assured results, and will lead to many happy patients and grateful parents.

With great appreciation,

Dr. Nandkishore S. Laud

FOREWORD

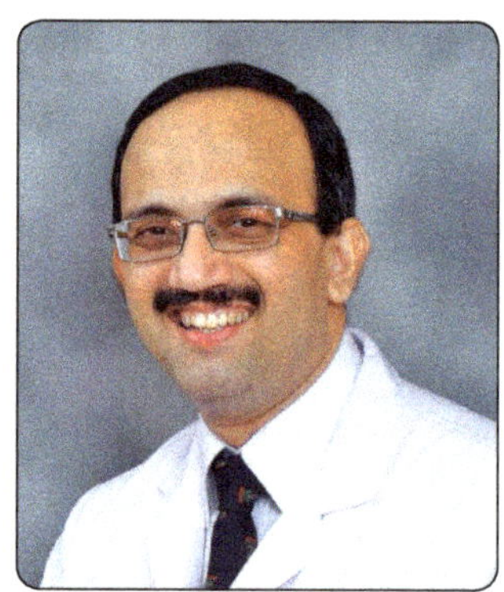

Dr. Sandeep Patwardhan
Paediatric Orthopaedic surgeon
Professor, Orthopaedics
Sancheti Institute for Orthopaedics and Rehabilitation
Director (IFICS) International Fractures in Children Symposium Foundation

Paediatric fractures? Why does one need a text book? They all heal and remodel well!!!!

This would be the common response from most Orthopaedic Surgeons for long and it was no different when I did my Post graduate training in 1992-1995.

But as time passed and I specialised in Paediatric Orthopaedics, I realised the importance of treating Paediatric fractures well.

The fractures came in all shapes and sizes, from neonates to adolescents, from Intra articular to Physeal, from diaphyseal to metaphyseal, from normal bones to pathological bones, from operative to conservative, from acceptable to unacceptable, from rural to urban, from fresh to neglected and so on.....

It was imperative that we discussed them and rationalised treatment plans for the Indian situation.

Inspired by Dr. Kaye Wilkins the 1st attempt was via IFICS started in 2013 where we conducted a conference on Children's fractures the 1st time in India and realised that it was important to train practising General Orthopods as well as Pedipods in nuances of Paediatric Trauma care.

The next step was a comprehensive text on Paediatric Orthopaedic trauma, a need which is fulfilled by this beautiful textbook compiled by my friends Mandar, Sandeep and Binoti.

I am honoured to be writing a foreword to this superb textbook.

It was a pleasure to read the well thought out textbook, replete with charts, diagrams and pictures highlighting all aspects of Children's fractures put together in a simple and concise way.

It gives the reader a complete approach to identifying, examining and treating all Paediatric fractures, with tips and tricks to avoid complications.

This text book fulfils a long standing void in Orthopaedic literature of an Indian text with a universal appeal, useful for PGs, as well as consultants.

I congratulate Dr. Mandar Agashe, Dr. Sandeep Vaidya and Dr. Binoti Sheth for producing this masterpiece, and predict that it will become a best seller and THE reference book for Children's fractures.

Best wishes and happy reading.....

Dr. Sandeep Patwardhan

ACKNOWLEDGEMENTS

Writing, collating, coordinating and finalizing a book of this nature is never easy and requires help from various quarters. Over the course of a year and a half, that we spent writing this book, we were helped by many people in various ways, whom we would like to thank personally...

- Our Illustrator, Ms. Rayee Satyabodh, for the amazing work she has done in putting forth our ideas and concepts in pictures. All the beautiful and self-explanatory illustrations which you can see in all the chapters are her creation. A special thanks to her for tolerating our whims and fancies and innumerable changes over countless zoom calls.
- Our editorial team Mr. Rajesh Bhalani and Mr. Rushabh Bhalani from Bhalani Publishers and Mrs. Harsha Shah from M/S National Medical Book House along with the DTP typesetter who were excellent and supportive from the start and helped us in realizing what sort of textbook will be appropriate and best suited for the readers.
- Our colleagues who helped us in some of the chapters- Dr. Mihir Patel (Intra-articular injuries of the knee), Dr. Ashok Rathod and Dr. Arjun Dhawale (Cervical spine injuries and Thoracolumbar injuries) and Dr. Maulin Shah (Humeral shaft fractures). They were of great help in revising, re-organising and modifying certain parts of the chapters as well as provided a few images for the same.
- Our respective families who tolerated us typing away to glory for many days, (and in some cases, even helped during a few zoom calls).... The Sheth family (Dr. Arun and Divyanshu), the Vaidya family (Dr. Mitali, Om and Janhavi) and the Agashe family (Dr. Prachi and Vyom)...... we will be forever grateful to you....
- Our greatest source of inspiration and help- our patients without whom we will not be where we are and we won't have the luxury of this experience..... a big Thank you to them.....
- And finally and surprisingly.... The COVID-19 pandemic and the lockdown, which gave us some breathing space and time away from our busy clinical schedules and practices and helped us in taking this endeavor to fruition......

ABBREVIATIONS

AAD	:	Atlanto-Axial Dislocation
ABC	:	Aneurysmal Bone Cyst
AC	:	Acromio-Clavicular
ACL	:	Anterior Cruciate Ligament
ADI	:	Atlanto-Dens Interval
AE	:	Above-Elbow
AFO	:	Ankle Foot Orthosis
AIIS	:	Anterior Inferior Iliac Spine
AK	:	Above-Knee
AP	:	Antero-Posterior
ASIS	:	Anterior Superior Iliac Spine
ATLS	:	Advanced Trauma Life Support
AVN	:	Avascular Necrosis
BE	:	Below-Elbow
BK	:	Below-Knee
BMD	:	Bone Mineral Density
BMI	:	Body Mass Index
BPBI	:	Brachial Plexus Birth Injury
C Spine	:	Cervical Spine
CBC	:	Complete Blood Count
CC	:	Cannulated Cancellous
CCS	:	Cannulated Cancellous Screw
CMC	:	Carpo-Metacarpal
CML	:	Classic Metaphyseal Lesion
CNS	:	Central Nervous System
CORA	:	Centre of Rotation of Angulation
CPT	:	Congenital Pseudoarthrosis of Tibia
CRIF	:	Closed Reduction Internal Fixation

CRP	:	C-Reactive Protein
CRPP	:	Closed Reduction Percutaneous Pinning
CS	:	Compartment Syndrome
CT	:	Computed Tomography
DCP	:	Dynamic Compression Plate
DHS	:	Dynamic Hip Screw
DIP	:	Distal Inter-Phalangeal
DRUJ	:	Distal Radio-Ulnar Joint
e.g.	:	For example
ECRB	:	Extensor Carpi Radialis Brevis
ECRL	:	Extensor Carpi Radialis Longus
EDL	:	Extensor Digitorum Longus
EHL	:	Extensor Hallucis Longus
ENT	:	Ear Nose Throat
EPL	:	Extensor Pollicis Longus
ESIN	:	Elastic Stable Intramedullary Nailing
ESR	:	Erythrocyte Sedimentation Rate
FABER	:	Flexion Abduction External Rotation
FAI	:	Femoro-Acetabular Impingement
FCD	:	Fibrous Cortical Defect
FDP	:	Flexor Digitorum Profundus
FDS	:	Flexor Digitorum Superficialis
FPL	:	Flexor Pollicis Longus
GA	:	General Anaesthesia
GCS	:	Glasgow Coma Scale
GT	:	Greater Trochanter
HO	:	Heterotopic Ossification
IF	:	Internal Fixation
IM	:	Intra-Medullary
IP	:	Inter-Phalangeal
ISS	:	Injury Severity Score
IV	:	Intra Venous

LA	:	Local Anaesthesia
LCDCP	:	Limited Contact Dynamic Compression Plate
LCL	:	Lateral Collateral Ligament
LLD	:	Limb Length Discrepancy
M/3	:	Middle Third
MAD	:	Mechanical Axis Deviation
MCL	:	Medial Collateral Ligament
MCP	:	Metacarpo-Phalangeal
MPFL	:	Medial Patello-Femoral Ligament
MRSA	:	Methicillin Resistant Staphylococcus Aureus
MRI	:	Magnetic Resonance Imaging
MUGA	:	Manipulation Under General Anaesthesia
MVA	:	Motor Vehicle Accident
NAT	:	Non-Accidental Trauma
NIRS	:	Near-Infrared Spectroscopy
NOF	:	Non-Ossifying Fibroma
NWB	:	Non-Weight Bearing
OPD	:	Out-Patient Department
OR	:	Operating Room
ORIF	:	Open Reduction Internal Fixation
OT	:	Operation Theatre
PALS	:	Paediatric Advanced Life Support
PCL	:	Posterior Cruciate Ligament
PEER	:	Pronation Eversion External Rotation
PET	:	Positron Emmision Tomography
PFLCP	:	Proximal Femur Locking Compression Plate
PICU	:	Paediatric Intensive Care Unit
PIN	:	Posterior Interosseous Nerve
PLC	:	Posterior Ligament Complex
POP	:	Plaster OF Paris
PP	:	Percutaneous Pinning
PSIS	:	Posterior Superior Iliac Spine

PTS	:	Partially Threaded Screw
ROM	:	Range Of Motion
SAC	:	Space Available for Cord
SBC	:	Simple Bone Cyst
SC	:	Sterno-Clavicular
SCFE	:	Slipped Capital Femoral Epiphysis
SCI	:	Spinal Cord Injury
SCIWORA	:	Spinal Cord Injury Without Radiographic Abnormality
SER	:	Supination External Rotation
S-H	:	Salter-Harris
SI	:	Sacro-Iliac
SI	:	Supination Inversion
SLIC	:	Subaxial Cervical Spine Injury Classification
SLR	:	Straight Leg Raising
SOMI	:	Sternal Occipital Manubrium Immobiliser
SPF	:	Supination Plantar Flexion
TA	:	Tendo Achilles
TAL	:	Transverse Acetabular Ligament
TBW	:	Tension-Band Wiring
TEN	:	Titanium Elastic Nailing
TFCC	:	Triangular Fibro-Cartilaginous Complex
TFL	:	Tensor Fascia Lata
TLSO	:	Thoraco-Lumbar Spinal Orthosis
TMT	:	Tarso-Metatarsal
UCL	:	Ulnar Collateral Ligament
VAC	:	Vacuum Assisted Closure
VIC	:	Volkmann's Ischaemic Contracture
VMO	:	Vastus Medialis Obliquus
WB	:	Weight Bearing

CONTENTS

Feedback

Help Us Improve

Scan the QR code
and give your feedback
Or
You can email us your feedback on

☞ bhalanipublishers@gmail.com
☞ cleverpen9@gmail.com

1 Special Features of Children's Fractures

Introduction and epidemiology

- Children's fractures result in a period of temporary disability, hospitalization, sometimes permanent disability and rarely, even death. Epidemiological studies have reported an annual incidence of paediatric fractures of 1.6 to 2.1%.
- There is a significant variation in the incidence of fractures between boys and girls, with boys outnumbering girls by a ratio of 1.8:1. About 40% girls and 60% boys are likely to have sustained at least one fracture by the age of 16 years.
- Fractures of the upper limb are commoner than lower limb fractures in children. In the upper limb, radius is the most commonly fractured bone. Distal radius fractures are commoner than shaft or proximal radius fractures. Hand (phalanges/metacarpals), clavicle and distal humerus fractures are next most commonly fractured bones. In the lower limb, tibia is the most commonly fractured bone.
- Presence of physis is a unique feature of children's fractures, and incidence of physeal fractures across various studies ranges from 14 to 30% of all fractures. Open fractures are relatively rare in children and constitute about 1% of all paediatric fractures.
- There is a linear relationship between age and incidence of fractures. The peak age of fracture occurrence is seen in adolescence. Age also influences the incidence of specific fractures. So, some fractures are early peak fractures (e.g. fracture supracondylar humerus, fracture lateral condyle humerus), whereas some fractures are late occurring (e.g. fracture distal forearm, fracture proximal humerus). Some fractures exhibit a bimodal incidence pattern (e.g. fracture clavicle, fracture femur), with fractures in younger age typically occurring after low energy trauma such as fall from height, and fractures in older age occurring following high energy trauma like Motor Vehicle Accidents/contact sports.
- There is a direct correlation between Body Mass Index (BMI) and fracture incidence with obese children found to be at higher risk of sustaining fractures. Also, low Bone Mineral Density (BMD) and low serum levels of Calcium and Vitamin D have been found with higher frequency in children who sustain fractures.

Aetiology

Aetiology of children's fractures can be broadly classified as:

- Accidental trauma
- Non-accidental trauma (discussed in a later section of this chapter)
- Pathological fractures (discussed in chapter 4)

Accidental trauma is the commonest cause of fractures in children. Common accidental injuries include:

- Household and school injuries
- Sports injuries
- Motor vehicle accidents

Household and school injuries are generally low energy injuries and occur mainly in toddlers and juveniles. Greenstick fractures, torus fractures, toddler's fractures of the tibia occur commonly after household or school injuries. Injuries following contact sports and motor vehicle accidents may be high energy injuries and are more commonly seen in adolescents.

Anatomy

The growing bone consists of following parts **(Fig. 1.1)**:

- **Epiphysis**

  Epiphysis is seen at the ends of long bones. It is covered by articular cartilage either wholly (e.g. femoral head) or partially (e.g. distal femur). At birth, except for the distal femur and proximal tibia, the epiphysis is entirely cartilaginous. As the child grows, ossification centre appears in the epiphysis. The ossification centre slowly grows in size and at the end of skeletal growth, fuses with the metaphysis as the intervening physis disappears. The appearance, increase in size and fusion of each ossification centre follows a specific pattern and helps us to estimate the skeletal age and timing of skeletal maturity of the child **(Tables 1.1 and 1.2)**.

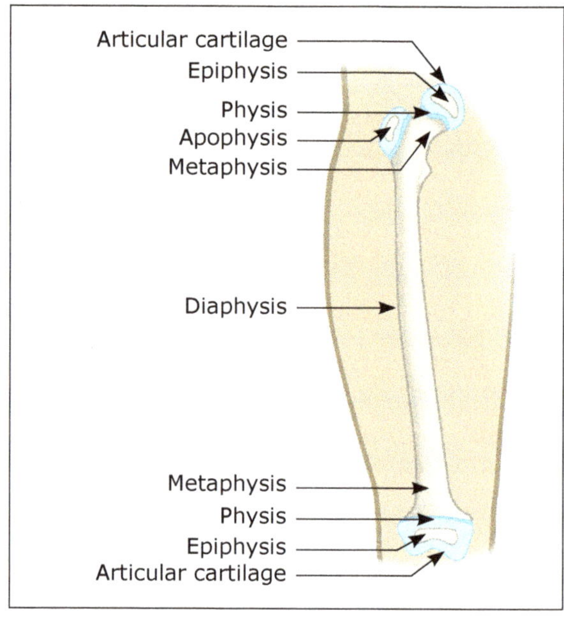

Fig. 1.1: *Anatomy of skeletally immature bone.*

Table 1.1: Timing of appearance and closure of secondary centres of ossification of the upper limb

Ossification Centre	Appearance	Closure
Humeral head	3 months	18 to 20 years
Capitellum	1 year	14 to 15 years (girls), 15 to 17 years (boys)
Radial head	3 to 6 years	14 to 15 years (girls), 15 to 17 years (boys)
Medial epicondyle	5 to 7 years	15 years (girls), 17 years (boys)
Olecranon	4 to 10 years	14 years (girls), 17 years (boys)
Trochlea	7 to 9 years	14 to 15 years (girls), 15 to 17 years (boys)
Lateral epicondyle	11 to 12 years	14 to 15 years (girls), 15 to 17 years (boys)

Table 1.2: Timing of appearance and closure of secondary centres of ossification of the lower limb

Ossification Centre	Appearance	Closure
Femur head	4 months	16 to 17 years (girls), 17 to 18 years (boys)
Iliac crest	puberty	20 years
Distal femur	36th fetal week	17 years (girls), 18 to 19 years (boys)
Proximal tibia	40th fetal week	16 to 17 years (girls), 18 to 19 years (boys)
Distal tibia	6 months	17 to 18 years

The progressing ossification of the epiphysis is also responsible for the changing patterns of injury seen at different ages. An apophysis is extra-articular, usually has muscle/ligament attachments and is susceptible to avulsion fracture. Like the epiphysis, the apophysis has an ossification centre and a physis separating it from the parent bone. The ossification centre grows in size during skeletal growth and eventually fuses at skeletal maturity with disappearance of the growth plate.

- **Physis**

  The physis is a highly dynamic structure composed of chondrocytes. It is sandwiched between the epiphysis and metaphysis. It is responsible for the increase in length of children's bones.

  The physis is composed of 4 zones **(Fig. 1.2)**:

- *Resting (germinal) zone:* As the name suggests, chondrocytes in this zone are in a resting state. Damage to this zone of the physis as occurs in Salter Harris Type 3, 4 and 5 injuries can result in growth disturbances (see Chapter 2).
- *Proliferative zone:* In this zone, the chondrocytes undergo active replication.

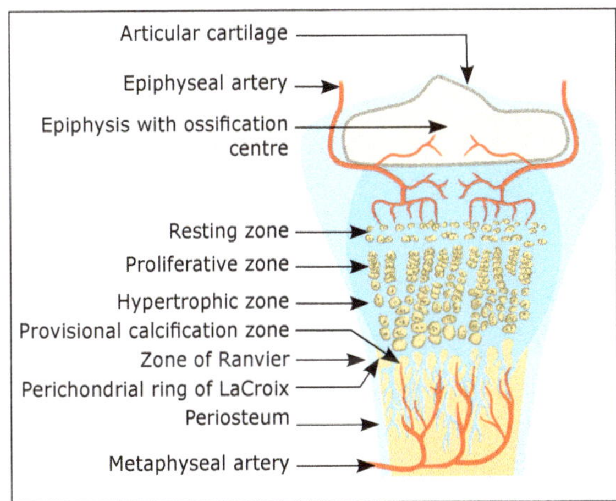

***Fig. 1.2**: Organisation of physis.*

- *Hypertrophic and provisional calcification zones:* In these zones, the chondrocytes secrete extracellular matrix which is then embedded with calcific deposits. The chondrocytes undergo hypertrophy, invasion by proliferating blood vessels and eventual apoptosis. The collagen content of the hypertrophic zone is lower and orientation of fibres is vertical in contrast to the germinal zone where the collagen fibres are horizontally oriented. This makes the hypertrophic zone mechanically weak and therefore physeal injuries generally propagate through this zone of the physis.
- *The perichondrial ring of LaCroix* is a circumferential ring of fibrous tissue which connects the periosteum on the metaphyseal side with perichondrium on the epiphyseal side. It is firmly attached to the periphery of the physis and provides mechanical integrity to the physis against physeal seperations.
- *The zone of Ranvier* is a peripheral triangular zone underneath the LaCroix ring. It contains chondroblasts, osteoblasts and fibroblasts and is responsible for the increase in circumferential girth of the physis.

Each physis has variable contributions to the increase in length of bone, knowledge of which is important for estimation of effect of damage to a particular physis on the future growth of the bone **(Tables 1.3 and 1.4)**.

- **Metaphysis**

  The metaphysis is the flared portion of bone between the physis and diaphysis. The cortical thickness of metaphyseal bone is lesser than diaphyseal bone. Metaphysis contains high volume of spongy cancellous bone. Due to its composition, metaphyseal bone can undergo deformation without fracturing, explaining the incidence of torus fractures in this region.

Table 1.3: Contribution of physis to the increase in length of each long bone of the upper extremity

Ossification Centre	Contribution to increase in length of bone
Proximal humerus	80%
Distal humerus	20%
Proximal radius	25%
Distal radius	75%
Proximal ulna	80%
Distal ulna	20%

Table 1.4: Contribution of physis to the increase in length of each long bone of the lower extremity

Ossification Centre	Contribution to increase in length of bone
Proximal femur	30%
Distal femur	70%
Proximal tibia	55%
Distal tibia	45%
Proximal fibula	60%
Distal fibula	40%

- **Diaphysis**

  Diaphyseal bone constitutes the major part of each long bone. It is composed of mature lamellar bone. The centre of disphyseal bone contains marrow. The periosteum covering the diaphysis of children is much thicker than in adults. It is an important stabilising factor in preventing significant displacement in children's fractures. In children's diaphyseal fractures, it is usually incompletely torn and remains intact on the concave side, knowledge of which is important in treatment by closed reduction. Periosteum also plays an important role in remodelling of diaphyseal fractures and periosteum on the concave side deposits new bone whereas bone on the convex side is gradually resorbed resulting in gradual straightening of the diaphysis.

Unique fracture patterns in children

Children's bones have higher modulus of elasticity than adult bones and therefore can bend to a significant degree before eventually breaking. This feature results in unique fracture patterns in children like plastic deformation and greenstick fractures which are not seen in adults.

- **Buckle/torus fractures**

  Buckle/torus fractures occur most commonly in long bones at the junction of cancellous metaphyseal bone and cortical diaphyseal bone **(Fig. 1.3)**. Longitudinal force applied along the long axis of the bone results in compression of the thin cortex with bulging. Swelling is minimal as there is no extravasation of blood. Since only a part of the circumference of the cortex is buckled, it is a stable fracture and rigid immobilisation may not be needed. However, care should be taken not to misinterprete an undisplaced bicortical fracture as a torus fracture, as a bicortical fracture if not immobilised, can lead to late displacement.

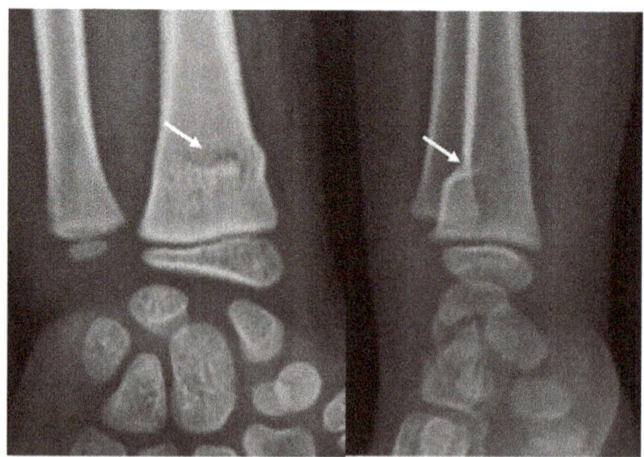

***Fig. 1.3**: X-ray wrist joint AP and Lateral views showing torus fracture of the distal radius.*

- **Plastic deformation**

When a bending force is applied to a long bone, initially elastic deformation occurs which reverses when the force applied is released. Beyond elastic limits, if the force applied is lesser than that needed to break the bone, plastic deformation occurs. It can result in significant angulation as well as rotational deformities. Microscopically, there is discontinuity at the junctions between osteon units. Pain and swelling may be minimal as there is no periosteal tearing or fracture hematoma.

Plastic deformation is most commonly seen in forearm. Plastic deformations have poor remodelling potential. Reduction of plastic deformation should be undertaken if the deformity is cosmetically visible, or forearm rotations are restricted. Closed reduction of plastic deformations is performed by applying sustained three-point pressure with fulcrum at the apex of the deformation on the concave side. Pressure may need to be applied for more than five minutes to effect a reduction. If closed reduction fails, osteotomy may be needed for correction of plastic deformation **(Fig. 1.4)**.

- **Greenstick fractures:**

If the bending force applied is beyond the limits of plastic deformation, but still not enough to create a complete fracture, a greenstick fracture will occur. Greenstick fracture is characterised by fracture of the cortex on the convex tensile side, whereas the concave compression cortex undergoes plastic deformation **(Fig. 1.5)**. Recent studies have proven that it is not necessary to complete a greenstick fracture before reduction. However, exaggeration of the deformity is recommended to unlock the fragments. Fracture is then reduced by three-point pressure. In the forearm, greenstick fractures of the radius and ulna at different levels are due to rotational injuries. They are reduced by derotating the fracture to the reduced position. (for details, see Chapter 15).

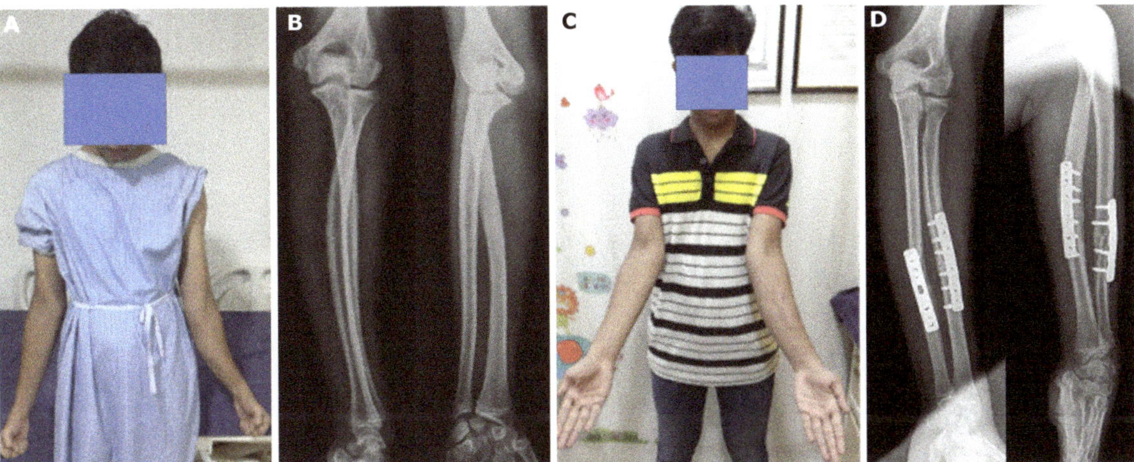

Fig. 1.4: *(A) 11-years-old boy presented with pain, deformity and restricted rotations of Left forearm following history of fall on the outstretched hand. (B) X-ray Left forearm AP and lateral views revealed plastic deformation of the radius and ulna. (C) Clinical picture and (D) X-ray Left forearm AP and lateral views following corrective osteotomy of the radius and ulna.*

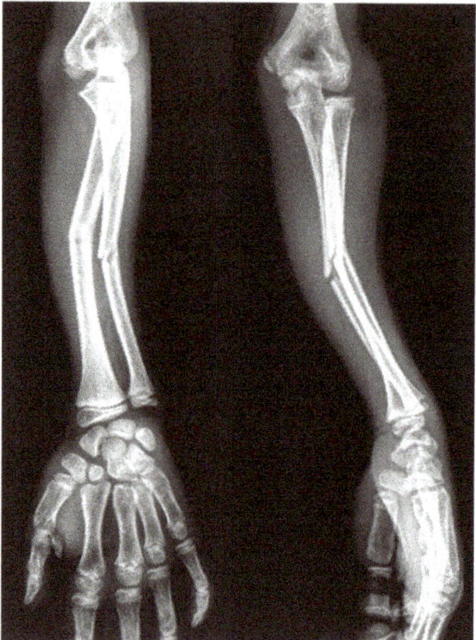

***Fig. 1.5**: X-ray forearm AP and lateral views showing fracture radius ulna greenstick with complete fracture of the convex cortex side with plastic deformation of the concave cortex.*

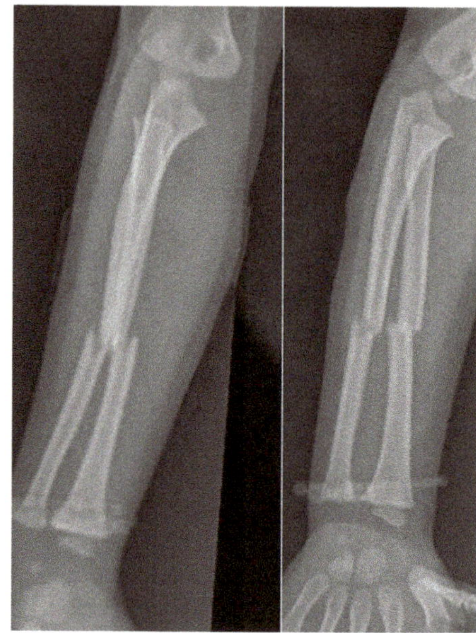

***Fig. 1.6**: X-ray forearm AP and lateral views showing complete fracture of the radius and ulna.*

Consolidation of greenstick fractures is usually delayed as compared to complete fractures and hence longer immobilisation of about 6 weeks is recommended in forearm greenstick fractures. Also refracture rate in greenstick fractures is higher than in other fracture patterns.

- **Complete fractures**

Complete fractures may occur due to bending forces (transverse fractures) or torsional forces (spiral fractures) or compression + bending forces (oblique/butterfly fractures) **(Fig. 1.6)**. Study of fracture pattern gives an idea of the mechanism of injury which indicates the reduction manoeuvre to be performed. In general, the deforming force is initially recreated to exaggerate the deformity and thereby remove interposed soft tissue (usually infolded periosteum). The deforming force is then reversed to reduce the fracture. The thick periosteal hinge is intact on the concave side and provides some degree of stability.

Remodelling of fractures

In paediatric fractures, malunion within acceptable limits undergoes spontaneous correction of residual deformity over a period of time. This phenomenon is called remodelling and is another special feature of children's fractures. Remodelling occurs most rapidly in the first year after fracture healing, but may continue to some extent upto 5 to 6 years after fracture healing.

- **Mechanisms of remodelling**

Asymmetrical growth of the physis is responsible for about 70% remodelling of a fracture malunion. This occurs in accordance with the *Hueter Volkmann law* which states that physis under compression grows to a lesser extent than physis under tension. So a physis adjacent to a fracture tends to realign itself with forces acting along the long axis of the bone.

Remainder remodelling occurs at the level of the fracture. It occurs as per *Wolff's law* which states that bone remodels according to the stress placed on it. It follows that in a malunited fracture, bone will be deposited on the concave side which is under compression, whereas on the convex side bone will be resorbed. This phenomenon is called *"bone drift"* **(Fig. 1.7)**.

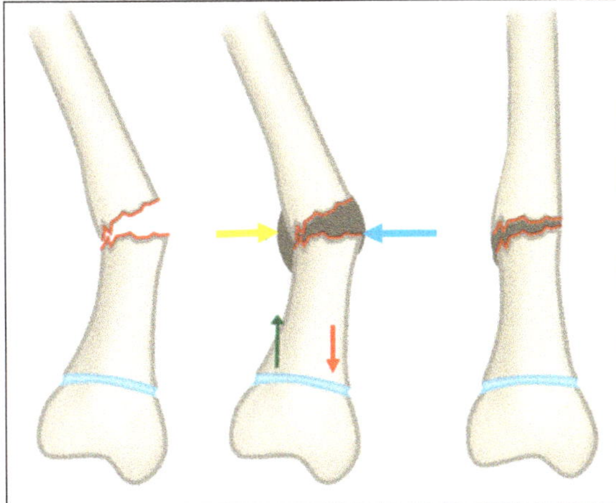

Fig. 1.7*: Remodelling of paediatric fractures occurs by two mechanisms. At the physis, the concave side is under tension and has accelerated growth (green arrow) as compared to the convex side which is under compression (red arrow). Also, at the fracture site, bone is deposited on the concave side (yellow arrow) and resorbed on the convex side (blue arrow).*

- **Deformities corrected by remodelling**

- Angulation and translation deformities within acceptable limits remodel well.
- Rotational deformities are not amenable to remodelling and so extreme care should be taken to achieve correct rotational alignment at the time of fracture immobilisation/fixation.

- **Factors determining remodelling:**

- Fractures in close proximity to the physis have better remodelling potential than diaphyseal fractures.
- Angulation in plane of motion of the adjacent joint remodels better. So in distal radius fractures, angulation in sagittal plane remodels better than a varus/valgus angulation.
- Fractures in proximity to growing ends of bones remodel better. So, fractures of proximal humerus, distal radius, distal femur and proximal tibia have better remodelling potential as these physes contribute majorly to the growth of the respective bones.
- Younger the child, better the remodelling potential **(Fig. 1.8)**. Remodelling potential is limited in children with less than 2 years growth remaining.

Overgrowth

- After fractures in children, there may be stimulation of bone growth leading to overgrowth.
- If bone heals with shortening, it may be compensated by the overgrowth. In that sense, it may be considered a type of remodelling.
- This overgrowth is believed to occur due to
  - Increased blood supply to the physis
  - Disruption of the periosteum with resultant loss of periosteal restraint on bone growth.
- Overgrowth is more likely if there is periosteal stripping as in Open Reduction-Plate fixation.
- Overgrowth is most common after femur fractures between the ages of

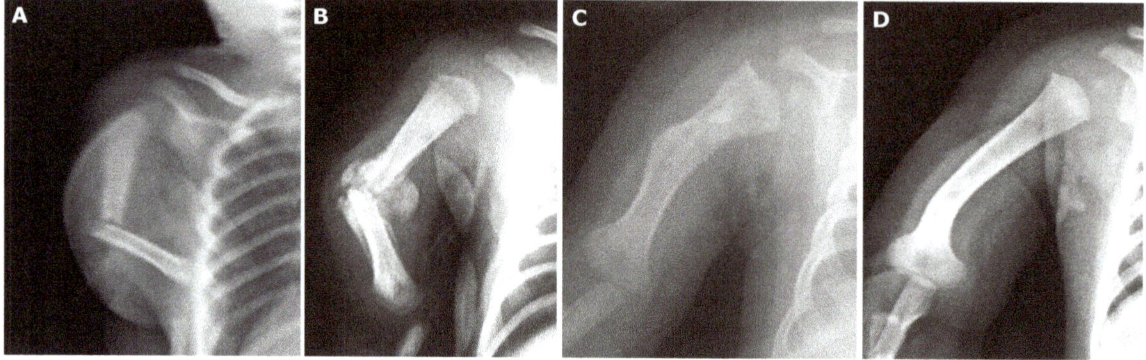

Fig. 1.8: *(A) X-ray humerus in a neonate reveals fracture humerus shaft. (B) At 4 weeks, the fracture healed with mal-union in varus. Subsequent X-rays at (C) 6 months and (D) 9 months revealed remodelling at the fracture site.*

2 to 10 years and occurs to an average of 1cm.

- Asymmetric growth stimulation can lead to angular deformities as seen in proximal tibial valgus deformity following proximal tibia metaphyseal fracture in a child (see Cozen's phenomenon in Chapter 25).

Non-accidental trauma

- Non-accidental trauma (NAT) is the recent terminology for Battered baby or child abuse syndrome.
- The incidence of NAT is highest in children less than 2 years age.
- The attending physician should be aware of the signs of NAT, and in cases of suspected NAT, should notify the concerned authorities, so that steps are taken to avoid re-exposure of the child to further trauma. In some cases, NAT can also lead to death.
- Studies have shown higher incidence of child abuse in households with marital discord, divorce, parental depression, job loss, recent family death, financial difficulties and adult substance abuse. Unrelated adult is the more likely perpetrator of child abuse. Poor care-giver supervision in day-care centres is another important setting for child abuse.
- Disabled children and stepchildren are more likely to face child abuse. Children who have faced physical abuse are also likely to have faced sexual abuse and should be evaluated for the same.

The following features should alert the attending physican to the possibility of child abuse:

- Delay in seeking treatment.
- Disparity between nature of fall and severity of injury. e.g. serious limb or head injury sustained after a household fall.
- Cluster of injuries.
- Injuries in various stages of healing.

Clinical features

- Suspected vicitms of child abuse, especially children less than 2 years age and children with special needs, should undergo thorough clinical evaluation to rule out other concomitant injuries. Apart from musculoskeletal system, skin, CNS, abdomen and genitalia should also be evaluated for injuries.
- External injuries indicating high probability of child abuse include external ear bruising, eye sub-conjunctival haemorrhage, tearing of frenulum of tongue and skin bruises/

lacerations/burns. Whereas skin bruises due to accidental trauma occur more often on bony prominences like eye-brows, chin, knees and shins, bruises occurring on back of head, neck, back, arms, legs, buttocks, cheeks and genitalia should be evaluated for non-accidental trauma **(Fig. 1.9)**.

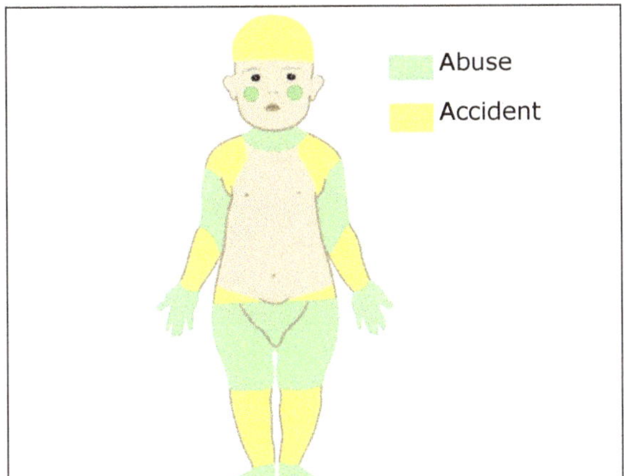

***Fig. 1.9**: Typical locations of bruising in accidental versus non-accidental trauma.*

- Internal injuries suggesting possibility of child abuse include rib fractures, intra-cranial haemorrhage and abdominal trauma.

Fractures in child abuse

- Children with child abuse may present with multiple fractures in different stages of healing.
- Few fractures are known to be highly specific indicators of probable child abuse and include:
- Classic metaphyseal lesions
- Posterior rib fractures
- Spinous process fractures
- Scapula fractures
- Sternal fractures

Diaphyseal fractures

- Traditionally, fractures secondary to child abuse have been thought to be more commonly fractures in tension (torsion) with a spiral oblique configuration, whereas accidental fractures were more commonly thought to be fractures due to physiological loading in compression (transverse/short oblique) as in falls/common childhood activities.
- However, recent studies have challenged this hypothesis, and in fact have proposed that transverse fractures due to violent bending force or direct blow to the extremities are more common in child abuse, than spiral oblique fractures which occur due to twisting injury during falls.
- In infants below walking age, spiral oblique femur fractures should raise suspicion of child abuse. Likewise spiral oblique humerus fractures in children less than 3 years age may indicate possibility of child abuse.
- Likewise, multiple fractures of metacarpals and phalanges of hands, and metatarsals of feet in infants less than one year age should raise suspicion of child abuse.

Classic Metaphyseal Lesions (CMLs) (Fig. 1.10 and Table 1.5):

- CMLs are pathognomic of Non-Accidental Trauma, and are seen in 15 to 30% cases.
- CMLs may be "corner fractures" or "bucket-handle fractures".
- Corner fractures are fractures at the edge of the ossified portion of zone of provisional calcification, which is the metaphyseal side of the physis.
- Bucket-handle fractures involve a more significant rim of the metaphysis. These are metaphyseal fractures occurring through the primary spongiosa just above the zone of provisional calcification.

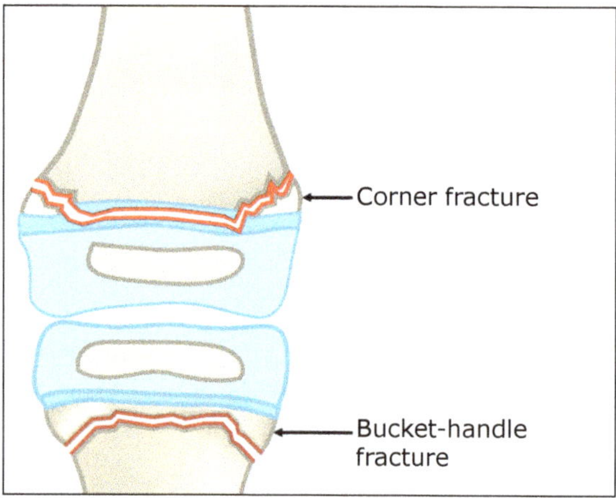

***Fig. 1.10**: Classic metaphyseal lesions of NAT: "corner fracture" of distal femur; "bucket-handle fracture" of proximal tibia.*

- CMLs are caused by violent shaking or traction applied to the child's extremities.

Radiographic evaluation

- If child abuse is suspected, radiological skeletal survey may be indicated to look for concomitant non-obvious fractures. A simple babygram has no role in the diagnosis of subtle fractures associated with child abuse.
- Lateral views of the involved joint are needed if Classic metaphyseal lesions are suspected but are not obvious on antero-posterior view.
- Lateral views of the spine are indicated for diagnosis of occult vertebral body fractures.
- Oblique views of the spine may reveal posterior rib fractures.
- Followup skeletal survey after 2 weeks may be ordered for diagnosis of occult fractures which are not visualised on primary radiographs. Rib fractures are often not diagnosed till callus appears, which can occur as early as one week post-trauma.
- Dating of child abuse fractures on the basis of radiographs is often inaccurate, even in the hands of experienced orthopaedic surgeons/radiologists.

Differential diagnosis

- It must be emphasized that before labelling every case of multiple injuries as a child abuse, normal variants and rare medical conditions need to be ruled out.
- Beaking of the metaphysis of the distal femur and proximal tibia should not be confused for CMLs.
- Fragmentation of distal femur metaphysis edge is a physiologic variant and should be differentiated from a corner fracture.
- A child with multiple bruises with inconsistent history of trauma may be suffering from a bleeding disorder like haemophilia.
- Likewise, there have been cases where children with Osteogenesis imperfecta presenting with multiple fractures have been thought to be victims of child abuse.
- Submetaphyseal lucencies seen in rickets or leukemia should be differentiated from CMLs.

Table 1.5: Pointers for possible child abuse

Medical and Social history	• Dysfunctional family • Children less than 2 years age • Children with special needs • Delay in seeking treatment • Disparity in mode, nature and severity of injury
Clinical examination	• Multiple injuries • Various stages of healing • Bruises on back of head, neck, back, legs, arms, cheeks, genitalia • Eye subconjunctival haemorrhage • Sexual abuse
Orthopaedic injuries	• Classic Metaphyseal lesions (corner and bucket-handle fractures) • Posterior rib fractures • Femur fractures in children of non-walking age • Multiple fractures in children of non-walking age

2 Physeal Injuries

Introduction

Physeal injuries are common and constitute 20 to 30% of all children's fractures. The microscopic anatomy of the physis has been described in Chapter 1. Histologically, physes are composed of the resting (germinal) zone, proliferative zone, hypertrophic zone and the zone of provisional calcification. Mechanically, hypertrophic zone is the weak link and physeal injuries propagate mainly through this zone. Post-traumatic physeal arrest, though rare, can lead to sequelae like limb length discrepancy and deformities.

Classification of physeal injuries

- **Poland's classification**

  Poland's classification was the first described classification of physeal injuries and consisted of four types **(Fig. 2.1)**

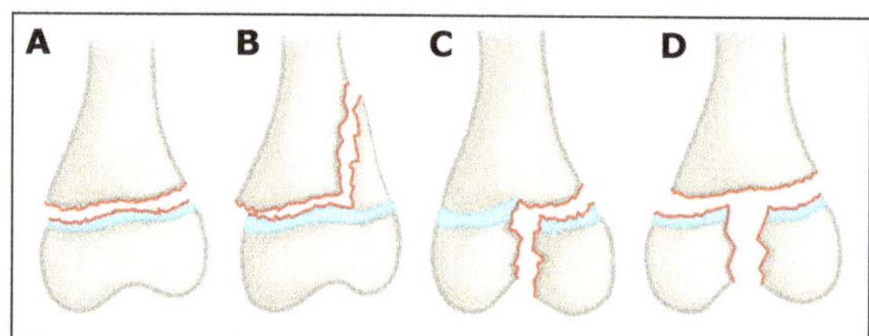

***Fig. 2.1**: Poland's classification of physeal injuries (A) Type 1: physeal fracture without metaphyseal or epiphyseal extension (B) Type 2: physeal fracture with peripheral extension into metaphysis (C) Type 3: Physeal fracture with extension to articular surface (D) Type 4: T-condylar fracture with articular surface extension resulting in two separate intra-articular fragments.*

- **Aitken's classification (Fig. 2.2)**

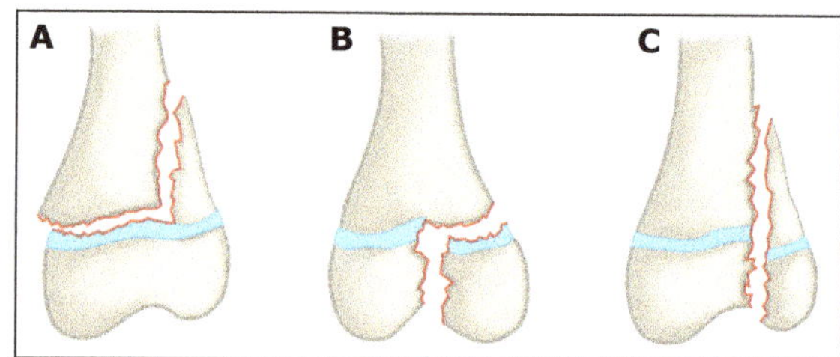

***Fig. 2.2**: Aitken's classification of physeal injuries. (A) Physeal fracture with peripheral extension into metaphysis (B) Physeal fracture with extension to articular surface (C) fracture line extending from articular surface to epiphysis, physis and exiting in the metaphysis.*

- **Salter-Harris classification**

  Salter-Harris classification is the most commonly used, 5 part classification system, first described in 1963. A sixth type was subsequently added by Mercer Rang.

Type 1 **(Fig. 2.3)**:

- Fracture line extends transversely through the physis with no extension into metaphysis/epiphysis.
- Injury can be missed, if undisplaced **(Fig. 2.4)**.
- Also in neonates, fracture can be mis-diagnosed if ossification centre has not yet appeared. e.g. distal humerus, proximal humerus, proximal femur. Advanced imaging (e.g. MRI/USG) may be needed to confirm diagnosis.
- Fracture line propagates through zone of hypertrophy, so there is low risk for growth arrest as germinal zone is not breached.

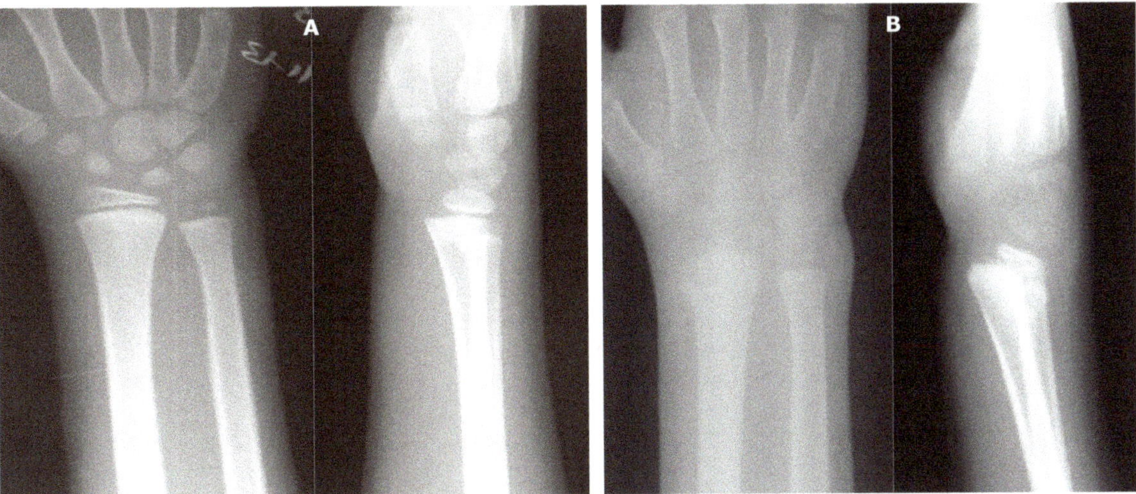

Fig. 2.4: *(A) AP and lateral X-rays of the Right wrist in a 7-years-old boy with fall on outstretched hand shows minimally displaced Salter Harris type 1 fracture distal radius, which was missed at initial presentation. (B) X-ray performed 3 weeks later showed late displacement with malunion.*

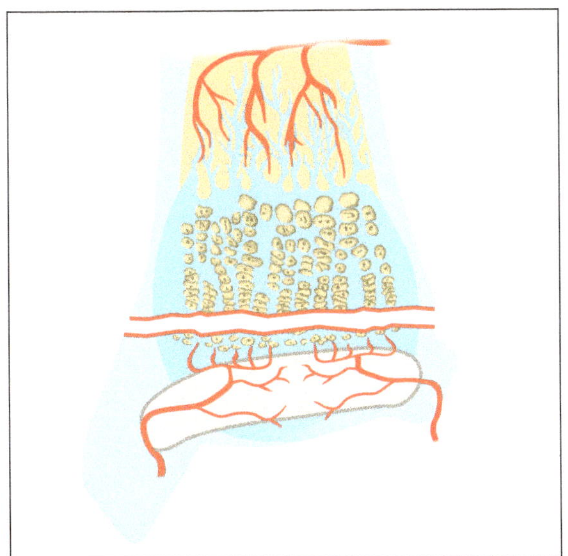

Fig. 2.3: *Salter Harris Type 1 physeal injury: transverse physeal fracture without metaphyseal or epiphyseal extension.*

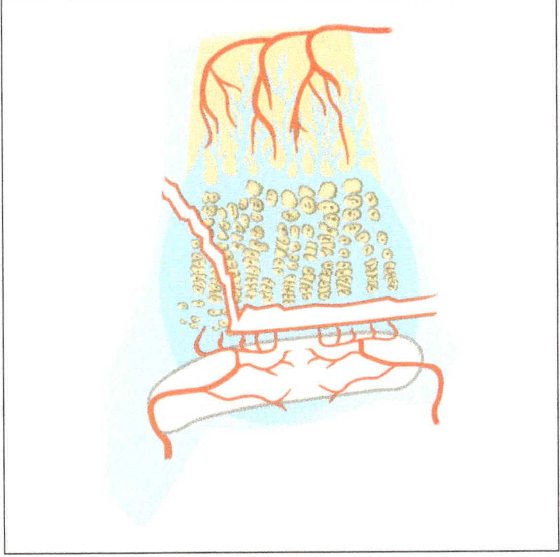

Fig. 2.5: *Salter Harris Type 2 physeal injury: fracture line extends transversely in the physis with peripheral extension into metaphysis.*

Type 2 **(Fig. 2.5)**:

- It is the commonest type of physeal injury.
- The fracture line extends transversely through the physis as in Type 1 but extends into the metaphysis at the periphery. The metaphyseal beak is called the Thurston Holland fragment **(Fig. 2.6)**.
- As in Type 1, risk of growth arrest is low as there is no breach of the resting/ germinal zone.

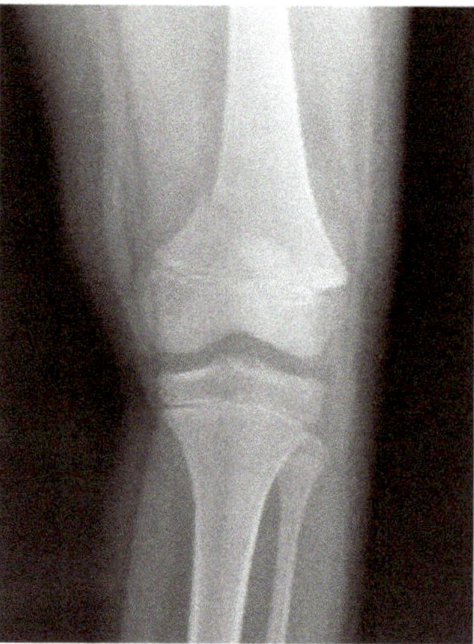

Fig. 2.6*: AP X-ray of knee showing fracture distal femur with large metaphyseal spike (Salter Harris Type 2).*

Type 3 **(Fig. 2.7)**:

- This is an intra-articular fracture in which the fracture line extends transversely through the physis and then extends vertically into the epiphysis and exits into the joint **(Fig. 2.8)**.

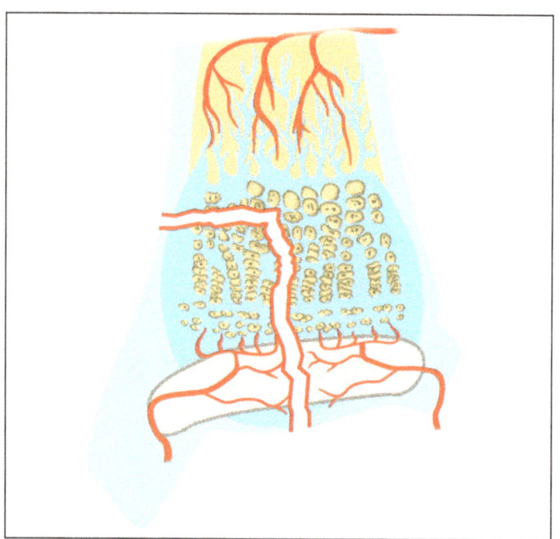

Fig. 2.7*: Salter Harris Type 3 physeal injury: fracture line extends from the physis to the articular surface resulting in an intra-articular fragment*

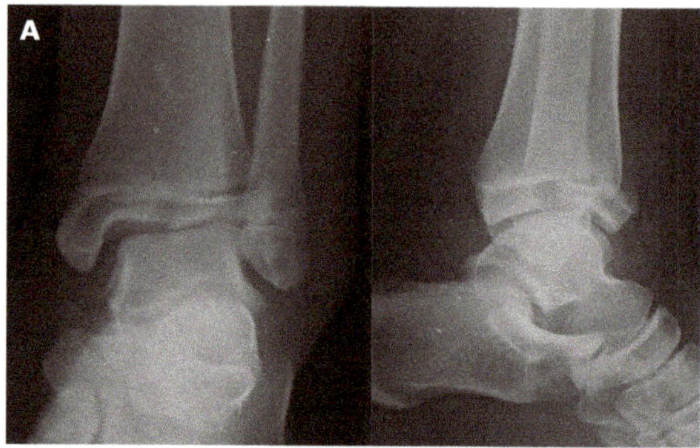

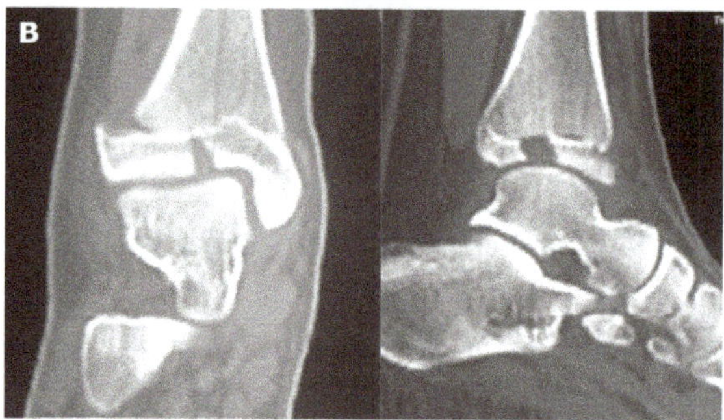

Fig. 2.8*: (A) AP and lateral X-rays of the Right ankle showing physeal injury of the distal tibia with the fracture line extending into the articular surface. This is Tillaux fracture of distal tibia, an example of Salter Harris Type 3 physeal injury. (B) CT scan delineates the fracture anatomy more accurately*

- The fracture line thus breaches germinal zone. These fractures are therefore at risk for growth arrest.
- Malunion of these fractures results in intra-articular incongruity.

Type 4 **(Fig. 2.9)**:

- These are also intra-articular fractures which commence in the metaphysis, extend vertically through the physis and then exit the joint surface through the epiphysis **(Fig. 2.10)**.
- Like Type 3 injuries, these injuries are at risk of growth arrest as the resting zone is breached.
- Malunion results in articular incongruity and also physeal malalignment which leads to growth arrest.

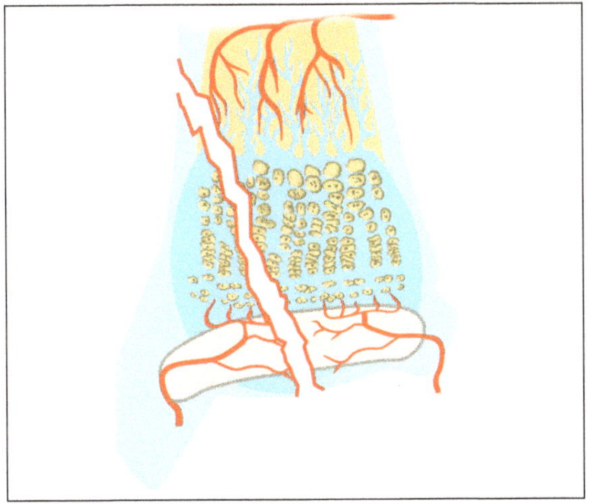

Fig. 2.9: Salter Harris Type 4 physeal injury: the fracture line extends vertically from the metaphysis, traverses the physis and epiphysis and exits distally at the articular surface.

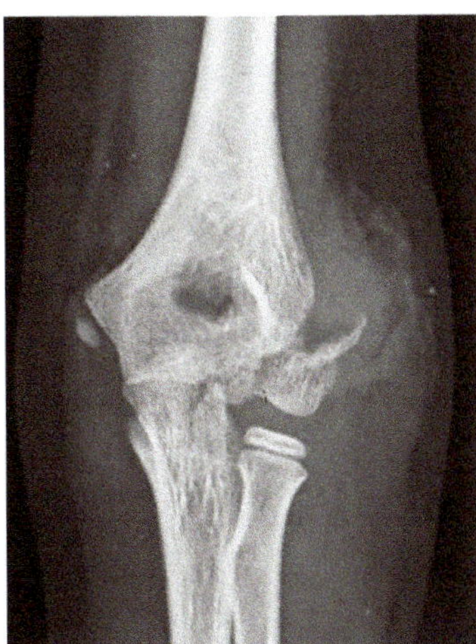

Fig. 2.10: Milch Type 1 Lateral condyle humerus fracture is an example of Salter Harris Type 4 physeal injury.

Type 5:

- It is an unrecognised physeal compression/ischemic injuries sustained at the time of primary trauma.
- In the acute setting, radiographs are normal and hence these injuries are only diagnosed later when premature physeal closure occurs with growth disturbances.

Type 6 (Mercer Rang):

- This type was subsequently added to the original classification and indicates injury to the peripheral zone of Ranvier, leading to subsequent growth arrest with deformities.

Peterson classification (Figs. 2.11)

Though Salter Harris classification is the most commonly used, Peterson pointed out two fracture patterns (Peterson Type 1 and Type 6) which could not be classified in the Salter Harris classification.

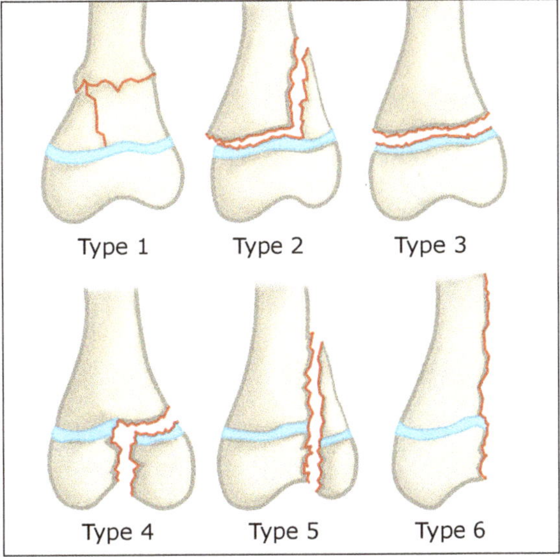

Fig. 2.11: Peterson classification of physeal injuries: Type 1 and Type 6 fracture patterns are not included in Salter Harris classification.

Peterson Type 1: Transverse metaphyseal fracture with vertical extension to the physis. This fracture pattern is known to occur in distal radius fractures **(Figs. 2.12)**.

Peterson Type 6: Partial loss of physis, can occur in open injuries.

Peterson Type 2,3, 4 and 5 correspond to Salter Harris Types 2,1,3 and 4 respectively

Peterson's classification does not recognise the occurrence of Salter Harris Type 5 injury.

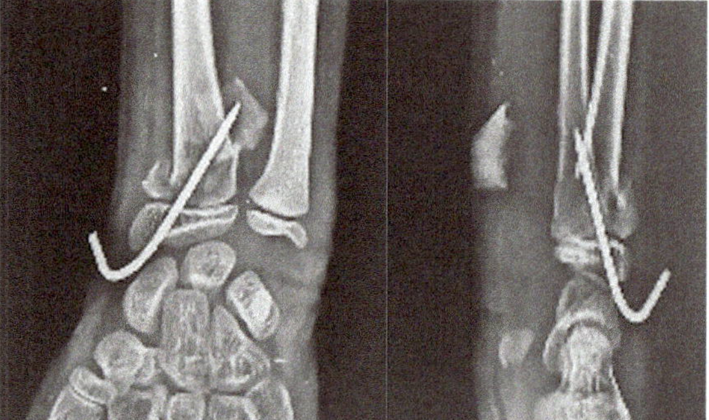

Fig. 2.12: *Peterson Type 1 distal radius physeal injury with a large metaphyseal fragment floating free on the volar aspect.*

Imaging of phyeal injuries

- X-rays: Standard AP and lateral views are usually sufficient for diagnosis. Undisplaced Type 1 fractures may be missed on plain radiographs **(Fig. 2.13)**.
- If the ossific nucleus is small or not yet ossified, Salter Harris Type 1 fractures may be missed or mis-diagnosed on plain radiographs **(Fig, 2.14)**.

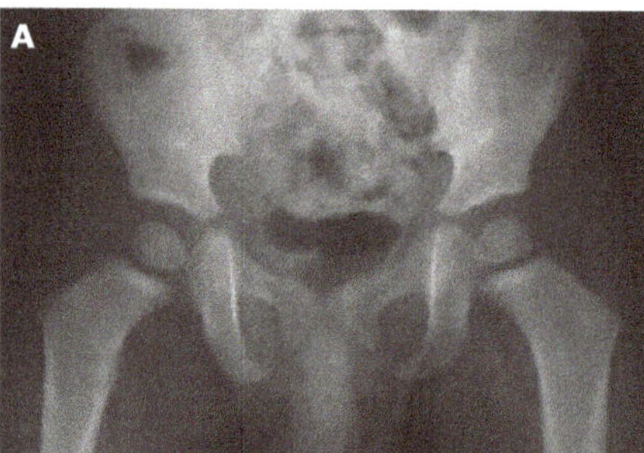

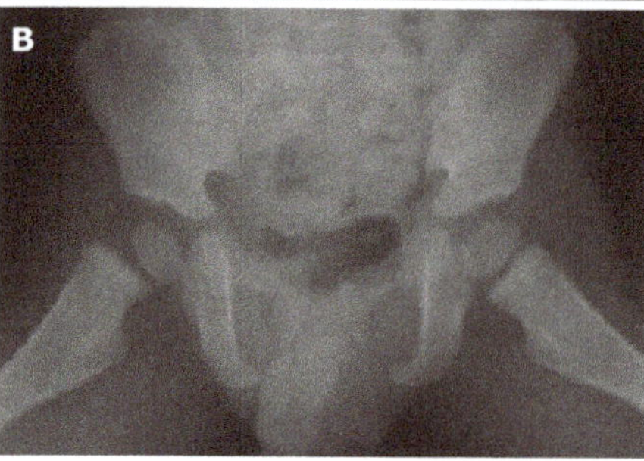

Fig. 2.13: *(A) X-ray of Pelvis with both hips AP view in a 3-years-old male with history of fall from height does not show any fracture. (B) Lateral view shows Salter Harris Type 1 (Delbet Type 1) fracture neck femur.*

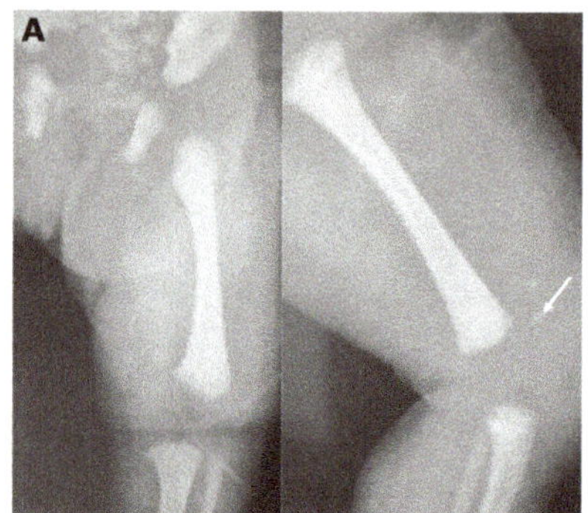

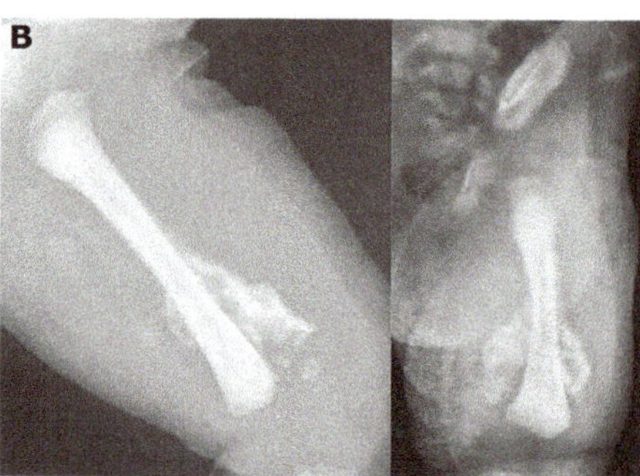

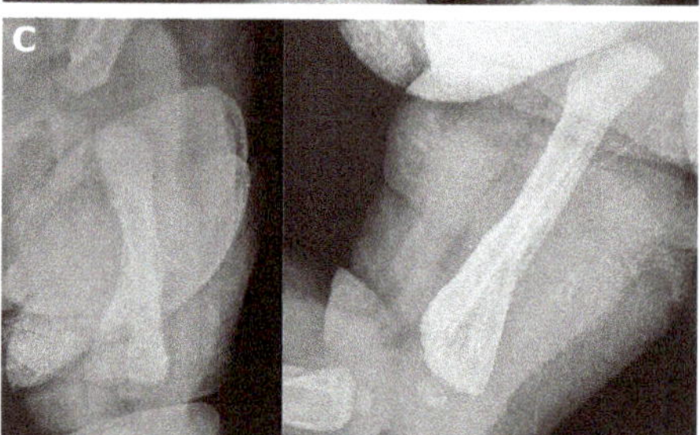

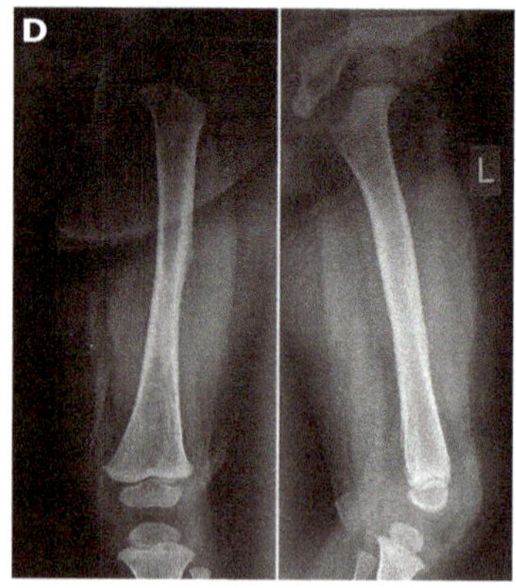

Fig. 2.14: *(A) X-rays of Right knee in a neonate born after difficult labour showing displaced distal femur Salter Harris Type 1 fracture (white arrow-head). Follow-up X-rays done at 2 weeks (B), 6 weeks (C) and 18 months (D) show fracture healing with callus formation and then complete remodelling of the fracture.*

In certain situations, fracture displacement may be underestimated on standard views and additional special views may be needed to assess true displacement. For example, in lateral condyle humerus fracture displacement can be best assessed on internal oblique view **(Fig. 2.15)**

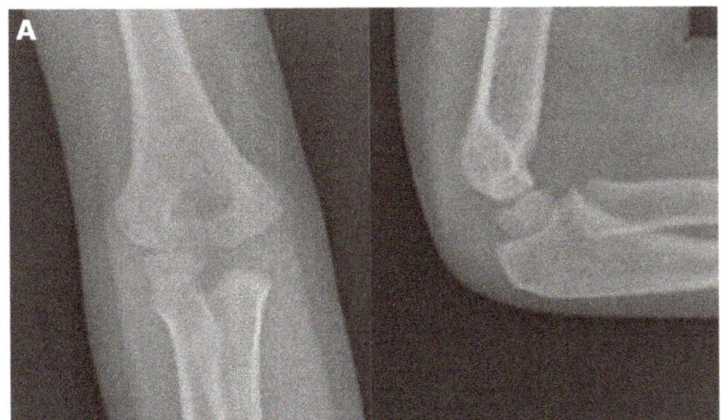

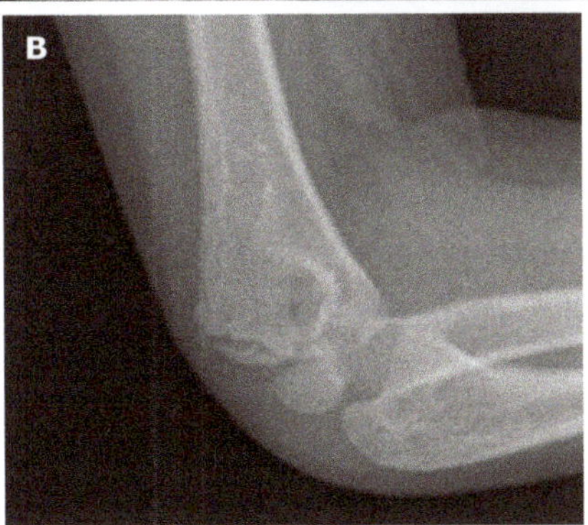

***Fig. 2.15**: (A) AP and lateral X-rays of the Right elbow in 6-years-old girl showing fracture lateral condyle humerus. The fracture appears undisplaced in these views. (B) Internal oblique view showing true extent of displacement.*

CT scan: It is useful in adolescents closer to skeletal maturity where ossification is almost complete. e.g. triplane fractures distal tibia **(Fig. 2.16)**

MRI: It is useful in younger children with largely unossified epiphyses where plain radiographs or CT scans cannot delineate the course of the fracture line through the largely unossified fracture fragments. e.g. in lateral condyle fractures to differentiate whether the fracture line is exiting the

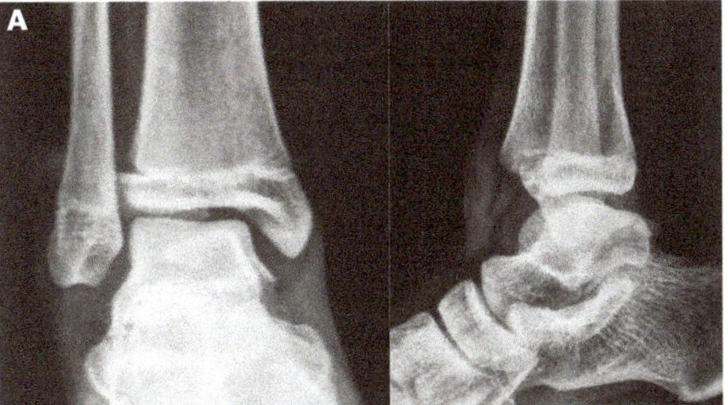

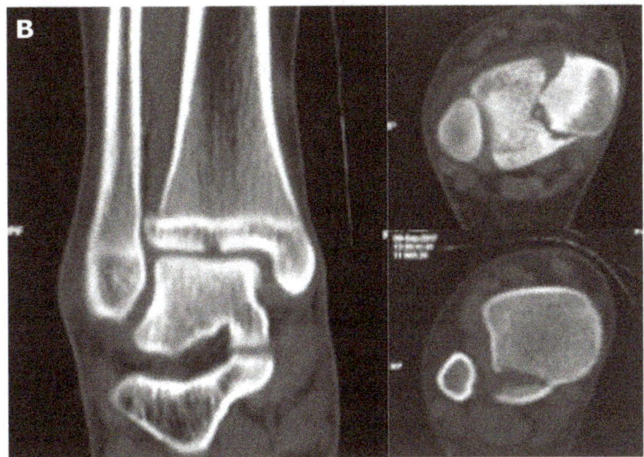

***Fig. 2.16**: (A) AP and lateral X-rays of the Right ankle showing triplane fracture of the distal tibia physis. (B) Fracture configuration can be better assessed on CT scan.*

articular surface (complete fracture) or stopping short of it (incomplete fracture) **(Fig. 2.17)**. MRI is also useful to evaluate unexplained widening of the physis following closed reduction of a physeal injury. In such instances, MRI has shown periosteal interposition in the fracture gap leading to incomplete fracture reduction.

Treatment of physeal fractures

Salter Harris Type 1 injuries

- These fractures are usually treated by gentle reduction and stabilisation as needed.
- The term "gentle" cannot be overemphasised, reduction should consist of 90% traction and 10% translation in order to disimpact the fragments and prevent the sharp metaphyseal edge from grinding against the physis.

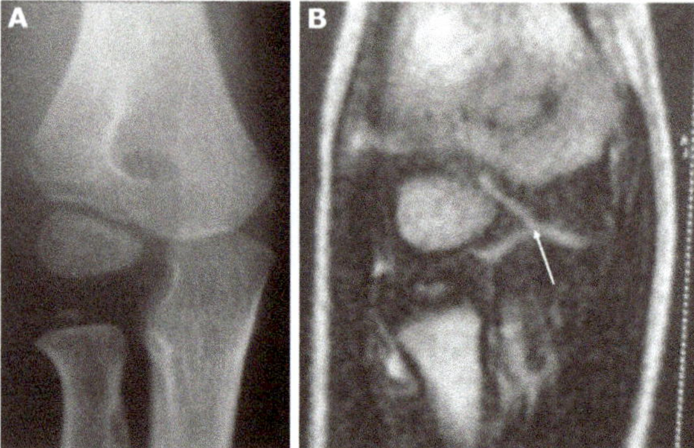

Fig. 2.17: *(A) AP X-ray of the Right elbow showing undisplaced fracture of the lateral condyle of humerus but the distal course of the fracture line through the unossified distal humeral epiphysis cannot be delineated; (B) MRI reveals fracture exiting into articular surface (arrow head) indicating complete fracture. Complete fractures are at risk of late displacement and non-union, so fixation is recommended in these cases.*

- In cases where the fracture reduction is deemed to be unstable, Type 1 injuries may be stabilised with internal fixation. Fixation across a physis runs the risk of causing iatrogenic growth arrest. To minimise the risk of growth arrest, following precautions may be followed.

- Avoid fixation across physes with small cross-sectional surface area. For example, it may be acceptable to fix distal radius physeal injuries, but fixation across distal ulna physeal injuries almost always results in growth arrest.
- Fixation across physis should be done with smooth K-wires of appropriate diameter.
- Multiple attempts at passage of K-wires across physis should be avoided.
- K-wires should be inserted with low torque drills and start-stop method to minimise heat generation and thermal necrosis of physis.
- K-wires should cross the physis in the central 2/4th portion rather than peripheral 1/4th as the peripheral physis is more susceptible to growth arrest.

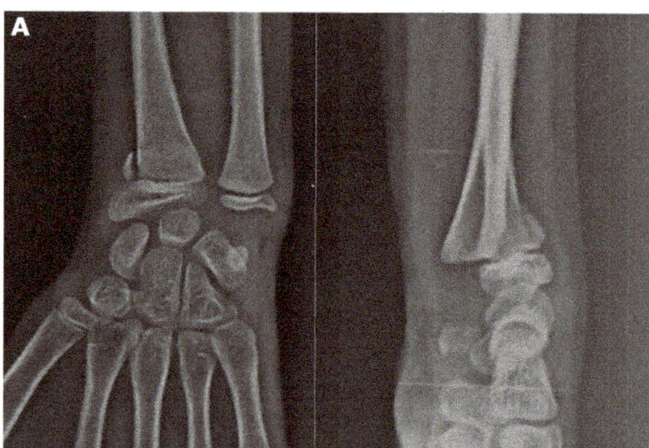

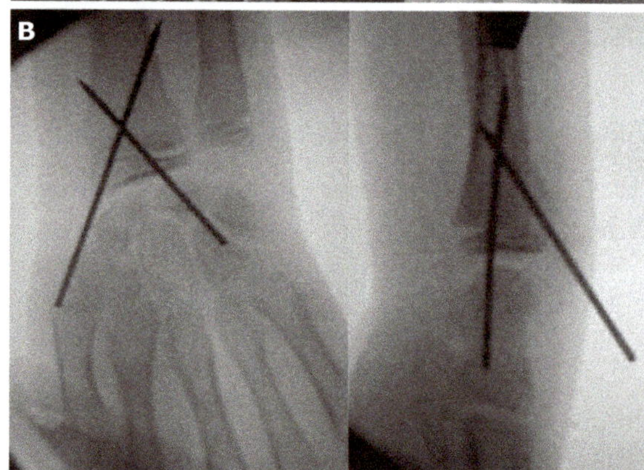

Fig. 2.18: *(A) AP and lateral X-rays of the Right wrist showing displaced fracture distal radius physeal Salter Harris Type 2 (B) AP and lateral intra-operative images following closed reduction and fixation with cross K-wires.*

- In certain anatomical locations (e.g. fracture neck femur, fracture lateral condyle) anatomical reduction and stable fixation gets precedence. In these locations, fixation must breach the physis. For example, fixation in Delbet Type 1 fractures of the femur neck must cross the physis. Fixation may be achieved with smooth K-wires in younger children, whereas in older children screws are used **(Fig. 2.19)**.

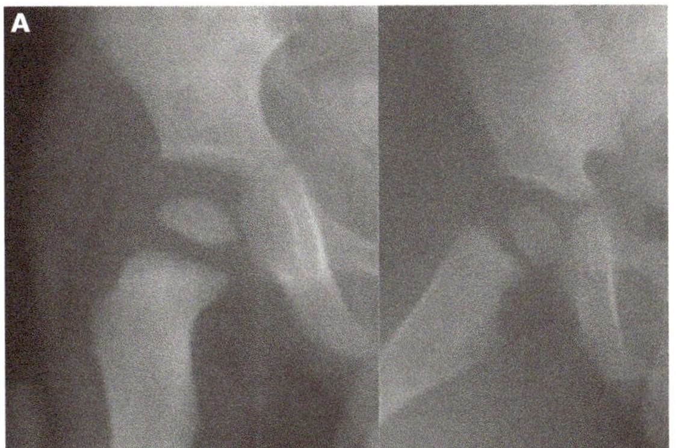

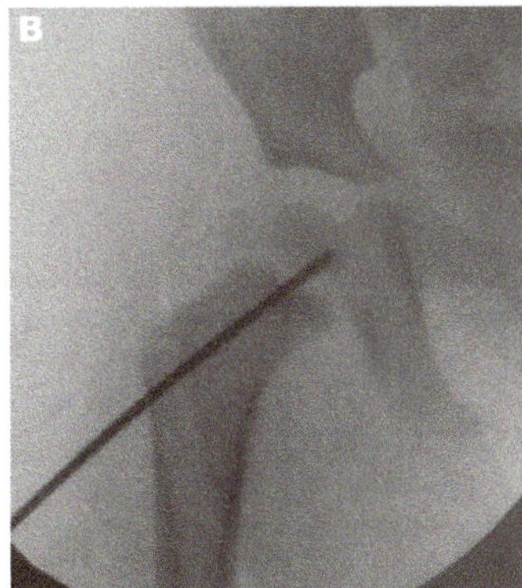

***Fig. 2.19**: (A) AP and lateral X-rays of the Right hip showing fracture femur neck, Delbet Type 1. (B) Intra-operative image following fixation with smooth K-wire.*

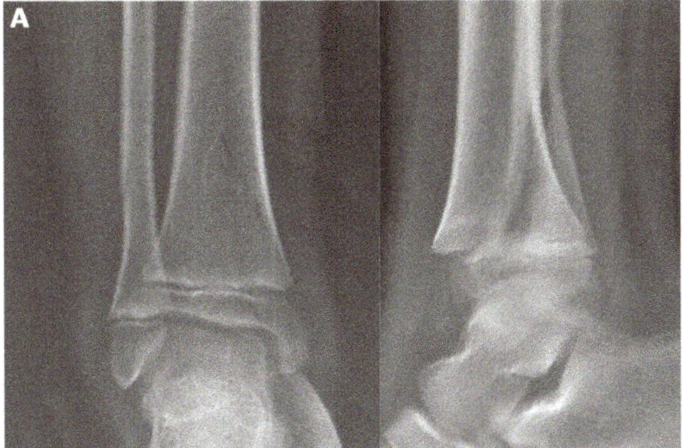

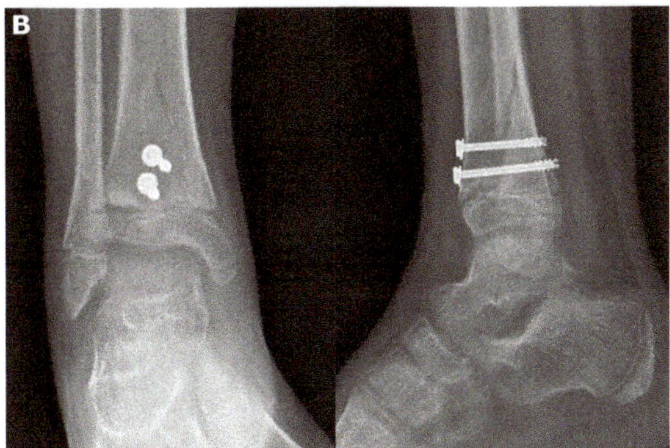

***Fig. 2.20**: (A) AP and lateral X-rays of the Right ankle distal tibia showing Salter Harris Type 2 physeal injury. (B) X-rays after fixation with transverse metaphyseal screws.*

Salter Harris Type 2 injuries:

- The general considerations for management of Type 2 physeal injuries are similar to Type 1 injuries.
- Most of the fractures are effectively managed with closed reduction and cast application.
- Fractures with large metaphyseal fragment can be effectively fixed with transverse metaphyseal screw, without the need to fix across the physis. This allows stable fixation while preserving integrity of the physis **(Fig. 2.20)**.

Salter Harris Type 3 and 4 injuries

- As mentioned earlier, Type 3 and Type 4 physeal injuries are intra-articular fractures. Malunion of these fractures leads to intra-articular incongruity as well as physeal malalignment resulting in physeal bar formation and growth arrest **(Fig. 2.21)**.
- It is imperative to achieve anatomical reduction and stable fixation to obtain optimal results in these injuries.
- Open reduction and internal fixation is needed to achieve this objective.
- Fixation of these fractures can be achieved by inserting transverse screws (in the epiphysis in Type 3 injuries; and in the epiphysis as well as metaphyseal beak in Type 4 injuries) **(Fig. 2.22)**.

Delayed presentation

- In case of Salter Harris Type 1 and 2 injuries presenting more than one

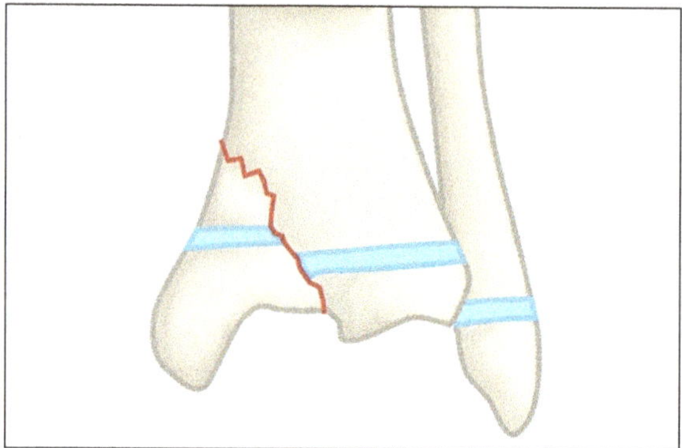

***Fig. 2.21**: Malalignment of growth plate and articular incongruity in a malunited SH Type 4 physeal injury.*

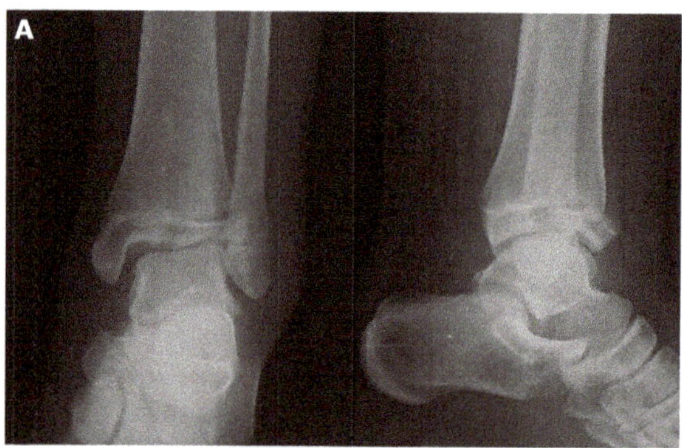

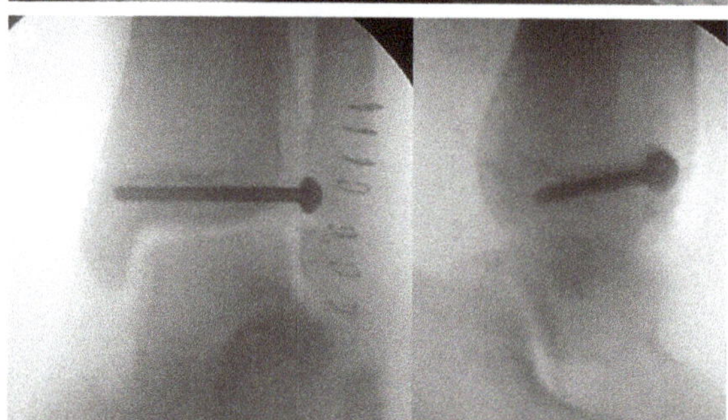

***Fig. 2.22**: (A) AP and lateral X-rays of the ankle joint showing distal tibia Tillaux fracture which is a Salter Harris Type 3 physeal injury (B) Intra-operative images following fixation with a single transverse epiphyseal screw*

week after trauma, reduction should not be attempted due to risk of causing iatrogenic growth arrest. These injuries usually have excellent remodelling potential and corrective surgery for residual malalignment, if any, can be undertaken at a later date.

- Salter Harris Type 3 and 4 injuries need to be anatomically reduced and fixed irrespective of delay in presentation due to risk of articular incongruity and growth arrest in malunited fractures.

Growth disturbance

Growth disturbance is a rare complication of traumatic physeal injuries.

- Growth disturbance may result in
  - angular deformity (if the physeal damage is eccentric)
  - shortening (if a central or large part of the physis is damaged) or both, angular deformity and shortening
  - distortion of the articular surface (by causing tenting of the epiphysis)
- Growth disturbance may occur
  - with physeal bar formation (in which case growth arrest is complete), or,
  - without physeal bar formation (in which case growth cessation may be incomplete).

Growth disturbance in a young child is extremely challenging to treat and often extensive and repeated surgical interventions are needed till skeletal maturity for correcting or preventing the shortening and deformities.

Apart from trauma, growth arrest may occur as a sequel of ischemia, infection, Tumour, irradiation, repetitive trauma or localised conditions like Blount's disease.

Diagnosis

- Physeal bar is characterised by bridge of bone traversing the physis, connecting the epiphysis with the metaphysis.
- The radiographic features of physeal growth disturbance without bar formation include

- loss of smooth contour and blurring of the sharp demarcation between the physis and metaphysis as well as epiphysis
- Sclerosis in the physis at the site of growth disturbance.
- The growth arrest lines of Park and Harris are transversely oriented radiodense lines seen in the metaphysis. These lines are seen after transient slowing/cessation of growth (generalised illness/localised infection or trauma), or, increased mineralisation (cyclical bisphosphonate therapy). The Park-Harris lines are usually parallel to the contiguous physis. However, lines which converge towards a part of the physis may be indicative of localised growth arrest and may occur even before angular deformity is seen.

- Angular deformity, shortening and epiphyseal distortions are effects of growth disturbances and will be noted on plain radiographs at a later stage.

Advanced imaging

- CT scan shows bony bars bridging the physis but cannot provide additional information in growth disturbance without physeal bar formation.
- MRI is the investigation of choice in growth disturbance, and is a sensitive method for assessing physeal architecture. Apart from frank bony bars bridging the physis, it also enables us to assess the architecture and growth potential of the residual physis thereby helping to predict the outcome of physeal bar resection.
- Bar mapping can be performed in an MRI which helps us to assess the surface area of the bar, and feasibility of resection.

Physeal bar

Physeal bar is a bridge of bone traversing the physis, connecting the epiphysis to metaphysis.

It is clinically manifested by joint distortions, angular deformities and limb length discrepancies.

Depending on their location and orientation, physeal bars are classified as **(Fig. 2.23)**:

- *Central bars:* Bony bar surrounded by a perimeter of normal physis
- *Peripheral bars:* Bony bar at the periphery of the physis
- *Linear bars:* occur due to malunited Salter Harris type 3 or 4 fractures with the bar traversing across the diameter of the physis. Linear bars typically occur following malunion of Type 4 physeal injuries.

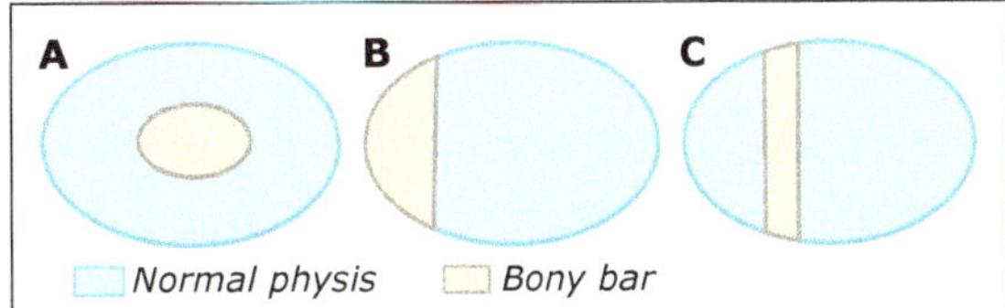

***Fig. 2.23**: Types of physeal bars (A) Central: the bar is surrounded circumferentially by normal physis (B) Peripheral: the bar is situated at the periphery of the physis (C) Linear: the bar traverses the diameter of the physis.*

Management

- Management of each case of growth arrest due to physeal bar formation needs to be individualised.
- Treatment plan for each case depends on:
  - age of the child
  - anatomic site involved
  - extent of physeal bar
  - clinical problems at hand which may include angular deformity and shortening.
- Treatment strategies employed for management of growth disturbances

may include one or more of the following:

Physeal bar resection:

- This procedure is aimed at growth restoration.
- It is also called physiolysis or epiphysiolysis.
- It consists of removal of bony tether between the epiphysis and metaphysis, and filling the void thus formed with inert material to prevent reformation of the bar.

♦ Indications for physeal bar resection are:

- Bars occupying less than 25% of cross-sectional area of the physis
- At least 2 years growth remaining

♦ Better results following physeal bar resection are seen in bars secondary to trauma/Blount's disease as compared to those following infection/ischemia/irradiation.

♦ There are better chances of growth restoration following resection of central and linear bars as compared to peripheral bars.

♦ Proximal tibia bars have best prognosis for growth restoration following resection followed by distal femur bars. Poor prognosis for growth restoration is seen in distal radius, distal humerus, proximal femur and proximal humerus bars.

Pre-operative evaluation

MRI is the investigation of choice.

Special "bar mapping" software enables us to assess cross-sectional surface area of the bar, and decide feasibility of bar resection.

Principles of bar resection **(Fig. 2.24)**

- Physeal bar resection may be combined with osteotomy if angular deformity exceeds 20°.

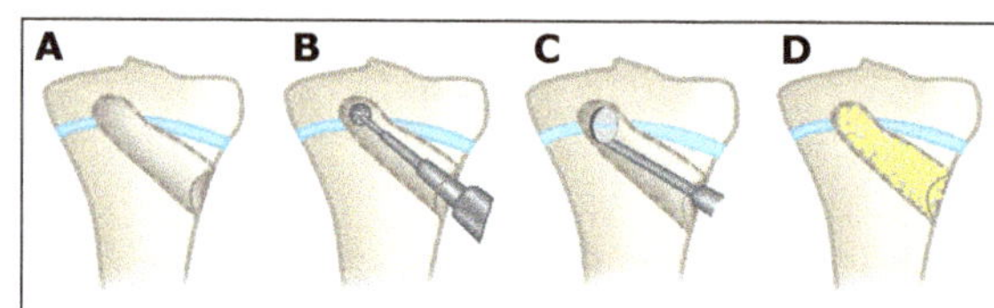

Fig. 2.24: *Steps in excision of central physeal bar. (A) The bar is approached through a window created in the metaphysis. (B) The bony bar is removed. (C) Completeness of resection is confirmed by circumferential visualistion of physis with dental mirror introduced into the tract created for inserting the burr. (D) The tract is then filled with inert material, most commonly fat to prevent reformation of physeal bar.*

- Central bars are approached either through window created in the metaphysis or, if simultaneous corrective osteotomy is performed, through the osteotomy site.
- Peripheral bars are approached directly with resection of overlying periosteum, in order to avoid reformation of bar.
- Bloodless field and good light source are essential.
- Bar resection is done under image intensifier control.
- High speed burr, good light source are needed to ensure completeness of bar resection.
- At the end of resection, a dental mirror or arthroscope inserted to the level of the physis helps to visualise the margins of the resected bar circumferentially and confirm completion of bar resection.
- Cavity created after bar resection needs to be filled up with inert material to prevent reformation of bar.
- Autologous fat graft harvested locally or from buttock, and methyl methacrylate are commonly used interposition materials.
- Metallic markers placed in epiphysis and metaphysis help to monitor growth resumption after bar resection.

- Growth restoration after physeal bar resection needs to be monitored till skeletal maturity.

Corrective osteotomy

- Osteotomy may be performed for correction of angular deformities greater than 20°.

Completion of epiphyseodesis

- After correction of angular deformities, completion of epiphyseodesis may be considered for prevention or recurrence of deformities, in cases where restoration of growth by bar resection is not feasible. This may occur in the following scenarios:

• When the physeal bar is > 30% of the cross-sectional surface area of physis.

• Less than 2 years of growth remaining.

• Failed previous bar resection

Bone length equalisation

- Where growth disturbance is creating limb length discrepancy of functional significance, procedures for equalising bone length are indicated. These procedures include:

• Lengthening of the affected bone

• Epiphysiodesis of the contralateral bone

- In two bone segments (forearm and leg), growth disturbance of one bone can create disparity between lengths of the two bones, and needs to be managed by lengthening of the affected bone or epiphysiodesis of the unaffected bone, e.g. in distal radius growth disturbance, the ulna outgrows the radius creating a positive ulna variance. Management options in this case include lengthening of the radius, shortening of the ulna and epiphysiodesis of the ulna.

3 Casts and Splints

Introduction

Over the past few decades, an increasing number of fractures are being managed surgically. However, in children, a significant number of fractures continue to be managed conservatively by cast application. For example, whereas adult forearm fractures are managed surgically, in children majority of forearm fractures are managed by cast application.

The purpose of casts is to maintain alignment till fracture heals. They may be used de novo, after closed reduction or after operative stabilisation.

However, even casts can be associated with complications, especially in children and it is essential that the treating clinician be well-versed with the technique of cast application, care after cast application and precautions to be taken during cast removal.

Types of cast materials and accessories (Fig. 3.1)

Plaster of Paris (POP)

- Advantages:
  - less expensive
  - easily mouldable
- Disadvantages:
  - less strength to weight ratio
  - poor resistance to water
- Chemical reaction involved in setting of POP:

  $2Ca(SO_4).H_2O$ (Plaster of Paris) + $2H_2O$ = $2[Ca(SO_4).2H_2O]$ (Gypsum)

Setting of POP is an exothermic reaction, and can cause thermal burns (precautions to avoid thermal burns are described later in the chapter).

Fiberglass cast

- Advantages:
  - Lighter
  - Curing generates lesser heat than POP
  - Water resistant
- Disadvantages:
  - Less mouldable
  - Edges sharp-jagged
  - Stiffer and potentially more constrictive

Softcast

- Non fiberglass synthetic cast
- Less rigid, ideal for stable fractures like torus fractures
- Easily removable; upto 3 layers can be unwrapped with hand/cut with bandage cutting scissors

Cast padding

- It is usually made of cotton.
- It may be wrapped directly on the skin or over underlying stockinette.
- Water-proof cast paddings are now available. If used with fiberglass cast, child can bathe over cast.
- Water-resistant cast liners made of polyester are available which prevent water seeping under edges of the cast.

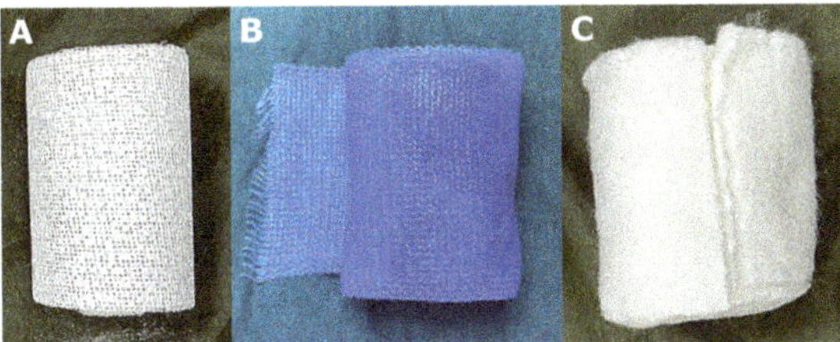

***Fig. 3.1**: Cast materials and accessories (A) Plaster of Paris (POP) cast (B) Fiberglass cast (C) Cotton Cast Padding.*

Cast application techniques

Ideal setting

Application of cast in an OPD setting should be done in a calm environment. The attending surgeon and assisting staff should speak in a soft voice. One parent should be allowed during the procedure. The procedure should be done after appropriate pain control with gentle handling of the injured part. The surgeon should sit at lower level in order to come across as less intimidating to the child. Some patients are "attenders", and, should be given more information about the procedure. Others are "distractors", and should be distracted with videos/music.

Position and extent of cast

Proximal and distal joints must be spanned by the cast. Position of immobilisation is specific to fracture and joint immobilised. e.g. in subtrochanteric femur fracture the proximal fragment is flexed and abducted, and therefore, the hip spica cast should be applied in flexion-abduction so that the distal fragment matches the alignment of proximal fragment. Hand injuries are generally immobilised in intrinsic-plus (safe position) with slight wrist extension, metacarpo-phalangeal (MCP) joint flexion to 70–90° and interphalangeal (IP) joint extension.

Cast padding

Cast padding should be 3 to 5 layers thick. Too many layers of cast padding can cause shearing at pad-skin interface, leading to loosening and slippage of cast. Disappearance of fingers/toes may be first sign of cast slippage **(Fig. 3.2)**. This can cause pressure sores due to mismatch between shape of cast and limb. In case of cast slippage, remove cast and reapply. Extra padding should be provided at bony prominences.

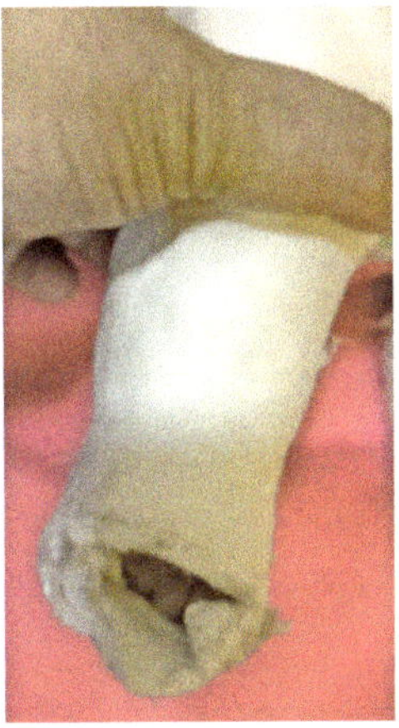

***Fig. 3.2**: Cast slippage with disappearing toes.*

Plaster of Paris cast application

Keep the plaster roll in contact with the limb to avoid wrapping the material too tight **(Fig. 3.3A)**. Plaster is unrolled with overlaps of 1/2 to 1/3 of the width of the plaster. Frequent rubbing and incorporation (initial moulding) is performed as the cast is applied. Plaster splints may be applied where additional reinforcement is needed (at joints). Position of the limb should not be changed after roll application, otherwise material will bunch up and cause pressure sores/thermal injury/vascular compression. e.g flexing elbow after applying initial layers of POP will cause compression in cubital fossa. Limb should be supported with broad surfaces like palm, and indentation with fingers should be avoided as the plaster sets. Terminal moulding is performed as the plaster starts warming up, but is still gently mouldable. Don't place limb on

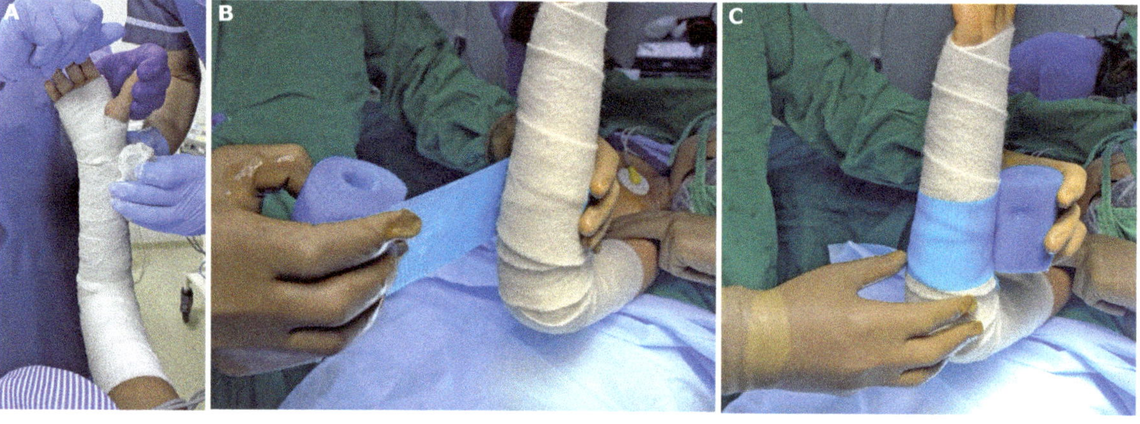

***Fig. 3.3**: Technique of cast application (A) Plaster of Paris roll is kept in contact with the cast padding as it is unrolled. (B) Fiberglass cast is applied by the stretch-relaxation technique in which short length is unrolled and (C) placed on the cast padding*

firm surface while setting. Heel should be hanging free as the plaster sets.

Fiberglass cast application

As the fiberglass cast is more rigid and can cause limb constriction, *"stretch-relaxation technique"* is applied during cast application. In this technique, short length is unrolled and then placed on the cast padding (unlike POP roll which is always in contact with the padding) **(Fig. 3.3)**.

- It is applied with 50% overlap of plaster width.
- 5 to 8 layers of fiberglass cast are applied.
- While applying in concavities like anterior elbow, relaxing cuts may be needed.
- Other precautions taken during application of POP cast are to be followed.

Location specific immobilisation

Below elbow cast/splint

The distal extent of below elbow immobilisation should be the metacarpo-phalangeal joint on the volar aspect (marked on the surface by the distal palmar crease of hand) and metacarpal heads on the dorsal aspect. This should allow free movements of the metacarpo-phalangeal joints of the fingers.

At the thumb, appropriate cutouts in the cast should allow free mobility of the metacarpo-phalangeal joint without impinging and injuring the skin. The wrist should be immobilised in 20^{0} dorsiflexion. The proximal extent of below elbow immobilisation should allow full flexion of the elbow joint **(Fig. 3.4)**.

The forearm portion of cast should be well moulded in order to achieve optimal stretch of the interosseous membrane. Hence in cross section, the cast should be oval shaped rather than round, with the cast index (ratio of antero-posterior to medio-lateral diameter) being less than

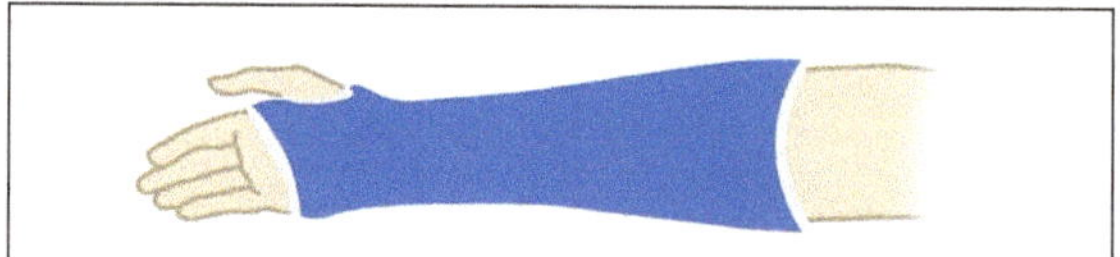

***Fig. 3.4**: Below elbow cast. Distal extent should be at the level of MCP joints indicated on surface by distal palmar crease to allow free movements of MCP joints of all fingers and thumb.*

0.7. Cast index is described in further detail in chapter on forearm fractures.

Above elbow cast/splint

- The distal extent of cast in above elbow immobilisation is as described for below elbow immobilisation.
- The forearm portion should be well moulded to achieve a cast index of less than 0.7 as discussed earlier.
- Moulding the ulnar border of the cast with the flat of the hand is important to prevent "banana-shaped" cast with dorsal angulation at the fracture site.
- While extending the cast above the elbow, care should be taken to prevent bunching of cast padding or cast material in the cubital fossa. Also for the same reason, after application of first layer of padding, avoid change in position of the elbow joint.
- The functional position of immobilisation for the radio-ulnar joints is 10–20° of supination. But this may be modified depending on fracture pattern and angulation. The concept of derotation in forearm fractures is described in further detail in chapter on forearm fractures **(Fig. 3.5A)**.
- The cast is preferably supported in a broad-arm sling rather than a cuff and collar, as there is a propensity to dorsal bowing of the ulna in a cuff and collar **(Fig. 3.5B)**.

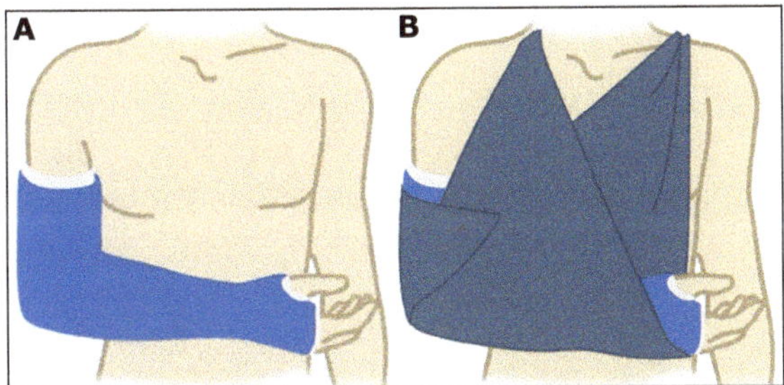

***Fig. 3.5**: Above-elbow cast (A) Extent. (B) Broad-arm sling.*

Thumb-spica extension cast

- While applying thumb spica extension, extra padding is provided in the anatomic snuff box and first web space to avoid pressure sores.
- Cast is applied till the tip of the thumb while the thumb is maintained in neutral abduction and opposition.

U slab/cast

- U slabs or casts are a popular method of immobilisation of middle and lower third humerus fractures.
- The slab extends from the medial aspect of the arm (need not be too high to reach the axilla), extends distally and curves underneath the elbow joint and then along the lateral arm to reach the tip of acromion process **(Fig. 3.6)**.
- As the slab sets, it is tightly wrapped with a bandage so as to obtain a good mould. During moulding, lateral pressure should be applied at the fracture site to counteract the tendency of the fracture to angulate into varus. Once the slab has set, the bandage is removed and is replaced with a lighter fitting bandage or is wrapped over with a casting material to convert it to a U cast.
- Common pitfalls in the application of U slab is keeping the medial edge of the slab too thick or too high into the axilla, or, keeping the lateral edge of the slab too low so that the slab ends at the level of the fracture and in fact acts as a deforming force.

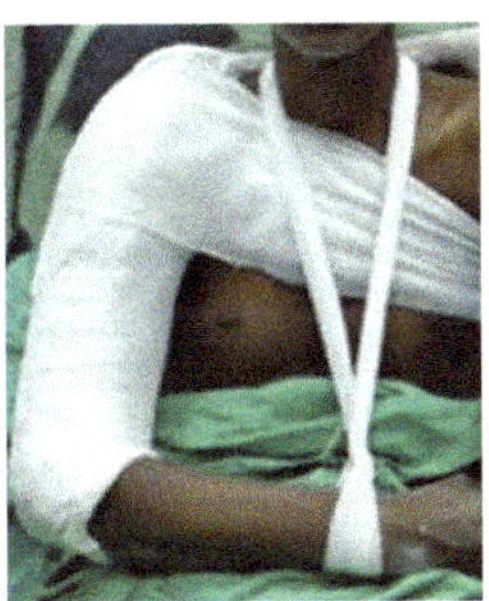

***Fig. 3.6**: "U" slab for fracture humerus shaft.*

Hanging arm cast

- A hanging arm cast is an alternative for immobilsation of proximal third and surgical neck humerus fractures.
- Hanging arm casts don't extend across the fracture. In fact, they don't immobilise the fracture, but instead function on the principle of maintaining fracture reduction by virtue of gravity and weight of the cast.
- Following application of hanging arm cast, the child needs to sleep in upright position for several weeks till the fracture is gummy **(Fig. 3.7)**.

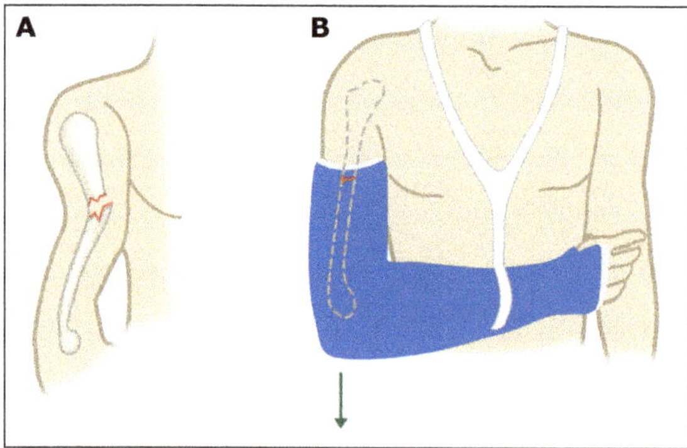

***Fig. 3.7**: (A) Fracture shaft humerus. (B) Hanging arm cast. The weight of the cast helps in fracture reduction. The position of the sling is vital to prevent angulation at fracture site.*

- The cuff and collar applied to a hanging arm cast is attached to the mid-forearm. Cuff and collar attached closer to the wrist tends to create posterior angulation, whereas one attached closer to the elbow creates anterior angulation at the fracture site.

Short leg cast

- A short leg cast should be applied with ankle in neutral flexion.
- The ankle should be held in neutral flexion throughout the process of cast application either by an assistant or by supporting the foot with the surgeon's torso.
- Failure to do so will lead to equinus and attempts to correct the equinus in the later stages of cast application will lead to bunching of plaster on the dorsum of the ankle which can cause skin complications or in rare cases, vascular compromise.

Long leg cast

- The long leg cast should be applied in two portions, short leg cast first followed by the above knee portion.
- The knee should be immobilised in 10 to 20° flexion.
- Fiberglass or hybrid POP/fiberglass cast is preferred since POP only long leg casts tend to be heavy.

Complications of casts

Thermal burns

Curing of casts is an exothermic reaction and therefore thermal burns can occur. Curing of fiberglass cast is less exothermic than POP, so lesser chances of thermal burns. The following precautions should be taken to minimise risk of thermal burns during cast application:

- Temperature of water used for cast dipping should be less than 50°C.
- Do not allow the cast to rest on a pillow while curing, because this does not allow the heat to dissipate and may cause thermal injury.
- Cast layers > 24 is a risk factor for thermal injury. Casts are rarely more than 24 layers thick, but inadvertent increase in number of layers beyond the safe limit can occur in concavity of joints (e.g. cubital fossa, dorsum of ankle) or if slab prepared is too long and is folded back on itself thereby doubling its thickness.

- Some surgeons apply a layer of fiberglass cast over POP cast in order to achieve higher cast strength. Before applying the fiberglass cast, care must be taken to ensure that the underlying POP cast is fully set and the heat generated is fully dissipated to minimise risk of thermal burns.

Pressure sores

Increased pressure underneath a cast leads to ischaemia of the localised area which in turn leads to skin necrosis and pressure sores. Following precautions must be taken to avoid pressure sores underneath a cast:

- Bony prominences should be adequately padded before cast application.
- During cast setting, surgeon/assistant must avoid creating dimples or finger tip indentation points.
- During cast setting, limb should not be resting on firm surfaces. Bony prominences like heel should be hanging free.
- Casts should be well moulded so as to avoid cast slippage which is an important causative factor for pressure sores. Well moulded casts should conform to contours of the limb. For example, in the forearm, casts should be oval rather than spherical with cast index less than 0.7.
- Insertion of foreign objects/coins in the cast should be strictly avoided. In case foreign object is inserted, the cast should be removed and skin inspected **(Fig. 3.8)**.
- If pressure sores occur, superficial erythema may resolve with removal of cast. Eschars which are intact, non draining, non fluctuant and separate from underlying bone should not be disturbed as they serve as biological dressing. On the other hand, deep sores may need debridement, and formal wound management in the form of graft/flap.

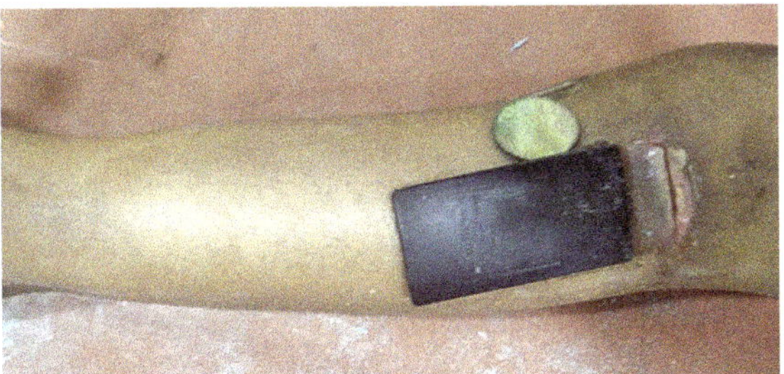

***Fig. 3.8**: Pressure sore following insertion of a coin and foreign object into the cast.*

Infection

- Pressure sores left unattended can get secondarily infected.
- Also, wet POP casts left alone can lead to skin breakdown and infection.
- Small spots of wetting can be dried with hair dryer taking care that the dryer temperature is not too warm.
- If wetting is more extensive, POP casts should be changed.
- Parents should be instructed about change of diapers with hip spica.
- Parents are instructed to look for warning signs of infection which include foul smell/soakage/excess crying/fever.

Compartment syndrome

- Compartment syndrome is undoubtedly the most disastrous complication of a cast.
- Diagnosis and management of compartment syndrome is discussed in detail in Chapter 5.
- Early diagnosis is the key to a good outcome. In children, look for 3 'A's (anxiety, agitation, need for increased analgesia). Remember "there are no hypochondriacs in a cast".

- Children with impaired sensations like spina bifida/neuromuscular injuries or fractures with associated nerve palsy and children with altered sensorium/ small children are especially susceptible to late diagnosis.
- If compartment syndrome is suspected, emergent splitting of cast and padding down to the skin is mandatory. There should be no circumferential bandage encircling the limb. In fiberglass casts, bivalving (splitting of cast on two diagonally opposite sides) is needed. (See section on cast splitting later in this chapter)

Localised acquired Hypertrichosis

- It is characterised by increased hair growth noted after cast removal.
- Incidence is directly proportional to duration of cast.
- It spontaneously resolves in 6 to 12 months after cast removal, no intervention is needed.

Joint Stiffness

- Joint stiffness can be prevented by removing cast and commencing mobilisation as soon as feasible.
- Early restoration of range of motion can be ensured by maintaining joint in functional position during cast immobilisation. (e.g. ankle should be immobilised in neutral position; hand with MCP joints in 70-90^{0} flexion and IP joints in extension).

Cast Cutting

- Cast is removed with oscillating saw which uses high frequency, small amplitude blade oscillations.
- In contact with hard stationary material like cast, the shear forces generated by the oscillating saw cut the fixed material.
- However in contact with skin, it allows the soft tissues to move back and forth with the blade thereby dissipating the shear forces and preventing injury.

Cast saw injuries

- Cast saw injuries can be thermal or abrasive or both.
- Risk factors for thermal cast saw injuries are dull blade, thick cast, thin cast padding and cutting in concavities of joints.
- Risk factors for abrasive cast saw injuries are sharp blade, thin cast padding and cutting over bony prominences.

Avoiding cast saw injuries

- Cast should be perforated rather than cut.
- "In-out" technique which implies firm pressure into cast material, then withdrawal, then reinsertion at adjacent location prevents prolonged contact of cast saw with skin.
- "Dragging" of saw blade may pull the skin taut, thereby cutting it **(Fig. 3.9)**.

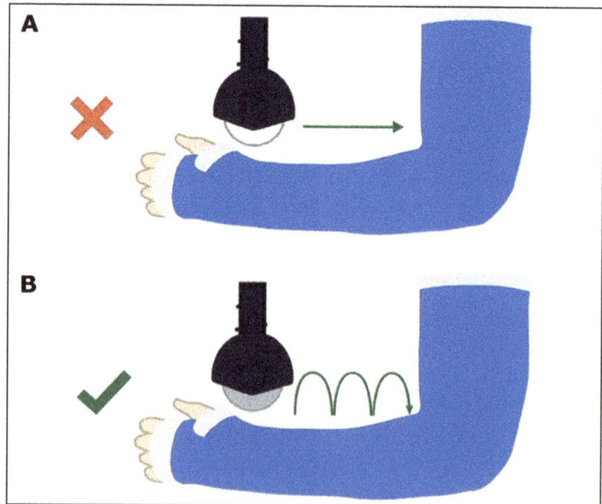

***Fig. 3.9**: (A)Cast saw should not be dragged linearly. (B) Rather it should be perforated by in-out technique.*

Table 3.1: Cast complications and preventive measures

Thermal burns	- Water temperature < 50°C - Cast thickness < 24 layers - Allow POP to cool before reinforcing with fiberglass layer
Pressure sores	- Adequate cast padding, especially at bony prominence - Avoid cast indentation during cast setting - Well moulded cast to avoid slippage - Avoid insertion of foreign bodies in cast
Compartment syndrome	- Identify at risk patients - High index of suspicion (3 'A's) - Cast splitting down to skin at earliest
Hypertrichosis	- Spontaneously resolves
Joint stiffness	- Immobilise in functional position - Remove cast as soon as feasible
Cast cutting complications	- Cast should neither be too thick nor thin - Cast padding should be adequate - Saw blade should neither be too sharp nor too dull - Cast should be perforated by in-out technique - Saw should not be thrust too deep - Avoid cutting in joint concavity - Avoid cutting over bony prominences - Periodically check blade during cast cutting to avoid over-heating

- Avoid firm pressure deep into the skin as it renders the soft tissues immobile and increases chances of injures.
- Water proof cast padding is less heat resistant than cotton padding, so higher risk of cast saw burns.
- Fiberglass cast cutting generates more heat than POP cast cutting and so higher risk of cast saw burns.
- Dull blade generates more heat, so change saw blade periodically.
- While cutting, intermittent checking of blade temperature to look for overheating.
- Intermittent pause to allow cooling of saw blade.
- Cast thickness should be lesser than 10mm. Casts are invariably thicker in the concavities of joints and therefore cutting in concavities should be avoided **(Fig. 3.10)**.
- Cast padding should be adequately thick.
- Newer safety strips are now available for insertion between padding and skin.
- Skin relatively more immobile overlying bony prominences like malleoli, ulnar styloid, olecranon and therefore avoid cutting over these prominences.

Cast Wedging

- Cast wedging is usually employed for fractures less than 2 weeks old, where the reduction is deemed to be unsatisfactory.
- Wedging should be done under image intensifier control for accurate

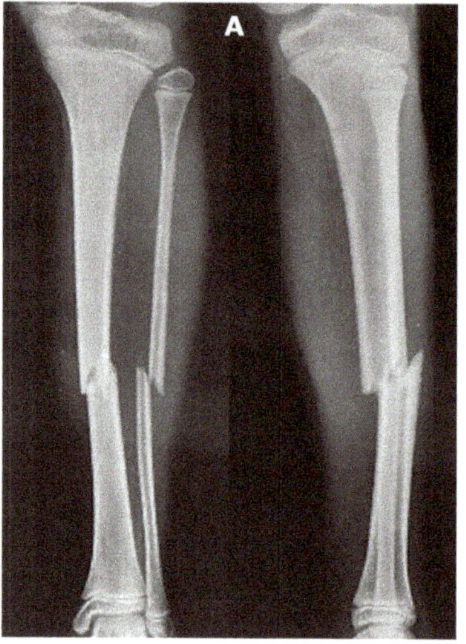

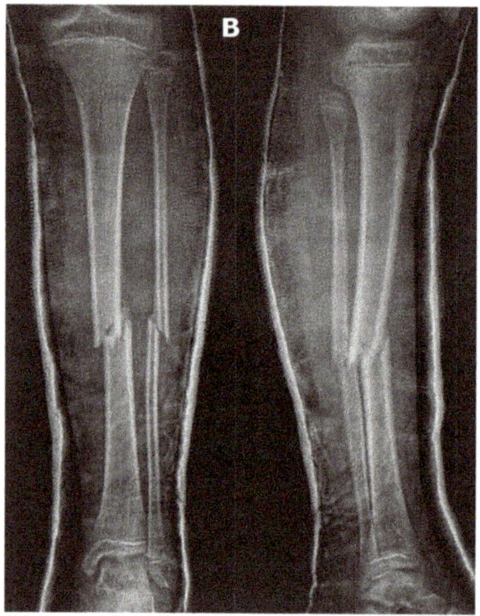

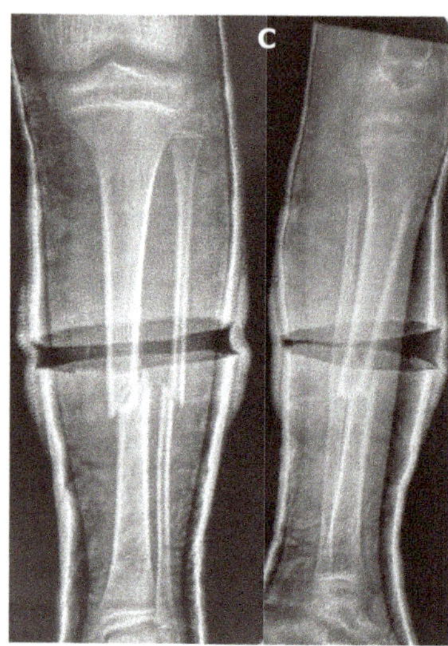

***Fig. 3.10**: Cast wedging: (A) X-ray Left tibia-fibula AP and lateral views showing fracture tibia and fibula (B) This was primarily treated by closed reduction-cast. Recurvatum angulation noted at follow-up radiograph. (C) Angulation was corrected by open cast wedging at the apex of the deformity.*

localisation of fracture level. Cast is cut circumferentially leaving a bridge at the convex apex. Deformity is then corrected till the line becomes straight. The opened edge of the cast is held open by inserting a wedge of the appropriate size. The wedge may be obtained by cutting the central plastic tubing of a plaster roll, or from the plunger of a syringe.

- Closing wedge correction may be employed especially during correction of valgus-procurvatum deformity of tibia, but care taken to avoid pinching of skin on the convex side **(Fig. 3.10)**.
- After cast wedging, child is observed to ensure no pressure effects on underlying skin/neuro-vascular structures.
- In case of failure of cast wedging to obtain satisfactory fracture alignment, remove cast and reapply new cast

Cast Window

- Cast window can be created to inspect an area of concern within a cast. This may be required when cast is applied over wounds, or after surgery or to inspect K-wire insertion sites.
- The window created should be round or oval to avoid creating stress risers and weakening of the cast which may occur with the sharp edges of a rectangular cast window.
- Once the area of concern is inspected, padding of equal depth should be placed and the removed window should be replaced and tied with tape or reinforced with additional cast roll. Failure to do so may cause swelling through the cast window.

Cast Splitting

- A cast may be split if there is concern regarding increased compartment pressure
- Some surgeons perform cast splitting prophylactically after Closed/Open reduction
- Cast splitting must be performed only after cast has set and cooled.
- In case of POP cast, univalve splitting

suffices. Splitting the cast decreases the pressure by 50 to 60% and splitting underlying cast padding further decreases pressure by 10 to 20%.

- In case of fiberglass cast applied without using stretch-relaxation technique, univalve splitting does not suffice and bivalve splitting should be performed.
- In case of fiberglass cast applied using stretch-relaxation technique, univalve splitting may suffice but the split should be held open by inserting a wedge, otherwise the cast may spring back to its original position.

4 Pathological Fractures in Children

Introduction

- Pathological fracture is one that occurs through weakened bone.
- The underlying pathology may either be a localised or generalised disease.
- Treatment of a pathological fracture includes treatment of the underlying pathology in addition to treatment of the fracture itself.

Causes of pathological fractures in children

Common causes of pathological fractures in children include:

- Congenital and genetic diseases e.g. osteogenesis imperfecta, congenital pseudarthrosis of tibia, osteopetrosis.
- Metabolic bone disease
- Neuromuscular disease
- Infections, i.e. osteomyelitis.
- Benign tumours, e.g. Simple bone cyst, Aneurysmal Bone Cyst, Fibrous dysplasia, eosinophilic granuloma, enchondroma, etc.
- Malignant tumours, e.g. osteosarcoma, Ewing's sarcoma, metastases from neuroblastoma/Wilm's tumour, etc.

Clues to diagnosis

The following features may offer a clue to the diagnosis of underlying pathology in pathological fractures in children:

- *Age of the child*
  - 0 to 5 years: Osteomyelitis, Osteogenesis Imperfecta, Eosinophilic Granuloma.
  - 5 to 10 years: Simple Bone Cyst, Aneurysmal Bone Cyst, Fibrous Dysplasia.
  - 10 to 15 years: Simple Bone Cyst, Aneurysmal Bone Cyst, Fibrous Dysplasia, Osteosarcoma.
- *Location of lesion* ***(Tables 4.1 and 4.2)***
  - Diaphysis: Fibrous Dysplasia, Eosinophilic Granuloma, Ewing's sarcoma.
  - Metaphysis: Most tumours.
  - Epiphysis: Chondroblastoma, Brodie's abscess.
  - Spine posterior elements: Aneurysmal Bone Cyst.
  - Spine anterior body: Infections usually Tuberculosis, Eosinophilic Granuloma, Haemangioma, Leukemia.

Fig. 4.1: Distribution of bone lesions in long bones of children

Location	Pathology
Diaphysis	Fibrous Dysplasia
	Eosinophilic granuloma
	Adamantinoma
	Leukemia
Metaphysis	All tumours
	Infections
Epiphysis	Chondroblastoma
	Brodie's abscess

Fig. 4.2: Bone lesions in paediatric spine

Location	Pathology
Posterior elements	Aneurysmal Bone Cyst
	Osteoid Osteoma
	Osteochondroma
Anterior elements	Infection
	Eosinophilic granuloma
	Haemangioma
	Leukemia

- *What is the lesion doing to the bone?*
- Lytic: Most tumours and infections.
- Blastic: Osteoblastoma.
- *How is the bone reacting?*
- Reactive bone formation: Slow growing tumours.
- *Is there an associated soft tissue mass:*
- Usually aggressive, perhaps malignant lesion.

General Principles of Treatment

- Establishing diagnosis is necessary before embarking on definitive treatment in pathological fractures. Work-up of a child with a pathological fracture through a suspected malignant lesion must include advanced imaging (MRI of entire bone segment) followed by biopsy and PET scan (if malignancy is confirmed).

Imaging

- In addition to plain AP and lateral X-rays of the affected bone, imaging in pathological fractures of uncertain aetiology should include MRI of the entire bone, with contrast enhancement. Points to be noted on imaging include the location, extent, nature of lesion, zone of transition between the lesion and surrounding normal bone; and periosteal reaction. Lesions which appear entirely lytic on plain radiographs may reveal solid component on MRI indicating more sinister nature of pathology. Also intra-osseous and peri-osseous soft tissue component should be carefully studied on MRI to obtain a clue to diagnosis.

Biopsy

- Histopathological confirmation of diagnosis with J-needle biopsy should be obtained in pathological fractures with suspected neoplastic aetiology. All principles of biopsy in malignant bony lesions should be meticulously observed. Biopsy should preferably be performed by the surgeon who would perform the definitive surgery if the lesion is shown to be neoplastic. The trajectory of needle insertion should avoid violation of multiple muscle compartments. Also the needle tract should be located within the definitive surgical approach so that it can be excised with sufficient margins at the time of definitive surgery. Location of soft tissue component of the neoplasm should be carefully studied on MRI and biopsy should be obtained from this region for most accurate histopathological diagnosis. The dictum "Culture every biopsy, and biopsy every culture" should be followed, and samples obtained should be sent for histopathological examination, aerobic culture and investigations for Mycobacterium Tuberculosis.

Specific Pathologies

Simple Bone Cyst (Unicameral Bone Cyst)

Introduction

- Simple Bone Cyst (SBC) is a benign, solitary cystic lesion that involves the metaphysis or metadiaphysis of long bones.

Clinical Features

- SBC occurs mostly in the first two decades of life.
- The commonest locations include proximal femur, proximal humerus and proximal tibia.
- In 80% cases, initial presentation is with a pathological fracture.
- The cyst may heal along-with the fracture in 10% cases.

Imaging

Plain radiographic characteristic features of SBCs include:

- Well defined, centrally located, radiolucent/cystic lesion in metaphysis/meta-diaphysis.
- Cortical thinning and mild expansion.
- Fractures through simple bone cysts are usually incomplete or undisplaced.
- If pathological fracture is of some duration, mild periosteal reaction may be seen.
- *Fallen leaf/fragment sign:* may be seen in some cases of pathological fracture wherein the fragment of bone is seen floating within the cyst fluid.
- MRI with contrast is performed to rule out other differential diagnoses.

The red flag signs which suggest that the lesion under consideration may not be a SBC include:

- Eccentric location in bone.
- Significant expansion beyond the limits of the original bone.
- Significant periosteal reaction.
- Soft tissue component and fluid-fluid levels on MRI.

Biopsy

- Histopathological confirmation of the diagnosis of SBC is obtained in cases with atypical radiographic characteristics. All principles of biopsy of bone tumour as mentioned earlier are meticulously observed. The inner linings of the cyst wall are scraped with the bevel tip of the J-needle. This procedure is a combination of minimally invasive curettage and biopsy and hence is called "curopsy". In addition to providing material for diagnosis, curopsy induces an inflammatory healing response which may increase healing rates and improve healing time in SBC.

Treatment

Non-operative treatment:

Non-operative treatment of pathological fracture through SBC is indicated in following scenarios:

- Pathological fractures through SBCs of the upper limb, especially those involving less than 80% bone diameter.
- Undisplaced or minimally displaced fractures through SBCs in the lower limb (except around the hip) may also be treated non-operatively.
- Non-operative treatment consists of immobilisation, nature of immobilisation depending on anatomical site.
- Fractures through SBC usually heal uneventfully.
- The cyst may heal along with fracture in about 10% cases.

Operative Treatment:

Operative treatment of pathological fractures in SBC is indicated in following scenarios:

- Fractures around the hip.
- Displaced fractures in the lower limb.
- Fractures through upper limb SBC involving more than 80% canal diameter.

- Surgery consists of curettage, bone grafting and internal fixation.
- Prophylactic fixation may be indicated in cysts around the hip, those with cortical thinning and those occupying more than 50 to 80% of bone diameter **(Figs. 4.1 and 4.2)**.

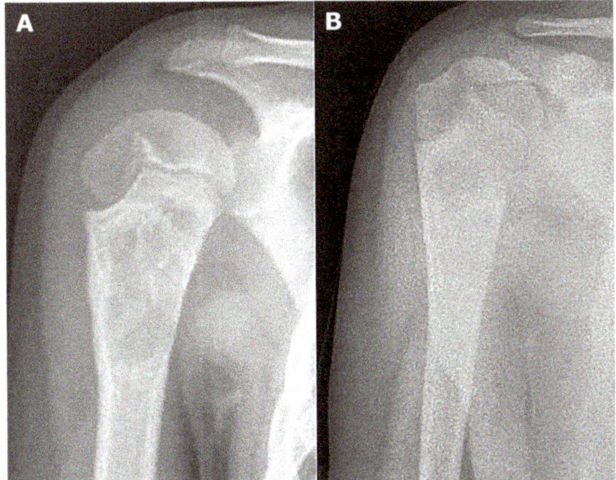

Fig. 4.1: *(A) AP X-ray of the Right shoulder in a 13-years-old male adolescent, presenting with pain Right proximal humerus of acute onset following history of trivial trauma, shows lytic lesion Right proximal humerus which was diagnosed to be a Simple Bone Cyst after MRI and needle biopsy. (B) X-ray following treatment with curettage of inner walls of the lesion with needle bevel tip and steroid injection shows complete healing of the lesion at 6 months followup.*

There are various modalities for management of SBC after fracture healing, including:

- Intra-lesional steroid injection.
- Curettage-excision of cyst lining-packing of cyst cavity with bone graft or calcium sulfate pellets.
- Intra and extra-medullary decompression of cyst cavity.
- Insertion of TENS nail as prophylactic fixation as well as to provide continuous intra-medullary decompression.
- A detailed discussion of these treatment modalities is out of scope of this book.

Aneurysmal Bone Cyst (ABC)

Introduction

- Aneurysmal Bone Cyst (ABC) is a benign but locally aggressive bone tumour.
- Most of the ABCs are primary, but a third of them are secondary and associated with underlying benign or malignant lesions.

Clinical Features

- Common sites involved are femur, tibia, humerus and spine posterior elements.

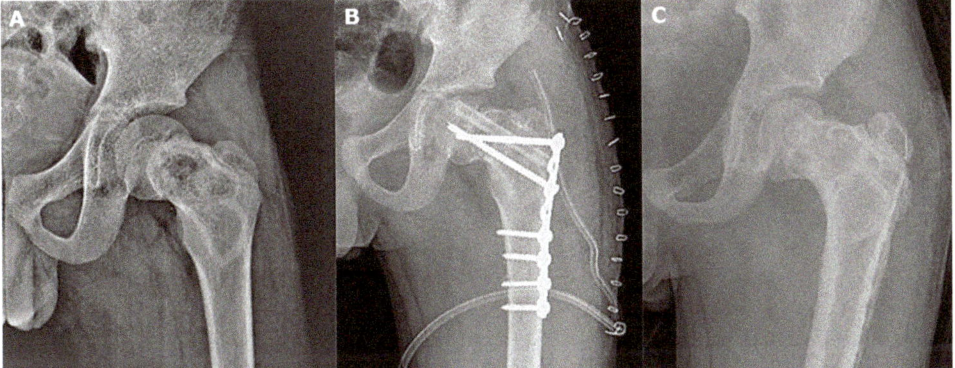

Fig. 4.2: *(A) X-ray Left hip AP view showing Left proximal femur central, non-expansile lytic lesion in a 9-years-old male child presented with vague pain Left proximal thigh and limp of few months duration. MRI and needle biopsy was diagnostic of a simple bone cyst. (B) X-ray Left hip AP view following surgical treatment with curettage, bone grafting and fixation with plate and screws. (C) X-ray Left hip at 1.5 years followup shows complete healing of the lesion.*

Imaging

- On plain radiography, Aneurysmal Bone Cyst is seen as an eccentric, expansile, multiloculated lesion, which may occasionally extend into adjoining epiphysis.
- MRI reveals classic fluid-fluid levels in Aneurysmal Bone Cyst. Evaluation of contrast images is essential to identify solid components which indicate the possibility of ABC being secondary to an underlying benign or malignant lesion.

Biopsy

- Biopsy is essential for diagnosis and to rule out underlying pathology (secondary ABC). Histopathology in an Aneurysmal Bone Cyst reveals blood filled clefts within bony trabeculae with osteoid tissue within the stromal matrix.

Treatment

- In the setting of a fracture, minimally displaced ABCs are treated conservatively. Fracture heals with immobilisation. However ABCs don't heal with fracture healing and need to be independently treated at a later stage.
- Preoperative embolization helps to shrink the size of the tumour, and may be used in large neoplasms prior to definitive surgery.
- After fracture heals, intralesional sclerotherapy by injecting sclerosants like Polidocanol or Doxycycline has emerged as first line treatment for management of ABCs.
- Open surgery consists of four-step resection consisting of curettage of inner walls of the cyst, followed by use of high speed burr, then electrocautery and finally thorough lavage with 5% phenol. The cyst is then packed with bone graft and internal fixation is performed. Titanium implants are preferred for fixation of ABCs so as to facilitate MRI, should recurrence occur in the future.

Fibrous Dysplasia

Introduction and Clinical Features

- Fibrous dysplasia is a condition characterised by replacement of normal bone and marrow with fibro-osseous tissue which is susceptible to undergo deformation and pathological fracture.
- The disease may be monostotic or polyostotic. McCune Albright syndrome is a condition characterised by polyostotic fibrous dysplasia, café-au-lait spots and endocrine dysfunction.
- Bones commonly involved are femur, humerus and tibia.
- Many times, diagnosis of fibrous dysplasia is made after occurrence of pathological fracture. Microfractures may present with insidious onset of pain and swelling in the absence of radiologically visible fracture. Repeated micro-fractures lead to slowly progressive bowing deformities of long bones. Shepherd crook deformity of proximal femur is an example.

Imaging

- Radiologically, fibrous dysplasia is a well-defined, lytic, central lesion in the diaphysis of long bones. The characteristic "ground glass" appearance is due to the woven bone content of the lesion.

Biopsy

- Histopathology of fibrous dysplasia reveals fibrous stroma surrounding irregularly woven bony trabeculae which are arranged in a pattern referred to as "resembling Chinese letters".

Treatment

- Fractures through fibrous dysplasia heal with immobilisation but are frequently associated with progressive deformities.
- In the setting of acute pathological fracture, surgical intervention is indicated in displaced fractures or fractures in significantly deformed bones, especially of the lower extremity.
- Bone grafting of fibrous dysplasia lesions is not indicated as there is a high propensity to graft resorption. However strut cortical grafts may be used to provide temporary structural support in large lesions till such time that the fracture heals.
- For internal fixation of pathological fractures in fibrous dysplasia, intramedullary nails are preferred so as to provide whole bone stabilisation and avoid stress risers at the tip of the implant. Deformities may be corrected with additional corrective osteotomies at the same sitting or may be deferred to a later stage **(Fig. 4.3)**.

Fibrous Cortical Defect (FCD) and Non Ossifying Fibroma (NOF)

- Fibrous Cortical Defect (FCD) and Non Ossifying Fibroma (NOF) are cortical based lytic lesions of the metaphysis and are surrounded by a sharp sclerotic border **(Fig. 4.4)**.
- FCDs are small (< 2cm in diameter) whereas NOFs are larger and can be multiple in a third of patients.
- In most cases, FCDs and NOFs are incidentally detected on radiographs

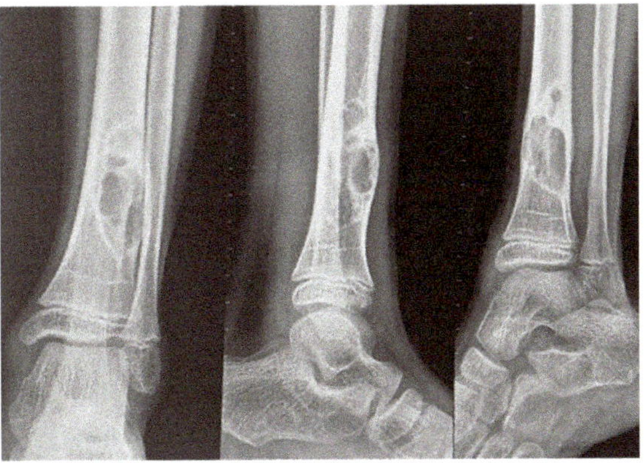

***Fig. 4.4**: X-ray showing lytic lesion distal tibia, with sharp sclerotic margin suggestive of Non ossifying fibroma*

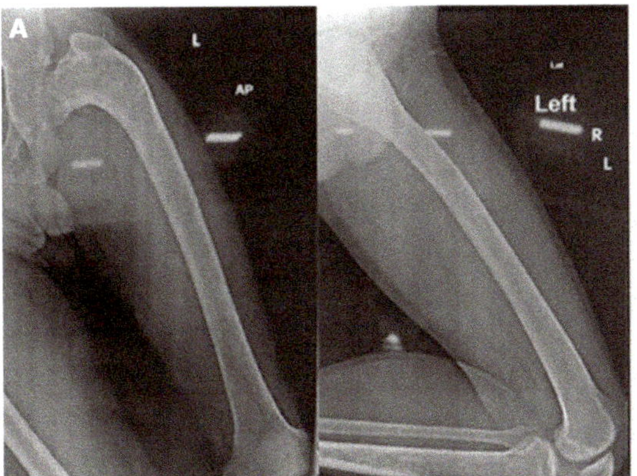

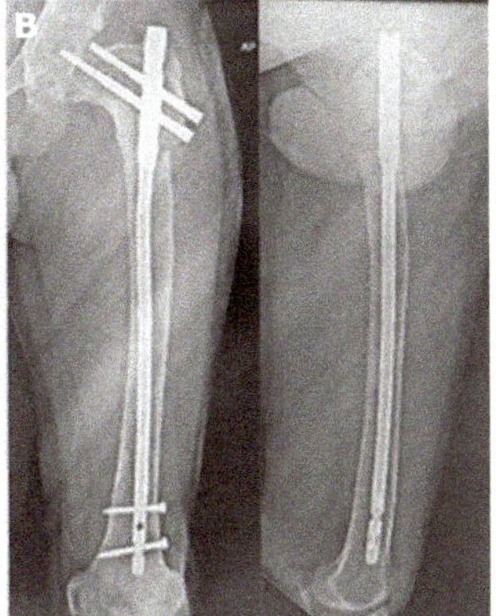

***Fig. 4.3**: (A) X-ray Left hip AP and lateral views in a 16-years-old adolescent boy presenting with Left lower limb Trendelenberg gait and chronic pain of insidious onset of five years duration showing central, well-defined lytic lesion with ground glass appearance and "Shepherd crook" deformity of Left proximal femur. Biopsy and skeletal survey revealed the diagnosis of polyostotic fibrous dysplasia. (B) X-rays following deformity correction and fixation with intramedullary interlocking nail.*

obtained for unrelated causes. However, lesions exceeding 50% transverse diameter of bone are at risk for fracture. Age group 6 to 14 years and lower extremity lesions are other risk factors for fracture.

- Fractures through FCD or NOF are treated with immobilisation. Fractures usually heal uneventfully but lesions usually persist and may need definitive treatment if at risk for recurrent fractures.
- However prophylactic fixation for lesions which have never fractured is not indicated irrespective of the size of the NOF.

Enchondromas

- Enchondromas are benign cartilaginous tumours most commonly seen in the phalanges of hands and feet, metacarpals, metatarsals, humerus and femur. Multiple enchondromas are seen in Ollier's disease **(Fig. 4.5)**.

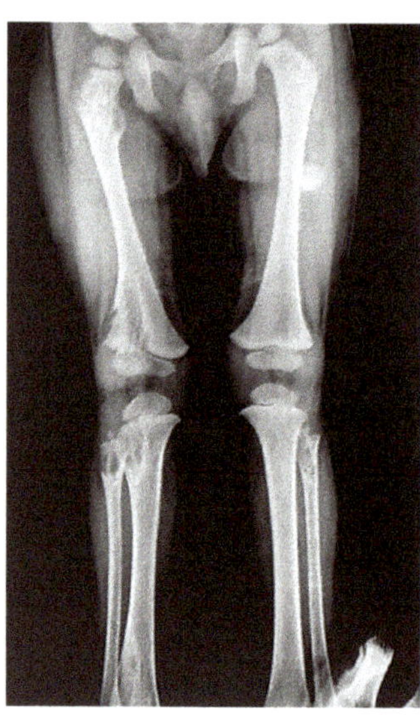

Fig. 4.5*: X-ray both lower limbs showing typical linear translucent streaks extending from metaphysis to diaphysis in Right proximal femur, distal femur, proximal tibia and distal tibia suggestive of multiple enchondromatosis (Ollier's disease).*

- Radiographic characteristics of enchondroma are as follows:
  - Central intramedullary lesions with stippled calcification.
  - In large lesions, cortical thinning and scalloping.
  - Linear radiolucent streaks extending from metaphysis to diaphysis.
- Lesions in small bones with typical radiographic features of enchondroma need not be biopsied but histopathological confirmation of diagnosis must be sought wherever there is doubt regarding diagnosis.
- Acute and impending pathological fractures with pain are treated with curettage and bone grafting. Fixation is not needed for lesions in small tubular bones of hands and feet, but should be performed for large lesions through long bones, especially of the lower extremity.

Malignant/Metastatic Lesions

- The most common malignant bone tumours in children are osteosarcoma and Ewing's sarcoma.
- Rarely, diagnosis of malignant bone tumours may occur after a pathological fracture.
- Work-up of a child with a pathological fracture through a suspected malignant lesion must include advanced imaging (MRI of entire bone segment) followed by biopsy and PET scan (if malignancy is confirmed).
- With advent of neo-adjuvant chemotherapy, limb salvage is possible in malignant bone tumours even in the setting of pathological bone fracture.
- Definitive management of pathological fractures should be done by surgeons with sufficient training and experience in Orthopaedic oncology.

Congenital Pseudarthrosis of Tibia

- Congenital Pseudarthrosis of Tibia (CPT) is a rare condition occurring in 1/150000 live births.
- It is frequently associated with underlying neurofibromatosis type 1.
- It is a disease of the periosteum rather than bone. Hamartomatous periosteum surrounding pseudarthrosis site is shown to have decreased osteogenic potential (limited response of osteoblasts to Bone Morphogenic Protein) and increased osteoclastic activity (responsible for increased bone resorption). The periosteum surrounding the pseudarthrosis site is also weakening of bone due to decreased vascularity.
- Congenital Pseudarthrosis of Tibia is characterised by anterolateral bowing of tibia which eventually fractures, typically before the age of 3 years.
- Achieving and maintaining union in CPT requires combined redressal of both biological and mechanical issues at hand.
- Biological treatment consists of combination of peri-operative bisphosphonates (to inhibit increased osteoclastogenesis) and intra-operative implantation of Bone Morphogenic Protein at the pseudarthrosis site (to stimulate osteoblastic activity). Also radical circumferential excision of hamartomatous periosteum at the pseudarthrosis site is essential.
- Mechanical treatment consists of correction of the anterolateral bow and rigid fixation of the tibia and fibula with intramedullary implants (may be supplemented with external fixator/plate and screws). Additionally, increasing the cross-sectional surface area of union by bone grafting to achieve tibia-fibula cross-union has been shown to increase the rates of primary union as well as decreasing the incidence of re-fractures **(Figs. 4.6)**.

Osteopetrosis

- Osteopetrosis is a rare congenital disease characterised by decreased osteoclastic activity. Decreased osteoclastic resorption of bone leads to increased bone density seen on X-rays. Though dense, these bones are brittle and are at risk for pathological fractures.

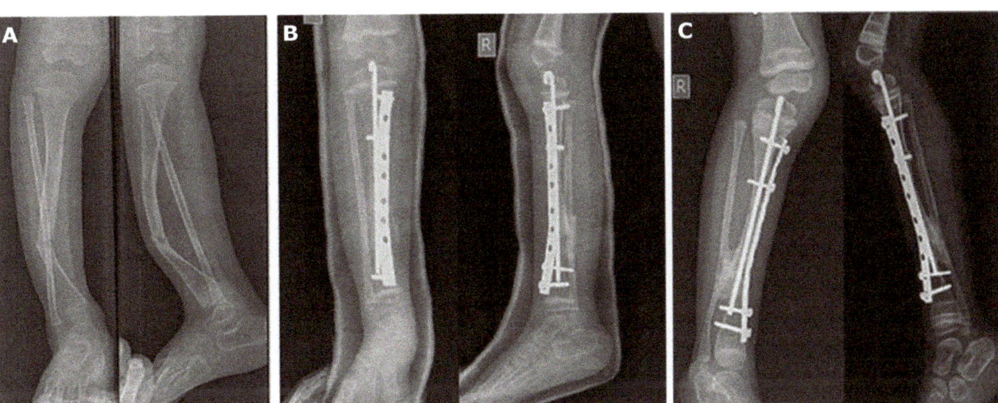

Fig. 4.6: *(A) X-ray Right tibia-fibula AP and lateral views in a 9 years old female child with underlying neurofibromatosis Type 1 showing antero-lateral bowing with Congenital Pseudarthrosis of Tibia (B) X-rays following treatment with hamartomatous periosteum excision, fixation of the tibia with plate and screws, rush rod and bone-grafting (C) X-rays at one year follow-up show cross-union between the tibia and fibula.*

- Additionally these patients have decreased haematopoietic activity due to encroachment of the medullary canal by bone.
- Bone marrow transplant offers best chance of cure.
- Fractures in osteopetrotic bone can heal with conservative measures, but due to decreased osteoclastic activity, bone resorption is limited which in turn leads to decreased remodelling capacity.
- Intramedullary nailing is extremely difficult.
- Fixation with plate and screws can lead to stress risers and fractures at the tip of the implant.

Osteogenesis imperfecta

Introduction

- Osteogenesis imperfecta is a congenital bone disorder occurring due to defect in the collagen component of extra-cellular matrix. The genetic defect in osteogenesis imperfecta has been localised mainly to COL1A1 and COL1A2 genes. Mutation of these leads to either defective or deficient production of collagen Type 1.

Classification

- Osteogenesis imperfecta was originally classified by Sillence into four types with Type 2 being most severe and lethal type. Amongst children who survive, Type 3 is most severe type, followed by Type 4 and Type 1 in order of decreasing severity. Advances in genetics have identified additional types of Osteogenesis imperfecta leading to expansion of the original Sillence classification, and as of now 18 different types are identified.

Clinical Features

- Clinical features of osteogenesis imperfecta include fractures with trivial trauma, blue sclerae of eyes, dentinogenesis imperfecta and deafness due to auditory nerve compression in the auditory canal. Spine involvement in the form of kyphoscoliosis or basilar invagination may further complicate the picture.
- Children with osteogenesis imperfecta either present with acute fractures or with bowing of bones of both upper and lower limbs. The bowing may occur due to malunion of fractures or more commonly it may occur due to repeated micro-fractures which heal with progressive bowing.

Treatment

Non-operative treatment:

- Medical treatment consists of bisphosphonates which inhibit osteoclastic activity and bone resorption. Usually cyclical therapy with intravenous bisphosphonates (Pamidronate/Zolendronate) is preferred. Before bisphosphonate infusion, hypocalcemia should be ruled out, as serum levels of calcium can decrease following bisphosphonate infusion and in rare cases, this can even lead to hypocalcemic tetany. Children with osteogenesis imperfecta should receive adequate calcium- Vitamin D supplementation.

Operative treatment:

- Surgical treatment in osteogenesis imperfecta consists of fixation of fractures, correction of bony deformity and stabilisation with intramedullary nails. Bones are often bowed and more than one osteotomy is usually needed for deformity correction and nail insertion.
- These children usually undergo their first surgery at a young age (around 5 years), and therefore choice of implant

should take into account the future growth of the bone. For this reason, telescoping nails which expand in length with bone growth are preferred. Fassier Duval nails are the current generation telescopic nails being used and they are an improvement over the previous generation nails in that both male and female components of the nail can be inserted through a single end of the bone. So incisions and arthrotomies at both ends of the bone are avoided. **(Fig. 4.7)**

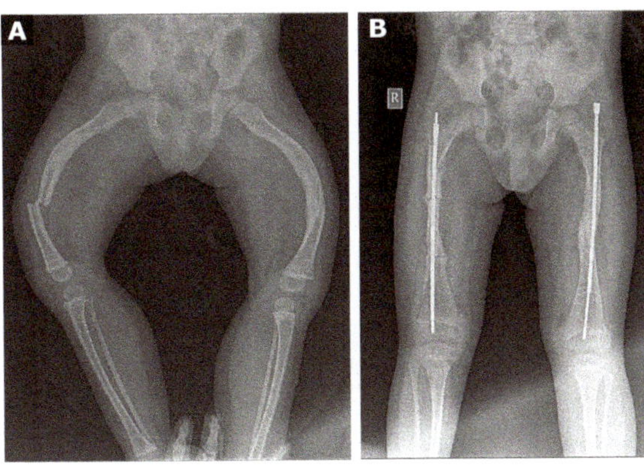

***Fig. 4.7**: (A) X-ray both lower limbs in a child with osteogenesis imperfecta shows bilateral femur bowing with Right side fracture (B) After deformity correction and intra-medullary nailing with telescoping Fassier-Duval nails.*

- Plates as solitary mode of fixation in osteogenesis imperfecta should be strictly avoided, however along with nail, they may be used as accessory fixation to provide rotational stability at fracture/osteotomy site.
- Technical details of surgery in osteogenesis imperfecta are out of scope of this book and readers are referred to textbooks of Pediatric Orthopaedics for a more detailed reading of the same.

Infections

Introduction

- Pathological fractures in bones affected by osteomyelitis can occur once bone demineralization exceeds 50%. This typically occurs in infections presenting late, or infections not responding to medical/surgical treatment or once infection has progressed to stage of chronic osteomyelitis.

Clinical Features

- Children with pathological fracture following osteomyelitis may have variable presentation.
- In acute osteomyelitis, children may present with acute onset pain, fever, swelling and inability to use the affected limb.
- In late presentations or partially treated cases, children may present with discharging sinus. Occasionally there may be history of extrusion of bone fragments through the sinus tract indicating sequestration.
- In some cases, the infection may be completely quiescent following previous medical/surgical treatment and the fracture may occur as a consequence of weakening of bone due to the previous infection.
- In some cases, resorption of bone or extrusion of sequestrated bone may result in significant gap at the fracture site. Such gap non-unions result in considerable shortening and instability at the fracture site. **(Fig. 4.8)**.

Imaging

- Plain radiographs are usually sufficient for diagnosis of pathological fractures following osteomyelitis. Since fractures usually occur late in the course of infection, the radiographic changes of osteomyelitis are usually well established by the time fracture occurs.
- Advanced imaging in the form of MRI is reserved for acute presentations where the changes of osteomyelitis are not yet

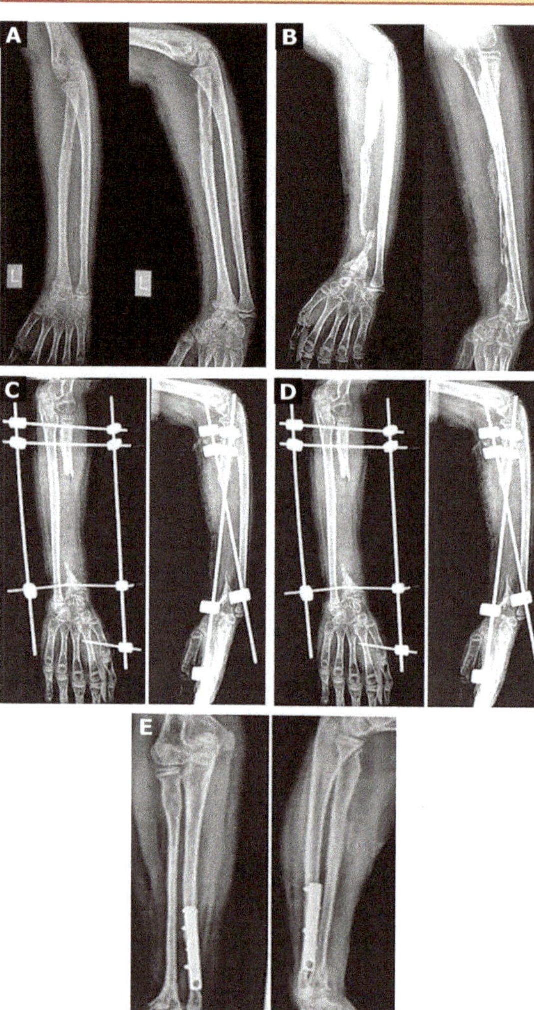

***Fig. 4.8**: An 8 years old girl presented with pain, swelling Left forearm which was diagnosed elsehwhere as an abscess and treated with incision and drainage. (A,B) X-rays Left forearm AP and lateral views in the post-operative period revealed osteomyelitis of the Left radius which progressed to a pathological fracture. (C) Extrusion of the sequestrated fragment resulted in a gap non-union. (D,E) The child was treated with serial debridements, and after infection control, the gap non-union was reconstructed by interposition of fibula strut graft.*

well established. MRI is also useful for obtaining more information regarding the extent and spread of intra-osseous and peri-osseous abscess. MRI must also be done if there is any possibility of the lesion under consideration being neoplastic in nature.

Blood Investigations

- Complete Blood count (CBC), Erythrocyte Sedimentation Rate (ESR) and C-Reactive Protein (CRP) should be obtained to identify persistence of active infection and to track response to treatment.

Bacteriological Investigations

- Blood cultures are positive in only about 40% cases of acute osteomyelitis. Positivity rate is further decreased in the setting of chronic osteomyelitis with pathological fracture, wherein the children may already have been treated with a course of antibiotics.
- In cases presenting with discharging sinus, we avoid obtaining specimens for culture from the sinus tract as these are almost always contaminated. Deep cultures obtained at the time of definitive surgery are more reliable to guide the choice of antibiotics in these scenarios.

Treatment

Prevention of pathological fracture:

- In the setting of acute osteomyelitis, every attempt must be made to prevent pathological fracture. This is done by adequate control of infection (medical treatment with/without surgical treatment) and adequate immobilisation and protection of the affected part till bone strength is restored. Immobilisation may be achieved with simple slab/splint or an external fixator may be applied in the event of an impending pathological fracture.

Non-operative treatment:

- If the pathological fracture is detected

early, there is no gap at fracture site and periosteal cover is intact, the fracture may heal with simple immobilisation in plaster cast provided the infection is well-controlled by administration of appropriate antibiotics.

Operative treatment:

The priniciples of surgical management of pathological fracture following osteomyelitis are:

- Infection control: This consists of medical treatment (antibiotics), and thorough surgical debridement of dead, devitalised tissue and sequestrated bone. In addition, high dose local antibiotic delivery may be achieved with antibiotic mixed Calcium sulfate granules or antibiotic mixed cement spacer.
- Reconstruction of bony defect: This may be achieved with:
  - Acute docking at fracture site
  - Internal bone transport
  - Bone graft: cancellous/fibula strut graft (complete control of infection is essential before bone grafting)
- Stable fixation: Fixation may be achieved with
  - External fixator: This is preferred in case of active infection. Fixator may be a monolateral fixator or ring fixator.
  - Internal fixation: Internal fixation is performed only after infection is adequately controlled. This can be assessed by absence of fever, absence of local signs of inflammation, quiescent sinuses for at least 6 to 8 weeks and normalisation of haematological parameters. Internal fixation may be performed with plate and screws/ intramedullary fixation devices/K-wires.

Fractures in Children with Cerebral Palsy

- Children with cerebral palsy are at risk for fractures due to reduced mobility leading to disuse osteopenia, poor nutrition due to impaired swallowing leading to Calcium/Vitamin D deficiency, and, oral anti-convulsant therapy leading to impaired Vitamin D hydroxylation in the liver. Non-ambulatory children with cerebral palsy are at higher risk for fractures than ambulatory children.
- Majority of fractures in children with cerebral palsy occur in the lower limb. Fractures of the distal femur are especially common and vigorous manipulation of knee flexion contractures is a common cause for the same. Fractures also commonly occur after seizure episodes.
- Fractures of the distal pole of patella may occur in children walking with flexed knee crouch gait for a prolonged period. Overactivity of the quadriceps with patella alta leads to fatigue fracture of the distal pole patella. These fractures spontaneously heal after correction of crouch gait pattern and don't need fixation.
- Vitamin C deficiency leading to scurvy is a common cause for physeal seperations and should be suspected when these occur spontaneously at multiple sites in the absence of any antecedent trauma, accompanied by bleeding gums.
- More awareness needs to be raised towards prevention of fractures in children with cerebral palsy. Measures for fracture prevention include nutrition to avoid Calcium deficiency, sunlight exposure to satisfy Vitamin D requirements and physical activity to build bone/muscle mass. Calcium and Vitamin D supplements may be prescribed if dietary intake is inadequate to satisfy daily requirements. Also for high-risk children, bisphosphonates are recommended to improve bone density.

- Treatment of fractures in children with cerebral palsy needs to be individualised, and should be aimed at restoring the child to pre-fracture level of activity.
- Many of these can be successfully treated conservatively, but care should be taken to provide adequate cast padding to prevent pressure sores in spastic children.
- Physeal fractures secondary to scurvy heal dramatically following administration of oral Vitamin C supplements. **(Fig. 4.9)**

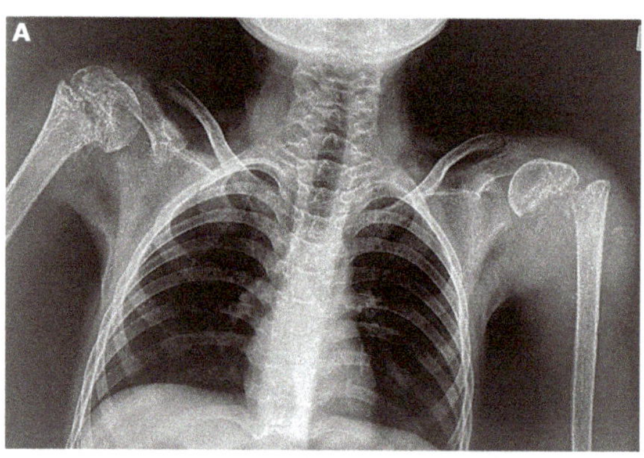

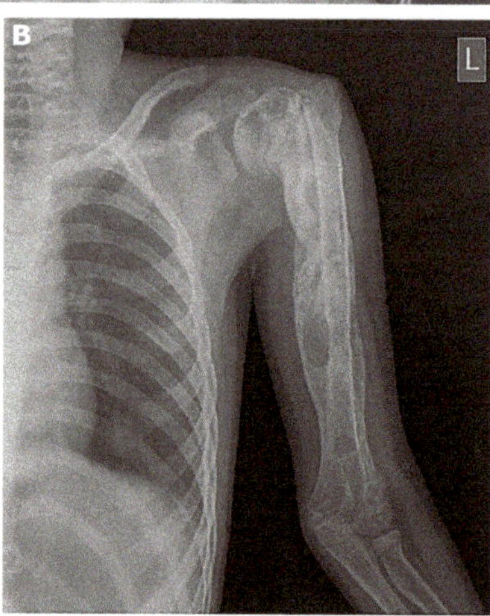

Fig. 4.9: *(A) X-ray Bilateral proximal humerus shows physeal fracture due to scurvy in a child with cerebral palsy (B) Fracture healing with ossification of sub-periosteal hematoma following treatment with oral Vitamin C supplements.*

- Fractures of neck femur should be treated surgically, with the same diligence as in a neuro-typical child.
- Fracture of the femur in an older child is usually treated surgically. The implant used for fracture fixation should ideally be an intramedullary nail, as plate fixation is associated with a high rate of implant failure and fractures through stress-risers at the tip of the implant.

Fractures in Children with Meningo-myelocele

- Children with meningomyelocele are at risk for fractures due to disuse osteopenia caused by decreased mobility, abnormal stresses on the lower limbs while walking due to dragging and twisiting of the legs, and, absent pain perception leading to lack of trauma awareness.
- Risk of fractures increases with increasing levels of neurological deficit. Fractures most commonly occur in the lower limbs, mainly the femur **(Fig. 4.10)**.

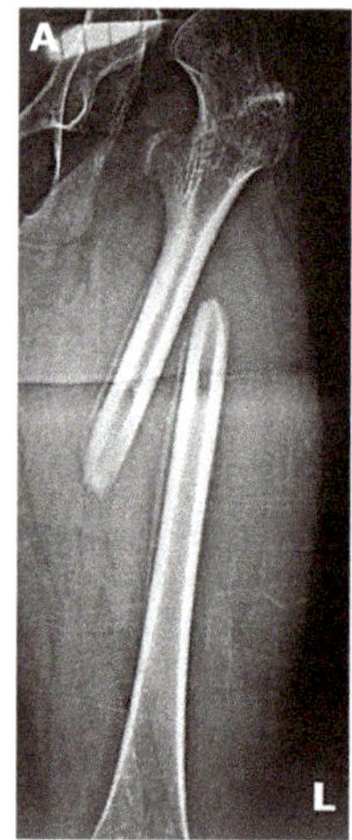

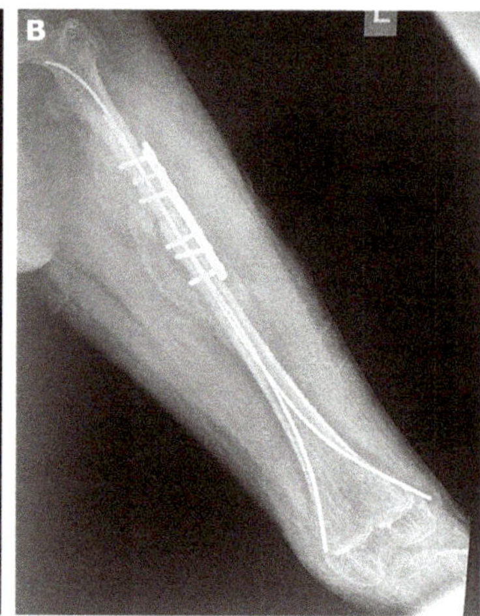

Fig. 4.10: *(A) X-ray Left femur in a child with meningomyelocele showing Left fracture femur with severe over-riding (B) Following surgical treatment with femoral shortening and fixation with TENS nails supplemented with plate.*

- Children with meningomyelocele are also prone to sustain physeal injuries. In the acute stages, physeal injuries are often confused for infections due to presence of overlying soft tissue oedema, erythema and warmth, and, elevated cell counts and C-Reactive Proteins. These injuries respond dramatically to two to three days of immobilisation. During healing phase, physeal injuries exhibit physeal widening with exuberant callus formation for which reason they may be mistaken for infections or malignant neoplasms.
- Fractures in children with myelomeningocele may be treated conservatively or surgically depending on location and patient profile. Undisplaced low energy fractures may be treated conservatively. Mobilisation should be commenced as early as possible to minimise disuse osteopenia. If surgical management is chosen, intramedullary nails are the preferred implants, since plate fixation run the risk of causing stress fractures at the implant tip.
- On the other hand, physeal injuries in children with meningomyelocele have prolonged healing time, and hence require immobilisation for a longer period.

5 Compartment Syndrome

Introduction

- Compartment syndrome is sustained increased pressure within a closed osteo-fascial compartment resulting in circulatory compromise, tissue ischaemia, and eventually tissue death.
- If not identified and treated expeditiously, it can result in severe and irreversible disability.
- Compartment syndrome occurs most commonly as a complication of fractures or due to constricting casts applied for the treatment of fractures.
- In the upper limb, supracondylar humerus and both bones forearm fractures, and, in the lower limb, tibia fractures are most commonly complicated by compartment syndrome.
- High risk injuries include "floating injuries", e.g. "floating elbow" which is a combination of ipsilateral fracture supracondylar humerus with fracture both bones forearm.
- Even in the absence of fractures, compartment syndrome can occur in the setting of severe soft tissue injuries, insect/snake bites and underlying bleeding disorders. A high index of suspicion is needed to make a diagnosis in these conditions.

Pathophysiology

- Normal tissue pressure within a closed osteo-fascial compartment is about 10mm Hg, whereas the capillary filling pressure is essentially the diastolic arterial pressure. The difference between the tissue pressure and diastolic pressure is called Muscle Perfusion Pressure.
- Muscle oedema leads to increase in tissue pressure within a closed osteo-fascial compartment leading to progressive decrease in the Muscle Perfusion Pressure. When the tissue pressure reaches within 30mm Hg of the diastolic pressure, capillary filling and subsequently tissue perfusion is significantly impaired.
- Simultaneously, increased venous pressure due to obstructed venous drainage further worsens the capillary filling and tissue perfusion.
- Decreased tissue perfusion leads to tissue ischaemia, which if sufficiently prolonged and severe, leads to muscle cell necrosis. This leads to release of histamine and other intracellular inflammatory mediators, which increase vascular permeability with further worsening of muscle oedema.
- Thus, this sets in motion a self-perpetuating cycle of increasing oedema, worsening tissue perfusion and tissue necrosis, which unless broken by timely and appropriate management leads to irreversible tissue death and functional sequelae **(Fig. 5.1)** .
- The ability to withstand ischaemia depends on type of tissue. Whereas muscle shows functional loss after 2 to 4 hours of ischaemia, irreversible damage occurs after 4 to 12 hours of unrelieved ischaemia. Nerve tissue on the other hand, exhibits functional loss after 30 minutes of ischaemia and irreversible damage after 12 to 24 hours.

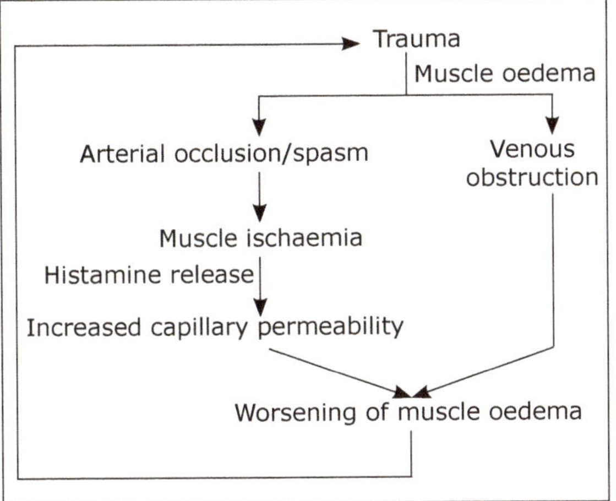

Fig. 5.1: *Pathophysiology of compartment syndrome depicted by the Eaton-Green's cycle.*

Clinical Features

- A high index of suspicion is essential for early diagnosis.
- Classically, the 5'P's (pain, pallor, paresthesia, paralysis, pulselessness) have been described as clinical signs of compartment syndrome. However, these signs may be unreliable in children and may be delayed in appearance.
- In children, the 3'A's, *anxiety* (restlessness), *agitation* (excess crying) and increasing *analgesia* requirement are more reliable clinical signs.
- Out of proportion pain must raise the suspicion of developing compartment syndrome. The pain is aggravated by stretching the muscles in the involved compartment.
- Clinical evaluation of increased compartment pressure is subjective and unreliable.
- Paralysis and pulselessness are late clinical signs and intervention should not be delayed till the appearance of these signs.
- Similarly, pulse oximetry should not be relied on for the diagnosis of compartment syndrome.

Investigations

- Measurement of compartment pressure by manometry is an objective modality for diagnosis of compartment syndrome. The pressure is measured by inserting the needle at different sites and to different depths. Compartment pressure closer to fracture site is considered most reliable.
- There is controversy regarding the threshold level for diagnosis of compartment syndrome. In adults, while some studies mention compartment pressure above 30 to 40mm Hg to be diagnostic, other studies have recommended a threshold level of within 30mm Hg of the diastolic pressure or mean arterial pressure.
- There is further controversy in children. Children have a baseline compartment pressure lower than adults and so it is proposed that the threshold for diagnosis of compartment pressure should be lower in children than in adults.
- A careful correlation of the measured pressures with clinical findings is essential for diagnosis of compartment syndrome in children.
- Near Infrared Spectroscopy (NIRS) is a non-invasive method of assessment of tissue perfusion. It is not yet widely available or used, but holds promise for the future.

Pitfalls in diagnosis

- Clinical diagnosis of compartment syndrome may be easily missed in certain clinical scenarios.

- Pain may not be significant in fractures associated with nerve deficits. e.g. fracture supracondylar humerus with median nerve palsy.
- Also clinical assessment cannot be relied on in children with altered sensorium

(polytrauma with head injury) or altered sensations (e.g. congenital insensitivity to pain, meningomyelocele).

- Children who have been given regional anaesthesia may be difficult to evaluate clinically. e.g. children with fracture supracondylar humerus who have been administered brachial block for closed reduction- K wire pinning will not report pain for several hours. So, in children with impending compartment syndrome it would be advisable to avoid regional anaesthesia if any surgical intervention is performed.

Treatment

- Early recognition and intervention are essential to prevent irreversible sequelae of compartment syndrome.
- First step consists of removal of all extrinsic circumferential casts/ bandages. The cast padding/bandage should be cut down to the skin. The limb should be elevated to the level of the heart. Excess elevation of the limb should also be avoided due to risk of decreasing arterial perfusion.
- Additionally, in polytrauma cases, optimal management of shock, correction of hypoxia and hypovolemia helps to improve peripheral tissue perfusion.
- In cases of impending compartment syndrome, these measures may suffice, however in established compartment syndrome, emergent surgical intervention in the form of fasciotomy is necessary.

Fasciotomy

- Fasciotomy is a surgery in which fascia overlying the affected compartments is released. Additionally, epimysium overlying the individual muscles is also released. Obviously necrotic muscles should be excised as they can be a nidus for infection, and later contracture of these muscles can lead to deformities and disabilities. However, in children, muscles with doubtful viability may be preserved and decision on excision may be taken during a second look debridement performed 24 hours after the primary fasciotomy.
- Additional surgical interventions are performed as warranted. So, vascular injuries should undergo appropriate vascular intervention, and fractures should be reduced and stabilised. Nerves are explored if indicated, and if nerve injuries are observed, the nerve ends should be tagged to surrounding soft tissues. Definitive nerve repair with/without nerve grafting should be delayed till the time of definitive wound closure.
- Options for wound management after fasciotomy include sterile dressings, VAC dressings, primary skin grafting or loose primary partial closure. Tissue viablility, risk of infection, muscle oedema, exposure of neurovascular structures and bone and need for nerve reconstruction are some of the factors which dictate the choice of primary wound management option following fasciotomy.
- Second look debridement of tissues of doubtful viability which have been preserved during the primary fasciotomy surgery should be performed within 24 hours. At this stage, partial delayed primary closure may be performed to cover any exposed neurovascular structures and bone.
- Definitive closure should be delayed till the tissue oedema has completely subsided and infection is definitively ruled out. If feasible, the wound may be sutured or skin grafting may be performed. In rare cases, with exposed bones, flap closure may be needed.

- Irreversible tissue damage occurs if compartment pressure has remained elevated beyond the threshold for a prolonged time period. Additionally, late fasciotomy is associated with significant risk of infection. For these reasons, many authors don't recommend fasciotomy for presentation more than 24 hours after the onset of compartment syndrome. However in children, the tissues are more resilient to irreversible damage and there is one study which recommends fasciotomy for upto 72 hours after onset of compartment syndrome in children provided the limb is still in the acute swelling phase.
- In addition to the limb complications, compartment syndrome is associated with systemic complications like myoglobinuria, hyperkalemia and metabolic acidosis with resultant renal failure, cardiac arrhythmias. Adequate hydration and expert medical management are necessary to prevent and manage these complications.

Post-operative care

- All skin incisions are left open.
- If vessels and nerves are not exposed, VAC dressing can be applied at the time of fasciotomy. If exposed, gauze dressings are applied.
- Dressing is done in the Operation Theatre under anaesthesia 24 hours after the fasciotomy. If muscles with doubtful viability have been left behind at the time of fasciotomy, they should be reassessed and debrided if needed. Partial delayed primary wound closure may be performed at that time to cover exposed vessels/nerves if any.
- Definitive closure is performed only after swelling has subsided. At the time of definitive closure, nerve reconstruction if needed is performed. If skin closure is tight, skin grafting is performed.
- Splintage to maintain all joints in optimal position is commenced immediately after the fasciotomy.

Regional Considerations

Thigh

- There are three compartments in the thigh:
  - Anterior: quadriceps
  - Posterior: hamstrings
  - Medial: adductors
- Compartment syndromes of the thigh are extremely rare.
- A single lateral incision suffices for adequate decompression of anterior and posterior compartments. If the medial compartment is also involved, an additional medial incision is needed. **(Fig. 5.2)**

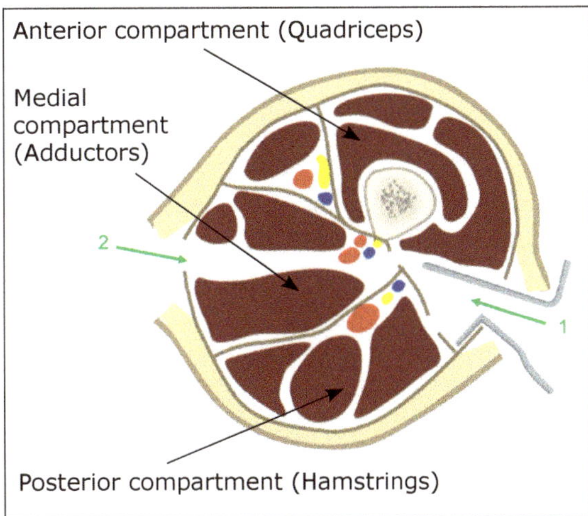

***Fig. 5.2**: Two-incision fasciotomy for release of all three compartments of the thigh. The anterior and posterior compartments are released through a single lateral incision (arrowhead 1). The medial incision is released through a separate medial incision (arrowhead 2).*

Leg

- The leg consists of four compartments:
  - Anterior

- Lateral
- Posterior superficial
- Posterior deep

- The leg is the commonest site of compartment syndrome in the lower extremity.
- Leg compartment syndromes are commonly seen after tibia- fibula fractures, or after derotation/ angulation osteotomies of the tibia-fibula. Distal femur and proximal tibia physeal fractures are high risk injuries and are known to be associated with vascular injuries and compartment syndrome.
- Compartment syndrome of the leg can be released by either a two-incision or one incision technique.

Two-incision technique

- The anterior and lateral compartments are released through an anterolateral incision
- An additional incision along the posterior-medial border of tibia is used to decompress the posterior-superficial and posterior-deep compartments.
- Through a sufficiently long postero-medial incision, the posterior-superficial compartment is released in the proximal half and soleus is detached from its origin on the tibia. The posterior-deep compartment is released in the distal half of the incision. **(Fig. 5.3 A)**

Position

- Supine (radiolucent table if fracture fixation is planned)

Technique

- The first incision is placed on the anterolateral aspect of the leg, half-way between the lateral border of fibula and anterior border of tibia. Longitudinally, the incision extends from the level of the fibula neck to ankle joint.
- The subcutaneous tissue is under-mined to expose the fascia overlying the anterior and lateral compartments of the leg.
- A small transverse incision is placed to identify the intermuscular septum between the anterior and lateral compartments.
- The superficial peroneal nerve lies just posterior to the septum, and is protected and retracted, following which the fascia overlying the peroneal muscles is incised from the proximal to distal extent of the incision.
- The fascia overlying the anterior compartment is incised along the whole extent of the incision along the course of underlying tibialis anterior muscle and tendon.
- The second incision is placed on the posteromedial aspect of the leg about 2cm behind the posterior border of tibia, along the same longitudinal extent as the first incision.
- The great saphenous vein with accompanying saphenous nerve is protected and retracted.
- The subcutaneous tissue is undermined to expose the fascia covering the superficial and deep muscle compartments of the leg.
- A small transverse incision is made in the fascia in the mid-third of leg to identify the intermuscular septum seperating the superficial and deep posterior compartments.
- The superficial posterior compartment is released by incising the fascia overlying the gastrocnemius in the whole extent of the incision.
- Similarly, the deep posterior

compartment is released by incising the fascia overlying the flexor digitorum longus. In the proximal third, the origin of the soleus may need to be released off the medial border of tibia in order to achieve this.

- Obviously necrotic muscle is excised. Meticulous haemostasis is achieved.
- Wound is covered with sterile saline or VAC dressings.
- Plaster slab is applied with ankle in neutral and knee in slight flexion.

One-incision technique

- All four compartments of the leg are released through a single incision along the lateral border of fibula.
- In this technique, initially the septum between the anterior and lateral compartments is visualised and the anterior and lateral compartments are decompressed.
- Elevation of muscles of the lateral compartment allows access to the posterior intermuscular septum, which is released to allow decompression of both the posterior compartments. **(Fig. 5.3B)**

Foot

- The foot consists of nine compartments:
  - four interossei
  - one adductor
  - two central
  - one medial
  - one lateral
- Compartment syndromes of the foot are usually caused by run-over injuries. Lisfranc's fracture dislocations may be associated with foot compartment syndrome.
- All compartments can be effectively released by two incisions centered on the second and fourth metatarsals. An additional medial incision may be

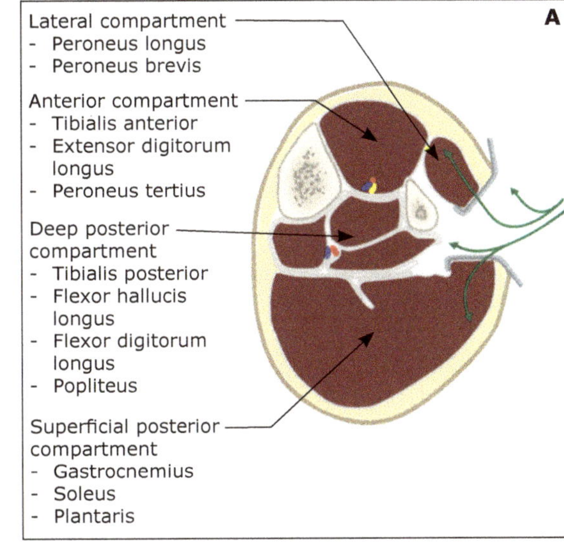

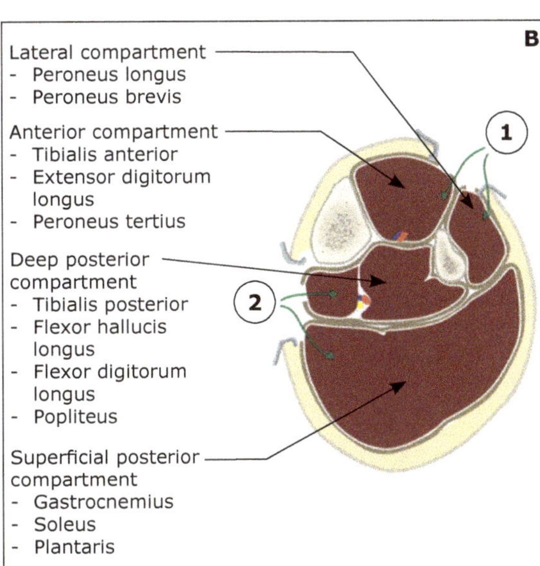

***Fig. 5.3**: Fasciotomy for leg compartment syndrome: (A) One incision technique: anterior, lateral, posterior superficial and posterior deep compartments are released through a single lateral incision (B) Two incision technique: anterior and lateral compartments are released through an antero-lateral incision (arrowhead 1). The posterior-superficial and posterior-deep compartments are released through a separate postero-medial incision (arrowhead 2).*

placed to decompress the adductor compartment **(Fig. 5.4)**.

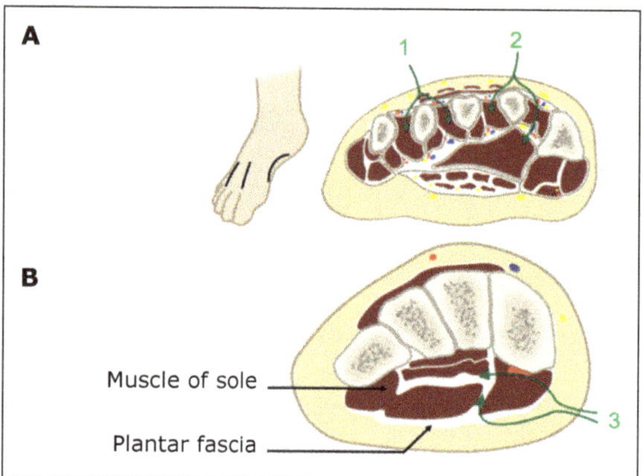

***Fig. 5.4**: Fasciotomy for compartment syndrome of the foot. (A) Two incisions are centered on the dorsum of the foot overlying the second and fourth metatarsals (arrowheads 1 and 2). (B) If needed, an additional incision may be placed on the medial aspect of the foot at the midtarsal level to decompress the muscles of the sole (arrowhead 3).*

Arm

- The arm consists of two compartments:
- • Anterior
- • Posterior
- Release of these compartments may be accomplished by placing two seperate anterior and posterior midline incisions.
- When exploration of neurovascular structures is to be performed, compartment decompression may be performed through a single medial incision **(Fig. 5.5)**. The medial intermuscular septum is excised to allow release of both anterior and posterior compartments.
- If indicated, compartment release of the arm may be extended distally into the forearm.

Forearm

- Forearm is the commonest site of compartment syndrome. The forearm consists of four compartments:

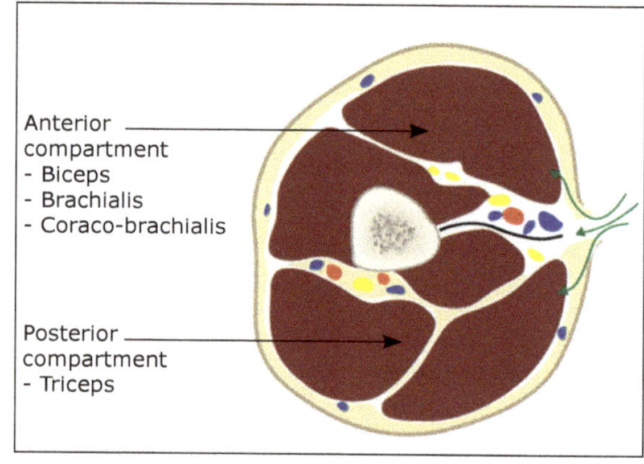

***Fig. 5.5**: Fasciotomy for compartment syndromes of the arm. A single incision placed on the medial aspect of the arm allows decompression of both anterior and posterior compartments of the arm, and also allows exploration of the neurovascular bundle.*

- • Superficial flexor compartment consisting of superficial flexors
- • Deep flexor compartment consisting of the flexor digitorum profundus, flexor pollicis longus and pronator quadratus
- • Extensor compartment consisting of the wrist and finger extensors
- • Mobile wad of Henry: Brachioradialis, Extensor Carpi Radialis Longus and Extensor Carpi Radialis Brevis
- The deep flexor compartment is first and most severely affected in compartment syndrome.
- Release of compartment syndrome of the forearm should extend from the lacertus fibrosus proximally to the carpal tunnel distally.

Surgical technique

Position:

- Supine with the affected limb on side-arm table (radiolucent if fracture fixation is planned).

Pre-operative preparation:

- We prefer to avoid tourniquet during fasciotomy for compartment syndrome, though other authors have described use of tourniquet without exsanguination.
- Keep adequate blood cross-matched and reserved as fasciotomy is associated with significant blood loss during surgery and in the post-operative period.
- Avoid regional anaesthesia to facilitate monitoring of neurological status in the post-operative period.

Technique

- An incision is placed on the volar aspect of forearm. The incision commences above the elbow joint crease, from the medial aspect of biceps tendon. It crosses the elbow joint at an angle. It then extends in a curvilinear fashion on the volar aspect of the forearm. Distally, the incision crosses the wrist joint at an angle, to faciliate release of the carpal tunnel **(Fig. 5.7)**.
- Proximally, the antebrachial fascia and lacertus fibrosus is released.
- The fascia of the forearm is incised along its entire extent to release the superficial flexor compartment of the forearm.
- Then, starting at the mid forearm, the plane between the flexor carpi ulnaris and flexor digitorum superficialis is developed to approach the deep flexor compartment consisting of the flexor digitorum profundus and flexor pollicis longus.
- The fascia overlying the flexor digitorum profundus, flexor pollicis longus and pronator quadratus is then incised to release the deep flexor compartment.
- Distally the carpal tunnel is released by incising transverse carpal ligament.
- The epimysium overlying individual muscles is also released.
- The subcutaneous tissue is undermined and fascia overlying the mobile wad of Henry is released.
- The brachial artery is explored and repaired if indicated.
- Median nerve exploration is done if indicated. If nerve is exposed in distal forearm, it is covered with tag sutures in overlying muscles.
- The dorsal compartment is checked, and if found to be tense, it is released through an incision extending from the lateral epicondyle distally for 10 cm.
- Wounds are covered with moist sterile dressings.
- Slab is applied in less than 90^{0} flexion **(Figs. 5.6 and 5.7)**

Post-operative:

- Management of fasciotomy wound in the post-operative period is as described earlier in the section on general principles of fasciotomy.

Hand and fingers:

- The hand consists of ten compartments:
- • Hypothenar
- • Thenar
- • Adductor
- • Carpal
- • Four dorsal interossei
- • Three volar interossei
- It is rarely necessary to release all, decision regarding the compartments to be released is based on clinical judgement and measurement of compartment pressures.
- The superficial and deep palmar spaces are released through an extended

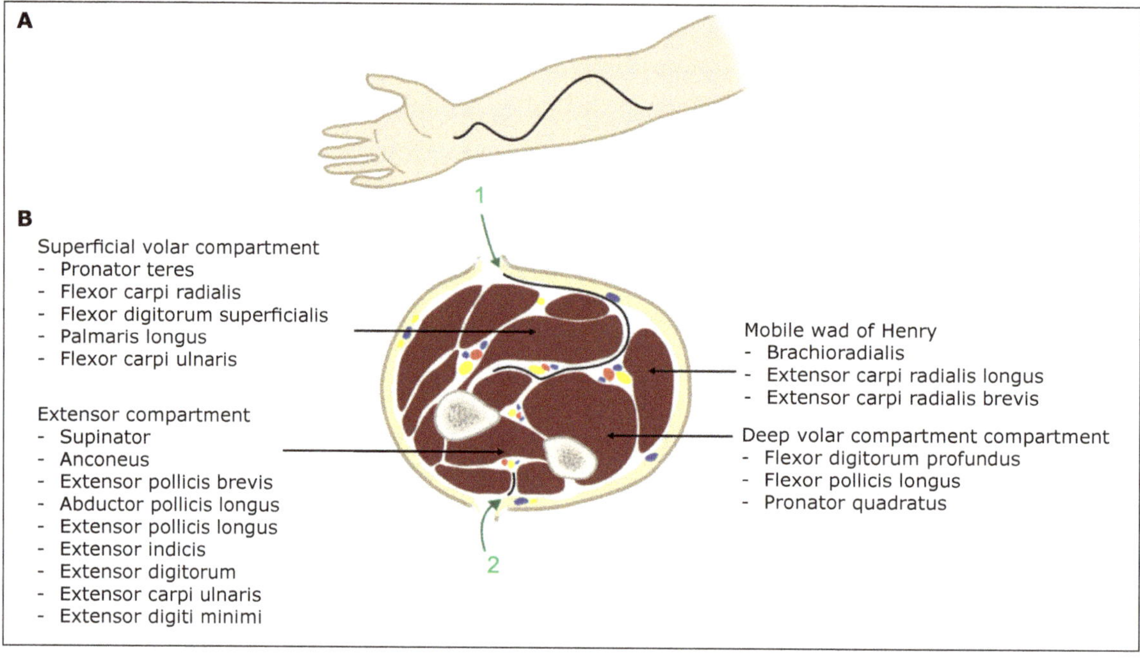

***Fig. 5.6**: Fasciotomy for release of compartment syndrome of the forearm: (A) Curvi-linear incision on volar aspect of forearm; (B) Two incisions for release of all compartments of forearm. The superficial flexor, deep flexor and mobile wad of Henry are released through a volar incision (arrowhead 1). If extensor compartment is involved, a separate dorsal incision is placed (arrowhead 2).*

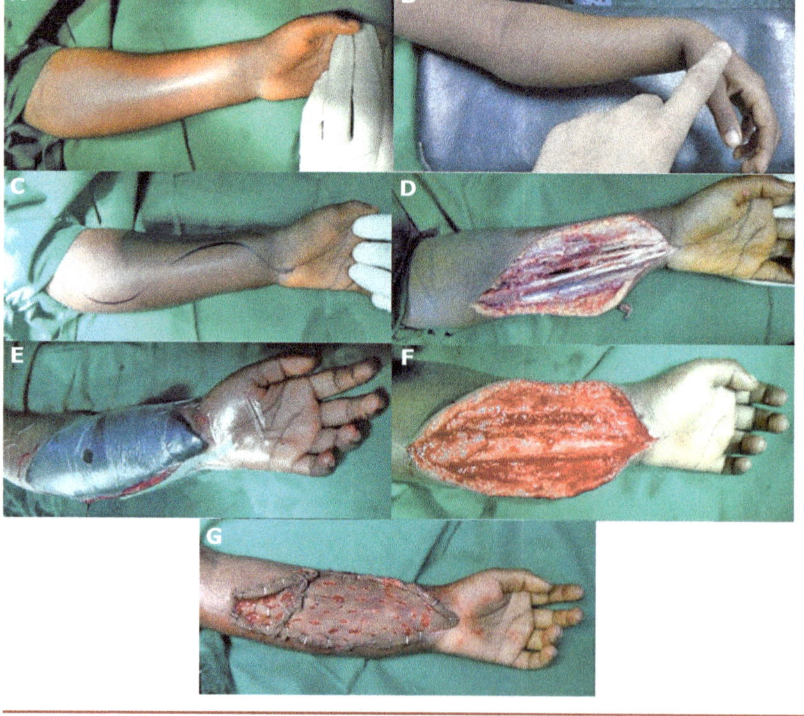

***Fig. 5.7**: (A) 6 years old female child presented with compartment syndrome of the Right forearm following blunt trauma and soft tissue injury. (B) The wrist and fingers were held in an attitude of flexion, and any attempt to extend elicited severe stretch pain. (C,D) Emergency fasciotomy was performed to release the superficial and deep flexor compartments of the forearm. (E) The fasciotomy wound was covered with VAC dressing. (F) After two more debridements, the wound bed was seen to be healthy and granulating with no evidence of infection. (G) At this stage, wound closure was achieved by covering the raw area with Split-Thickness Skin Graft.*

carpal tunnel release incision. This incision also adequately decompresses the Guyon's canal with the ulnar neurovascular structures. Distally, the fascia covering the adductor pollicis and volar interosseous muscles are released. The thenar and hypothenar muscles are released through separate incisions.

- The dorsal interosseous muscles are released through incisions placed in the first webspace (first dorsal interosseous), between second and third metacarpals, and between fourth and fifth metacarpals. Through these incisions dorsal fascia of the volar interossei and adductor pollicis can also be released.
- In compartment syndrome involving fingers, dermotomies in the mid axial plane helps to release the Cleland and Grayson's ligaments which can constrict the digital vessels. Incisions are placed on the side where scar irritation will be least. So, for the index and middle fingers, dermotomies are performed laterally, while for the ring and little fingers, incisions are placed medially **(Fig. 5.8)**.
- Post-operative care of fasciotomy wound is as described earlier. Definitive closure is performed only after swelling has subsided. In the hand, only the carpal tunnel incision needs to be closed, rest of the incisions heal by secondary intention.
- Physiotherapy and splintage to maintain all joints in optimal position is commenced immediately after the fasciotomy. Physiotherapy may be temporarily discontinued while the skin grafts heal, but is resumed immediately thereafter. Rehabilitation needs to be continued till the joints and scars are supple.

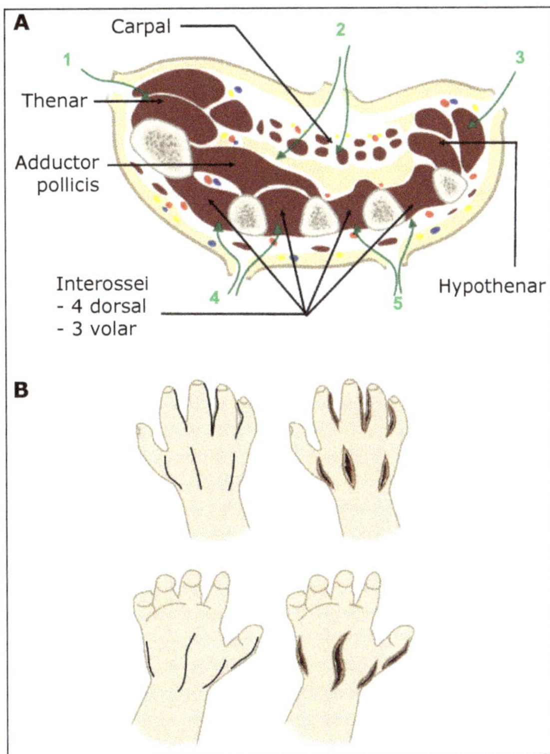

***Fig. 5.8**: Incisions for release of compartment syndrome of the hand (A) The thenar, hypothenar, and, superficial and deep palmar spaces are released through volar incisions (arrowheads 1,2,3). The dorsal interossei compartments are released through two separate dorsal incisions placed in the 2nd and 4th inter-metacarpal spaces (arrowheads 4,5). (B) Skin incisions for release of compartment syndrome of hand.*

Outcomes

- The main determinant of outcome of compartment syndrome is the timing of surgical decompression. In children, compartment syndrome decompressed within 12 hours of onset can be predictably expected to have full recovery within first 6 months.
- Complications include

• Volkmann's Ischemic Contracture with muscle contractures, loss of useful muscle function and nerve deficits (motor + sensory)

- Cosmetic deformity
- Growth arrest
- Infection
- Loss of limb (rare)
- Rare systemic effects include rhabdomyolysis, multi- organ failure and even death

Volkmann's Ischemic Contracture (VIC)

- VIC is the end result of prolonged tissue ischaemia, resulting in irreversible tissue necrosis and contractures.
- Forearm is the commonest site of VIC. Forearm VIC is classified as mild, moderate and severe (Tsuge).

- Mild VIC: Mild VIC selectively affects the deep flexor compartment of forearm (flexor digitorum profundus and flexor pollicis). There is no nerve involvement. Fingers can be fully extended with wrist flexion.
- Moderate VIC: In addition to deep flexor compartment, superficial flexor compartment is partially affected with variable degrees of flexor digitorum superficialis (FDS) contracture. Nerve involvement is always present with median nerve more affected than ulnar nerve and intrinsic-minus hand.
- Severe VIC: This category includes cases with involvement of deep flexor, superficial flexor and extensor compartment and all three nerves of the forearm. Cases complicated by fixed joint contractures, scarred soft tissues and previous failed surgeries are also included in this category.

Treatment

- Though Tsuge's classification provides a rough guide for the treatment of VIC, treatment for each case needs to be individualised according to the problems at hand. Factors to be considered while deciding treatment for VIC include: extent and severity of contractures, residual motor and sensory deficits, and the patients' needs. Surgical treatment for VIC should be undertaken only after all scars and soft tissues have completely healed.

Non-operative treatment

- Non-operative treatment should commence even before VIC is established. Physiotherapy and splintage form the mainstay of non-operative treatment.
- Physiotherapy should be directed towards keeping the joints supple by moving them through the range of motion, and strengthening the remaining muscles.
- Splintage helps to maintain the joints in their optimal position. In case of established contractures, static progressive splintage or serial casting should be employed in an attempt to stretch out the deformities.
- In case of mild VIC with no nerve involvement, non-operative treatment may suffice. In moderate and severe VIC, surgery should be proceeded with as soon as the soft tissues and scars have healed, supple fingers have been achieved by a period of rehabilitation and adequate time has been allowed for recovery of nerves and muscles.

Operative treatment:

Operative treatment of VIC includes bony and soft-tissue procedures

Soft Tissue surgeries:

For muscle contractures, soft tissue surgeries include:

- muscle slide operations (flexor-pronator origin slide, Page)

- excision of scarred, fibrotic muscles
- fractional lengthening of muscles

For residual nerve deficits, surgeries performed include:

- neurolysis
- tendon transfers
- functional free muscle transfers
- Excision of scarred, fibrotic nerves with nerve grafting (to restore distal sensations)

Fixed joint contractures are released by

- soft tissue release
- capsulectomy
- collateral ligament excision/recession

Bony surgeries:

- Bony surgeries in VIC are of two types: bone shortening procedures and arthrodesis.
- Bone shortening procedures are used to correct the imbalance between muscle and bone lengths. In the forearm, radius-ulna shortening can be performed in cases of severe VIC where there is shortening of both flexor and extensor compartment muscles. This is rarely employed in children, as the forearm is usually already shortened due to ischaemia to the growth plates.
- Arthrodesis may be used as a means of shortening, or to stabilise joints. Arthrodesis should be done only after skeletal maturity. The joints commonly arthrodesed include wrist, first carpo-metacarpal and metacarpo-phalangeal joints.

According to severity of VIC, treatment decision making is as under:

- Mild VIC → Page flexor-pronator muscle slide
- Moderate VIC → Page flexor-pronator muscle slide + neurolysis of median and ulnar nerves + SOS tendon transfer
- Reconstruction of thumb function: Brachioradialis/ECRL to FPL transfer; Extensor indicis proprius to opponens pollicis transfer
- Reconstruction of finger flexion: gracilis free muscle transfer
- Nerve reconstruction: excision of fibrotic nerve segments with nerve grafting (to restore useful sensations)
- Severe VIC: gracilis free muscle transfer

Post-operative

Therapy and splintage are needed till skeletal maturity.

Flowchart 5.1: Algorithm for management of established Volkmann's ischemic contracture

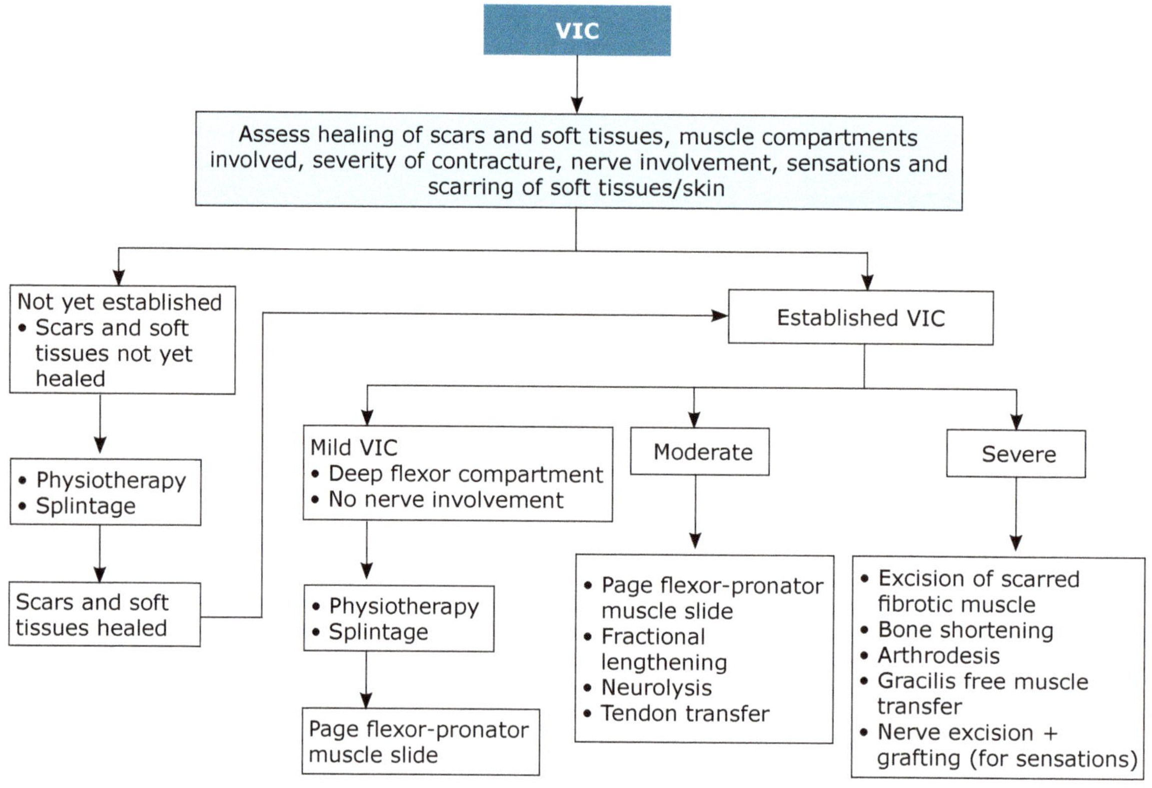

6 Care of the Child with Multiple Injuries

Introduction

The incidence of polytrauma in children is lesser than in adults. Children with polytrauma need specialised care which commences at the site of injury, is maintained during transfer of the child to nearby hospital, followed by care at the hospital, and then if needed, referral to specialised tertiary care center plays a key role in minimising morbidity and mortality in children with multiple injuries.

Initial Evaluation and Resuscitation

The Advanced Trauma Life Support (ATLS) or Paediatric Advanced Life Support (PALS) protocols are followed for the initial evaluation and resuscitation of children with multiple injuries. ABC of resuscitation includes assessment and maintenance of Airway (A), Breathing (B), Circulation (C), administration of appropriate Drugs (D) and adequate Exposure (E) of body parts.

Clearing the airway and maintaining the breathing at the site of accident can make the difference between life and death. Special care should be taken to stabilise the cervical spine during transfer to the nearby hospital. It should be borne in mind that due to larger head size in children less than 6 years age, placing the child on a flat board will induce flexion of the cervical spine **(Fig. 6.1 A)**. To avoid this, a board with cutout to accommodate the occipital area of the head should be used to transfer these children with polytrauma **(Fig. 6.1 B)**. Alternatively, the shoulders may be slightly elevated by placement of folded sheets to avoid cervical spine flexion.

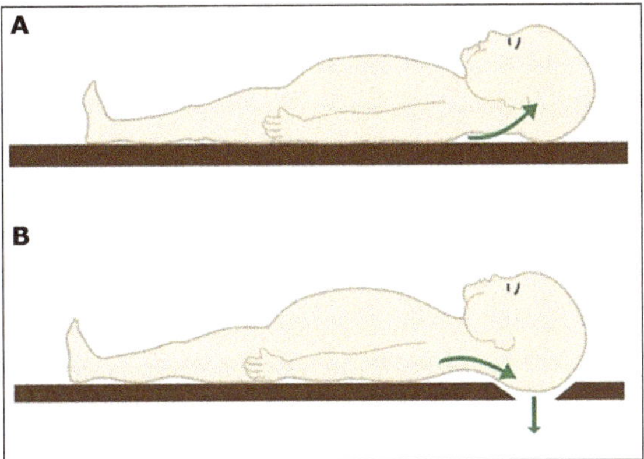

***Fig. 6.1**: (A) Placing a child on a flat board will induce flexion of the cervical spine due to larger head size. (B) To prevent this, a board with cut-out is used to transport a child with suspected cervical spine injury.*

Once airway and breathing is secured, hypovolemia due to internal or external haemorrhage is replenished by adequate fluid resuscitation. Prolonged hypoperfusion of vital organs due to prolonged hypovolemia can induce systemic inflammatory response in the form of acidosis, hypothermia and coagulopathy, and is an important cause of mortality if the child survives the initial few hours after major trauma. In case adequate peripheral intravenous access is not available due to vessel collapse, wide bore needle inserted into the proximal tibial metaphysis may be used for fluid replacement. Crystalloids are preferred for fluid replacement in children. Care should also be taken to avoid excess fluid administration, as it can cause internal fluid shifts and exacerbate cerebral and pulmonary oedema in the setting of underlying head and chest trauma. Adequate fluid replenishment is monitored through central venous pressure after insertion of central venous catheter, and urine output.

After the initial resuscitation, trauma rating scales are applied for assessing trauma severity. Glasgow Coma Scale (GCS), Injury Severity Score (ISS) and Paediatric Trauma Score (PTS) have all been validated for the paediatric population. GCS is the most commonly used scale in head injury **(Table 6.1)**. GCS less than 8 has been shown to be correlated with a significantly increased mortality in the paediatric age group. Serial assessment of GCS helps to monitor the course of neurologic injury, with the 72 hour score correlating with the risk of permanent disability. However GCS has been found to be unreliable for use in pre-verbal children.

Table 6.1: Glasgow Coma Scale (GCS)

Response	Action	Score
Best motor response	Obeys	5
	Localises	4
	Withdraws	3
	Abnormal flexion	2
	Extensor response	1
	Nil	0
Verbal response	Oriented	4
	Confused conversation	3
	Inappropriate words	2
	Incomprehensible sounds	1
	Nil	0
Eye opening	Spontaneous	3
	To speech	2
	To pain	1
	Nil	0

At this stage, a throrough secondary assessment from head to toe is done for evaluation of other injuries. Upper and lower extremity fractures which are closed and with intact distal vascularity are low priority injuries and may be managed with temporary splinting for pain relief till such time that other life threatening injuries are evaluated and stabilised. However, pelvis fractures with haemodynamic instability can be life-threatening and may need emergency surgical treatment. Major intra-abdominal injuries may be revealed externally by abdominal wall ecchymosis and guarding/rigidity on palpation. Chest injuries should be suspected in case of breathing difficulty. Tension pneumothorax can be life threatening in the absence of emergent treatment. Loss of consciousness, ENT bleed and vomiting are signs of head injury. In the presence of head injury with unconsciousness, great care should be taken to avoid missing other injuries.

Imaging

Plain X-rays

Initial screening X-rays classically obtained in a case of multiply injured child include lateral X-rays of the cervical spine and anteroposterior X-rays of the chest and pelvis. In the presence of neck pain with suspected instability, if lateral X-rays of the cervical spine are normal, carefully supervised flexion views are obtained in a conscious child. X-rays of the limbs and the dorso-lumbar spine are obtained based on findings of clinical examination.

CT scan

CT scan of the head is obtained in head injuries and helps to identify skull fractures and intracranial bleeds. CT scan of the abdomen with IV contrast is a good modality to identify injury to intra abdominal organs and to quantify haemorrhage. CT scan with serial measurement of haematocrit is an important determinant of surgical treatment of spleen, liver and kidney lacerations. CT scan of the pelvis helps to identify pelvic fractures not seen on plain radiographs and also aids to plan fixation of pelvic fractures. Contrast studies help to locate source of continuing intrapelvic haemorrhage and associated injuries to urinary bladder and other intrapelvic structures. CT scan in dorsolumbar spine fractures aid in decision making regarding stability of these fractures and need for surgical stabilisation.

MRI

In an acute setting, MRI is useful mainly in head and spine injuries. In the paediatric age group, increased flexibility of the spine can lead to injuries to the spinal cord without injury to the bony vertebral column. These injuries are called SCIWORA (Spinal Cord Injury Without Radiographic Abnormality) and can only be identified on MRI. MRI may also be useful in knee injuries to identify meniscal and cruciate ligament tears.

Ultrasonography

The primary utility of ultrasonography in a child with polytrauma is for evaluation of intra abdominal injuries. Though CT scan with contrast is the preferred imaging modality, ultrasonography can be quickly obtained in settings where CT scan may not be readily available.

Non Orthopaedic injuries

Head injuries

Severity of head injury is often the most important determinant of mortality and morbidity in a child with polytrauma. Treatment of head injury is directed primarily towards the normalisation of raised intra cranial pressure and includes elevation of head end of the bed, lowering of pCO_2 which may need ventilator assistance, and fluid restriction. Surgical intervention may be needed for evacuation of intracranial haematoma.

Prognosis for motor recovery from severe head injury is much better in the paediatric age group as compared to adults. pO_2 at admission and Glasgow Coma Score at 72 hours are prognostic factors for recovery from head injury. For this reason, orthopaedic injuries in a child with severe head injury are treated with the assumption that the child will have full neurological recovery. Pain caused due to movement at the fracture site can raise the intracranial pressure. For this reason, extremity fractures are adequately immobilised by splintage at presentation. Circumferential cast is best avoided in the unconscious child due to risk of missing compartment syndrome. In cases where surgical stabilisation of fractures is warranted, the same may be proceeded with after primary stabilisation of the general condition of the child, even if the child is in coma. Surgery may be in the form of internal fixation, or external fixation in situations where shortening surgical duration is an important consideration.

Orthopaedic effects of Head Injury

- Spasticity:

  Spasticity can set in within a few days after head injury. This can lead to angulation and shortening at the fracture site despite splintage. Early recognition is important as fractures heal faster in head injury leading to malunion. Early surgical treatment of fracture is indicated if medical management and splintage fail to control the malalignment at the fracture site.

- Contractures:

  Joint contractures set in and progress early in the course of head injury. Early institution of passive physiotherapy is important to attempt prevention of this complication. Frequent change in position of hip and knee joints should be a part of the nursing protocol. Ankles tend to rest in an attitude of equinus with extension posturing of the hips and knees. For this reason, hips and knees should be periodically flexed by placing pillows under the knee to relax the gastrocnemius muscle. Ankle Foot Orthosis (AFOs) may be given to apply sustained stretch to the gastrocnemius muscle and prevent ankle equinus contractures. Despite these measures, joint deformities and contractures can occur, and need to be managed by Botulinum Toxin injections in the affected muscles in the early stages when the deformities are passively correctable, and by muscle lengthening surgeries in fixed contractures.

- Heterotopic bone formation:

  Heterotopic ossification (HO) is a common occurrence in severe head injuries, and occurs if comatose state persists beyond few weeks. Peri-articular tissues around the hips and elbows are the commonest sites for HO. Rising alkaline phosphatase levels may be seen in evolving heterotopic ossification. Although pharmacological prophylaxis with Salicylates (40 mg/kg/day in divided doses for 6 weeks) and NSAIDs may have a role in the prevention of heterotopic ossification, in most cases, by the time diagnosis is made HO has already progressed beyond the inflammatory stage and medication has no role. However, pharmacologic and local low-dose radiation prophylaxis should be routinely given post-operatively to children with head injury undergoing surgical fracture treatment.

  Options in case of HO include observation versus early surgical excision. In case of post head injury HO, if it is interfering with rehabilitation, early surgical excision is preferred to waiting for 12 to 18 months for HO maturation.

- Faster fracture healing rates:

  Fractures typically heal faster in children with head injury. This may be related to elevated serum calcitonin levels after head injury.

Abdominal injuries

Abdominal injuries occur in about 25% of polytrauma paediatric patients. The incidence is even higher in the presence of pelvic fractures. Splenic and liver lacerations are the most commonly seen intra abdominal injuries. Genitourinary injuries are commonly seen in association with pelvic fractures. CT scan with contrast is the most commonly used investigation modality to diagnose intra abdominal injury. Treatment is usually conservative with monitoring of serum haematocrit and serial ultrasound evaluation. Once the child's general condition has stabilised, non-operative abdominal injury should not delay surgical fracture management.

Fat and pulmonary embolism

Fat embolism is rarer in children than in adults. The signs of fat embolism include hypoxemia, axillary petechiae and radiographic pulmonary infiitrates typically occurring few hours after trauma. Altered sensorium, in the absence of head injury and narcotic administration, can occur due to fat embolism. Early stablisation of fracture with splintage should be done to decrease risk of fat embolism. Treatment of established fat embolism consists of endo-tracheal intubation, positive pressure ventilation and adequate hydration.

Deep Vein Thromosis and Venous Thrombo-embolism is rare in children. It is more likely to occur in adolescents, pelvic and lower limb fractures, and severe head injury. Role of pharmacologic prophylaxis in children is unclear.

Management

Nutrition

In the polytraumatised child on ventilator support in the PICU, the daily nutrition requirements are 50% over and above the baseline requirements for his/her age and weight. Special care should be taken to fulfill these requirements. If it is anticipated that the child won't be able to acquire daily nutritional requirement through oral intake beyond a few days, nutrition should be provided through a feeding tube or central venous catheter to avoid catabolism, to promote early healing and to prevent complications.

Management of orthopaedic injuries in child with polytrauma

As mentioned in an earlier section, in a child with polytrauma, emergency management of life threatening injuries gets precedence over surgical management of closed orthopaedic injuries without distal vascular deficit. These injuries should be adequately splinted and immobilised to relieve pain. Once the life-threatening injuries are stabilised, if the fractures merit surgical intervention, surgery should preferably be performed within the first 72 hours to decrease the length of hospital stay, to facilitate early mobilisation, and to decrease the incidence of complications like chest infections.

Pelvis fractures with haemodynamic instability, compound fractures, fractures with vascular injury and compartment syndrome are orthopaedic injuries which need emergency surgical treatment.

Pelvic fractures

Pelvic fractures can be life threatening due to severe haemorrhage from the fracture site itself or shearing of the iliac vessels by vertical displacement of the hemi-pelvis. Additionally, pelvic fractures have a strong association with other life-threatening injuries like genitourinary injuries, intra abdominal visceral injuries, chest injuries and head injury which contribute significantly to mortality. Pelvic fractures may initially be stabilised with simple pelvic binder applied in the Casualty Department to close the retro-peritoneal dead space and control bleeding by tamponade effect. However, if the child continues to be haemodynamically unstable, CT-angiogram may be performed to identify the source of haemorrhage, and in centres where the facility is available, embolization of the bleeding vessel may be performed. In children with persistent haemorrhage, external fixator is applied to more effectively tamponade the bleeding vessels. At this stage, no aggressive attempt should be made to reduce and fix the fractures or sacroiliac joint dissociations, which can be deferred to a later date.

Compound fractures

The incidence of compound fractures in children with polytrauma is about 10%. Conversely, in children with compound fractures, additional injuries to the chest/ abdomen/ head/ other extremities is seen in about 25 to 50% cases.

Compound fractures are classified by the system of Gustilo and Anderson which takes into account the size of the wound, the extent of soft tissue injury and contamination **(Table 6.2)**.

Management of compound fractures

The principles of management of compound fractures are:

(1) Initial stablisation and infection prevention
(2) Soft tissue management
(3) Bony reconstruction

Initial stablisation and infection prevention

The ABCs of resuscitation are followed

Table 6.2: Gustilo and Anderson classification of compound fractures

	Size of wound	Soft tissue injury	Contamination
Grade 1	• < 1cm	Minimal	Minimal
Grade 2	• > 1cm • With skin flaps or lacerations • Can be managed with primary/delayed primary closure; no skin grafts/flaps needed	Moderate crushing	Minimal
Grade 3A	• Extensive • Skin graft/ flap needed for wound coverage	Extensive soft tissue crushing, but soft tissue coverage of bone maintained	Significant
Grade 3B	• Extensive • Skin graft/ flap needed for wound coverage	Loss of soft tissue coverage of bone with periosteal stripping	Significant
Grade 3C	Compound fracture with major arterial injury, needing vascular repair		

as described earlier. In the casualty department, a sterile povidone-iodine dressing is applied and fracture is temporarily splinted. Injection Tetanus Toxoid is given if the child's immunization status is not known or if it's been more than 5 years since the last dose.

Intravenous antibiotics are commenced as early as possible. For Grade 1 fractures, first or second generation Cephalosporins (Cefazolin at 100 mg/kg/day in three divided doses, maximum daily dose 6 gm) is administered. In more severe Grade 2 and 3 injuries, aminoglycosides (Gentamicin at 7.5 mg/kg/day in three divided doses) and MRSA coverage (Clindamycin or Vancomycin) are added. After the initial trauma, intravenous antibiotics are continued for 24 hours in Grade 1 injuries, and for 72 hours in more severe Grade 2 and 3 injuries. Intravenous antibiotics are peri-operatively repeated for 48 hours around repeat interventions like debridement/ delayed closure/ open reduction- fixation of fractures. A course of oral antibiotics may be given in the presence of soft tissue erythema.

Soft tissue management

Though studies have shown no significant difference in complication rate if wound debridement is performed within 6 hours versus within 24 hours following trauma, it is desirable to perform the initial surgical debridement as early as possible. The principles of surgical debridement of compound fractures are:

1) Excision of necrotic skin till healthy bleeding wound edges.
2) Surgical extension of the original wound to allow adequate exposure and debridement of the fracture ends.
3) Excision of non-viable skin, sub-cutaneous fat, fascia and muscle: Though in adults, muscle of doubtful viability is aggressively excised due to risk of infection, in children, excision of doubtful muscle may be delayed till second look debridement is performed 48 hours after the initial debridement.
4) Fracture ends and medullary canal are adequately exposed and cleaned. Clinical judgement is exercised to arrive at a decision regarding bone fragments

lying loose at the fracture site. Grossly contaminated fragments without any soft tissue attachments are excised. Also, fragments which are small and would not complicate later bone reconstruction are excised, whereas large fragments are preferably preserved if not significantly contaminated.

5) In the absence of vascular injury, debridement of compound wound may be performed under tourniquet control. However, the tourniquet should be released at the end of the debridement to confirm healthy, bleeding, viable wound edges.

6) Thorough wound lavage should be performed at the end of the procedure. Normal saline with or without soap solution (6 litres for the upper extremity, 9 litres for the lower extremity) is preferred. High pressure pulse lavage should preferably be avoided due to some concern regarding occurrence of compartment syndrome after use of these systems.

7) Exposed neurovascular bundles, bone and tendons should be covered with muscle or fascia. If adequate coverage is not available, either local muscle flap may be performed or Vacuum Assisted Closure (VAC) dressing may be applied.

8) At the end of debridement, portion of the wound which has been surgically extended to provide adequate exposure is primarily closed. If the remaining wound can be primarily approximated, it is closed over drains. Otherwise, VAC or sterile saline/ Povidone-iodine dressings are applied.

9) The child is returned to the operating room for a second look irrigation and debridement within 48 hours. Once the wound is confirmed to be clean and tissues viable, the wound is closed. If the wound edges can be approximated without tension, delayed primary closure is performed. If not, options for wound coverage are skin grafting or flap coverage depending on tissues in the wound bed. Wound coverage should be preferably provided within a week following the initial trauma.

Bony stabilisation

Bone stabilisation in compound fractures depends on multiple factors:

1) In Grade 1 fractures with minimal soft tissue contamination, options for fracture stabilisation are guided by patient age, fracture site and fracture configuration. Fractures which merit closed reduction and cast immobilisation, e.g. Grade 1 compound radius-ulna fractures in children less than 10 years old, Grade 1 compound tibia fractures, are treated conservatively. Inspection of compound wound is done through a cast window, which is closed once the wound heals. On the other hand, fractures which deserve operative intervention. e.g. completely displaced Grade 1 compound radius-ulna fractures in older children should be treated surgically. Usually elastic stable intramedullary nails are the implants of choice, but depending on the situation, K-wires/ plates/ screws/ rigid intramedullary interlock nails may be used for fixation of Grade 1 compound fractures.

2) Grade 2 and 3 compound fractures with more extensive soft tissue injury and contamination should be surgically stabilised in order to facilitate easy access to the wound for dressings and debridements.

In Grade 2 and 3 fractures, at the end of initial debridement, if the risk of wound infection is perceived to be unlikely, internal fixation may be primarily performed for fracture stabilisation. In some situations, e.g. intra articular fractures, combination of internal and external fixation may be performed, where the intra articular fracture is fixed with K-wires or screws, and a neutralising external fixator is applied to span and immobilise the joint in optimal position. Once internal fixation is deemed appropriate for a compound fracture, the choice of implant is dictated by the site and configuration of the particular fracture.

Though internal fixation is more comfortable for the patient and family, external fixation should be preferred in cases with significant initial contamination where infection risk persists despite thorough surgical debridement.

Another situation where external fixation may be preferred is where the child is systemically unstable, and "damage control orthopaedics" in the form of quick fixator application is considered safer than to perform definitive open reduction-internal fixation which may prolong the operative time. Once a fixator is applied, it may be used as definitive fixation till the fracture heals, or may be converted to internal fixation once the general condition of the child permits and the wound is confirmed to be clean with no risk of infection.

External fixation is also preferred in cases with circumferential bone loss and shortening. In children, in such cases, if the intervening periosteum is intact and vascularity is reasonably well-preserved, bone may regenerate to some extent if kept distracted with the fixator, and the extent of later reconstruction may be lesser than estimated at initial evaluation.

There are various options for secondary reconstruction of post-traumatic bone defects. In case of small defects, acute docking of fracture site with or without bone grafting and bone lengthening through a corticotomy placed at a distant site may be opted for. In case of larger defects, options include Masquelet induced membrane technique, or vascularised fibula graft, or internal bone transport.

Due to tremendous recovery potential in children, amputations in paediatric compound fractures should be rarely performed. The Mangled Extremity Severity Score in children does not correlate accurately with the need for amputation. If amputation is absolutely necessary, attempts should be made to preserve the physis even if it means a short stump. If the physis is preserved, the stump can increase to a functional length with growth. This is in contrast to the consideration for amputation performed in congenital limb deficiencies where trans-articular amputations are preferred to trans-osseous amputations to avoid the complication of stump overgrowth.

Flowchart 6.1: Sequence of assessment and management of injuries in a child with multiple injuries

CHILD WITH MULTIPLE INJURIES

↓

ATLS/PALS protocols

- Assess and maintain Airway (A), Breathing (B), Circulation (C), Drugs (D), Exposure (E)
- Protect and stabilize cervical spine pending clearance
- Emergent management of life threatening injuries like tension pneumothorax

↓

Secondary survey

- Glasgow coma score to assess Head injury
- Head to toe assessment and appropriate investigations to identify head/chest/abdomen injury and Orthopaedic injuries

↓

Emergency management

- Head/Chest/Abdomen injury
- Orthopaedic injuries: Pelvis fractures with haemodynamic instability, Compound fractures, Compartment syndromes
- Other non emergency orthopaedic injuries: Splintage and pain relief

↓

Preferably within 72 hours

- Non emergency orthopaedic injuries which need operative management

7 Clavice Fractures

Introduction and Relevant Anatomy

- Clavicle fractures are common childhood injuries and represent around 10-15% of all childhood fractures.
- Clavicle is an "S" shaped bone connecting the axial skeleton with the appendicular skeleton.
- Important muscles attached: Sternocleidomastoid (medially) and trapezius (laterally) on the superior border and Pectoralis major (medially) and Deltoid (laterally) on the inferior border along with a small subclavius attached all along the inferior border **(Fig. 7.1)**.
- Dangers involved in the dissection: The subclavian neurovascular bundle is just postero-inferior to the clavicle and can be injured during fracture fixation of the clavicle. The brachial plexus is also posterior to the clavicle and passes near the lateral third of the clavicle into the axilla.

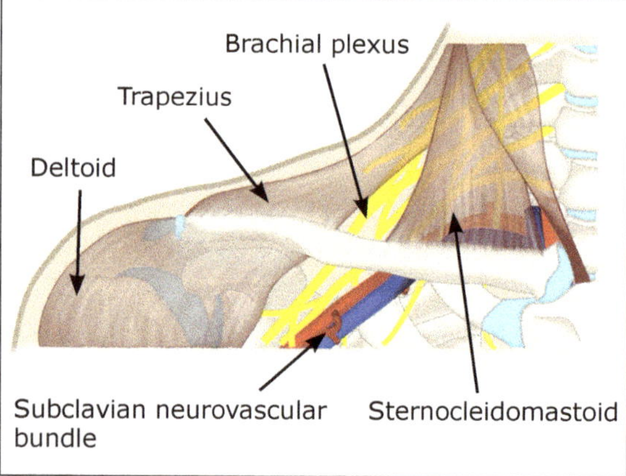

***Fig. 7.1**: Anatomy of the clavicle with respect to neurovascular structures and muscles.*

- Clavicle fractures occur in three groups of patients- Neonates, infants and school-going children, and adolescents.

Neonatal clavicular fractures:

- Clavicle is the most commonly fractured bone in obstetric trauma and the etiology is related to forceps delivery, obstructed labour as well as shoulder dystocia.
- The common mode of injury is indirect force during the passage of the shoulder girdle through the maternal pelvis, through a narrow birth canal.

  The other etiology which is slightly less common is massage, which is commonly performed in Indian households due to cultural traditions.

Clavicular fractures in infancy and early childhood:

- These are some of the commonest childhood fractures and are usually a result of indirect trauma with a fall on the edge of the shoulder being the commonest mechanism of injury, followed by direct trauma and then followed by fall on outstretched hand.
- These are usually low energy injuries and are not commonly associated with other injuries.

Adolescent clavicular fractures:

- Adolescent fractures are seen more and more with high energy trauma or with high impact injuries especially with adolescents participating in professional high contact sports. These may be associated with other injuries like chest wall or rib injuries.

Clinical Features

Neonatal fractures:

- The clavicular fracture due to obstetric causes is usually an undisplaced one and as such, in a large proportion of cases, is not diagnosed immediately after birth.
- It is in fact diagnosed after around 10-15 days by the formation of a small bump at the fracture site, which is usually the junction between the middle third and lateral third of the clavicle. This bump is pathognomonic of the fracture and is a sign of good union. In some cases, the child can present with pseudoparalysis or an asymmetric Moro's reflex.
- Pseudoparalysis (or painful paralysis) can be due to other causes also, such as obstetric brachial plexus palsy, humerus fractures, septic arthritis of the shoulder etc. It should be noted that these causes can in fact co-exist and hence it is always necessary to rule out the others.

Infantile fractures:

- These are usually brought on by trivial fall on the shoulder and as such present with a swelling and pain on movements. The child is usually not in severe pain, though in some of them they may present as pseudoparalysis.
- Just like in neonates, it is the bump which forms in about ten days, that brings the child to the clinician.

Adolescent fractures:

- Clavicle fractures in adolescents are usually associated with high energy trauma such as fall from bicycle and road traffic accidents etc.
- Though most of them are isolated injuries, care should be taken not to miss other associated injuries like rib fractures, scapular fractures, etc.

Imaging

- For most clavicular fractures, just a plain AP X-ray of the clavicle and shoulder is enough. It usually shows the actual displacement well and oblique views are usually not needed.
- Only in suspected fractures at the ends of the bone and especially in adolescents are special views required. For suspected fractures of the medial end of clavicle, a 45^{0} cephalad AP view centred on the sternoclavicular joint known as the *Serendipity view* is recommended. This view shows the exact orientation of the medial end of the clavicle along with the sternoclavicular joint.
- The second special view is for lateral end of clavicle fractures or suspected AC joint dislocations. Here an erect AP view of the shoulder with weight on the ipsilateral hand is recommended to know the exact dynamic displacement of the acromion with respect to the clavicle.
- Special investigations like CT scans or MRI are rarely needed in case of clavicular fractures unless associated with other injuries like rib fractures, etc.

Treatment

- The most common method of treatment of clavicular fractures in children is conservative management. There have been a number of methods described in conservative management like figure of 8 bandage, clavicular strapping, chest arm bandage and a simple arm pouch or a cuff and collar sling. A number of review articles have shown no significant difference between any of these means and it is best left to the experience of the clinician as well as the comfort of the child in deciding the mode of conservative management.

- It usually shows exuberant callus on plain X-rays in about three weeks **(Fig. 7.2)**.
- Velpeau stockinette method for neonates (Refer chapter 8).
- The most important tip about management of these fractures is good counselling of the parents as regards the possibility of a bump at the clavicle which will take a few months to disappear. It is also important to counsel the parents that amount of displacement is not important and almost all clavicle fractures irrespective of displacement heal completely and remodel without any residual deformity.

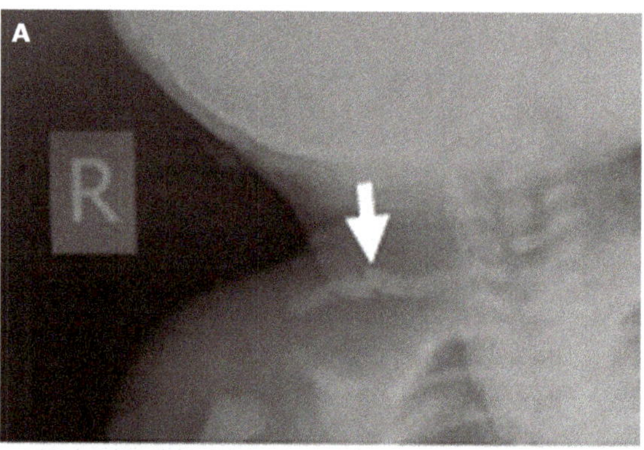

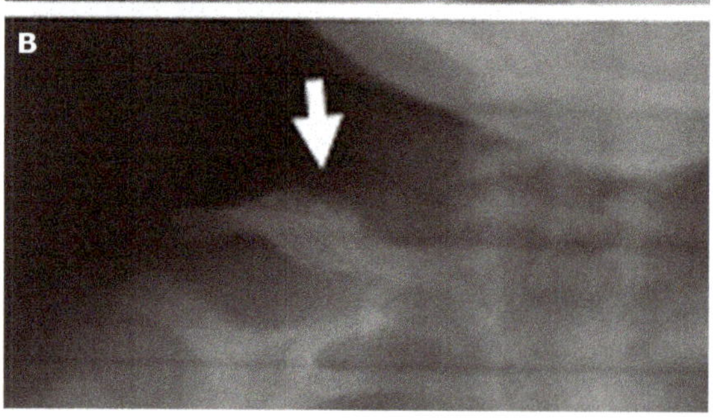

***Fig. 7.2**: (A) AP X-ray of a neonate with birth trauma with fracture clavicle (B) Healed fracture with exuberant callus in about 4 weeks.*

Operative treatment:

The very few indications of operative management of clavicular fractures in children are:

1) High energy injuries in adolescents especially with a segmental fracture (so called Z fracture)
2) Fractures associated with floating shoulder
3) Displaced fractures in a dominant hand in an adolescent.

   In such cases, the treatment is similar to adults, with plate or nail fixation.

Surgical procedure:

Clavicular plate fixation:

- Position:

  Supine with a bump under the scapula
- Incision:

  Along the subcutaneous border of the clavicle or slightly superior to it
- Special precautions:

  Cutaneous nerves need to be isolated and kept intact during the exposure as injury can lead to hypoaesthesia over the nipple and chest area.
- It is a direct exposure of the clavicle and the clavicle is reduced using towel clip clamp taking care not to go more inferior due to the danger to the subclavian vessels.
- Plate fixation is performed using either a reconstruction plate or a special clavicular locking plate, using three screws medially and three screws laterally **(Fig. 7.3)**.
- Closure is performed in a routine manner preferably taking sub-cuticular sutures.

Clavicular intramedullary nailing:

- Indication:

  Same as for plating, though this can be used in a person who would like a more cosmetically appealing procedure.

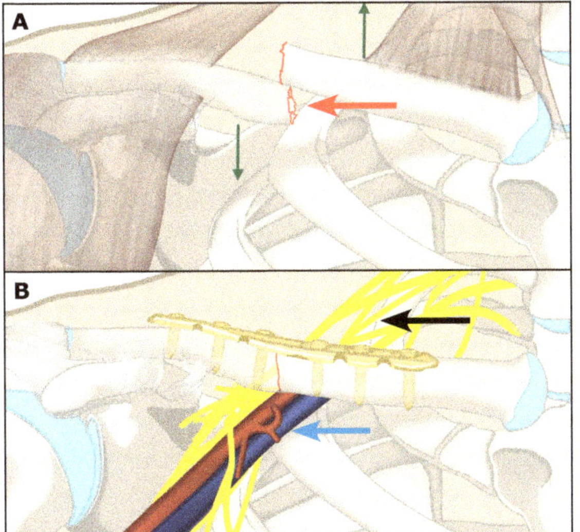

***Fig. 7.3**: Open reduction and plate fixation of displaced mid-shaft clavicular fracture in an adolescent. (A) Classical displacements which are commonly seen (Red and green arrow). (B) Proximity of the plate and ends of the screws to the neurovascular bundle (black and blue arrows)*

- Position:

  Supine with bump under the scapula, with C-arm on the ipsilateral side **(Fig. 7.4)**.

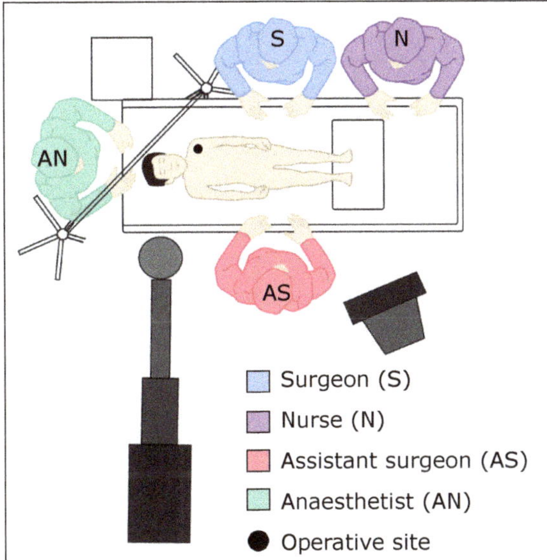

***Fig. 7.4**: Position of the patient and the operating team for clavicular nailing.*

- Entry point:

  The entry point of the nail is medial – just lateral to the SC joint, on the most prominent part of the metaphysis of the clavicle. Entry is to be taken with a curved awl taking care that it does not plunge.

- Nailing is performed in a routine manner towards the lateral clavicle using an elastic nail, with gentle rotatory movements.

- Reduction can be performed closed or using a small mini-open method and holding the reduction using a towel clip clamp.

- The typical manoeuvre for closed reduction of clavicular fractures is in-line traction with external rotation of the shoulder. This usually brings the fracture fragments close, after which they can be accurately reduced by manipulation of the nail ends.

- If the reduction is not obtained closed, then one can perform a mini-open clamp assisted reduction by clearing off the interposed soft tissue.

- The nail is completely seated on the lateral end of the clavicle and then cut flush to the bone on the medial side.

In both the methods, no immobilisation is required, only an arm pouch is enough and the child is allowed gentle shoulder mobilisation early in the first week.

Uncommon Clavicular Injuries

Most clavicular injuries are mid-shaft injuries. The uncommon injuries are as under:

- Medial clavicular fractures and Pseudo-sternoclavicular joint dislocations
- Lateral end clavicular fractures
- Acromioclavicular joint injuries

Medial Clavicular Fractures and Pseudo-sternoclavicular Dislocations

Introduction

- Medial clavicular fractures and dislocations are very rare injuries especially in children and account for only about 5% of all clavicular fractures.
- The sternoclavicular joint capsule is extremely thick and stronger than the metaphysis of the medial clavicle and hence once a particular force is applied to the medial clavicle, the metaphysis fractures more easily than the capsule. Also the medial clavicular physis is one of the last to fully fuse (at almost 22-24 years of age) and hence this injury can occur till that age also. Hence medial clavicular type 1 and type 2 physeal injuries are more common than the very rare "true" sternoclavicular dislocations.

Mechanism of Injury

- Medial clavicular fractures and pseudodislocations occur by two specific mechanisms. One is by a medially directed force from the point of the shoulder which forces the medial clavicle anteriorly or posteriorly with respect to the sternum.
- The other is a direct force to the medial clavicle from the anterior aspect, such as a direct kick from the front in physical sports, which as a rule is a posterior clavicular dislocation/ fracture.

Clinical Features

- Pain and swelling at the medial aspect of the clavicle following a direct or indirect trauma.
- The symptoms of its complications are more important than the injury itself and include dysphagia, dysarthria, respiratory distress, and/ or distension of the neck veins (due to compression of oesophagus, recurrent laryngeal nerve, trachea or major vessels of the neck respectively).

Imaging

- Routine plain AP X-ray may not be very conclusive for medial clavicular injury

The *"Serendipity view of Rockwood"* (which is a 45° cephalad view centred on the sternum) is very important in diagnosing the condition and can aid in the diagnosis

CT scans are of utmost importance and have become the gold standard for management of these injuries **(Fig. 7.5)**.

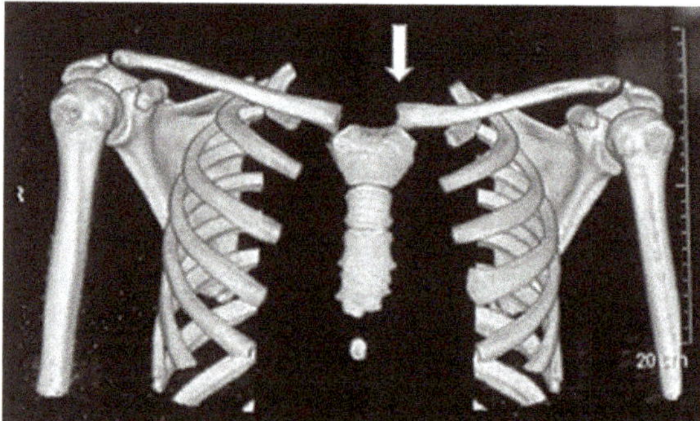

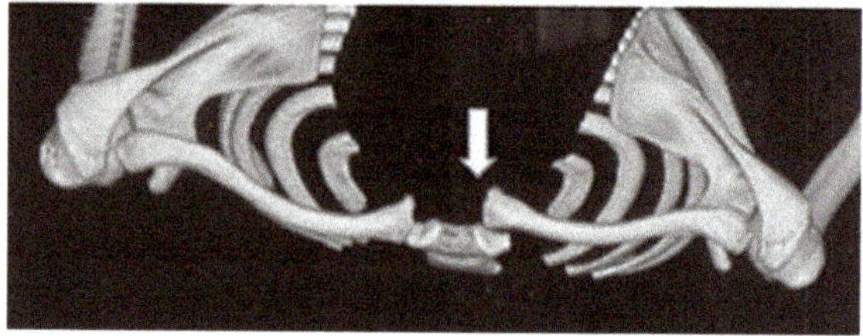

***Fig. 7.5**: CT scan of a 15-year-old boy with left sided medial clavicular fracture with posterior displacement (White arrows).*

Treatment

Almost all medial clavicular injuries can be managed conservatively with either an in-situ figure of 8 bandage with a sling or with closed reduction. Usually anteriorly displaced fractures can be left alone. Posteriorly displaced fractures need to be looked into with detail and treated if there are associated complications like oesophageal and tracheal compression, etc. In some cases, a small mini-open approach can be taken with the help of a thoracic or cardiothoracic surgeon, the medial clavicle is pulled back in place with the help of towel clip clamps and the overlying periosteum sutured back in place.

Lateral End clavicular fractures and Acromioclavicular joint injuries

Introduction

- These are also uncommon injuries and account for only about 10% of all clavicular injuries.
- Their mechanism of trauma and pathogenesis is similar to the medial end clavicle injuries where the AC joint capsule is much thicker than the metaphysis of the lateral clavicle.

Classifications

Dameron and Rockwood classification of Distal end clavicular fractures:

Type A: Undisplaced fractures

Type B: Displaced but non-articular fractures

Type C: Displaced fracture-dislocations of the AC joint.

Allman's classification of AC joint injuries:

I- Mild sprain with no dislocation

II- Sprain of the Acromioclavicular ligaments with subluxation but with no disruption of the coracoclavicular ligaments

III- Disruption of both ligaments with subluxation of joint which is obvious on the AP X-ray of the chest.

Clinical Features

- Pain, swelling and prominence of the lateral end of the clavicle.
- Inability to abduct or restriction of abduction of shoulder

Imaging

- Usually a plain AP X-ray of the shoulder with the clavicle is sufficient to diagnose these injuries.
- In case, we need to exactly diagnose this injury, a "weight-bearing radiograph" may be important for diagnosing the exact amount of displacement.

Treatment

Considering the tremendous amount of remodelling potential in this region, the commonest treatment modality even for displaced fractures and dislocations is conservative. A number of splint supports and braces have been used- from simple arm pouch to shoulder immobiliser to figure of 8 slings with equivalent results.

The very few indications for operative intervention are older children and adolescents, especially those in high level contact sports with fracture involving dominant hands. These injuries are treated like in adults.

Flowchart 7.1

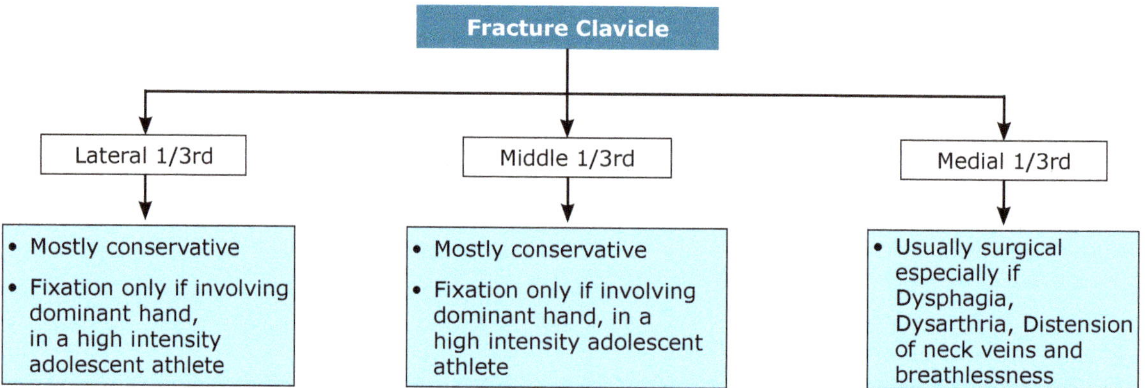

8 Proximal Humerus Fractures

Introduction

Proximal humerus fractures are uncommon injuries constituting around 0.5% of all children's fractures. The characteristic feature of fractures of this region is the great propensity for healing and remodelling with the result that most of these fractures are treated non-operatively in children.

Developmental and Applied Anatomy (Fig. 8.2)

The proximal humerus is composed of a tent-shaped curvilinear physis which has a very high growth potential. Almost 80% of all the growth of the humerus takes place in the proximal humeral physis. The metaphysis is intra-articular in some portions, which has importance for the potential of an osteomyelitic focus to cause septic arthritis. The other important point of the physis is its shape which is undulating and tent-shaped, which itself is many a time mistaken for a fracture and treated as such **(Fig. 8.1)**. In such a case, an opposite side X-ray is very important.

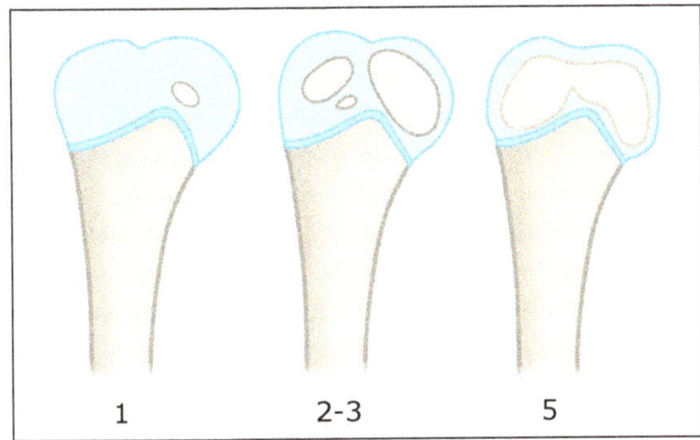

Fig. 8.1: *Ossification of the proximal humeral physis at various ages (in years).*

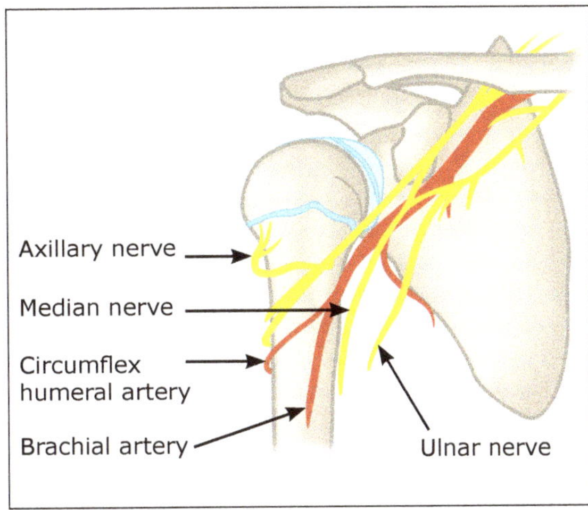

***Fig. 8.2**: Proximal humerus anatomy and the various nerves and vessels in relation to it.*

Epidemiology

The proximal humerus fractures contribute about 0.5% of all childhood fractures and around 3% of all physeal injuries. Fractures in the neonatal and early infantile period are typically type I Salter-Harris injuries (which in fact, seem similar to shoulder dislocations since the proximal humeral epiphysis is not ossified at this young age). The second common age is between 5 to 11 years in which metaphyseal fractures are quite common. Fractures in the adolescent age group are typically higher velocity sporting injuries which are Salter-Harris type 2 injuries.

The other known aetiologies of physeal injuries in the proximal humerus are post-Scurvy epiphyseal slips in nutritionally poor chronically ill children like those with severe cerebral palsy or a similar debilitating neurological disorder. These are typically non-traumatic and are associated with a large sub-periosteal haematoma, which sometimes even requires blood transfusion.

Mechanism of Injury

Neonatal fractures of the proximal humerus are associated with a difficult labour and shoulder dystocia, though hand prolapse and difficult extraction of the hand with abduction and external rotation are also associated mechanisms. The mechanism of injury in older age children is usually indirect with fall on outstretched hand being the commonest. However metaphyseal fractures of the humerus are seen in direct trauma to the upper humerus with a blunt object or fall at the point of the shoulder.

There are six distinct mechanisms by which proximal humerus fractures can be produced (as described by Williams):

- Forced flexion
- Forced extension
- Forced extension with lateral rotation
- Forced extension with medial rotation
- Forced flexion with lateral rotation
- Forced flexion with medial rotation.

The other point of interest in proximal humerus fractures is that they are common sites for pathological fractures. Fractures associated with cystic conditions (unicameral bone cysts or aneurysmal bone cysts), malignant lesions like osteogenic sarcoma, or metastatic bony lesions or even post-radiotherapy fractures are seen commonly in the proximal humerus.

Proximal humerus is also a common site for other causes of pathological fractures like those seen in neuropathic conditions like Arnold-Chiari malformations, Syringomyelia and myelomeningocele.

The final mechanism can be due to non-accidental trauma and child abuse. In this case, a comprehensive history and detailed local and systemic examination is needed to rule out such cause.

Classification

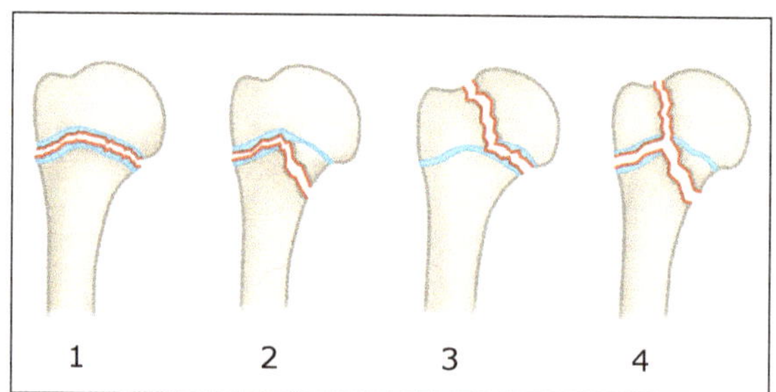

***Fig. 8.3**: Classification of Proximal humeral fractures in children- according to the Salter-Harris classification.*

Proximal humerus fractures are commonly classified according to the Salter-Harris classification itself **(Fig. 8.3)**.

Type 1: S-H type 1 injuries are the commonest, seen in children less than 5 years of age (mostly a birth trauma).

Type 2: S-H type 2 injuries are second-most common injuries with a posteromedial Thurston Holland fragment. They are commonly seen in adolescents.

Type 3: Type 3 injuries are relatively rare intra-articular injuries which are usually seen in association with shoulder dislocations.

Type 4: Type 4 injuries are extremely rare and are associated with open fractures.

The commonest two fractures can be further sub-classified into four types depending on the amount of displacement based on the Neer and Horowitz classification.

Grade 1: <5mm of displacement

Grade 2: < 1/3rd of displacement of width of shaft

Grade 3: 1/3rd- 2/3rd of displacement of width of shaft

Grade 4: Displacement of more than 2/3rd of width of the shaft including total displacement.

Clinical Features

- Pain, swelling and deformity is usually obvious around the shoulder.
- In infants and very young kids, there is usually pseudoparalysis with inability to abduct the shoulder with marked tenderness around the upper humerus.
- The diagnosis in neonates is not easy and is often confused with other causes of pseudoparalysis of the upper limb like clavicular fractures, Obstetric Brachial plexus palsy and neonatal septic arthritis of the shoulder. Since the proximal humerus epiphysis is unossified in neonates, a displaced proximal humerus fracture is diagnosed as a shoulder dislocation.
- Metaphyseal fractures are also sometimes confused due to the undulant nature of the proximal humerus physis. Hence as mentioned before, it is best if an opposite X-ray is taken to compare the shape of the physis versus the fracture
- In older kids with high velocity injuries, there is significant contusion around the medial aspect of the shoulder which can track down till the elbow.
- Neurovascular injury is very rare and is seen only with very high velocity injuries in older kids and adolescents where axillary nerve or brachial artery can be injured.

Imaging

- Plain X-rays for proximal humerus fractures are usually adequate though there are some special points to be noted in certain circumstances.
- The proximal humerus epiphysis is not ossified below 6 months of age and hence the relation of the proximal humeral metaphysis in relation to the glenoid needs to be evaluated to diagnose these fractures.
- In older children, with displaced type I physeal injuries, with a posteriorly displaced epiphysis, with the metaphysis overlapping the epiphysis, the epiphysis may be seen to be "absent", in the so-called *"vanishing epiphysis sign"* which is pathognomonic of proximal humeral type I injuries.

Theoretically, two orthogonal views are important in the diagnosis and management of any bony injury. However in the proximal humerus fracture, in a young irritable child, it is extremely difficult to get a good axillary view for the perfect "orthogonal" position for the AP view. Hence there are a number of modifications of this view which are: the transthoracic scapular Y view, apical oblique view, Velpeau view, etc, which help in easier positioning of the patient for the second view.

Treatment

The treatment of proximal humerus fractures in children in general is conservative, considering the tremendous growth and remodelling potential of the proximal humeral physis. Neonatal and childhood fractures can be treated with just a simple arm pouch or a chest arm bandage, whichever is comfortable to the child. The question arises basically in the adolescent fractures whether to accept some (usually varus) angulation which may remodel or correct it and keep it reduced by conservative or surgical means. It depends on the degree of displacement and the amount of growth left in the child. In adolescence, in case of an unstable reduction or if the reduction is possible only in particular positions which are quite difficult to maintain, it is better to fix with K-wires and hold it till union.

The acceptable criteria for various ages are as follows:

Age	Acceptability criteria
0-5 years	70° angulation, 100% displacement
5-12 years	40-70° angulation, 100 % displacement
➤12 years	<40° angulation and 50 % displacement

Operative Technique

There are basically two procedures which need to be considered in proximal humerus fractures- closed reduction and K-wire fixation and closed/open reduction and intra-medullary nailing. The operative steps of the two procedures are as follows:

1) ***Closed reduction and K-wire fixation* (Fig. 8.4):**

   Indications:

   SH type 1/ 2 fractures of the proximal humerus with angulation of more than 40° in an adolescent or floating shoulder fractures.

   Position and Anaesthesia:

   Supine position with the patient under general anaesthesia with or without a brachial plexus block. Arm/shoulder on the arm board if the child is big or within the table if the child is small. The C-arm in the first case will be from the side and if it is a small child, then it will come from across the table.

   Operative technique:

   - The typical displacement in proximal humeral physeal fractures is varus, with over-riding and apex anterior angulation. Hence the method of closed reduction is traction, abduction, external rotation and applying anterior pressure to correct the apex-anterior angulation.
   - Once the reduction is obtained, fixation is performed using two 2.5 mm K-wires placed retrograde from the metaphysis into the epiphysis.
   - The entry of the K-wires has to be marked about 5-8 cm from the physis with the trajectory marked at around 20-25° to the shaft of the humerus. This entry point has to be through a small incision which is placed slightly distal to the entry point so as to account for the trajectory of the wire. The subcutaneous tissue and muscle is bluntly dissected with an artery hemostat to reach the bone. This keeps the axillary nerve safe and also helps in achieving the correct direction of the K-wire.
   - The wire is initially directed perpendicular to the bone in order to gain a good entry and then it is directed towards the physis in the desired direction. This is to ensure that the wire doesn't skid on the bone. Always use a drill sleeve at this stage to prevent damage to the surrounding soft tissue. Before piercing the physis, good orthogonal views are taken to confirm the reduction as well as the position of the wire so as to minimise the surgical trauma to the physis.
   - The wire is passed into the epiphysis taking care that the chondral surface of the proximal humerus is not pierced by the wire **(Fig. 8.5)**.

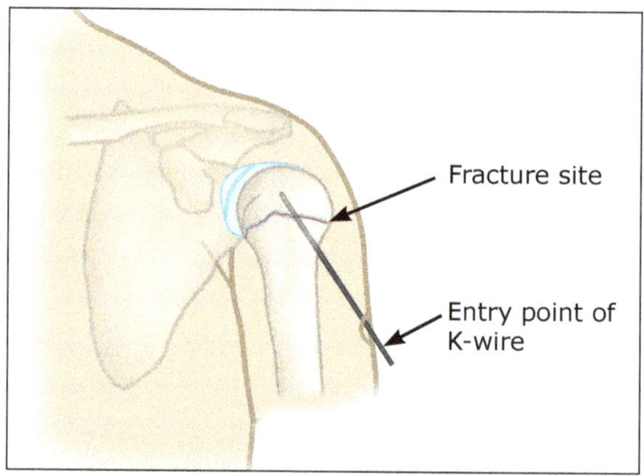

***Fig. 8.4**: Closed reduction and internal fixation with retrograde K- wire for Type I/ Type II proximal humeral fracture.*

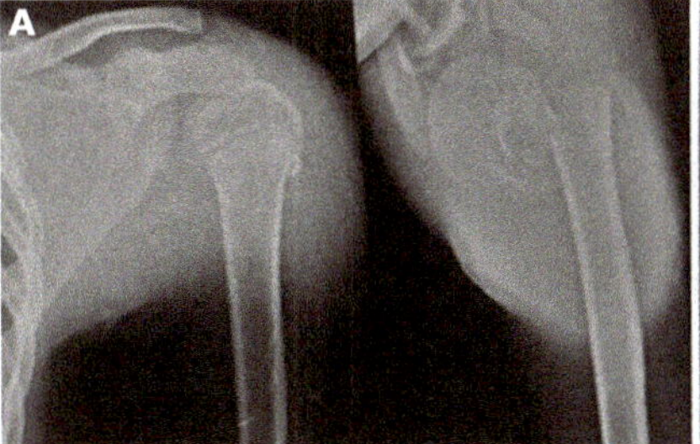

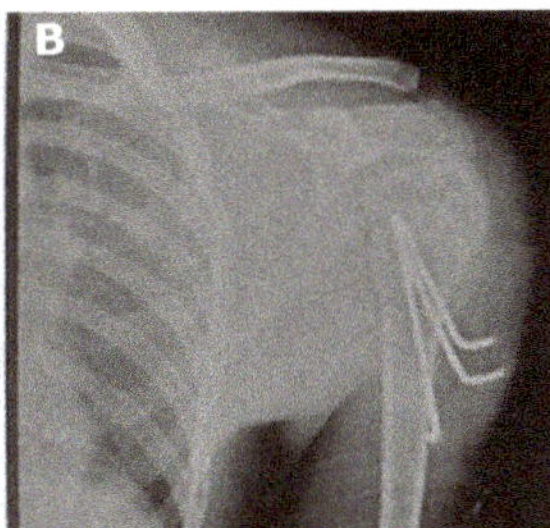

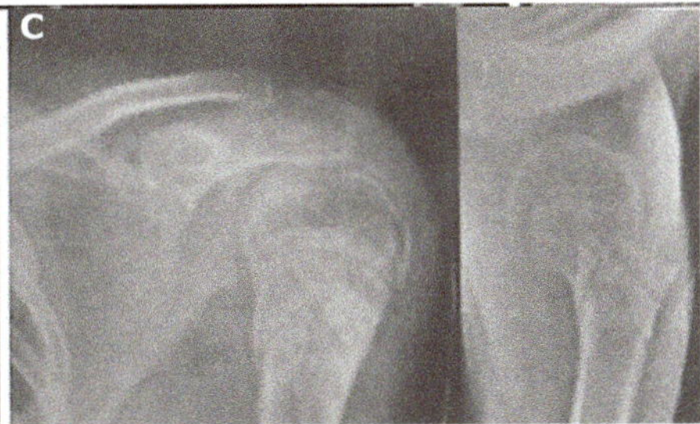

***Fig. 8.5**: (A) X-rays of a displaced Type II Proximal humeral fracture in a 10-year-old boy. (B) Post-operative X-ray showing fixation after closed reduction and K-wire fixation. (C) Six weeks post-op X-ray at the time of K-wire removal showing good healing and alignment.*

- One more wire is then placed, parallel or slightly divergent to the first wire taking the same precautions as the first.
- The wires are bent and cut above the skin taking care that the skin doesn't get puckered.
- The skin incision is closed around the wire with one or two stay sutures.
- Usually just an arm pouch is enough for immobilisation. This is kept for around 2 weeks followed by pendulum exercises for about 2-3 weeks after which full range of motion is allowed. K-wire removal can be done after confirmation of healing at around 4-6 weeks.

2) **Closed/open reduction and internal fixation with retrograde intramedullary nail (Fig. 8.6):**

- Position:

  Supine with arm on arm board with the child at the side of the OT table. It is very important to confirm that the entire humerus is visualised from the elbow to the humeral head on C-arm.

- Indication:

  Displaced metaphyseal fractures of the proximal humerus in older children and adolescents

- The entire limb is painted and draped free from the fingers to the axilla.
- Entry points on the bone are marked on both sides of the distal humerus just on the supracondylar ridge above the olecranon fossa.
- Incisions are made slightly distal to the marked entry points in order to accommodate for the trajectory of the nail.
- Alternatively both nails can be passed from only one side by slightly dilating the entry point.
- Entry is made with the help of a curved awl which is directed towards the centre of the canal.
- An appropriately sized elastic nail (0.4 x thinnest canal diameter) gently bent, is passed through this entry point and passed till the fracture site with to-and-fro rotatory movements or with gentle hammering.
- Both the nails are passed simultaneously till the fracture site after which the fracture is close or open reduced.
- The main concern with fixation of displaced metaphyseal fractures of the proximal humerus is achieving a satisfactory reduction. This is many a time difficult due to the interposed biceps tendon which makes it

extremely difficult to obtain a closed reduction. One method to do so is by widely abducting the shoulder at the level of the fracture site and trying to "milk" out the biceps tendon from the fracture site. In most of the cases, reduction is obtained by passing a thick 2-2.5mm K-wire through the fracture site, levering out the distal fragment and then keeping the reduction stable till definitive fixation **(Fig. 8.7)**.

- If the fracture is irreducible by closed means, then reduction is obtained by open reduction. This is performed through the delto-pectoral groove, keeping the cephalic vein intact and retracting it medially. The plane is developed between the deltoid and the pectoralis major and can be extended distally till the deltoid insertion. The interposed biceps tendon is retracted away from the fracture site and fracture is reduced using curved reduction clamps or Hohmann retractors.
- Once reduction is obtained, the nails are passed across the fracture site, with one nail directed medially and one nail laterally. The nails usually stop short of the physis and do not pierce it.
- Distally the nails are cut flush to the bone (they are *not* bent) and the skin is closed in a single layer over the nails.

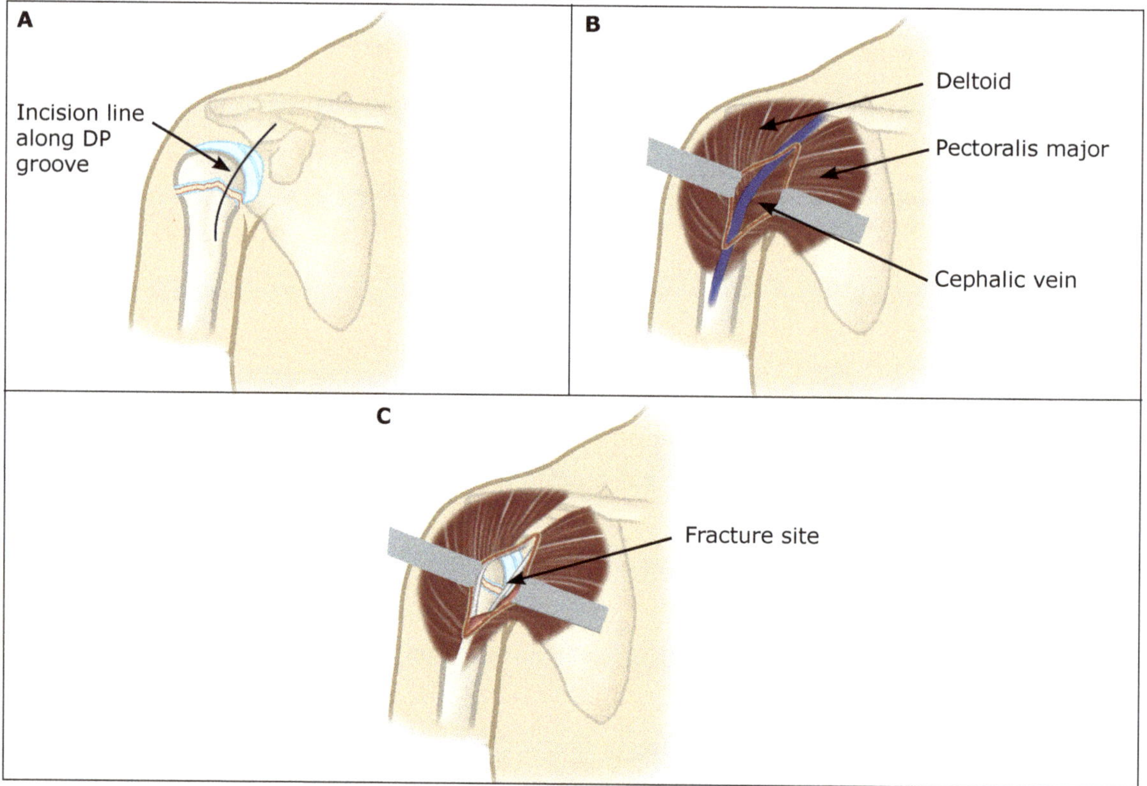

***Fig. 8.6**: Open reduction of proximal humeral fracture. (A) Incision is made through the delto-pectoral groove, (B) Deltoid and pectoralis major along the cephalic vein are retracted. (C) Fracture site is exposed in the deeper plane.*

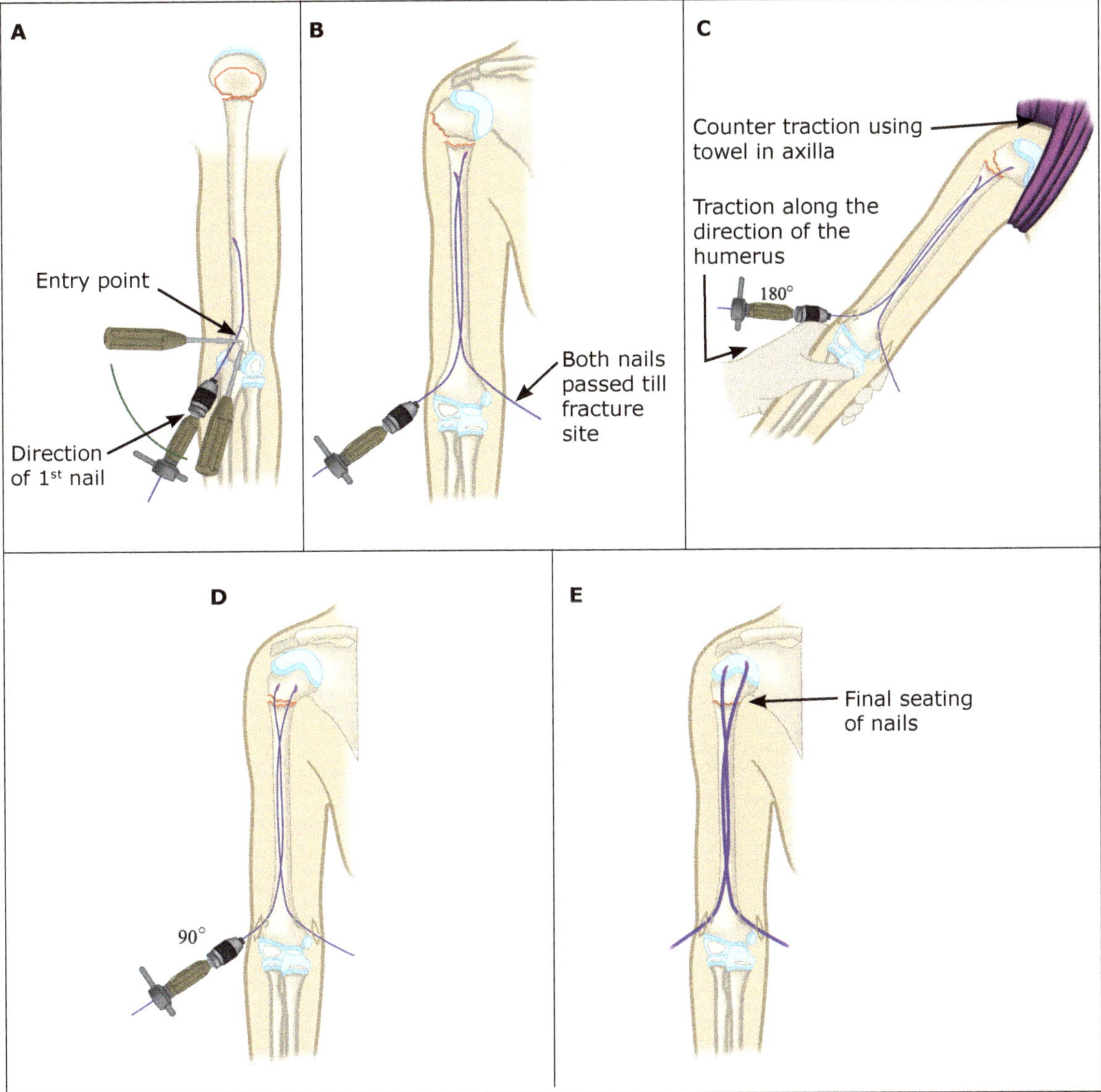

Fig. 8.7: *Closed reduction and internal fixation with 2 retrograde Titanium elastic nails (TEN) for displaced proximal humeral fracture. (A) Entry made using an awl followed by introduction of the nail. (B) Passage of both the nails till the fracture site (C) Reduction obtained using traction through the distal forearm and counter-traction using a towel in the axilla followed by passage of one nail across the fracture site. (D) Passage of both nails across the fracture site (E) Final seating of the nails.*

- Immobilisation in the form of an arm pouch or a U slab is given for around 3-4 weeks.
- The fracture starts consolidating by around 4 weeks and hence active and active assisted mobilisation can be started after that time. Nail removal can be performed at around 6 months **(Fig. 8.8)**.

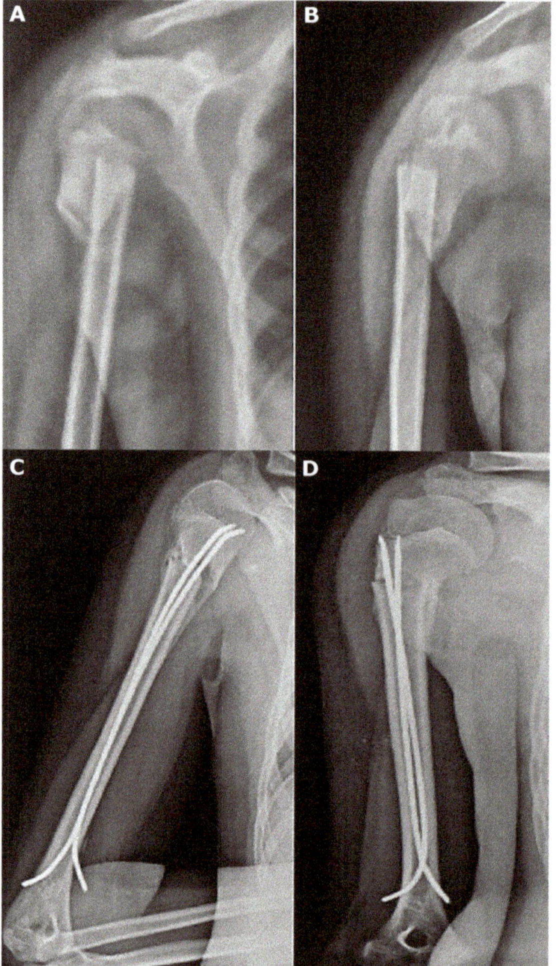

***Fig. 8.8**: Pre-operative (A and B) and Post-operative (C and D) X-rays of a 14-year-old boy with displaced fracture proximal humerus treated with closed reduction and internal fixation with Titanium elastic nails using retrograde manner.*

Complications

Since the growth and remodelling potential of proximal humerus fractures is so high, childhood proximal humerus fractures have a very low rate of complications. The common complications seen in proximal humerus fractures are:

1) Neurovascular injury:

   Grossly displaced proximal humerus fractures are known to rarely cause neurovascular injury by compression of the axillary artery and the brachial plexus. Surgical neck fractures can cause axillary nerve injuries, though its incidence in childhood is very less.

2) Humerus varus:

   Humerus varus is a potentially disabling complication of proximal humerus fractures characterised by a humeral neck shaft angle of less than 140°. This complication usually has an underlying pathology in the proximal humerus which can then angulate after a trivial trauma. This can cause significant restriction in abduction and usually requires a valgus osteotomy in order to correct the neck shaft angle as well as to bring the greater tuberosity more distally.

3) Limb length discrepancy:

   This is a rare complication seen more often in operatively treated proximal humerus fractures, where there were multiple attempts at passing trans-physeal wires or the wires have been kept for a long time. Usually limb length discrepancy of the upper limb is much less disconcerting than lower limb and no treatment is required unless the LLD is more than 3 cm.

4) Avascular necrosis of humeral head:

   Extremely rare complication seen typically in open fractures due to disruption of the anterolateral ascending branch of anterior circumflex humeral artery.

SHOULDER DISLOCATION

Introduction

Shoulder dislocation in the paediatric age group is an extremely uncommon injury with only less than 1% of all shoulder dislocations occurring in children in most series. However the incidence is slowly increasing due to increased involvement of adolescents in high energy sports like basketball and volleyball.

Mechanism of Injury

There are basically two major mechanisms- traumatic and atraumatic.

In case of traumatic causes of shoulder dislocations, the typical direction of dislocation is anterior. The usual force required to dislocate the shoulder is flexion, abduction and external rotation and is seen in many common sports injuries during the following actions:

1) Cricket: Forceful throwing of the ball, lunging and diving towards the side while fielding, lunging and diving while running between the wickets
2) Basketball: Vigorous throwing of the ball, "slam-dunk" activity, etc.
3) Volleyball: Forceful overhead serving
4) Tennis: Forceful serving

In case of the relatively rare posterior dislocation, the mechanism of injury and the force applied is different with a posteriorly applied force with the shoulder forward flexed, adducted and internally rotated. This commonly occurs in road traffic accidents, seizures, electric shock- either accidental or during electroshock treatment, etc.

Atraumatic shoulder instability has a totally different aetiology which includes syndromes with ligamentous laxity like Marfan's syndrome and Ehler-Danlos syndrome. Mild shoulder luxations are extremely common even without any demonstrable ligament laxity syndrome and are almost always painless and asymptomatic.

Shoulder dislocations which occur due to brachial plexus birth injuries are slowly developing posterior dislocations. These occur along with or following glenoid dysplasia which is due to the uncorrected muscular forces acting on the shoulder joint.

Classification

Shoulder dislocations can be classified in the following ways based on the mechanism, direction and duration of injury.

1) Mechanism:
   - Traumatic
   - Atraumatic

   Associated conditions like neuro-muscular disorders, brachial plexus birth injury, etc
2) Direction:
   - Anterior
   - Posterior
   - Inferior
   - Multi-directional
3) Duration of injury:
   - Acute
   - Chronic
   - Recurrent

Clinical Features

Traumatic anterior dislocations:

- Pain, swelling and severe deformity in the shoulder following a fall on outstretched abducted arm. The other typical injury can be a flexion, abduction, external rotation injury.
- The child/adolescent is unable to touch the opposite shoulder
- There is flattening of the rounded contour of the shoulder and one is able to place a flat object (wooden scale) from the acromion to the lateral epicondyle of the humerus.
- Hypoasthesia over the regimental badge area (lower third of the deltoid insertion) needs to be checked for, to look for axillary nerve involvement.

- In case of the rare subtype of the posterior dislocation of the shoulder, the arm is typically flexed, adducted and internally rotated and there is a concavity on the anterior aspect of the shoulder, denoting the absent humeral head in the glenoid cavity.

Posterior dislocations:

- The clinical deformity in a posterior dislocation is much less as compared to an anterior dislocation and the limb is held in the typical "sling" position of adduction internal rotation.
- Careful examination may show a small bony bulge near the posterior aspect of the shoulder representing the dislocated humeral head.

Inferior dislocations:

- Extremely rare in children and may be associated with laxity syndromes like Ehlers-Danlos or Marfan's syndrome.

Atraumatic dislocations:

- Atraumatic dislocations are typically painless and mostly have only mild discomfort. There is no predisposing history of trauma and usually it is the parents who notice something abnormal in the child's shoulder.
- Along with other signs of the ligamentous laxity, the pathognomonic feature is the *"sulcus"* sign on manual longitudinal traction to the limb.

Imaging

- Plain X-rays: Plain X-rays are usually diagnostic for traumatic anterior dislocations which are commonest. Typically only a shoulder AP view is taken due to the severe pain associated with acute anterior shoulder dislocation. In case another orthogonal view is required, a scapular "Y" view or Westpoint lateral view may be required as they are much less painful to the patient than the axillary view. The various views which can be taken for shoulder dislocation are:
- Velpeau axillary view: The child with a sling is inclined 45° backward and the beam is directed from above directed caudally orthogonally to the cassette.
- West Point axillary view: This view is for the anterior glenoid rim, with the patient prone, and the beam directed 25° off the horizontal and 25° medially.
- Hill-Sachs view: AP radiograph taken with shoulder in maximal internal rotation so as to visualize the Hill-Sachs lesion seen postero-laterally.
- MRI: MRI is typically indicated in recurrent dislocations or the atraumatic dislocations while they usually are not required in acute anterior traumatic dislocations. MRI in recurrent dislocations show the associated chondral, labral and capsular tears and is of utmost importance in planning surgical arthroscopic treatment for the same. This also shows the "Hill-sachs lesion" **(Fig. 8.9)** which is a depression

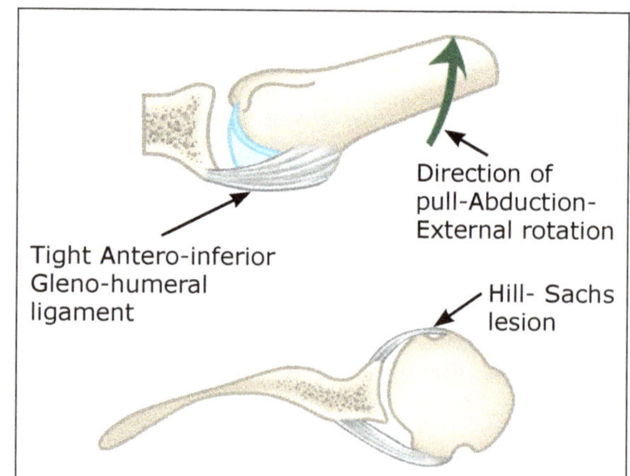

Fig. 8.9: *(A) Pathoanatomy of shoulder dislocation showing a tight antero-inferior gleno-humeral ligament after forceful abduction-external rotation force (B) Typical Hill-Sachs lesion seen posteriorly.*

or indentation of the posteroinferior portion of the humeral head.

CT scan: CT scan may be indicated in the rare fracture dislocations which are seen in adolescents and young adults. It may also be required in secondary shoulder dislocations like those in brachial plexus birth palsies to look for the associated glenoid dysplasia.

Treatment

A) ***Non-operative management***

- Non-operative treatment remains the most common method of management of traumatic anterior shoulder dislocations. Typically this is performed in a conscious child/ adolescent and very rarely requires some form of anaesthesia/ sedation to ensure painfree stable reduction. Over the years, a number of methods have been described to achieve reduction for anterior shoulder dislocation. They are:

1) ***Traction-countertraction method (Modified Hippocratic method)* (Fig. 8.10):** With child in supine position, a small towel or sheet is looped across the axilla and around the neck, and pulled by the assistant in line with the abducted arm. The surgeon holds the forearm and gives sustained traction, followed by external rotation, adduction and finally internal rotation. Here the counter-traction is provided by the assistant with the looped towel in the axilla instead of the padded foot in the axilla as described in the original Hippocratic method.

2) ***Stimson's method:*** The child lies prone with the arm lying free across the side of the bed with a small weight tied to the wrist. The weight along with gravity helps in distracting the shoulder joint, and the muscular fatigue helps to easily reposition the humeral head in the glenoid cavity by gentle manipulation.

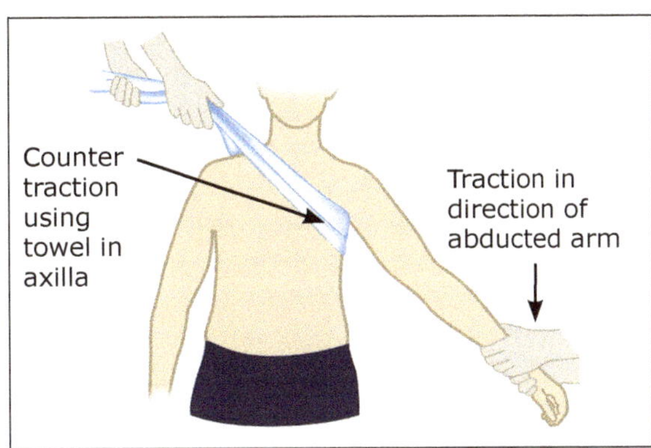

Fig. 8.10: *Reduction of anterior dislocation shoulder by the Hippocratic method.*

3) ***Milch method* (Fig. 8.11)*:*** In this method, with the child lying supine and the shoulder lying at the edge of the bed, gentle and slow abduction external rotation is performed holding the elbow. This helps in repositioning of the shoulder joint in a pain-free comfortable manner and can be easily performed without any form of anaesthesia.

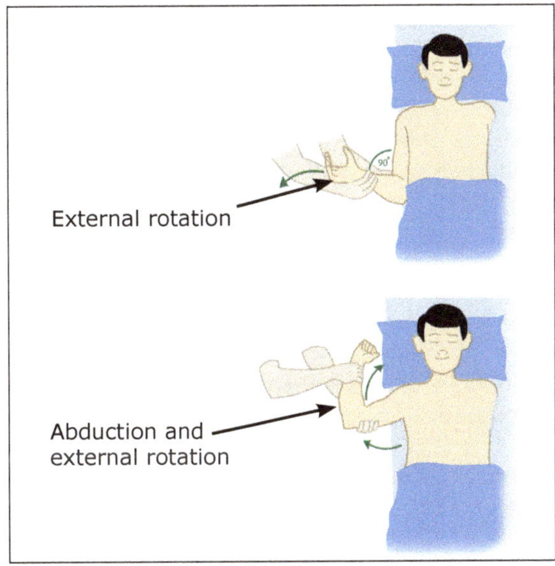

Fig. 8.11: *Milch method of reduction of shoulder dislocation.*

4) ***Thakur's method (Modified Kocher's method):*** Similar to the Milch method, except for gentle anterior flexion at the time of reduction.

5) ***Sustained external rotation (Fig. 8.12):*** With the child sitting on a stool, the shoulder is gently externally rotated, with a mild force of adduction applied. At one point of time, the humeral head slides over the anterior glenoid edge and falls back into the glenoid cavity. After this, the patient is able to internally rotate and touch the opposite shoulder.

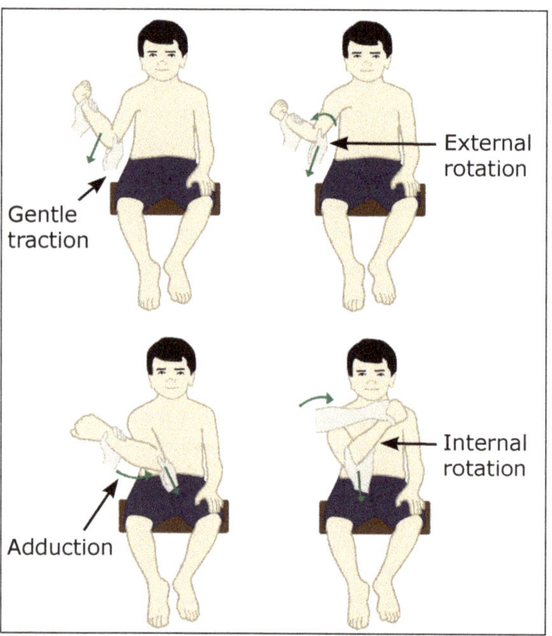

Fig. 8.12: *Sustained external rotation method for reduction of anterior shoulder dislocation.*

B) **Operative management:**

Operative management remains the cornerstone of treatment for recurrent traumatic and symptomatic atraumatic shoulder dislocations. With the advent and rapid development of arthroscopic shoulder surgery, all-arthroscopic repair of the torn labrum and capsule has become the treatment of choice for this condition. It is also indicated for first time dislocations in young high-level athletes with a high chance of recurrent dislocations. We will only be enumerating the different means of arthroscopic and mini-open treatment for recurrent shoulder instability as the details of these methods are outside the purview of this textbook.

- *Arthroscopic or mini-open Bankart repair:* This is the commonest surgery performed for recurrent dislocation shoulder. In this method the so-called Bankart tear (antero-inferior capsular tear) is sutured and fixed with suture anchors.
- *Latarjet procedure:* This is indicated when there is a bony defect in the anterior glenoid rim. The procedure entails restoring or augmenting the anterior glenoid by osteotomising the coracoid at its base with its attachment and re-attaching it to the anterior glenoid. This is an extremely robust procedure and is one of the treatments of choice for anterior shoulder instabilities.

Complications

1) Recurrent dislocations:

This is commonly seen in adolescent high energy high level athletes and are associated with the typical "Bankart's lesion". These usually require arthroscopic Bankart's repair.

2) Neurovascular injury:

Extremely rare injury usually seen with high impact injuries. Axillary nerve neuropraxia is seen in about 10% of cases which is almost always reversible.

Flowchart 8.1

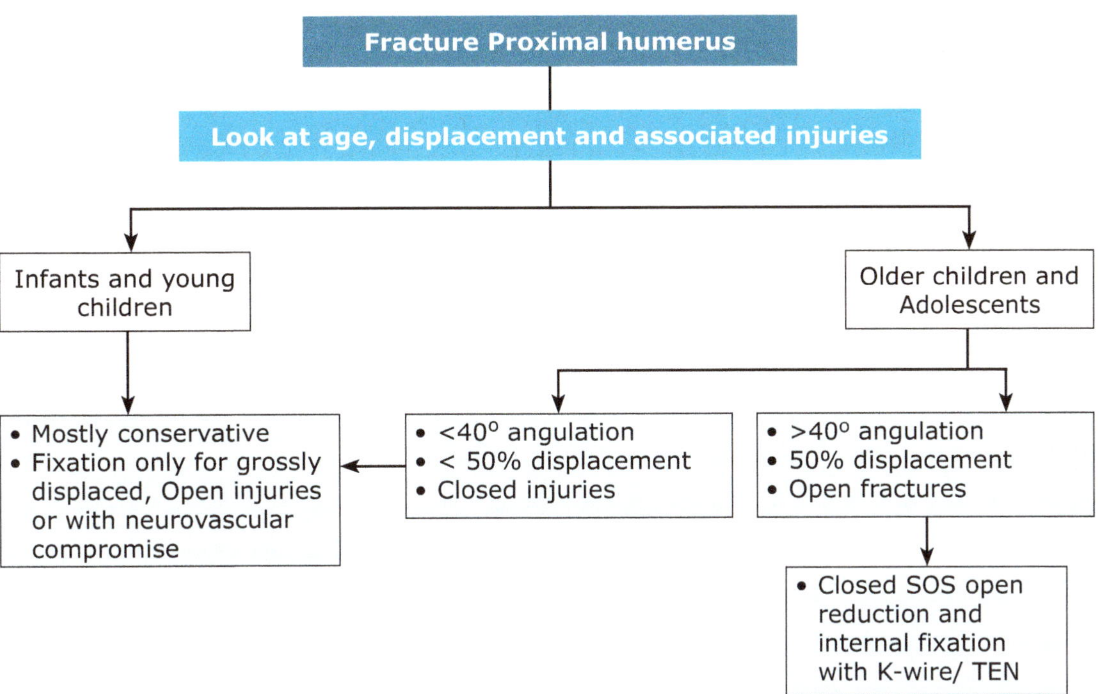

9 Humeral Shaft Fractures

Introduction

Humeral shaft fractures are common fractures in childhood and constitute about 4-6% of all paediatric fractures and about 20% of all paediatric humeral fractures. Humeral shaft fractures are unique due to the presence of a multi-axial, highly mobile joint proximally and a hinge joint distally, along with a very thick periosteal cover which gives a very high healing and remodelling potential to the bone.

Relevant Anatomy

The humerus is a long tubular bone having the proximal end as a spherical structure forming the shoulder joint with the glenoid and a flattened distal end articulating with the radius and ulna at the radio-capitellar and the ulno-humeral joint respectively. It is enveloped with large bulky muscles which give it relative safety from injury as well as help in making any deformity much less apparent. The muscular anatomy is also important for the deformities which can result after trauma as well as for the approaches for surgical exposures. The details of the muscular anatomy are provided in Figure 9.1.

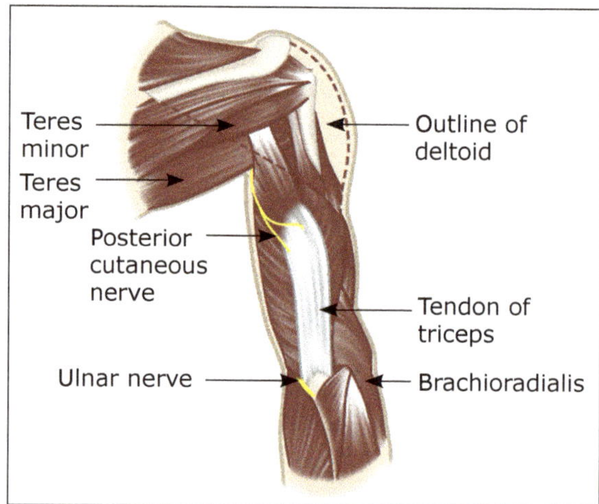

***Fig. 9.1**: Posterior view of the humerus showing the important muscles. The deltoid is the most important muscle proximally and covers the anterior, lateral and posterior parts of the proximal humerus till the level of the deltoid tuberosity. The rotator cuff muscles (subscapularis, supraspinatus, infraspinatus and teres minor) are attached on the proximal humerus near the humeral head. In the middle and distal third of the humerus, the coraco-brachialis, biceps brachii and the brachialis cover the anterior aspect and the three heads of the triceps brachii cover the posterior aspect.*

There are three nerves which are in close proximity of the humerus. From proximal to distal, these are- the axillary nerve near the surgical neck, the radial nerve along the spiral groove in the middle third and the ulnar nerve in the distal third. For the purpose of this chapter, we will be discussing the radial nerve in detail. The radial nerve arising from the posterior chord of the brachial plexus, enters the spiral groove at the level of the deltoid insertion, goes from proximal-medial to distal lateral and exits the posterior compartment by piercing the lateral inter-muscular septum at the level of the middle and distal third of the humerus. The radial nerve then exits the arm from the anterior aspect of the distal humerus.

Mechanism of Injury

Humerus fractures occur with a bimodal distribution with distinctly different mechanisms of injury. One peak is at birth and infancy, while the second is in adolescence and older children.

Humerus fractures are common injuries occurring as a result of difficult deliveries. This can occur when there is macrosomia, shoulder dystocia or when there is hand prolapse and forcible pulling of the abducted upper limb. It is also seen in Caeserian section deliveries when the hand gets stuck deep in the pelvis.

Humerus fractures are also seen as a result of non-accidental trauma when there is vigorous shaking of the child by holding on to the arm. In fact, humerus fractures are some of the commonest fractures seen in NAT.

Humerus fractures occurring in older children or adolescents are typically associated with higher energy trauma which can be direct or indirect. Indirect trauma occurs due to fall on outstretched hand usually on an abducted shoulder. Direct injuries can occur when there is a direct trauma to the side of the arm in high velocity motor vehicle accidents or in high impact sports injuries.

Typical displacements:

Due to the unique nature of the muscular attachments of the humerus, there are some specific deformities and displacements which develop according to the level of the fracture. In case of proximal humerus fractures (proximal to the attachment of the latissimus dorsi and the pectoralis major), the proximal segment will be abducted while the distal fragment will be adducted and proximally migrated. If the fracture is in the upper third-middle third junction just proximal to the deltoid insertion, then the proximal fragment will be adducted due to the pectoralis major and the distal fragment will be abducted due to the pull of the deltoid. On the other hand, if the fracture is in the middle third and distal third of the shaft, then the proximal fragment is abducted due to the deltoid and distal fragment is adducted due to the bulk of the triceps muscle **(Fig. 9.2)**.

Clinical Features

Humeral fractures seen in neonates following difficult deliveries typically cause pseudoparalysis and an asymmetric Moro's reflex. At this time, it is important to distinguish from other causes of pseudoparalysis namely brachial plexus birth injuries (BPBI), fracture clavicle and transphyseal injury of distal humerus. Children with birth fracture humerus usually have a significant deformity in the middle of the arm and have severe pain on passive movement as well as feeding from one side. The child is able to move

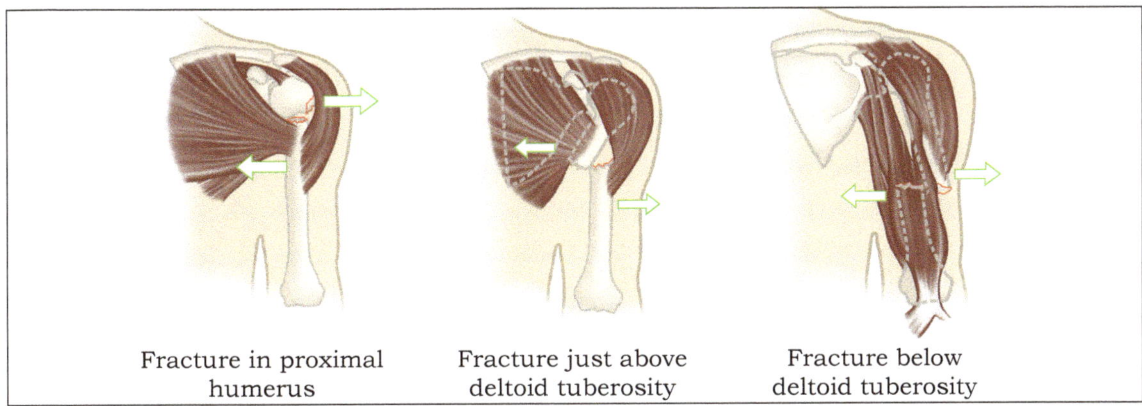

***Fig. 9.2**: Typical displacements seen with fractures at various levels in the shaft of humerus.*

his fingers and wrist which helps in distinguishing it from severe BPBI.

Children with non-accidental injury usually have other injuries like rib fractures, contusions as well as chronologically diverse fractures at different stages of healing. These injuries along with a careful social history will help in the diagnosis.

Older children with high velocity trauma have an obvious deformity in the middle third of the arm with or without a radial nerve palsy. Associated radial nerve palsy has to be looked for in detail especially in middle third-lower third junction fractures – at the time of injury or following manipulation.

Imaging

Plain X-rays – Antero-posterior and lateral views of the arm (including the shoulder and elbow) are usually sufficient to diagnose and plan management of shaft humeral fractures. Only in cases where pathological fractures are suspected is further imaging like MRI indicated.

Classification

There is no specific classification for fracture shaft humerus. Fractures of the shaft of the humerus are described variously, based on the site (upper third, middle third and lower third), type of fracture (transverse, spiral, oblique or comminuted) or soft tissue involvement (open or closed).

Treatment

A) Conservative management

A large proportion of humeral shaft fractures can be managed conservatively. A large multi-directional joint proximally, big bulky muscles around the shaft and a very thick periosteal layer, makes it a very appropriate bone for conservative management. The treatment options at different ages are as follows:

Neonatal fractures:

Neonatal fractures, irrespective of displacement heal very robustly and remodel completely over time. Hence the only aim of treatment is pain relief and comfort of the child and the mother while feeding. The options are:

Chest arm strapping:

The most commonly performed treatment modality, this involves strapping of the affected arm to the chest using soft sticking tape (Micropore®) taking care that the sensitive areas like nipples are covered with a soft gauze. The only disadvantage of this is the possibility of skin ulcerations or redness if the tapes are kept on for a long time.

Velpeau stockinette:

The Velpeau stockinette method is a very comfortable method for treating neonatal humerus fractures. Here a long roll of stockinnette is used to securely hold the arm to the chest, without any chance of skin issues **(Figs. 9.3 and 9.4)**. This also has the advantage of being quite easy to use and remove even to the parents.

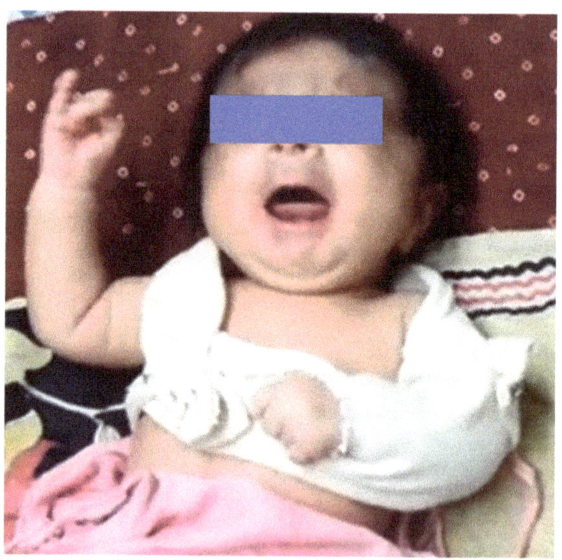

***Fig. 9.3**: Clinical picture of a 15-days-old child with fracture left humerus treated with Velpeau stockinette bandage.*

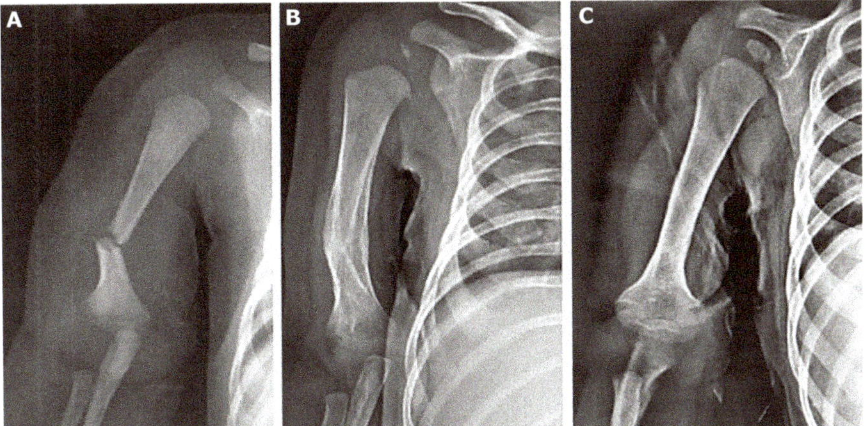

Fig. 9.4: (A) X-ray of a neonate with displaced fracture humerus following birth trauma, (B) Good healing at 3 months, (C) Complete healing and remodelling at 1 year.

Humerus fractures in older children:

A large proportion of humeral fractures in older children and adolescents can be conserved. The acceptability criteria are:

- 30° varus
- 20° apex anterior angulation
- 15° internal rotation
- Bayonet apposition (100% translation)
- 1-2 cm shortening

The three main methods of conservative management are:

1) "U" Slab:

The U slab or the Co-aptation slab is a very important method to treat humeral shaft fractures in older children. Here the requirements are- long stockinnete measuring slightly longer than the length of the arm, One roll of soft cast padding, some rolls of plasters and bandages. A slab is made which is equal to about twice the length of the entire arm. This is then applied to the fractured arm extending from the base of the neck to the outer side of the elbow, making a U around the elbow and then halfway up the arm on the inner side. This "co-apts" the fracture fragments together due to the "U" construct **(Fig. 9.5)**. The extension of the slab above the level of the acromion till the base of the

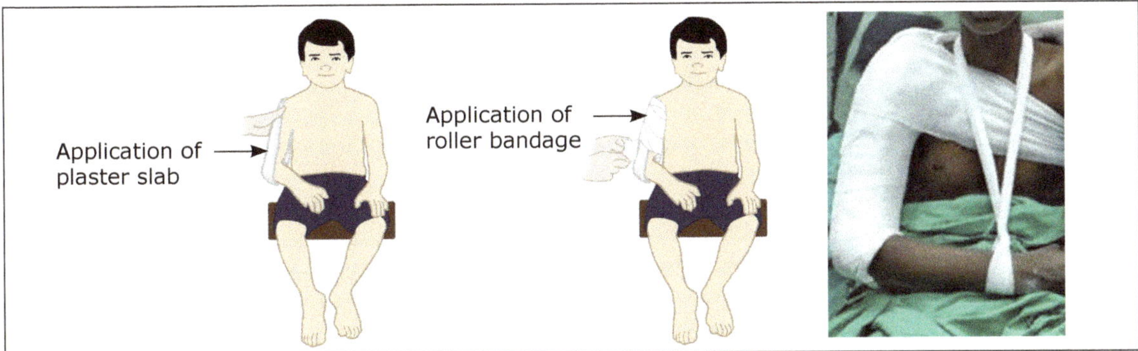

Fig. 9.5: Schematic diagram and clinical photo of a child with fracture shaft humerus treated with a "U" slab.

neck is important in preventing distal migration or loosening of the slab. This is then combined with an arm pouch for ease of usage. This is an extremely commonly performed method and is very comfortable to the child.

2) ***Hanging arm cast:***

This method can be used for middle and distal third humerus fractures. In this method, an above elbow cast is applied, till the level of the deltoid tuberosity, with the patient sitting, which helps in aligning the fracture fragments by traction and gravity **(Fig. 9.6)**. Though this method is widely used, loss of reduction due to inability to sit upright in some kids, and internal rotation contracture are known to occur in some cases.

3) ***Sarmiento functional bracing:***

The functional bracing method has been popularised by Sarmiento since the late 1970's and is widely used in many centres as a treatment of choice. In this method, well-moulded thermoplastic splints are made which help in converting hydraulic forces into compressive forces across the fracture site. This method has the advantage of being extremely patient friendly as well as very effective in trained hands.

B) Operative management

The indications for operative fixation of humeral shaft fractures are :

- Open fractures
- Floating elbow injuries
- Humeral fractures in which radial nerve palsy develops after manipulative reduction (Holstein- Lewis fracture)- relative indication
- Humeral fractures in adolescents involved in high impact or high energy sports who require early return to sports without any immobilisation.
- Displaced fractures in whom closed reduction cannot be maintained.

The various options for operative management of humeral shaft fractures are:

1) ***Closed/open reduction and internal fixation with elastic nails*** **(Fig. 9.7):**

- Position: Supine with arm on arm board with the child at the side of the OT table. It is very important to confirm that the entire humerus is visualised from the elbow to the humeral head on C-arm.
- Indication: Displaced fractures of the

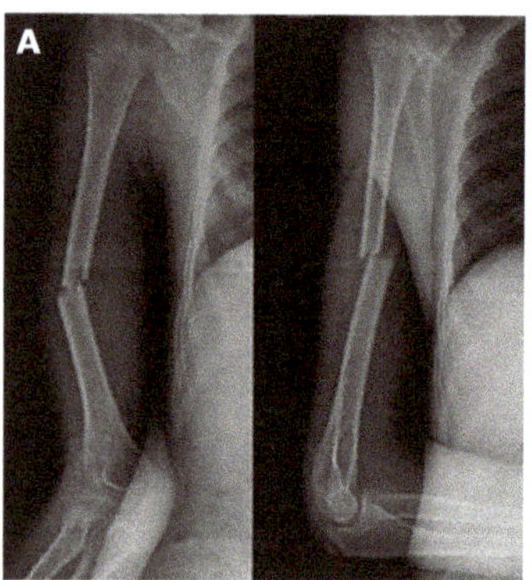

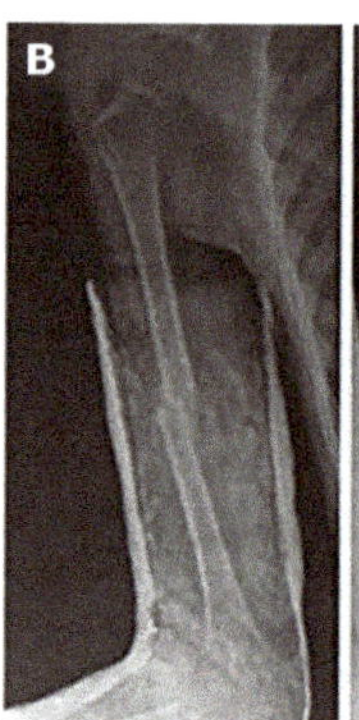

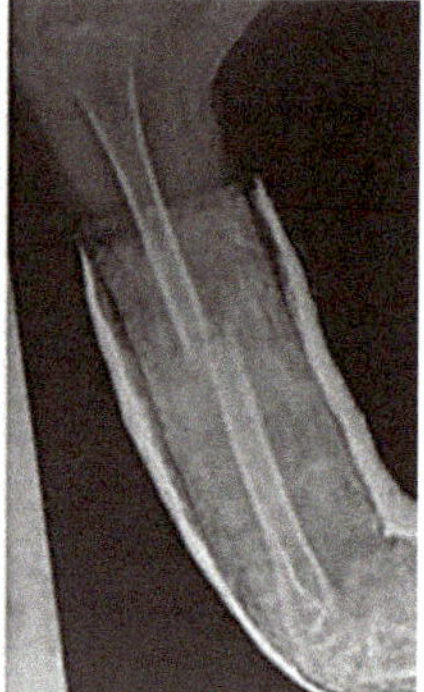
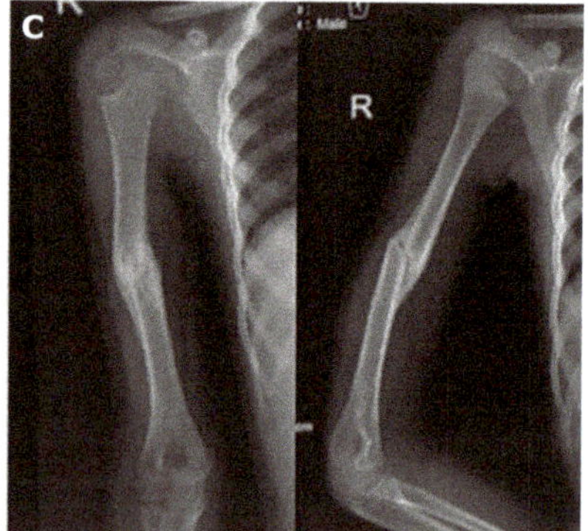

Fig. 9.6: *(A) AP and lateral X-ray of a child with middle third fracture shaft humerus, (B) Treatment with hanging arm cast showing good alignment in the immediate post-reduction X-ray, (C) Good healing and alignment in the X-ray taken at 3 months post-reduction.*

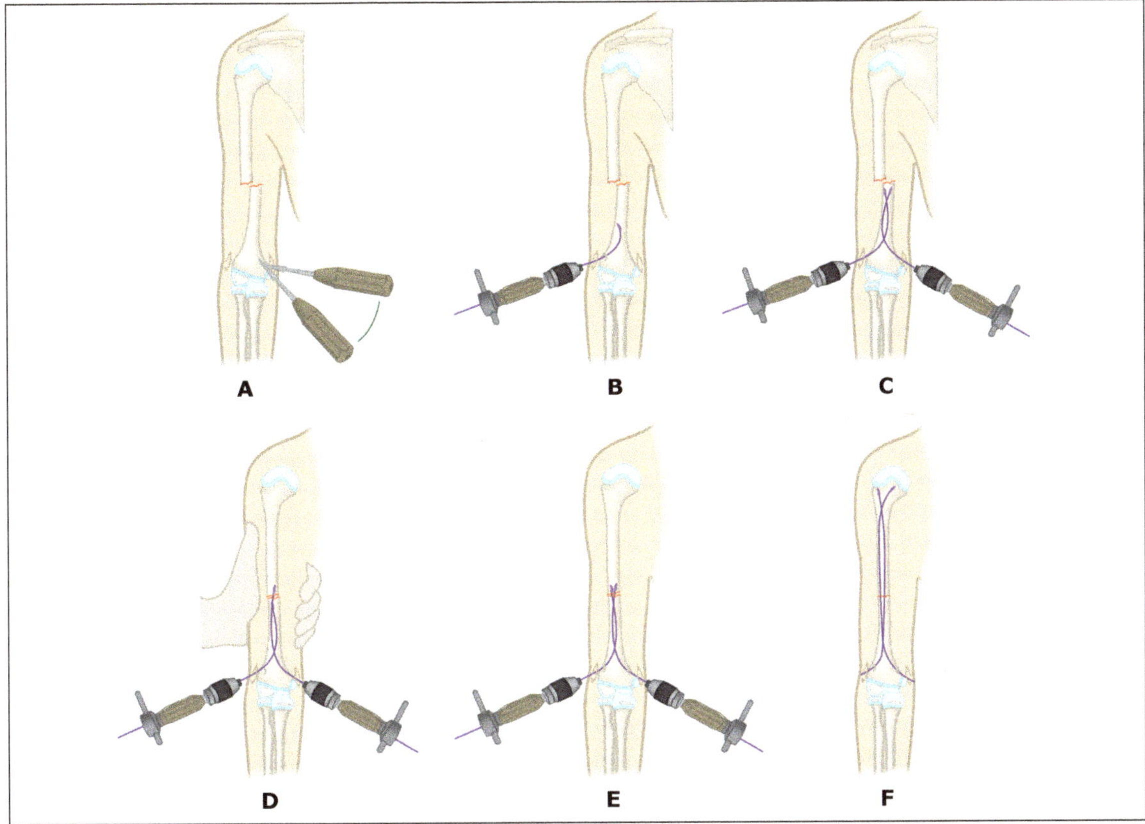

***Fig. 9.7**: Retrograde Titanium elastic nailing for fracture middle third shaft humerus. (A) Entry taken using Awl from the medial and lateral side (B) Nail is inserted with the help of the T-handle and (C) both nails inserted till the fracture site. (D) Reduction performed using manual pressure and traction-counter traction method (E) Nails passed across the fracture site and (F) Final seating of both nails performed till just distal to the physis of the proximal humerus.*

shaft humerus in older children and adolescents

- The entire limb is painted and draped free from the fingers to the axilla.
- Entry points on the bone are marked on both sides of the distal humerus just on the supracondylar ridge above the olecranon fossa.
- Incisions are made slightly distal to the marked entry points in order to accommodate for the trajectory of the nail.
- Alternatively both nails can be passed from only one side by slightly dilating the entry point.
- Entry is made with the help of a curved awl which is directed towards the centre of the canal.
- An appropriately sized elastic nail (0.4x thinnest canal diameter) gently bent with the apex of the bend at the level of the fracture site, is passed through this entry point and passed till the fracture site with to-and-fro rotatory movements or with gentle hammering.
- Both the nails are passed simultaneously till the fracture site after which the fracture is close or open reduced.
- Reduction is usually obtained by gentle longitudinal traction and mild

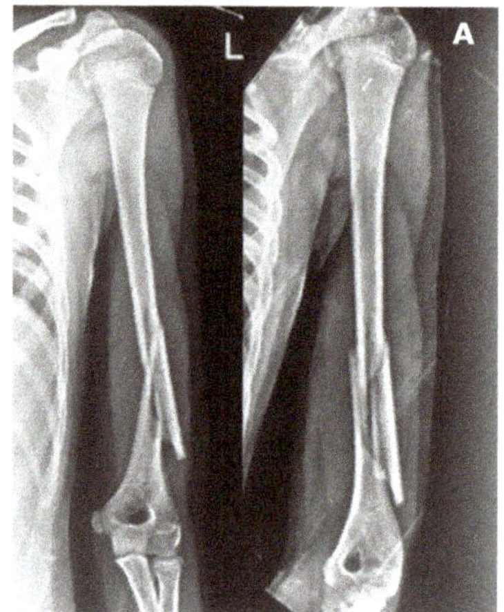

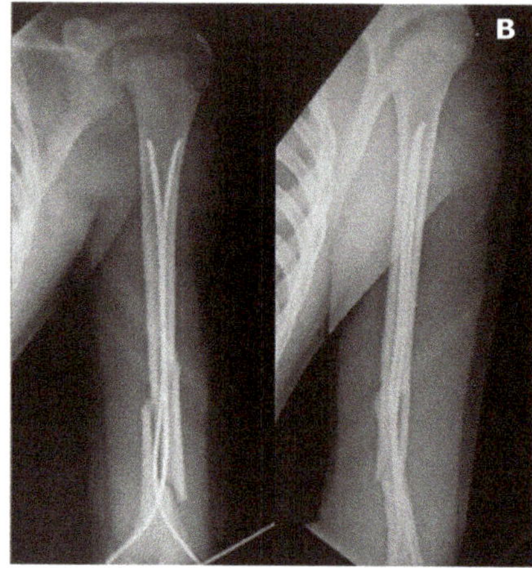

***Fig. 9.8**: (A) AP and lateral X-rays of an adolescent with comminuted fracture lower third humerus (B) Treatment with closed reduction and retrograde Titanium elastic nailing (TEN).*

abduction or by manipulating the nail so as to use the hockey stick end of the nail as a reduction tool. Care should be taken to obtain a good reduction without any soft tissue interposition due to the possibility of the radial nerve getting entrapped in the fracture site.

- If the fracture is irreducible by closed means, open reduction is performed. This is performed through the antero-lateral approach which is an extension of deltopectoral approach. This utilises the interval between the coracobrachialis and the brachialis and gives a good exposure of the fracture site without any danger to the radial nerve
- Once reduction is obtained, the nails are passed across the fracture site, with one nail directed medially and one nail laterally. The nails usually stop short of the physis and do not pierce it **(Fig. 9.8)**.
- Distally the nails are cut flush to the bone (they are *not* bent) and the skin is closed in a single layer over the nails.
- Immobilisation in the form of an arm pouch or a U slab is given for around 3-4 weeks.
- The fracture starts consolidating by around 4 weeks and hence active and active assisted mobilisation can be started after that time. Nail removal can be performed at around 6 months.

2) ***Open reduction and internal fixation with Plating:***

- Position: lateral position with arm over a radiolucent bump or supine position with the arm across the chest.
- Approach: The commonest approach used is the posterior approach though the anterolateral approach is also a popular approach. The authors' preference is the posterior incision through the extensile posterolateral approach so as to gain exposure of almost the entire humeral shaft **(Fig. 9.9)**.
- Incision: It is a long posterior midline incision extending from the level of the deltoid insertion to the top of the olecranon fossa.
- After initial subcutaneous dissection, the deep fascia is incised in the same line. In case a triceps splitting approach is utilised, the triceps is split in the middle at the lower third of the humerus. Proximally the interval between the long and the lateral head

is identified and the underlying medial head is split to expose the radial nerve in the spiral groove. In case of the extensile posterolateral approach, the entire triceps is retracted medially to expose the lateral intermuscular septum. The lower lateral cutaneous nerve of the arm is identified about 8-10 cm proximal to the lateral epicondyle piercing the lateral intermuscular septum. This is then traced distally in the anterior compartment and it is then seen with the radial nerve which also pierces the septum at around the same level. The radial nerve is then isolated and tagged with infant feeding tube and the entire triceps can be then retracted sub-periosteally on the medial side. The advantage of this approach is the excellent visualisation of almost the entire distal 4/5th of the humerus without any danger to the radial nerve.

- Reduction is obtained using bone-holding and reduction clamps and fixation is performed using 7-8 hole 4.5 mm Dynamic compression plate (DCP) or a limited contact DCP (LCDCP), fixed with minimum of 3 screws (with 6 cortices) proximally and distally.

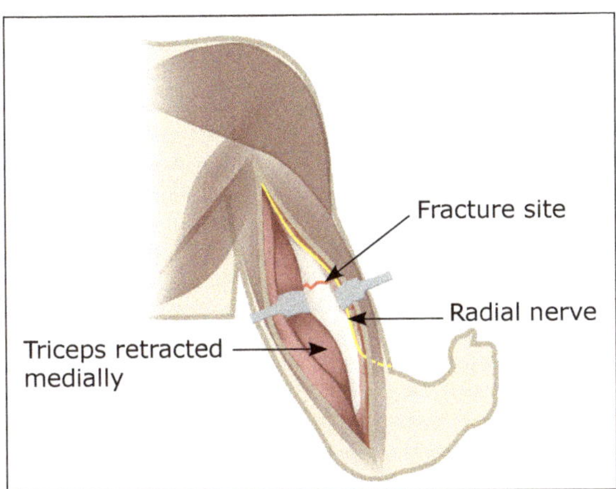

Fig. 9.9: *Schematic representation of the extensile posterolateral approach. As can be seen in the diagram, the radial nerve is isolated from the lateral intermuscular septum just where it pierces the septum and the entire triceps is retracted medially. This gives a very wide exposure of almost the entire lower 4/5th of the humerus.*

- Care should be taken that the radial nerve is away from the plate as well as the drill bit while drilling and usage of a drill sleeve is of utmost importance.
- Wound is closed in multiple layers in the usual manner.
- Usually no immobilisation is required and only an arm pouch makes the child comfortable. Mobilisation can be started after around 3 weeks or so depending on the reduction and the stability of fixation.

Complications

1) Radial nerve palsy:

Radial nerve palsy is the commonest complication of humeral shaft fractures which can be primary or secondary. Primary radial nerve palsy is the one which occurs at the time of injury and is almost always a neuropraxia which is reversible except in open injuries where transections of nerves can occur. The treatment of primary radial nerve palsy is usually conservative and full recovery can be expected in about 3-8 months. Radial nerve palsy can occur rarely as a delayed occurrence where the fracture callus can grow around the nerve and then have a small radiolucency on the X-ray where the radial nerve pierces. This so-called *"Matev's sign"* is pathognomonic and requires surgical exploration and release of the nerve from the callus. Secondary radial nerve palsy occurs following either conservative or operative treatment of humeral shaft fractures and the treatment is controversial. In radial nerve palsies occurring following manipulation and conservative management (the Holstein-Lewis fracture), the treatment is usually conservative in the form of undercorrection and re-casting.

For unacceptable deformities, open reduction can be performed. Secondary palsies following operative fixation may be neuropraxia due to excessive pull or traction or can be inadvertent transections during surgery. The treatment of this has to be individualised for every case.

2) Malunion:

Symptomatic malunion is extremely rare for humeral shaft fractures in paediatric age group. This occurs more commonly in adolescents where varus deformity is not well tolerated. The treatment depends on the degree of deformity and the growth remaining in the child.

3) Compartment syndrome:

Extremely rare complication

4) Vascular injury:

Extremely rare, can be seen in open fractures following road traffic accidents or gun-shot injuries.

Flowchart 9.1

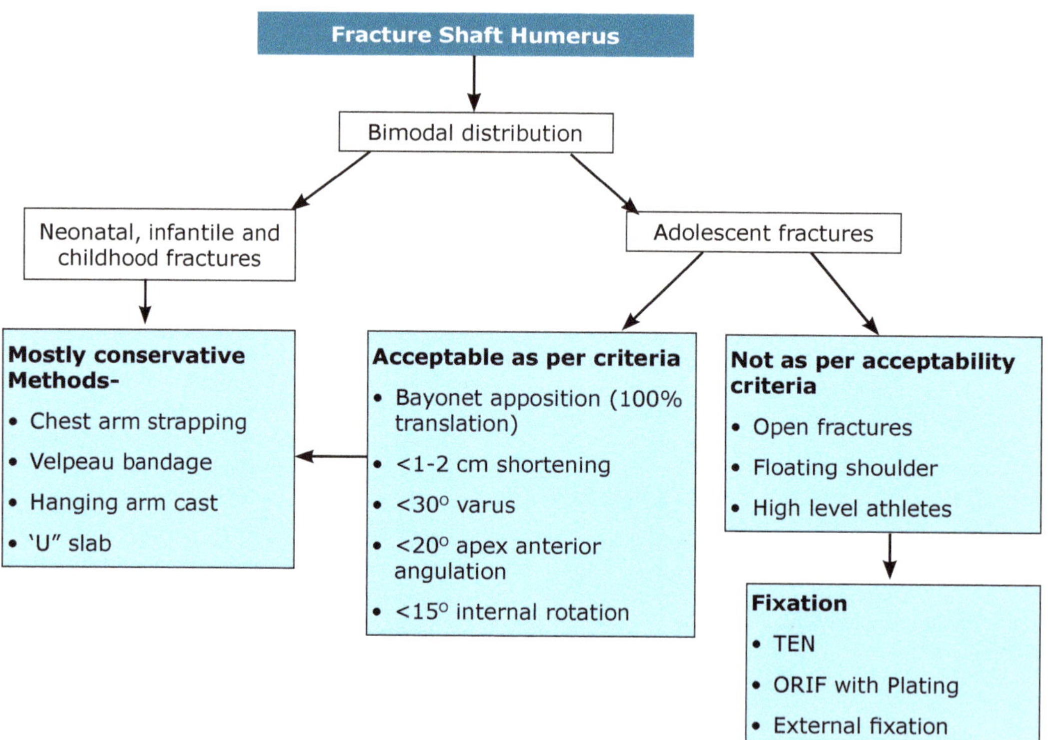

10 Supracondylar Humerus Fractures in Children

Introduction

- Supracondylar humerus fractures are some of the most common injuries around the elbow seen in children, and they account for 7-9% of all the fractures in children and about 86% of all fractures around the elbow.
- The most common age at which the fracture occurs is between 3-10 years of age. The fracture is more common on the left or the non-dominant side.
- Associated neurovascular complications range from 5-19% and open fractures constitute less than 1% of all fractures.
- They are the most common paediatric fractures requiring emergent surgical intervention.

Anatomy

The distal humerus is considered to be made up of two columns. The lateral column is made up of the lateral epicondyle and the lateral supracondylar ridge and the medial column is made up of the trochlea and the medial supracondylar ridge. The medial and lateral columns are connected by a thin wafer of bone between the olecranon fossa posteriorly and the coronoid fossa anteriorly **(Fig. 10.1)**.

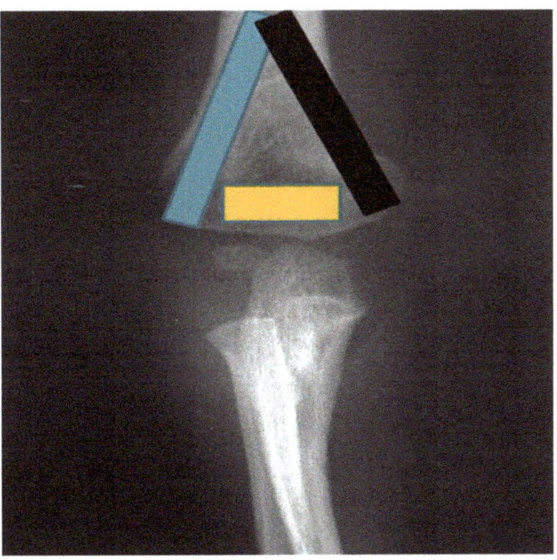

Fig. 10.1: *AP X-ray of the distal humerus depicting the two pillars. The lateral pillar (blue rectangle) starts from the lateral epicondyle and extends along the lateral supracondylar ridge till the humeral diaphysis. The medial pillar (black rectangle) starts from the medial epicondyle, extends along the sharp medial supracondylar ridge and reaches the shaft of the humerus. The two pillars are connected to each other distally with a thin wafer of bone between the coronoid and olecranon fossa (orange rectangle).*

Mechanism of Injury

Two common mechanisms:

When the elbow hyperextends forcibly in a fall on out stretched hand, the olecranon forcefully pushes into the olecranon fossa and acts as a fulcrum causing a fracture through the weakest region of the bone. Similarly, with forced elbow flexion the coronoid process is driven into the coronoid fossa creating a fracture at the level of the olecranon fossa.

Classification

Fractures of the supracondylar humerus are broadly classified into extension and flexion type **(Fig. 10.2)**.

Of the two, extension type supracondylar humerus fracture is more common accounting for 95-98% of all supracondylar humerus fractures leaving the flexion type as a rare injury amounting to only 2-5% of the supracondylar humerus fractures.

With extension type injuries, the distal fragment can be displaced either posteromedially (75%) or posterolaterally (25%).

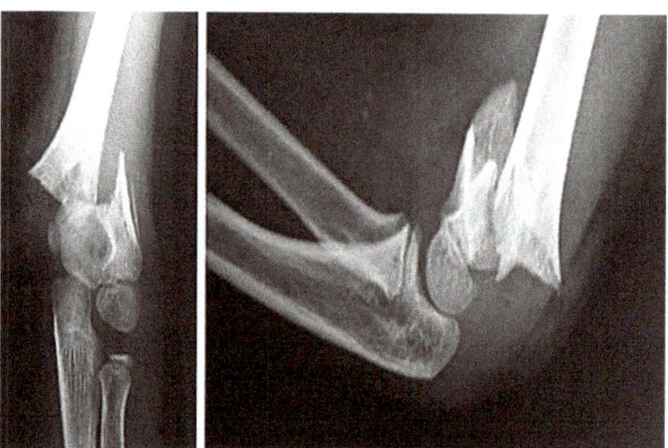

Fig. 10.2: *AP and lateral X-rays of the elbow showing a displaced flexion type of supracondylar humerus fracture. Note the posteromedial spike of the proximal fragment.*

Extension type supracondylar fractures are further classified by the Modified Gartland's classification **(Fig. 10.3)** into:

Type I includes undisplaced or minimally displaced fractures

Type II includes fractures with angulation with one cortex intact (posterior)

Type III includes completely displaced fractures

Type IV includes fractures which are highly unstable and distal fragment displaces into flexion and extension both **(Fig. 10.4)**.

The type III and IV fractures are paediatric orthopaedic emergencies and need urgent reduction and fixation in most cases.

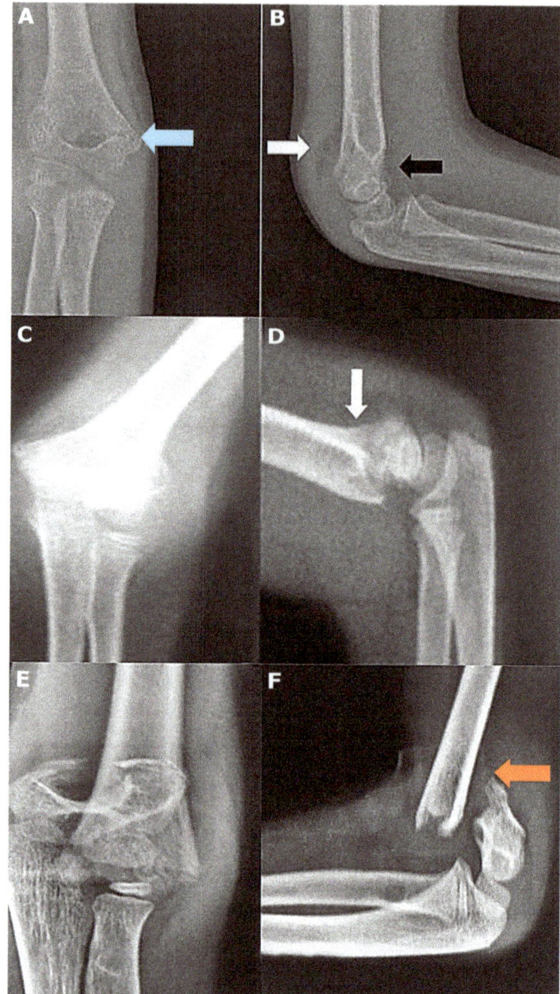

Fig. 10.3: *Figure showing type I (A,B), II (C,D), and III (E,F) Gartland fractures. Type I fractures show a faint (complete or incomplete) fracture line on the AP view (blue arrow) and positive posterior (white arrow) and anterior (black arrow) fat pad sign. Type II fracture has an intact posterior corical hinge (small white arrow). Type III fractures have complete discontinuity between the proximal and distal fragments (orange arrow).*

Bahk et al classification: Pattern based classification **(Fig. 10.5)**:

A) Sagittal fracture patterns:

1) Typical transverse fracture with <10^{0} of coronal obliquity

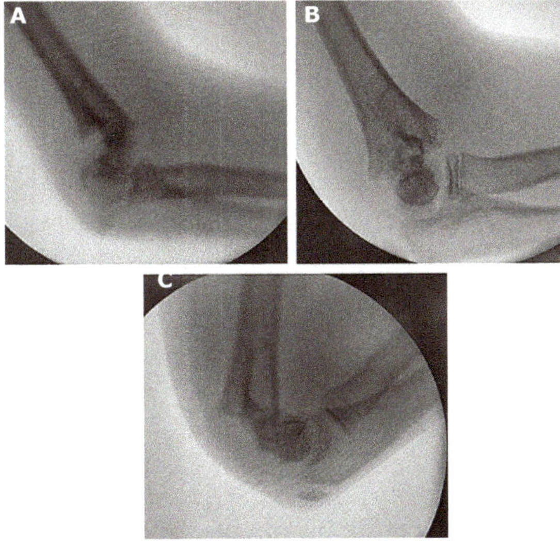

***Fig. 10.4**: Intra-operative C-arm images of a type IV fracture (described by Leitch et al) showing instability in extension (A), rotation (B) and flexion (C).*

2) Lateral oblique fracture pattern with more than 10° of coronal plane obliquity with the lateral fracture line exiting proximally
3) Medial oblique fracture pattern with more than 10° of coronal plane obliquity and with medial fracture line exiting medially
4) High supracondylar fractures: Fractures passing above the olecranon fossa but within the distal humeral metaphysis.

B) Coronal fracture patterns:

1) Low fracture patterns with the fracture plane directed less than 20°.
2) High fracture patterns with fracture plane directed more than 20°.

Clinical Features

- Children usually present to the emergency room with history of fall and a tense, swollen elbow with decreased movements of the elbow. However, the presentation may not always be dramatic making an accurate diagnosis difficult at times.

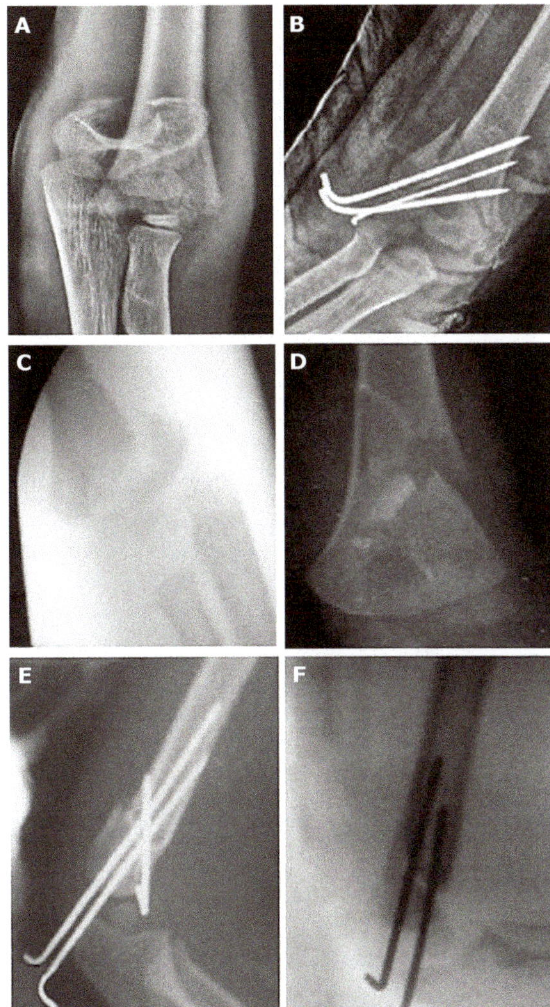

***Fig. 10.5**: X-rays showing fracture patterns according to Bahk classification. (A) Typical transverse fracture with less than 10° obliquity, (B) Lateral oblique fracture, (C) Medial oblique fracture, (D) High supracondylar fractures. (E) High sagittal fractures, (F) Low sagittal fractures.*

- Clinical examination reveals a swollen painful elbow and tenderness over the humeral condyles and supracondylar ridges.
- 'S' Shaped deformity of the elbow is sometimes evident in severely displaced

fractures and an anterior puckering may also be seen if the proximal fragment has impaled the brachialis and the anterior fascia of the elbow. Significant ecchymosis may be seen over the anterior aspect of the elbow in grossly displaced fractures **(Fig. 10.6)**.

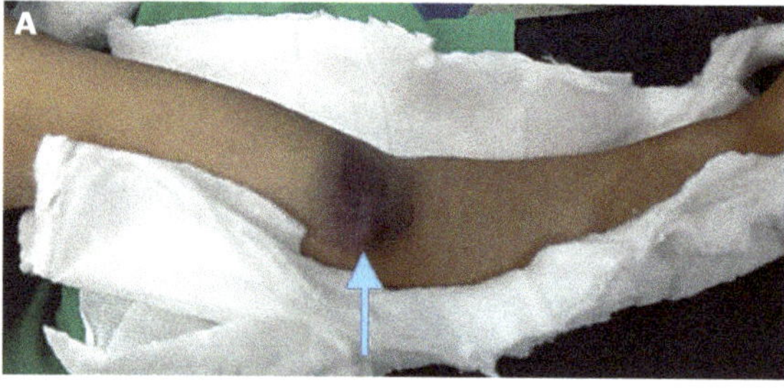

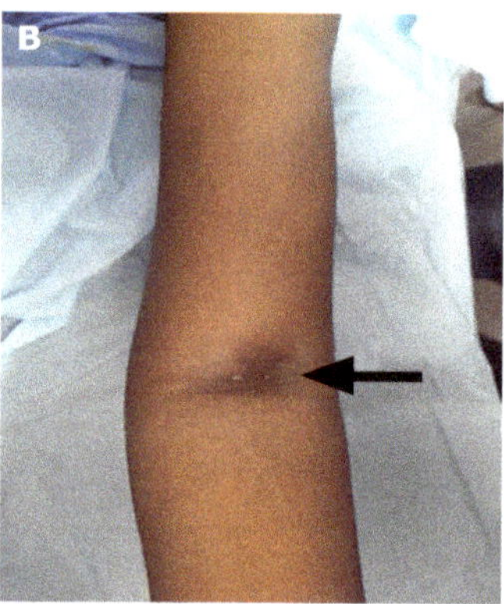

Fig. 10.6*: Clinical photo of the elbow of a child with a displaced supracondylar humerus fracture showing the typical signs of (A) severe bruising, swelling and contusion along the anterior and medial aspect of the elbow (blue arrow) and (B) Pucker sign (Black arrow)*

- Thorough neurological and vascular examination is mandatory due to association with neurovascular injuries. Sensory examination of the autonomous zones of the median, radial and ulnar nerves should be done. Motor examination including active wrist, finger and thumb extension (radial nerve) flexion of the thumb and index finger distal interphalangeal joint (median nerve) and examination of interossei (ulnar nerve) should be done.
- Vascular examination includes detail examination of the radial pulse, brisk capillary refill as well as the warmth and colour of the hand. Hand held Doppler examination is useful in the emergency setting and helps especially in grossly swollen hands. Pulse oximetry is also important and a good bounding waveform is a sign of good vascularity.
- Based on the vascular status, three patterns are usually present- warm with a good palpable pulse, warm and pink with absent pulse and good capillary refill and a white, pale cold hand with absent radial pulse and poor capillary refill.
- Carefully documented pre-manipulation exam findings and post manipulation neurovascular deficits can alter decision making.
- Compartment syndrome is a dreaded complication which can occur both before and after fixation. The signs and symptoms of CS need to be carefully looked at. The commonly quoted 5'P's (Pain, Paresthesia, Paresis, Pulselessness and Pallor) may not be very apparent in children and are replaced by the 3'A's which are Anxiety, Agitation and increased Analgesic requirement. A very high index of suspicion is required to diagnose and treat CS.
- Lastly the entire upper extremity should be thoroughly examined for any associated injuries.

Imaging

- Plain X-rays: Standard Anteroposterior and lateral radiographs are enough for diagnosis. They are assessed for evidence of fracture, degree of displacement; rotation and translation, degree of comminution of the fracture and evidence of intra- articular extension.

- In type I or occult fractures, when the fracture line is not clearly visible, the presence of the posterior fat pad sign is highly suggestive and should be taken as a surrogate sign of a fracture.
- Anterior humeral line should intersect the middle third of the capitellum. In cases of type II fractures, the line passes through the anterior third or in front of the capitellum.
- The Baumann's angle on the AP view is very important to confirm the reduction and prevent any varus. On the AP radiograph of the elbow the Baumann's angle formed by the line along the long axis of the humerus and the physeal line of the lateral condyle is useful to assess a coronal plane deformity.

Treatment

- Once the fracture has been diagnosed, treatment in the emergency room consists of splinting the fracture in a long arm posterior slab with the elbow in 20-40^{0} of flexion. It is advisable to avoid excess flexion or tight bandaging to prevent the development of vascular compromise.
- The distal circulation should always be checked before and after application of the splint.

Type I fractures

- These fractures are inherently stable due to intact periosteum and can usually be successfully managed conservatively.
- The child is given a long arm posterior splint for 5-10 days till the initial swelling subsides following which a check X-ray is taken to confirm that there is no further displacement of the fracture. Once it is confirmed that the fracture is stable, a long arm cast is given for two more weeks.

Type II fractures

In these fractures the intact posterior periosteal sleeve acts as a hinge and aids in reduction of the fracture. After reduction is achieved, the general consensus is to fix the fractures with K-wires inserted percutaneously followed by immobilisation in a long arm posterior slab in 30-60^{0} of elbow flexion for 3-4 weeks. At the 3-4 week follow up, radiographs are repeated, and the wires are removed in the office without any anaesthesia, immobilisation is discontinued, and range of motion exercises are encouraged.

Type III / Type IV fractures

These fractures are inherently unstable as the periosteum around the fracture is torn and there is no cortical contact between the two fracture fragments. These fractures are associated with significant soft tissue or neurovascular injuries.

Treatment options include open or closed reduction and fixation with K-wires.

Operative technique:

- Anaesthesia:

  The preferred method of anaesthesia is general anaesthesia especially in type III and IV fractures when full muscle relaxation is needed. Brachial plexus blocks- controversial- best avoided due to chance of masking the pain of compartment syndrome.

- Position **(Figs. 10.7)**:

  Supine with arm on arm-board draped free. The child is to be brought as near the edge of the bed as possible for better C-arm viewing. The C-arm is positioned in the axilla of the patient so that the lateral pinning is easier. There are a lot of different views about the ideal positioning of the child in a supracondylar pinning. Various authors have described different positions like prone, lateral, elbow

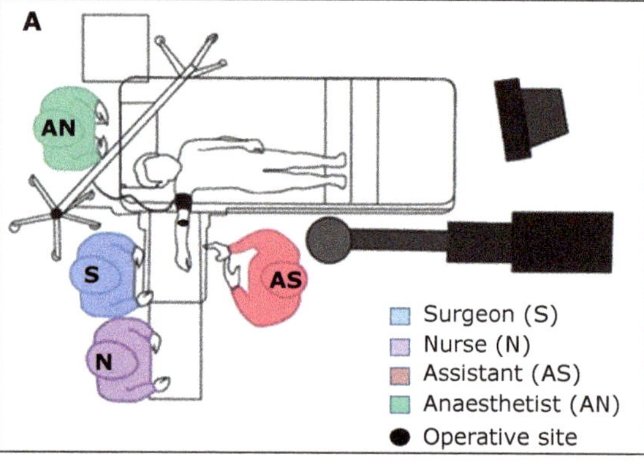

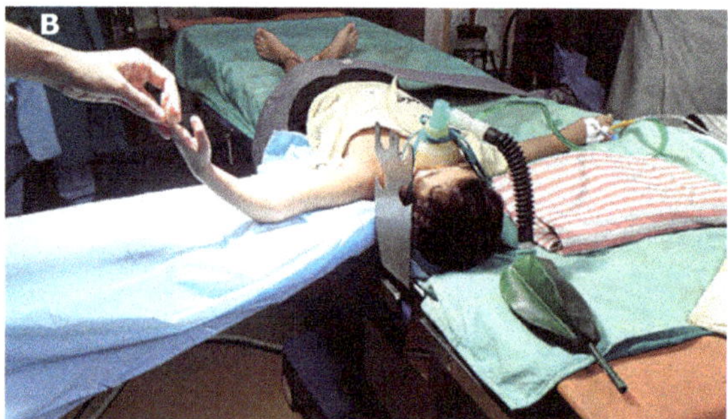

Fig. 10.7*: Positioning of the patient for fixation of a supracondylar humerus fracture. Note the child being placed right at the edge of the bed for maximal ease of visualisation under C-arm.*

strapped to a wooden plank, etc. There is also a controversy regarding whether the C-arm is to be swung for the lateral view or the arm can be rotated. The author's preferred method is rotating the elbow externally with full elbow flexion so as to lock the fragments and getting a lateral view.

- Manoeuvre of closed reduction includes the assistant holding the proximal fragment to apply counter traction while the surgeon applies axial traction to the distal fragment with the elbow extended. Once length is gained the varus/valgus alignment is corrected. Then the surgeon places the thumb of his dominant hand on the olecranon process to push the olecranon process anteriorly and the fore fingers on the anterior aspect of the proximal fragment to pull the fragment posteriorly **(Fig. 10.8).**

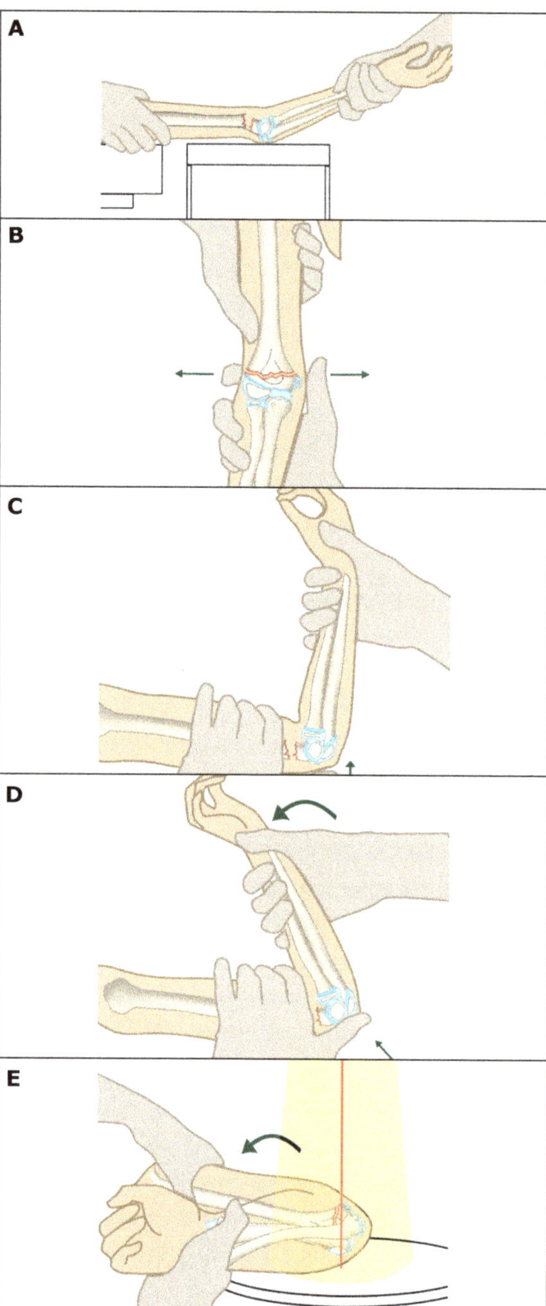

Fig. 10.8A-E*: Reduction of a supracondylar humerus fracture (A): Sustained traction in extension. (B): Correction of deformity in AP plane- varus and valgus. (C, D): Correction of extension by pressure on olecranon/ distal humerus and hyperflexing the elbow. (E): Obtaining a true lateral view by holding the proximal segment while externally rotating the limb, thus preventing mal-rotation.*

- Concurrently the non- dominant hand flexes the elbow and the forearm is either pronated or supinated depending upon the fracture displacement.

Once accurate reduction is obtained, it is confirmed under C-arm and pins are inserted percutaneously in one of the following configurations **(Fig. 10.9)**.

- two lateral pins
- two crossed pins
- three lateral pins
- two lateral pins and one medial pin

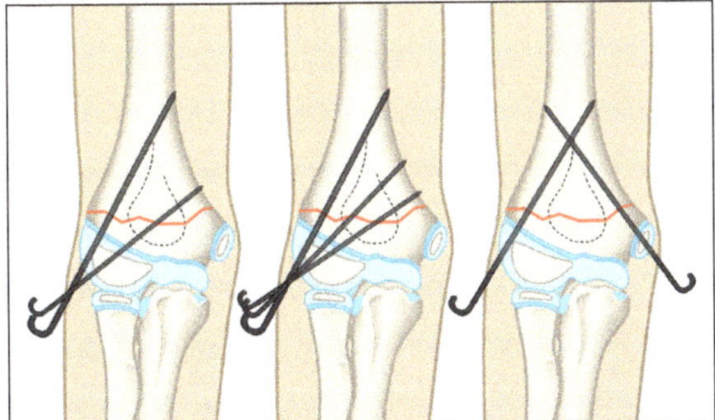

Fig. 10.9*: Schematic representation of different patterns of K-wire fixation which include- 2 lateral divergent, 3 lateral divergent and cross K-wire fixation.*

- 1st Pin is usually a lateral pin passing through the olecranon fossa thus getting a quadri-cortical hold and usually holding the medial pillar.
- The 2nd lateral pin is usually a parallel or divergent wire at a distance of around 8 mm from the first wire **(Fig. 10.10)**.
- If need be, a third wire can be put on the lateral side or an additional wire can be placed on the medial side.
- *Indications for Medial pinning:*
- Medial oblique fracture pattern
- Medial comminution
- Very high supracondylars (supra-supracondylars)

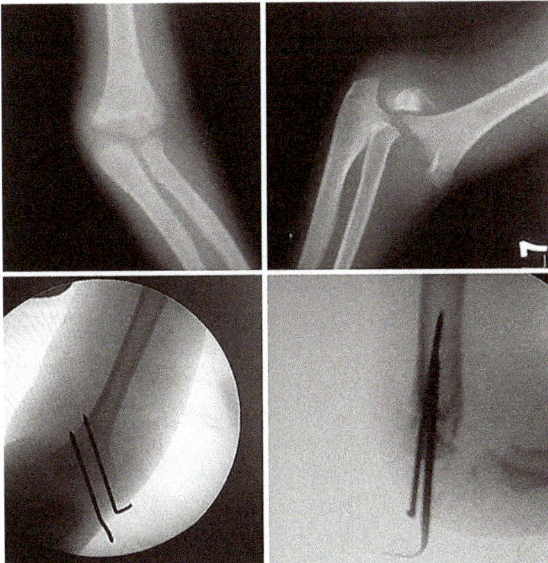

Fig. 10.10*: Standard fixation of a displaced supracondylar humerus fracture with 2 parallel lateral K-wires. Note the spacing between the two wires which is about 8-10 mm.*

- Very low supracondylars (transphyseals)
- *Steps to protect the ulnar nerve during medial pinning* **(Fig. 10.11)**:
- Pass the medial wire with the elbow in slight extension so that the ulnar nerve is displaced posteriorly.
- A small incision is usually made along the medial aspect of the elbow (around 0.5 cm in length) over the medial epicondyle, the bony prominence palpated and then the K-wire is passed.
- USG guidance can be used.
- Nerve stimulator guidance.
- Reduction and fixation is confirmed on AP and lateral views on C-arm and on dynamic views.

Fixation in specific fracture patterns:

- Unstable fracture pattern/ Type IV fractures: This type of fracture pattern is very unstable in all directions and

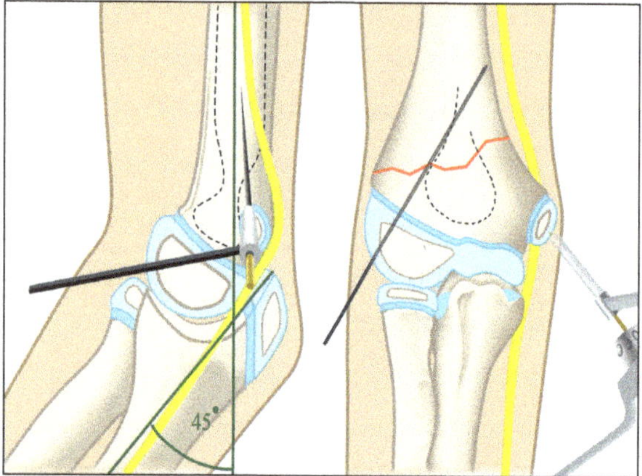

***Fig. 10.11**: Various methods to be undertaken while passing a medial wire and prevent injury to the ulnar nerve.*

may not remain stable even with 2 well-directed K-wires. In this case, a third wire can be added in a divergent manner so as to achieve additional stability **(Fig. 10.12)**.

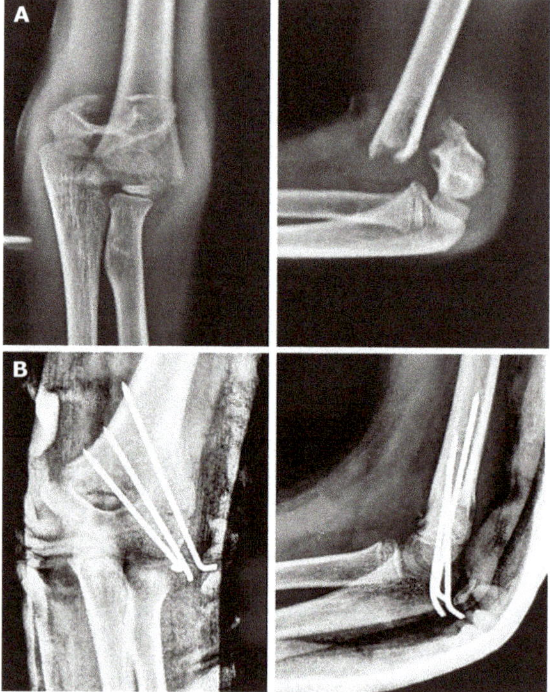

***Fig. 10.12**: (A) AP and lateral X-ray of a grossly displaced unstable supracondylar humerus fracture (B) Fixation using 3 lateral divergent K-wires with adequate spacing between the wires.*

- *Lateral oblique fracture pattern* **(Fig. 10.13):** In this case, the fracture line passes from proximal lateral to distal medial. It is important to prevent sliding and translation and achieve good reduction and fixation using 2 or 3 divergent wires from the lateral aspect which are perpendicular to the fracture site. Hence, it is not possible to pass a wire from the medial side as it will pass parallel to the fracture site and will not have any purchase.

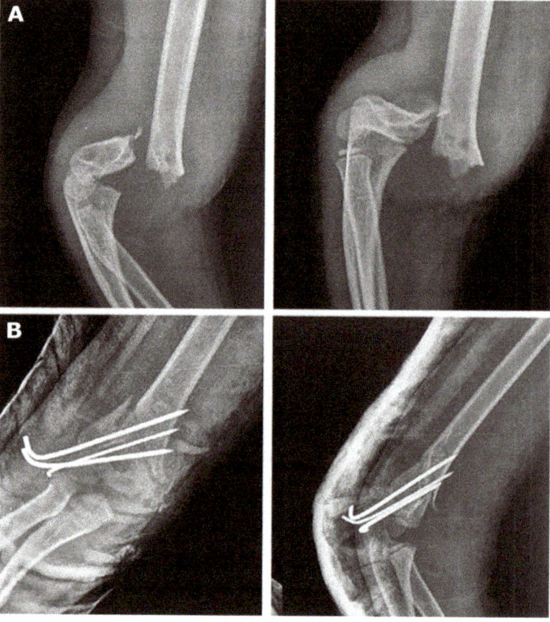

***Fig. 10.13**: AP and lateral X-ray of a displaced lateral oblique supracondylar humerus fracture (B) Fixation with lateral divergent wires which are perpendicular to the fracture site.*

- *Medial oblique fractures* **(Fig. 10.14)**: These fractures have their fracture line passing from proximal medial to distal lateral. Hence, it is not possible to pass 2 or sometimes even 1 wire from the lateral side as the wire would pass parallel to the fracture site. In this case, it may be required to pass 1 or 2 wires from the medial side keeping the ulnar nerve safe.

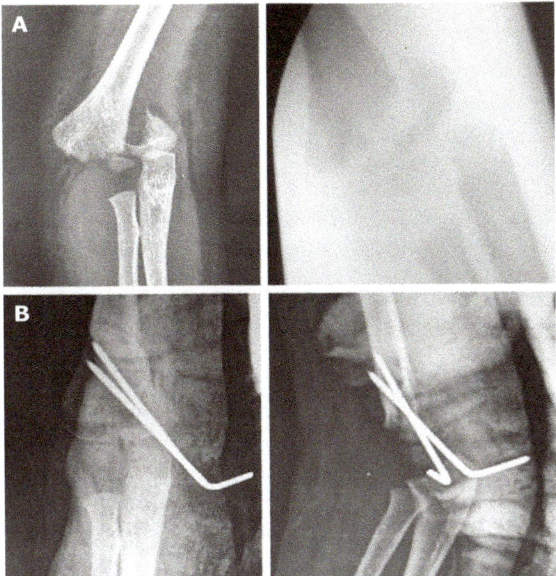

***Fig. 10.14**: (A) AP and lateral X-ray of a medial oblique supracondylar humerus fracture which had a big medial condylar piece extending laterally (B) Fixation with 2 medial K-wires.*

- *High supracondylar fractures (Supra-Supracondylars, or Meta-Diaphyseal fractures)* **(Fig. 10.15)**: This is another unique fracture pattern. In this case, the fracture line is above the level of the olecranon fossa at the meta-diaphyseal junction. Here it is not possible to pass two wires from either lateral side and it is not possible to have bi-cortical purchase of the wires as with the angle of the wire, it has a tendency to become intra-medullary. Hence in this case, intramedullary fixation using K-wires is an established method of treatment.
- The pins are usually kept outside the skin and bent at right angle so as to not entangle in the dressing and slab. The author's preference is to apply an above elbow slab, while some clinicians prefer to apply an above elbow cast which is then bi-valved to allow for post operative swelling.
- **Open reduction:**
- The indications for open reduction are:

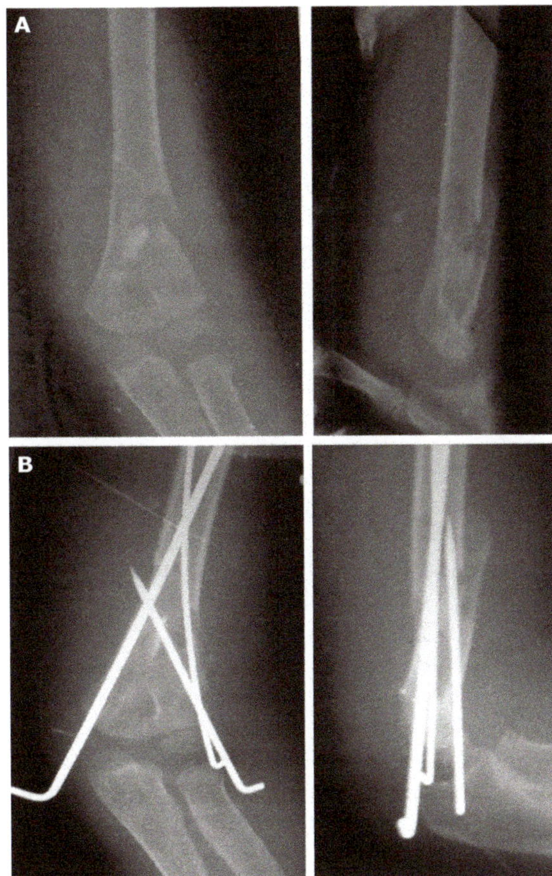

***Fig. 10.15**: (A) AP and lateral X-ray of a high supracondylar (supra-supracondylar) fracture (B) Fixation with intra-medullary K-wires.*

- Irreducible fracture after 3 attempts at closed reduction
- Open fractures
- Fractures associated with clear signs of vascular insult- Pulselessness with poor capillary refill (the so-called "white" pulseless hand)
- Pink pulseless hand with median or anterior interosseous injury (relative indication as such a combination is usually associated with a vascular entrapment and hence there should be a very low threshold for open reduction)
- Type IV supracondylar fractures which are very unstable

- **Technique of open reduction:**

- There are 4 basic approaches to open reduction- Anterior (Anteromedial or anterolateral), lateral, medial or posterior. The anterior approach is the commonest approach which is used and anteromedial or anterolateral is decided on whether the displacement is medial or lateral and the location of the proximal spike. The Anterior approach is also preferable in case of a suspected vascular injury with the help of a vascular surgeon, which gives easy and full access to the vasculature. The posterior approach is the least preferred, primarily because the displacement and the proximal spike is anterior and access to the proximal spike is very difficult in the posterior approach. Also, C-arm positioning as well as poor vascular access preclude the success of the posterior approach in paediatric supracondylar humerus fractures (unlike in adults). It has also been shown in various studies as well as meta-analysis that the chance of restricted range of motion is maximum in posterior approach as compared to other approaches.

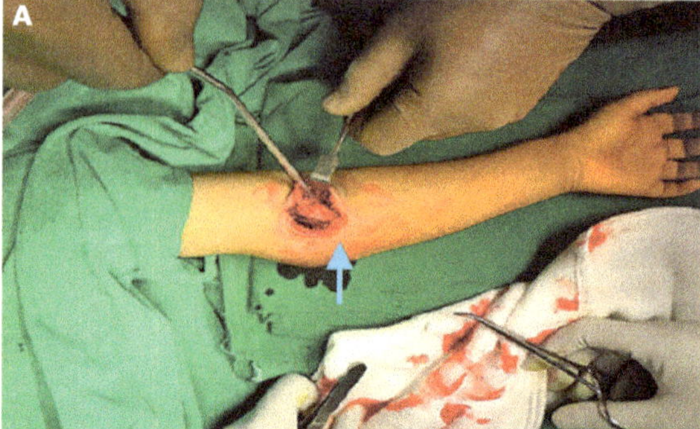

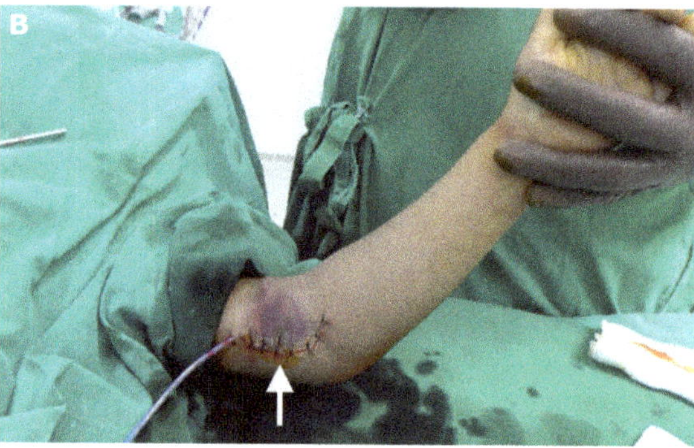

***Fig. 10.16**: (A) Clinical photos of anterior open reduction with the operative wound showing the proximal bony spike (blue arrow) in the subcutaneous plane of the wound and (B) the closure performed (white arrow).*

- **Anterior open reduction (Fig. 10.16):** The incision is a gentle curvilinear incision (C or S shaped) centred on the elbow crease. Usually in irreducible supracondylar humerus fractures, the proximal spike is subcutaneous and easily palpable. The neurovascular bundle (brachial artery and median nerve) is isolated and retracted and reduction is usually obtained after clearing off the soft tissue and by gentle digital pressure. Fixation is performed in the usual manner and wound is closed in single layer under negative suction drain.

Post-operative care:

- The child is usually kept admitted overnight to look for post-operative swelling, neurodeficit and compartment syndrome.
- The above elbow slab/cast is continued for a period of three to four weeks.
- X-rays are performed on the day of surgery post-operatively and at three weeks.
- The K-wires are pulled out in the clinic itself at around three to four weeks depending on the amount of healing seen on the X-ray.
- The child is allowed full movements after K-wire removal.
- Usually No physiotherapy is needed in kids with supracondylar humerus fractures and they usually get back their functional range in about three weeks and full range in about three to six months.

Complications

Early complications include neurovascular injury and compartment syndrome as discussed before. Delayed complications include malunion, elbow stiffness and myositis ossificans.

Management of early complications:

1) Pink Pulseless supracondylar humerus fracture:

   In some severely displaced fractures, the child presents with no palpable radial pulse but good capillary refill distally. This usually represents a spasm of the brachial artery distal to the fracture site and not an arterial injury. In a fracture supracondylar humerus with a pink pulseless hand, it is imperative to perform an urgent reduction and fixation of the fracture in order to relieve the pressure on the vasculature. In most cases, no other treatment is required and the vascularity remains intact. In case there is an inadequate reduction suggestive of interposition, or there is an anterior fracture gap seen on the C-arm or the hand turns white or avascular after reduction, then it is imperative to involve a vascular surgeon and explore the artery.

2) Supracondylar humerus fracture with vascular injury:

   This is an absolute emergency and this is diagnosed by the fact that along with pulselessness, there are other signs of avascularity like cold white limb or poor capillary refill. This requires exploration through the anterior approach with the help of a vascular surgeon and requires vascular repair/grafting. It is usually imperative to perform a wide fasciotomy after the procedure to prevent compartment syndrome which can develop after the vascular repair due to revascularisation injury. The details of the diagnosis and management of compartment syndrome are given in the chapter on Compartment syndrome.

3) Supracondylar humerus fracture with nerve injuries:

   The commonest nerve injuries in supracondylar humerus fractures are anterior interosseous nerve, radial nerve, median nerve and finally ulnar nerve injury (which is most commonly seen in flexion type supracondylar fractures). Most of the times the injuries are neuropraxia and usually recover in about 6 weeks to 3 months. Median nerve injury when it occurs in a pink pulseless supracondylar fracture needs to be looked at very carefully as it is very commonly associated with vascular injuries. When median nerve injury occurs with pulseless hand, there should be a very low threshold to open the fracture and explore the vasculature if required.

- Malunion leading to cubitus varus is one of the most common complications of supracondylar humerus fractures that are not treated appropriately. Cubitus varus is a painless deformity not affecting elbow range of motion. Cubitus varus requires a corrective osteotomy and fixation. A detailed discussion of this topic is beyond the scope of this book.

Flowchart 10.1

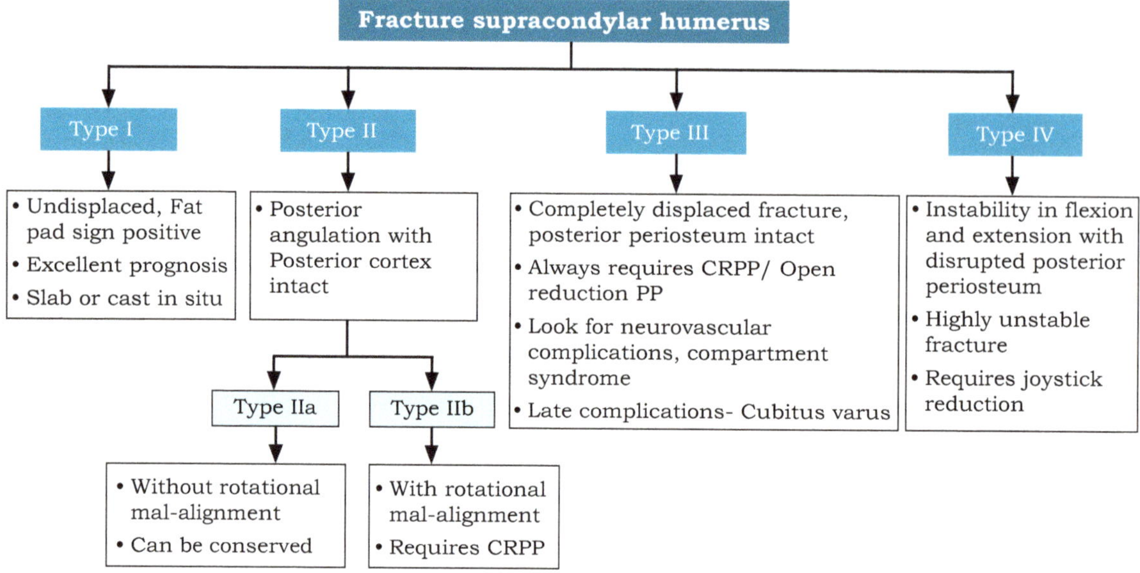

Flowchart 10.2

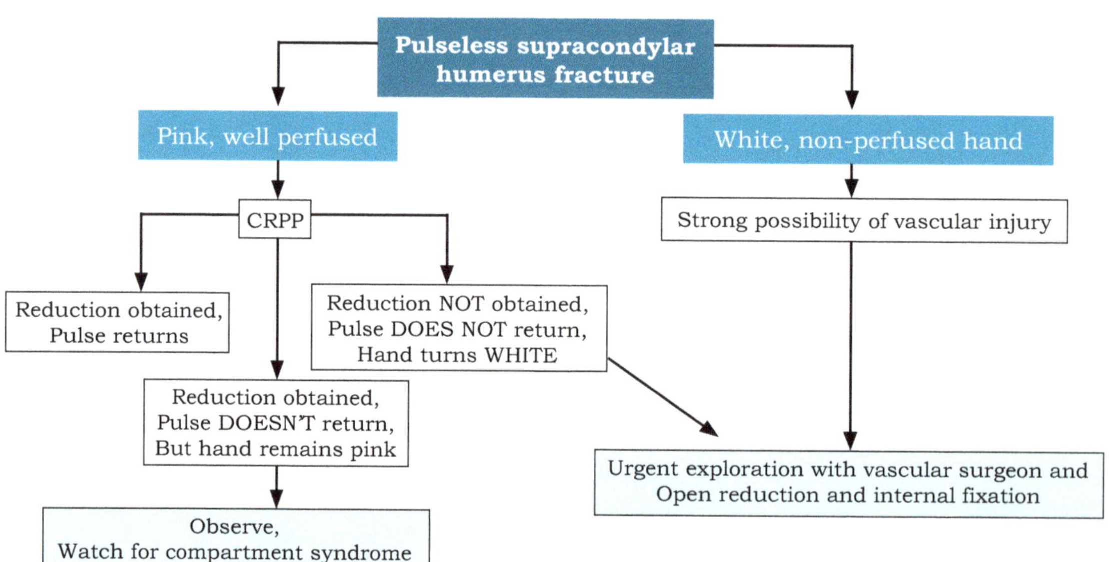

11 Lateral Condyle Humerus Fractures in Children

Introduction

Fracture of lateral condyle of humerus is one of the commonest fractures around the elbow in children constituting around 12-15% of all fractures around the elbow and one of the commonest fractures requiring surgical intervention. Conventionally, this is one of the "fractures of necessity" as surgical intervention is required in most of the cases and there are significant chances of complications if it is not done. There is also significant controversy as regards the diagnosis, classification as well as optimal management of this injury.

Relevant anatomy

Important muscles attached: The common extensor muscle group is attached to the lateral condyle and it is the main deforming force in lateral condyle fractures. The undisplaced lateral condyle humerus fracture can become displaced due to the constant overactivity of the common extensor group of muscles **(Fig. 11.1)**.

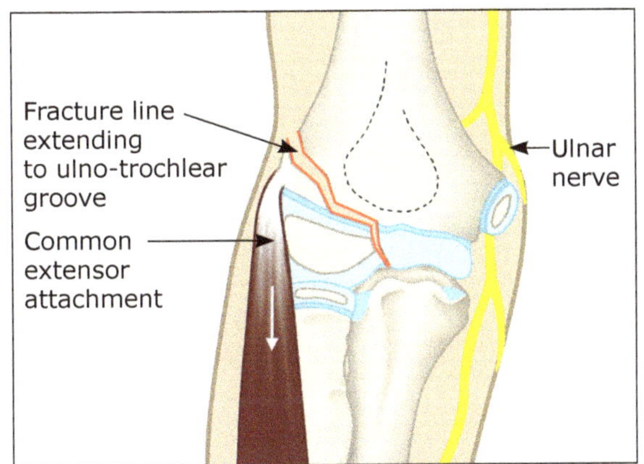

Fig. 11.1*: Anatomy of the lateral condyle showing attachment of the common extensors which results in displacement of the fracture.*

Classification

One of the most important aspects of lateral condyle fractures in children which affects management is its classification. There are a number of classifications of lateral condyle fractures and we are enumerating only the most important of them. The classifications can be grouped into:

1) Depending on the exit of the fracture line: Mirsky classification
2) Depending on the exit of the fracture line as well as its stability: Milch classification
3) Depending on the displacement: Jakob classification and the Song classification.

1) *Depending on the exit of the fracture line:* Mirsky's classification:

A) Exiting through or lateral to the trochlear groove
B) Exiting just medial to the trochlea
C) Exiting to the medial column

2) *Depending on the exit of the fracture and its stability*: The Milch classification:

A) Fracture exiting lateral to the trochlear groove- Stable injury (Salter-Harris type 4 injury)
B) Fracture exiting medial to the trochlear groove- Unstable injury (Salter-Harris type 2 injury)

3) *Depending on the displacement:*

A) Jakob's classification:

Grade I: Undisplaced fracture (*Crack)*

Grade II: Minimally displaced fracture (*Split)*

Grade III: Displaced and rotated fracture (*Tilt)*

B) Song's classification: By far the most comprehensive classification is the Song classification, which was described by Dr. Song from Korea and is the classification which guides current treatment **(Fig. 11.2)**.

Diagnosis

Clinical

The usual history is of fall on outstretched hand. The commonest age group is less than 6 years. Clinical examination shows tenderness on the lateral aspect of the elbow with restricted elbow flexion-extension.

X-ray

Plain X-ray examination of the elbow is the most important diagnostic step for lateral condyle humerus fractures. Along with simple AP and lateral views, an Internal rotation oblique AP view is of utmost importance in exact delineation of the displacement and should be an essential addition to all suspected lateral condyle humerus fractures **(Fig. 11.3)**.

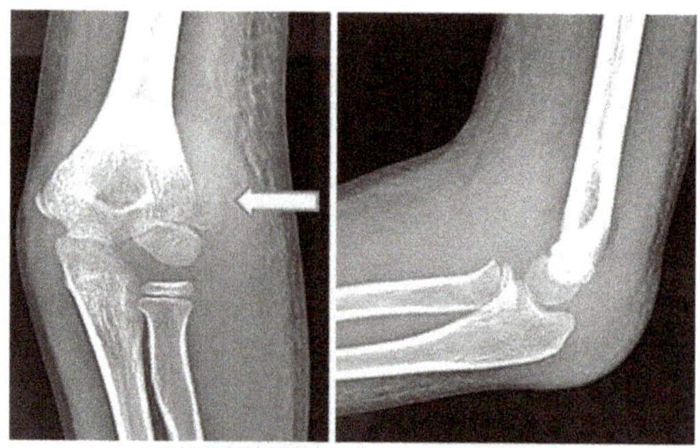

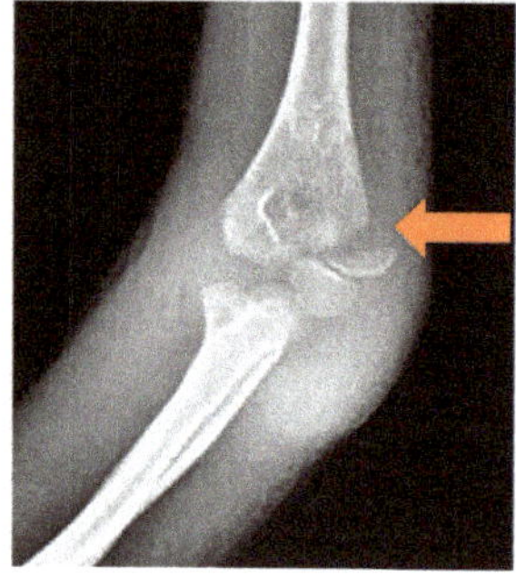

Fig. 11.3*: AP, Lateral and Internal rotation oblique view of a child's left elbow. White arrow shows the lateral condyle fracture which is not well visualized while the orange arrow shows the fracture which is well visualized and the displacement seen better.*

Arthrogram

Some clinicians have described the use of arthrogram as a diagnostic modality in order to decide on the need for fixation as well as whether open reduction is needed or closed reduction and fixation will suffice.

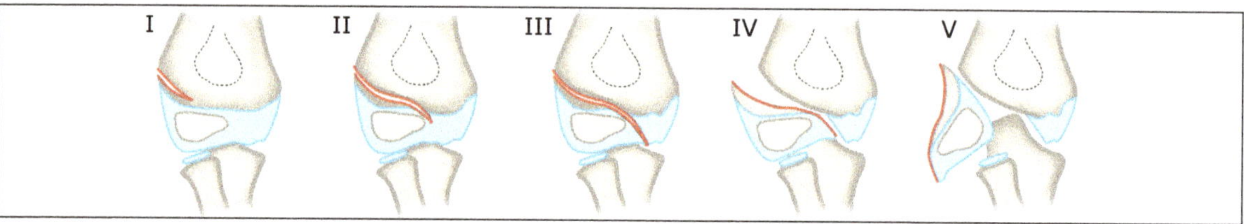

Fig. 11.2*: Lateral condyle fractures classified by the Song's classification into 5 types:*

I- Fracture line limited to metaphysis, Stable.

II- Fracture line extending to the physis, with gap only laterally. Indefinable stability.

III- Gap as wide laterally as medially. Unstable fracture.

IV- Displaced fracture but without rotation of the fragment. Unstable fracture.

V- Displaced and rotated fracture. Unstable fracture.

MRI

MRI is an excellent modality to exactly delineate the intra-articular extent of the fracture line so as to decide whether the present fracture is Song type II or III. However the need for general anaesthesia for small kids precludes the routine use of MRI in clinical practice.

Treatment

Conservative

- Above elbow plaster for 4-6 weeks- only if the displacement is below 2mm on all views including the internal rotation view and the fracture is not extending intra-articular.
- Closed watch is to be kept for secondary displacement with weekly X-rays of all three views.
- A low threshold is necessary for fixation of such fractures.

Operative treatment

A) **Arthrogram assisted closed reduction and K-wire fixation:**

This method is fast approaching to be the treatment of choice for Song II, III and sometime IV fractures.

However it is quite technically demanding and the surgeon should be well versed with the technique and the interpretation of the arthrogram.

Position: Supine with arm on the arm-board, with tourniquet applied to the upper arm.

- After anaesthesia, parts are prepared, painted and draped and tourniquet is elevated.
- Under C-arm control, a 22 gauge needle is passed in the "soft spot" in the radio-capitellar joint (in the triangle between the olecranon, lateral epicondyle and radial head) and assessed for the free passage of normal saline in the joint space.
- Urograffin dye is generally used in the dilution of 1:1. Usually only about 1-1.5 ml dye is required for the delineation of the articular surface **(Fig. 11.4)**.

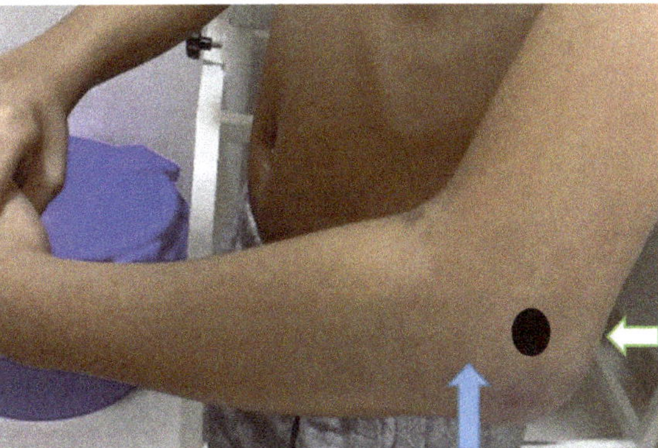

***Fig. 11.4**: Clinical photograph of the child with a displaced lateral condyle fracture with a swollen elbow. The black circle denoted the position of the lateral condyle while the two arrows denote the location of the needle placement for the arthrogram. Blue arrow denotes the radiocapitellar joint and the white arrow denotes the olecranon fossa.*

- The dye is then injected in the joint and checked under C-arm that it is not spilling over in the extra-osseous soft tissues.
- The other approach to the dye injection is the supra-olecranon space on the posterior aspect of the elbow **(Fig. 11.4)**.
- C-arm should be checked to ensure that the dye has entered the entire elbow joint.
- In fractures of the lateral condyle (Song III and IV), the intra-articular dye seeps into the fracture line and that is the confirmatory test for intra-articular extent of the fracture.
- The aim of the closed reduction is closing of the gap in the articular surface by manual pressure. This is really helped with arthrogram.

- Once it is confirmed that the intra-articular gap is closed by manual or instrumental pressure, K–wire fixation is performed with one wire from the metaphyseal fragment going along the lateral column and the other going towards the medial epicondyle parallel to the joint **(Fig. 11.5)**.
- The wires are bent and cut and above elbow plaster slab is given.
- Removal of wires is routinely performed after around 6-8 weeks depending on the state of union of the fracture.

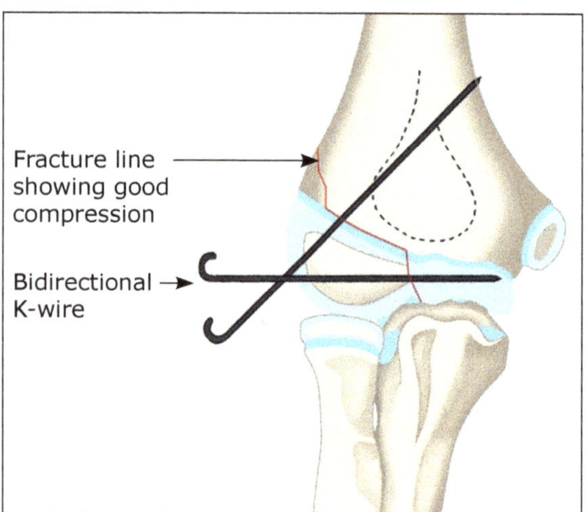

***Fig. 11.5**: Undisplaced lateral condyle fracture fixed with 2 bi-directional K-wires. Note the direction of the wires which help in good purchase and at the same time, give good compression at the fracture site.*

B) **Open reduction and internal fixation:**

- Open reduction and internal fixation of lateral condyle fractures is still the gold standard in management since there is still a significant chance of non-unions in lateral condyle fractures which are managed either conservatively or by closed reduction.
- Position:

  Supine with arm draped free on an arm board with tourniquet tied to the upper arm **(Fig. 11.6)**.

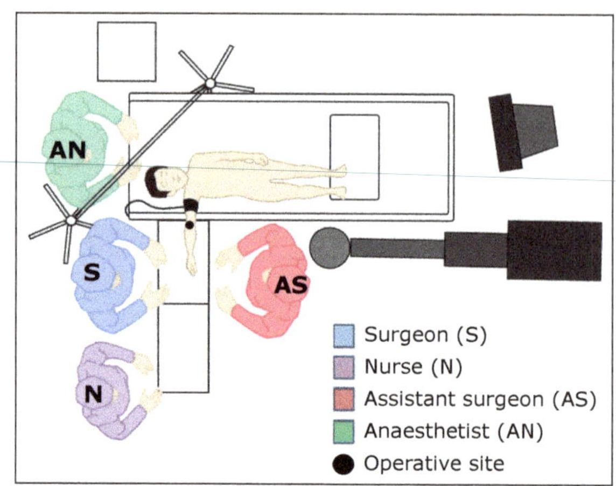

***Fig. 11.6**: Positioning of the patient and C-arm for closed or open reduction of lateral condyle humerus fractures.*

- Approach:

  The standard approach is the lateral approach which has the advantage of being easy to perform with no neurovascular risks and doesn't damage the precarious blood supply of the lateral condylar fragment. An alternative approach which is gaining popularity is the *posterolateral* approach. In this approach, the child is in lateral position and a posterolateral incision is made, and the fracture site is exposed between the lateral fibres of the triceps and the lateral intermuscular septum. The proponents of this approach believe that this approach protects the blood supply of the distal fragment and helps in better delineation of the articular reduction. For the purpose of discussion in this chapter, we will be describing only the lateral approach.
- Usually the haematoma guides the dissection and the fracture site is reached by gentle finger and blunt dissection.
- The fracture haematoma is thoroughly cleaned and irrigated and the interposed soft tissue is removed. Care should be taken to keep the dissection anterior as much as possible to prevent damage to the blood supply which comes from posterior aspect.

- Once the fracture fragments are cleared, reduction is obtained using manual force or with the help of a small towel clip clamp. It is important to check the articular alignment especially in fresh fractures **(Fig. 11.7)**.
- In case of grossly displaced and rotated fractures, it is necessary to derotate the fragment and align the articular surface as well as align the capitellar surface with the radial head.
- Keeping the manual pressure intact, fixation is performed using two to three K-wires (as described in the section on closed reduction) **(Fig. 11.8)**. In an older child and especially if the metaphyseal fragment is big, it may be better to put a 4 mm cannulated cancellous screw to achieve better compression **(Fig. 11.9)**. However, care should be taken to see to it that the screw is purely metaphyseal and it does not pass through the physis to avoid physeal damage.

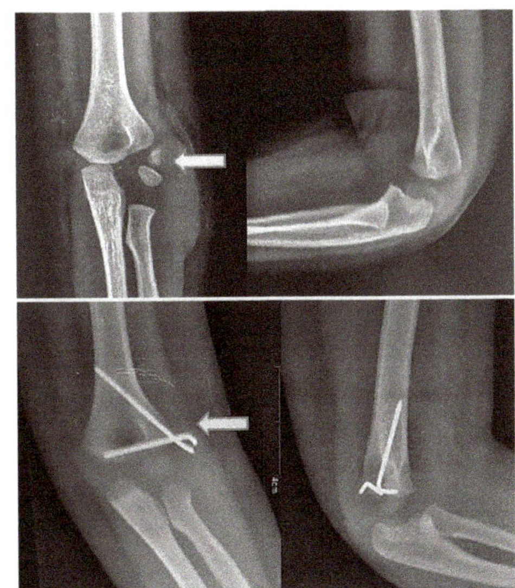

***Fig. 11.8**: AP and lateral X-rays of grossly displaced and rotated (Song type V) fracture lateral condyle humerus in a 5-year-old child treated with open reduction and Bi-directional K-wire fixation. Note the wires are only in the metaphyseal fragment which is usually big enough to allow adequate space for the wires.*

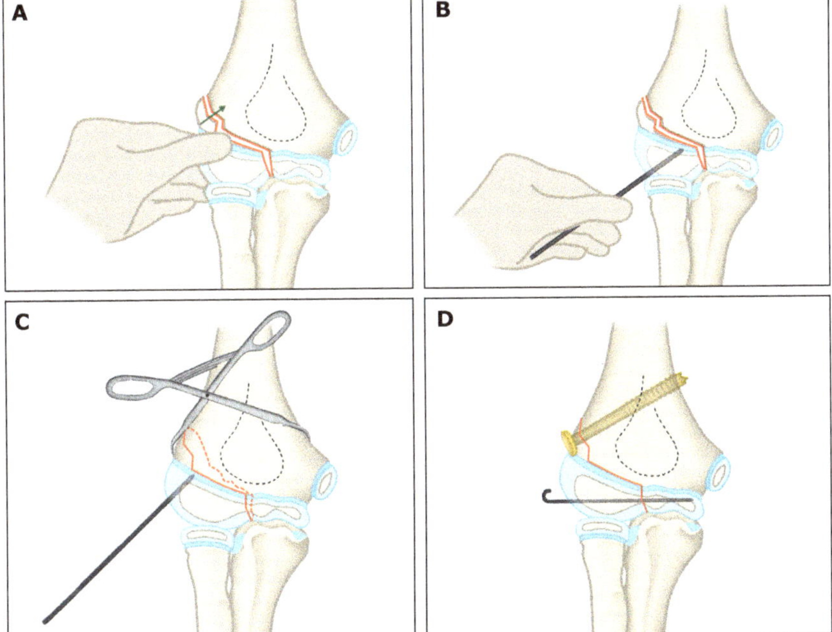

***Fig. 11.7**: Methods of manipulation of the lateral condylar fragment using either (A) hand compression or (B) by K-wire assisted manipulation. (C) Once reduction is achieved, compression can be obtained using a pointed towel clip clamp/ tenaculum clamp followed by (D) fixation using either one screw (passing through only the metaphyseal fragment) and one K-wire or two K-wires.*

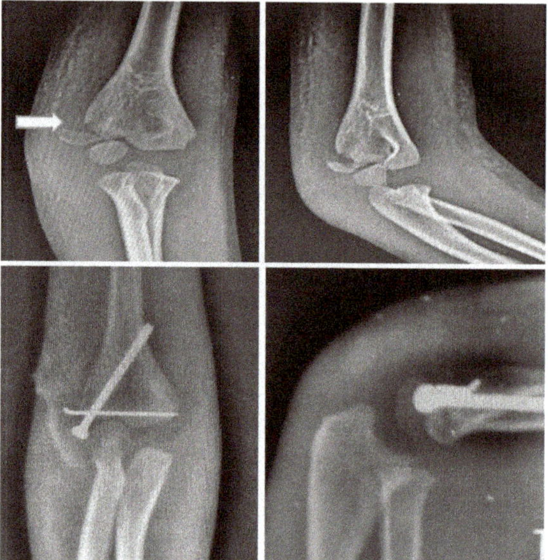

***Fig. 11.9**: AP and lateral X-rays of grossly displaced but not rotated (Song type IV) fracture lateral condyle humerus in a 10-year-old child treated with open reduction and Bi-directional fixation using one screw and one wire. Note the screw is holding and compressing only the metaphyseal segment (sparing the physis) and has achieved good compression.*

- The wires are cut, bent and buried in the skin and closure is performed in the routine manner.
- Above elbow slab/ cast immobilisation is continued for six weeks, after which, depending on the healing of the fracture, the wires are removed. The screw, if placed, is kept for a slightly longer period for around 3 months.

Complications

Lateral condyle fractures are prone for complications- especially non-unions and stiffness.

Non-union of lateral condyle humerus fractures is a dreaded complication not just in conservatively managed fractures but also in fractures in whom closed or open reduction and internal fixation is performed.

Lateral condyle non-unions can present either early or late and also can present either with or without deformity.

The easy way to classify non-union lateral condyle can be:

1) *"Early" lateral condyle non-union:* In this case, especially when the fragment is displaced but not rotated, the treatment of choice is in-situ screw fixation if the gap is less than 2-4 mm and good compression is achievable. In case the gap in the fracture fragment is more and adequate compression is not achievable, then open reduction, nibbling of the sclerotic bone ends and screw fixation with/without bone grafting can be attempted. The important principle to be noted in "early" lateral condyle non-unions is achieving metaphyseal union rather than attempting articular reduction. In case of displaced rotated fragments in kids who have presented late, an opinion should be given only after detailed counselling of the parents as reduction and fixation of the fragment can cause stiffness post-operatively.
2) *"Late" Lateral condyle non-union* with no obvious deformity with no ulnar nerve symptoms: This type can be left alone with watchful expectancy and the patient can be asked to come for yearly follow-up till skeletal maturity.
3) Non-union with obvious cubitus valgus without ulnar nerve symptoms: This child requires corrective osteotomy of the distal humerus for the cubitus valgus. If the child is about two years or more from skeletal maturity, it may be prudent to fix the non-union along with the osteotomy to prevent recurrence. However if the child is very near skeletal maturity, then it may not be necessary to perform fixation of the non-union.
4) Non-union with cubitus valgus with ulnar nerve palsy: In this case, along with the above, ulnar nerve transposition will be required.

Flowchart 11.1

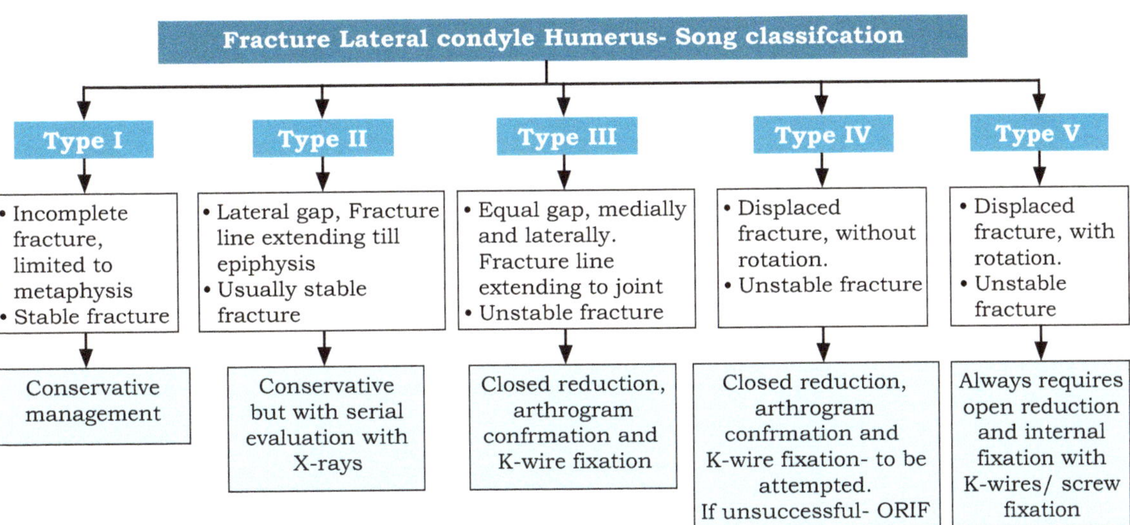

12 Radial Neck Fractures

Introduction

Radial neck fractures are rare childhood injuries and account for around 8% of all elbow fractures in children. Fractures of the proximal radius in children differ from those in adults in that the radial neck is more commonly injured as compared to the radial head in adults.

Classifications

A) *Judet classification (as per angulation):*

Type1: Undisplaced

Type II: < 30°

Type III: 30-60°

Type IVA: 60-80°

Type IV B: >80°

B) *Wilkin's classification:*

I-Valgus fractures

Type A: Salter-Harris types I and II

Type B: Salter- Harris type IV

Type C: Radius metaphyseal fracture

II-Fractures associated with posterior elbow dislocation:

Type D: Reduction injuries (Jeffrey type I)

Type E: Dislocation injuries (Jeffrey type II)

Diagnosis

Child with radial neck fracture presents with history of fall on outstretched hand with valgus stress on elbow. Clinical evaluation reveals pain, swelling and deformity along the lateral aspect of elbow.

The diagnosis of radial neck fractures is primarily radiological on plain X-rays. In some cases, the displacement is underestimated due to the significant overlap of the proximal epiphysis and the metaphysis. Hence an X-ray showing maximum amount of displacement (usually in about 40° of supination) is needed to exactly decide on the plan of management of radial neck fractures.

Radiocapitellar view

- Oblique lateral view is performed by placing the arm on the radiographic table with the elbow flexed 90° and the thumb pointing upward
- The beam is directed 45° proximally

Treatment

Acceptability criteria

The acceptable range depends on the age of the child and the degree of angulation and translation. As with most paediatric fractures, translation is much more accepted than angulation especially in children more than 9 years.

Need for reduction

An acceptable range of < 45° of angulation and 10% of translation is acceptable below 9 years of age while not more than 30° of angulation should be acceptable above 9 years of age.

Treatment

Any undisplaced or minimally displaced fracture can be treated with a long arm cast for around 3 weeks followed by range of motion exercises especially prono-supination.

Methods of reduction

There are basically four main groups of methods of reduction:

1) Closed reduction techniques
2) Assisted closed reduction techniques
3) Open reduction
4) Reduction of Jeffrey type II fractures

1) ***Closed reduction techniques:***

All the closed reduction techniques work on the principle that the mechanism of injury is a valgus force on the extended elbow. Hence the reduction manoeuvre should contain some traction and attempted varus force in order to realign the radial head fragment to the distal segment.

a) *Patterson manoeuvre:*

The elbow is held in extension and distal traction is applied with the forearm in supination. The forearm in then pulled into a bit of varus while direct pressure is applied over the radial head.

b) *Israeli (Kaufman) technique:*

In this technique, the flexed elbow is moved from supination to pronation, and direct pressure is applied on the radial head in order to squeeze it back in.

c) *Nehar and Torch technique:*

This technique is similar to the Patterson technique with some modifications. The elbow is in extension and traction is given, The assistant then pulls the radial shaft laterally while the surgeon applies direct medial force on the radial head fragment to achieve reduction.

d) *Elastic bandage technique:*

This is a very elegant technique where an elastic bandage starting at the wrist going along the forearm and the elbow from lateral to medial helps in achieving spontaneous reduction.

2) ***Assisted closed reduction techniques***

a) *Metazieu technique* **(Fig. 12.2)**:

This technique is one of the foremost methods of reduction and fixation used in displaced radial neck fractures. The method is as follows:

- Position- Supine with arm over an arm board with tourniquet applied over the upper arm **(Fig. 12.1)**.

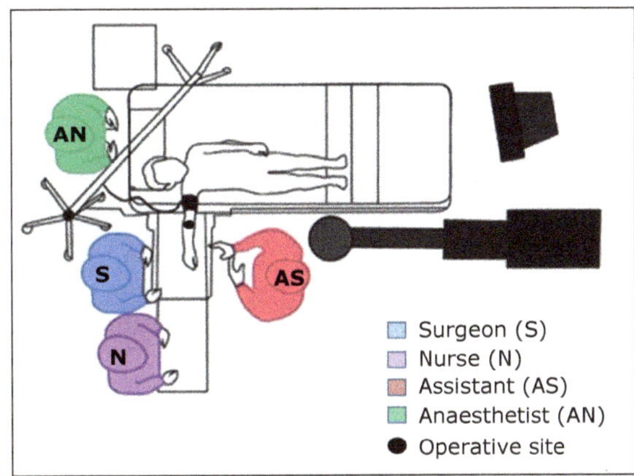

Fig. 12.1: *Position of the patient for fixation of displaced radial neck fracture with the help of intramedullary nail by the Metazieu technique.*

- The displaced radial head is seen in the position of maximum displacement (usually about 40° supination)
- A small incision is made on the radial aspect of the distal radius for the entry point of the titanium elastic nail.
- The nail of appropriate size is introduced and passed retrograde till just distal to the radial neck.
- The proximal radial head fragment is allowed to be engaged (in the displaced position) with the help of the hockey stick bend of the nail.
- Once the head fragment is engaged

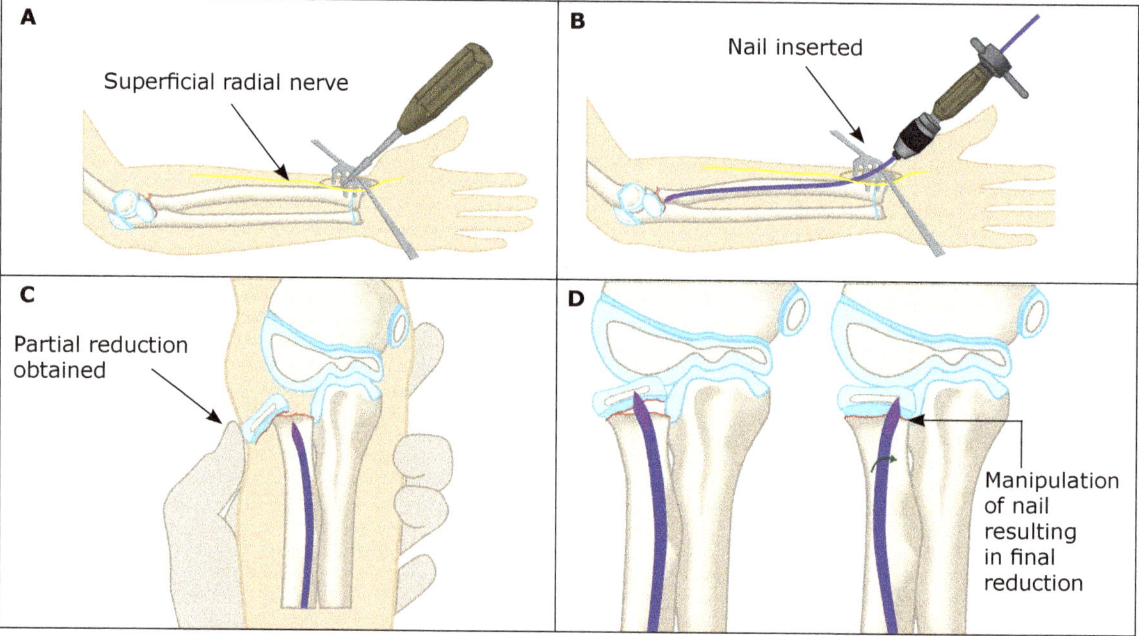

***Fig. 12.2**: Metazieu technique for fixation of displaced radial neck fracture. A) Entry taken from the dorsal side of the radial styloid, retracting the superficial radial nerve and the extensor tendons. B) Titanium elastic nail inserted using a T-handle and passed till fracture site. C) Judet type IV fracture converted to Judet type II-III with the help of thumb digital pressure. D) Nail passed across the fracture site in the un-reduced position and the tip of the nail turned 180° so as to achieve good reduction.*

well, the nail is rotated 180°, so that the hockey stick bend is turned medially.

- If the radial head fragment is held and engaged well with the nail, then reduction is usually achieved with this manoeuvre as well as with gentle manual pressure on the radial head.
- Reduction is confirmed on all views as well as on the fluro shot, and the nail is hammered a few turns in order to seat it well in the radial head.
- An above elbow plaster slab is given in 90° flexion and supination for about three weeks.

b) *Intra-focal reduction technique* **(Figs. 12.3 & 12.4)**:

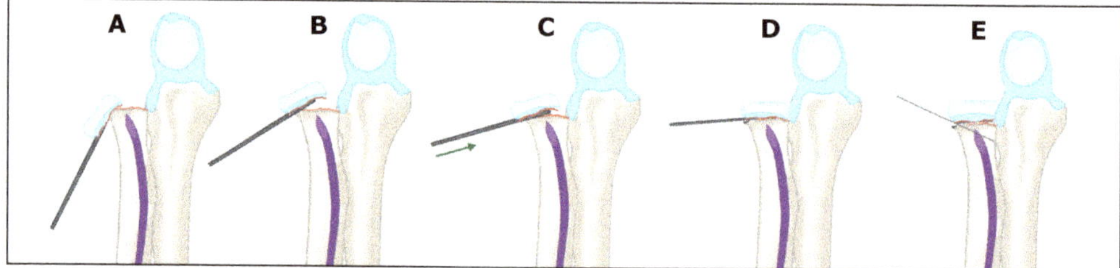

***Fig. 12.3**: Intra-focal reduction using K-wire for a displaced radial neck fracture. K-wire passed along the axilla of the radial head-neck junction (A). The radial head fragment manipulated in place (B,C,D) with the help of the K-wire and then inserted across the medial cortex (E). The intra-medullary elastic nail can then be passed across the fracture site.*

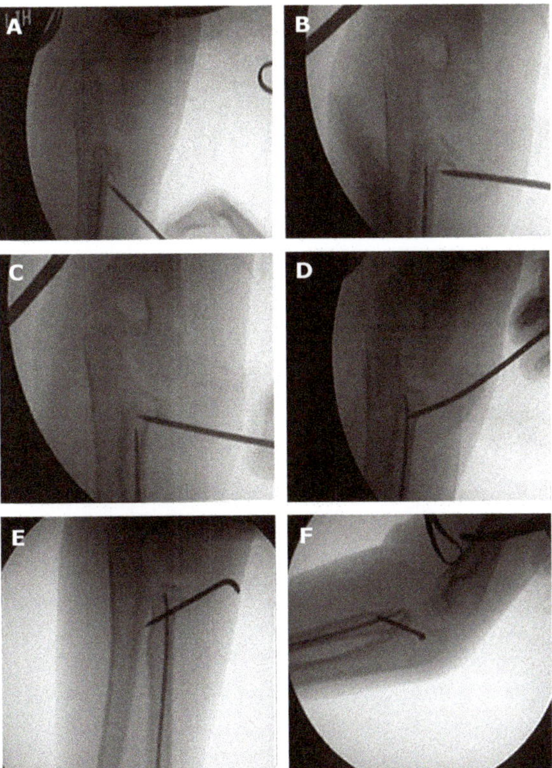

***Fig. 12.4**: Method of intra-focal reduction for a displaced radial neck fracture (Judet type IV). (A) K-wire passed in the axilla of the radial neck, (B,C,D) Radial head fragment elevated, and reduced in place, (E,F) K-wire drilled into the medial cortex and intra-medullary nail advanced for added stability.*

This is another technique which is very commonly used especially in severely displaced fractures (with initial angulations 80° and more).

- Position- Supine with arm on arm board with tourniquet applied over upper arm
- As with previous method, the fracture is visualised in the position of maximum displacement.
- A 2-2.5 mm K-wire is introduced from distal to proximal in the *axilla* of the radial head-neck junction and the K-wire is hitched in the fracture gap.
- The risk to the posterior interosseous nerve is minimised by keeping the forearm in mild pronation.
- The radial head fragment is then levered into position by manipulating the K-wire so that now the wire is directed distally.
- Usually with this manoeuvre, the radial head flips back in place.
- A drill is then applied to the K-wire and the K-wire is then advanced into the *medial cortex of the radius metaphysis.*
- The last step is an optional step and some clinicians do not put any wire once reduction is achieved and the K-wire is removed.
- The other option is to combine the Metazieu and the intrafocal reduction techniques by using the intra-medullary nail to achieve the final reduction and then keeping the intra-medullary nail rather than the intrafocal wire.
- An above elbow slab is applied for about three weeks.
- The intrafocal wire if kept can be removed early by around 3 weeks.

3) ***Open reduction:***

Open reduction is only resorted to if satisfactory reduction is not achieved by any of the techniques described. In fact, it is sometimes better to leave a fracture slightly less reduced rather than doing an open reduction and ending up with stiffness. Open reduction if at all attempted needs to be done with utmost care and with very delicate soft tissue handling.

- Position- Supine with arm on arm board with tourniquet applied over upper arm
- A small 3-4 cm incision is made over the lateral aspect of the upper forearm starting from the lateral epicondyle and extending distally towards the radial styloid.

- The interval between the anconeus and the extensor carpi ulnaris (ECU) is identified and the muscles are retracted in the direction of the fibres **(Fig.12.5)**.

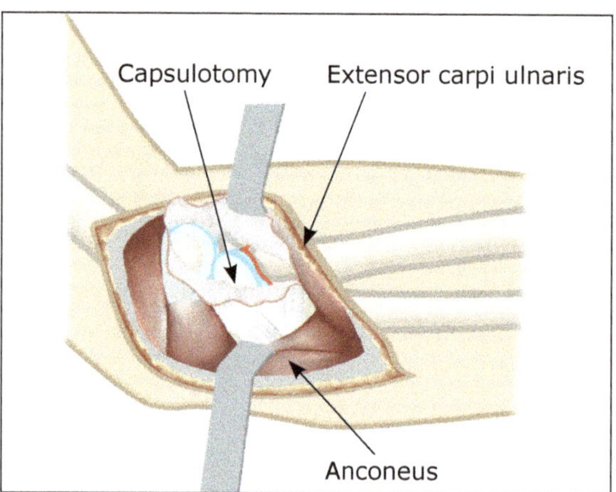

Fig. 12.5: *Open reduction for a displaced radial neck fracture through the Kocher's approach. The interval is between ECU and anconeus keeping the forearm in full pronation so as to protect the posterior interosseous nerve.*

- The forearm is kept in full pronation in order to protect the posterior interosseous nerve.
- Capsulotomy is performed and the radial neck fragment is exposed.
- The periosteal sleeve (which is generally intact medially) is preserved as much as possible and the radial head is gently repositioned over the radial neck.
- An intramedullary wire which has already been passed retrograde till the radial neck is then advanced into the radial head fragment.
- Trans- capitellar wires are strictly avoided.
- Above elbow plaster slab given in the usual manner.

4) *Management of radial neck fractures associated with elbow dislocation: (Jeffrey type 2 injuries):*

- These injuries are caused during spontaneous or iatrogenic reduction of the elbow dislocation and are characterised by displacement of the radial head fragment posteriorly and proximally. These fractures are extremely difficult to manage and usually require open reduction.
- Closed reduction can be attempted in a specific manner as follows: The surgeon and assistant attempt to recreate the subluxation of the elbow first so as to disimpact the fracture as well as remove the interposition of the capitellum between the epiphysis and the metaphysis of the radial neck (**Figure 12.6** - Black arrow). Once the fragments are dis-impacted, the surgeon then applies an anteriorly directed force with the help of thumb pressure, so as to re-position the radial head fragment (**Figure 12.6** - Blue arrow). The elbow subluxation is gently reduced, keeping a close watch under C-arm control, so as to prevent the radial head from displacing again.

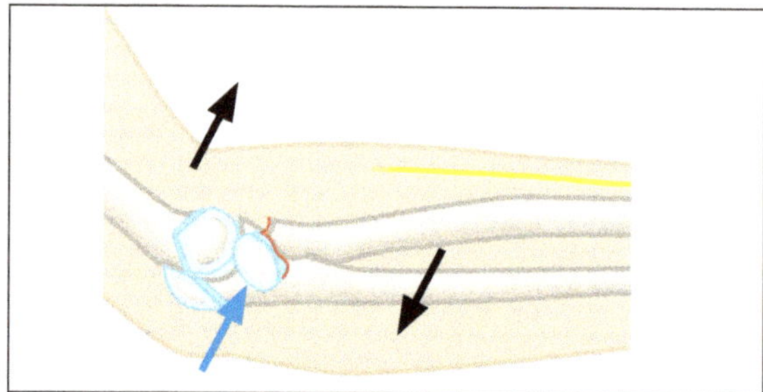

Fig. 12.6: *Reduction manoeuvre for a Jeffrey type 2 radial neck fracture.*

- A similar manoeuvre can be performed using a K-wire inserted in the radial head and used as a joystick to reduce it.
- Once the radial head is reduced, usually it remains stable and requires

only a plaster. If there is any instability, then fixation can be performed using a K-wire or with an intra-medullary nail in the usual manner.

Complications

1) *Decreased range of motion:*

   This is the most common complication of radial neck fractures which needs to be avoided as much as possible. Loss of pronation is more common than loss of supination. Early mobilisation, meticulous soft tissue care and no massage are the keys to prevent loss of ROM.

2) *Radial head overgrowth:*

   A very common complication, though this is one which has least effect on overall function.

3) *Avascular necrosis of the radial head:*

   This is quite common especially in open reduction (almost 70% of all AVNs are caused after open reduction). It is best that the periosteal sleeve is left intact while performing open reduction.

4) *Posterior interosseous nerve injury:*

   This complication can be an iatrogenic one which is relatively commonly seen in intra-focal reduction technique. Thankfully, this is usually reversible and usually corrects by itself by around 3 months.

5) *Synostosis:*

   This is the most dreaded complication and is more related to the initial soft tissue injury rather than being iatrogenic. It is extremely difficult to treat and once set, it becomes very difficult to correct.

Flowchart 12.1

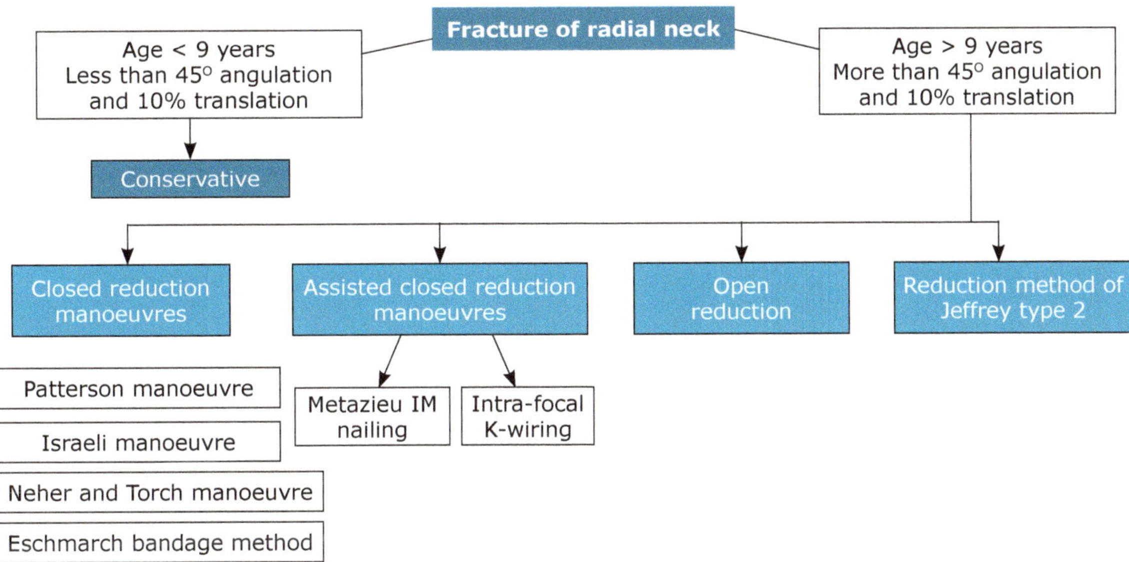

13 Monteggia Fracture-Dislocations and Equivalents

Introduction

- Monteggia fractures were described first by Giovanni Monteggia in 1814 (long before X-rays were discovered) and have now been described in great detail by many authors.
- Monteggia fracture-dislocation is basically an ulnar fracture with dislocation of the radial head (though there is significant variability in terms of the type of the ulnar fracture as well as the direction of the radial head dislocation).

Classification

Bado in 1971 published his now-famous classification for all Monteggia fracture dislocations and is now widely used **(Fig. 13.1)**.

- Type I: Ulnar fracture with *anterior* dislocation of the radial head
- Type II: Ulnar fracture with *posterior* dislocation of the radial head

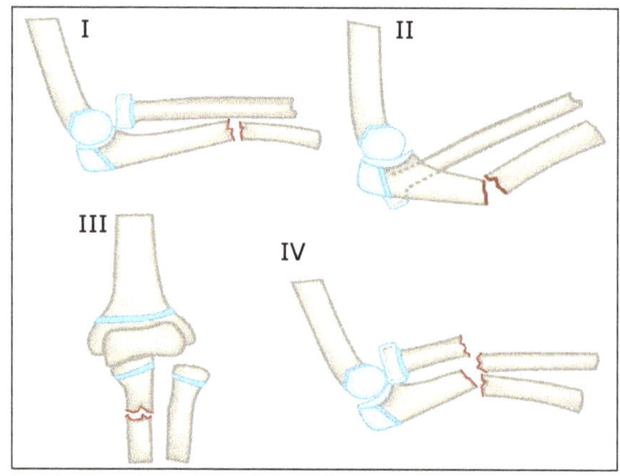

Fig. 13.1: *Bado classification.*

- Type III: Ulnar fracture with lateral dislocation of the radial head
- Type IV: Ulnar fracture with proximal radial fracture at the same level as the ulnar fracture with dislocation of the radial head (usually anterior).

In addition, he also put forth some injuries to the proximal radiocapitellar complex which have similar soft tissue injuries and are clubbed together as *Equivalents.* They are:

1) Plastic deformation of the ulna with anterior dislocation of the radial head.
2) Fracture of the ulna diaphysis with Proximal radius physeal injury (usually type I or II)
3) Fracture of the ulna diaphysis with Radius fracture *proximal* to the ulna
4) Fracture of the olecranon with Ulna shaft with radial head dislocation
5) Ulnar metaphysis fracture with radial neck fracture
6) Elbow dislocation with Ulna fracture and proximal radius fracture.

Hume's fracture

Hume's fracture is a very unique entity which consists of a fracture of the Olecrenon along with anterior radial head dislocation. The peculiarity of this injury is that the mechanism of injury of the two components of the injury are opposite (i.e. olecranon is due to sudden flexion of the elbow leading to an avulsion fracture while the radial head dislocation is primarily an extension injury) and hence the mechanism of reduction also is opposite to each other. This makes it a difficult fracture to treat.

Mechanism of injury

The mechanism of injury varies as per the Bado classification:

1) Type I: The type I injuries are the most common type in childhood. The type I injury occurs due to two mechanisms **(Fig. 13.2)**:

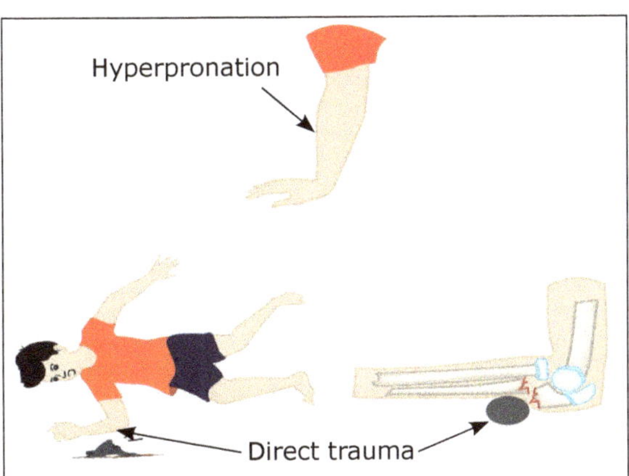

***Fig. 13.2**: Mechanism of injury in a Type I Bado Monteggia fracture dislocation.*

- Direct trauma to the ulna which forces the ulna anteriorly which pushes the radial head anteriorly.
- Fall on outstretched hand with the elbow in extension.

2) Type II: Direct trauma to the anterior aspect of the elbow forcing the radial head posteriorly
3) Type III: Direct trauma to the inner aspect of the elbow with some rotation **(Fig. 13.3)**.
4) Type IV: Fall on outstretched hand with forced pronation.

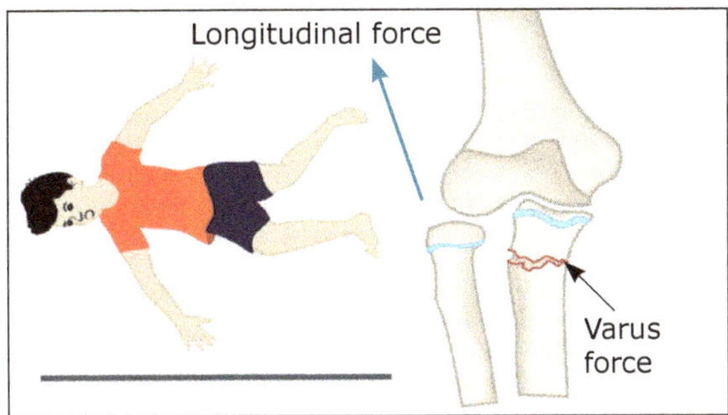

***Fig. 13.3**: Mechanism of injury of Type III Bado Monteggia fracture-dislocation.*

Clinical Features

- Monteggia fracture- dislocation is one of the most commonly missed orthopaedic injuries and needs to be diagnosed early and accurately for good result.
- The ulna fracture (if it is complete) is easily diagnosed, but the radial head dislocation or subluxation is something which gets missed.
- This is most common when the ulnar fracture is not complete but a greenstick or a plastic deformation.
- Usually the child comes with pain, swelling and tenderness over the upper aspect of the ulna, along with tenderness on the radial head. Any child with an upper third ulna fracture should be evaluated for radial head dislocation.
- In some types, especially the type I and type III Bado, the radial head is easily palpable anteriorly or laterally, respectively. However, this sign can be easily missed.

Imaging

- Plain X-rays of the elbow as well as full length X-rays of the entire forearm are essential for the diagnosis of the radial head component of the injury.
- Good quality AP and lateral views are of utmost importance.
- On the lateral view, along with the ulna fracture, the radial head position with respect to the capitellum is very

important. The radio-capitellar line has to be drawn in every lateral X-ray of the elbow and it has to pass through the capitellum, in all positions of the elbow.

- However, this may not be entirely true especially in children younger than 8 years, where around 16-20% of all radiocapitellar lines pass anterior to the capitellum. In this case, the line passing through the metaphysis of the radial neck has to be drawn and evaluated for subluxation.
- The other important radiological sign is that described by Lincoln and Mubarak about the *"Ulnar bow sign"* in minimal Monteggia fractures (or the Plastically deformed ulna with the radial head dislocations). For this sign to be seen, it is essential to get a long forearm X-ray- lateral view where a gentle plastic bow is seen. If a line is passed from the two most prominent parts of the ulna (at the proximal metaphysis and the ulnar styloid), then ideally the ulnar shaft (which is usually convex) intersects this line somewhere in the middle third. However, when there is a plastic deformation of the ulna with an anterior dislocation of the radial head, the ulna becomes *concave*, the shaft of the ulna *does not* intersect this "ulnar Bow line" or the *"Mubarak's line"* **(Fig. 13.4)**.

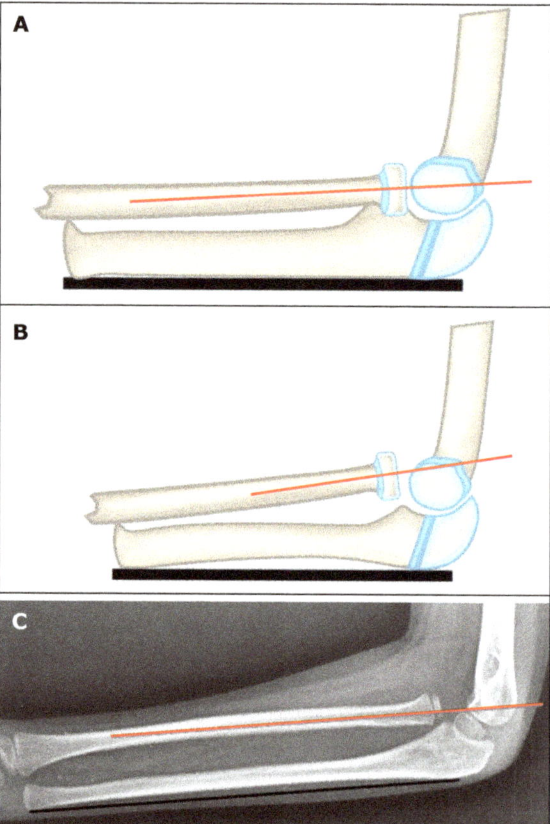

***Fig. 13.4**: (A) Schematic figure of a normal proximal elbow and radius-ulna complex with the radiocapitellar line passing through the centre of the capitellum and the "Mubarak's line" being along the dorsal border of the ulna and (B, C) a type I Bado Monteggia fracture dislocation with the radiocapitellar line passing anterior to the capitellum and a clear gap between the "Mubarak" line and the dorsal surface of the ulna due to the concavity of the ulna.*

Treatment

Treatment of acute injuries

The one issue of paramount importance in the management of Monteggia fracture dislocations is the maintenance of *Ulnar length.* The entire management of acute Monteggia injuries is directed towards achieving and maintaining ulnar length.

Conservative treatment

- Conservative management in form of closed reduction and casting has to be tried in only very young kids in whom regular follow-up is possible and in whom it is possible to get serial X-rays done.
- Weekly lateral X-rays are essential to look for radiocapitellar alignment and late radial head subluxation.
- In case of plastic deformation of the ulna with radial head dislocation, it is sometime very difficult to correct the ulnar bow. Hence it may be necessary

to give sustained posteriorly directed force on the front of the flexed elbow in order to achieve reduction of the radial head.

- Non-operative management can also be attempted in complete ulnar fractures especially the length stable ones. The method of closed reduction of various Monteggia lesions based on Bado types is as follows:
- Type I Bado: Here the ulna is angulated anteriorly and hence the reduction manoeuvre is longitudinal traction, correction of angulation by posteriorly directed force, followed by flexion and supination **(Fig. 13.5)**.

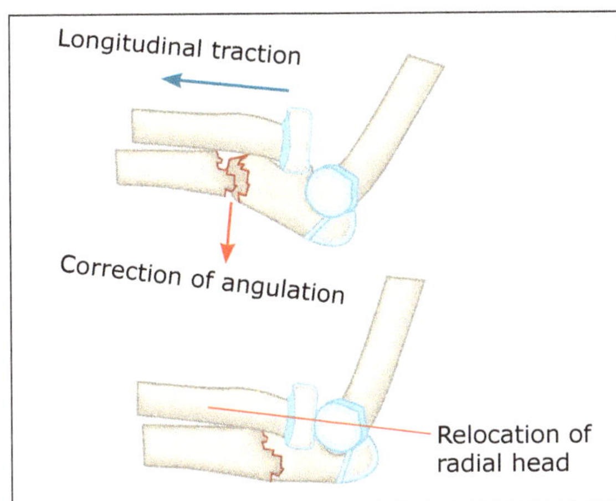

***Fig. 13.5**: Method of closed reduction of type I Bado Monteggia fracture dislocation.*

- Type II Bado: It is extremely difficult to closed reduce a type 2 Bado as the posteriorly dislocated radial head makes it almost impossible to achieve close reduction. Attempt can be made by giving longitudinal traction, anterior angulation and gentle thumb pressure on the radial head to push it anteriorly.
- Type III Bado: Type III Bado injuries require valgus force to correct the alignment of the ulna followed by digital pressure over the radial head to force it back in place **(Fig. 13.6)**.

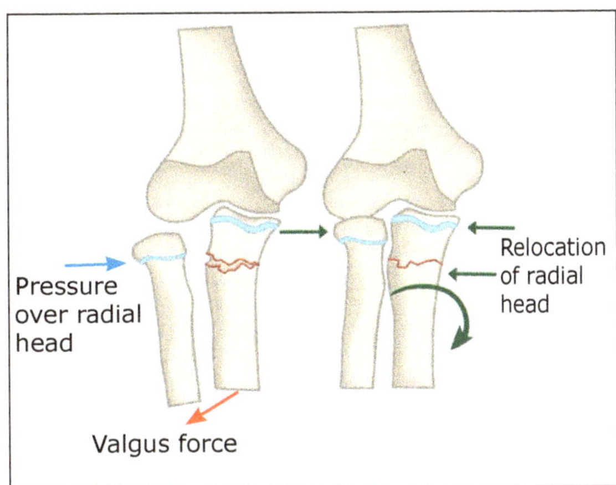

***Fig. 13.6**: Method of closed reduction of Bado type III Monteggia fracture dislocation.*

Operative treatment

- This is required in most cases of Monteggia injuries in order to maintain ulnar length. The indications of operative fixation of Monteggia fractures are open fractures, unstable fracture patterns, short oblique, spiral (length unstable fractures) or any fracture in which radial head reduction is not obtained. The method of fixation can be either an elastic nail from the proximal ulna or a plate for slightly older children. The fixation itself is standard like in any ulnar nailing or plating. The only caveat is that no malreduction should be accepted.
- The main issue comes when dealing with a type I Monteggia equivalent where there is a plastic deformation of the ulna and closed reduction is not possible by manual pressure. In this case, it is essential to pass a straight intramedullary nail from the olecranon, or in some cases, do a small percutaneous "osteotomy", break the ulna to straighten it and then pass the nail through.

Operative steps (Fig. 13.7)

1) Position: Supine with arm on arm board with tourniquet tied to upper arm.

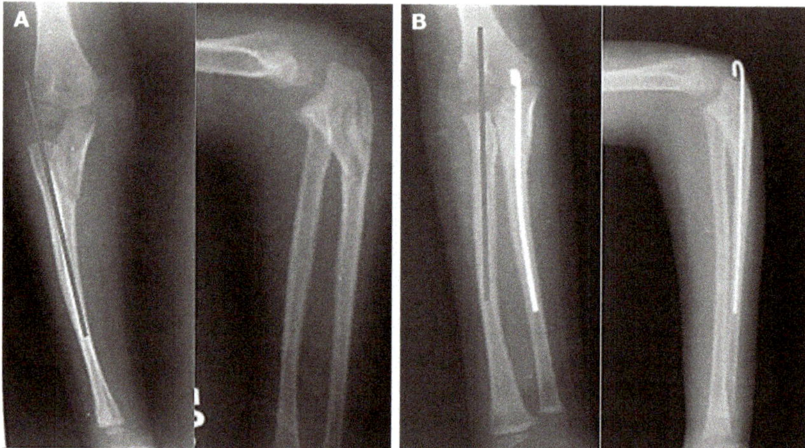

***Fig. 13.7**: (A) Pre-operative AP and lateral X-rays of a type III Bado Monteggia fracture dislocation showing a proximal third ulna fracture along with lateral radial head dislocation. (B) Post-operative X-ray of the same child after closed reduction and intra-medullary nail fixation showing excellent reduction of the radial head and restoration of the radiocapitellar alignment.*

2) After elevation of tourniquet, closed reduction is attempted of the ulna fracture and subsequently the radial head.
3) A small incision is made over the anconeus between the radius and ulna.
4) The entry is made just distal to the ulna apophysis through the anconeus muscle with a straight awl.
5) A 2-2.5 mm elastic nail is inserted through the entry point and closed reduction of the ulna is attempted.
6) If necessary, a small incision open reduction of the ulna is performed and the nail is negotiated.
7) It is of utmost importance that the length of the ulna is restored, which will help in reduction and stability of the radial head in the radiocapitellar joint.
8) In case, the radial head is not reducing closed, it is important to perform an open reduction of the radial head either through the Boyd's approach or through the Kocher's approach, clear the intervening soft tissues and stabilise the radial head. The details of the procedure are given in the section of Chronic Monteggia lesions.
9) Once it is confirmed, the nail is passed till the distal end of the ulna and cut short and hammered till the end.
10) Skin closure is performed in a single layer.
11) Above elbow plaster slab is applied for 4 weeks.

Complications

1) Chronic or missed Monteggia dislocations- Described in detail in the next section.
2) Nerve injuries:

   The commonest nerve injury associated is the posterior interosseous nerve which is seen characteristically in type III injuries. It is usually a neuropraxia and recovers in about three months.
3) Stiffness:

   Prono-supination is the movement which is mostly restricted in Monteggia fracture dislocations especially when reduction is attempted late or when open reduction of the radial head is performed.

Management of missed Monteggia fractures

Monteggia fractures are one of the commonest missed injuries especially in children where the radial head is not completely ossified and the ulna may not be fractured but plastically deformed in order to mask the severity of the initial injury.

The treatment of Missed Monteggia fractures is always operative.

- The principle here is also the maintenance of the ulnar length. However, this needs to be achieved with ulnar osteotomy which needs to be angulated in a direction opposite to the primary displacement.
- This may or may not be combined with an open reduction of the radial head along with annular ligament reconstruction if required.
- **Surgical procedure of Ulnar osteotomy/ Open reduction of radial head/ Annular ligament reconstruction:**
- Position: Supine with arm draped free on an arm board with a tourniquet tied to the upper arm.
- The author prefers to use the Boyd's extensile approach which helps in exposing both the proximal ulna as well as the proximal radiocapitellar joint and keeping the posterior interosseous nerve away from the surgical field.
- The incision is a long curvilinear incision extending from above the elbow near the lateral supracondylar ridge extending till the lateral epicondyle and then curving gently and extending distally towards the lateral aspect of the ulnar shaft.
- The ulna is exposed subperiosteally till the olecranon and the site of the osteotomy is marked, generally at the junction of the metaphysis and the diaphysis of the ulna.
- If open reduction of the radial head is also to be performed, then the anconeus is elevated off the lateral aspect of the olecranon. The common extensor origin is partially erased after taking tagging sutures for later reattachment. Once this step is performed, then the entire proximal third of the ulna, the radio-capitellar "joint" with the dislocated radial head and the distal part of the humerus is widely visible. The posterior interosseous nerve is in the anterior soft tissue and is not to be searched for.
- At this stage, the ulnar osteotomy is performed, and flexion and distraction is given to the osteotomy in order to reduce the radial head (in case of the commonest type I Monteggia). The author prefers to pre-drill one hole in the proximal segment, so that proximal control is obtained when the osteotomy is to be fixed.
- Once the radial head is seen to be reduced, the osteotomy of the ulna is fixed in the same position (usually in about 20^{0} of flexion and with around 8 mm of distraction) with the help of a 3.5 mm Reconstruction plate (or in older children- 3.5 mm DCP) **(Fig. 13.8).**
- The stability of the radial head at the radiocapitellar joint is checked in all movements including flexion extension and pronosupination.
- If the radial head is found to be unstable at this stage inspite of stable fixation of the radial head, an annular ligament reconstruction is performed using either the forearm or the triceps fascia, in order to achieve more stability to the radial head.
- Trans-radiocapitellar wires are strictly avoided.

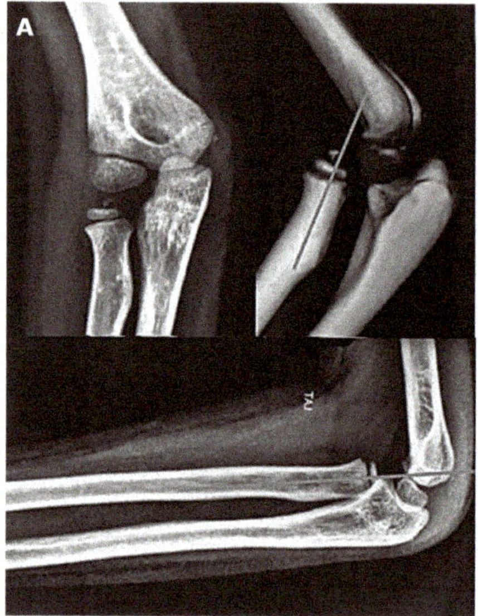

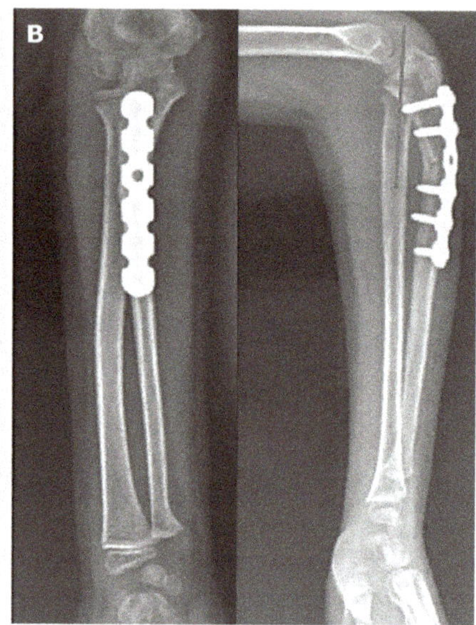

***Fig. 13.8**: (A) Pre-operative X-ray and CT scan of the elbow of a 8 year old child with missed type I Bado Monteggia fracture dislocation. (B) Post-operative X-ray of the same child after flexion distraction osteotomy of the ulna and open reduction of the radial head showing excellent alignment of the radiocapitellar line.*

- After closure, an above elbow slab is given in 90° of flexion and full supination.
- The Boyd's approach is a versatile approach which gives a full exposure to all components of the deformity without danger to the posterior interosseous nerve. The only complication which is reported by some authors is slightly increased chance of synostosis or stiffness.
- An alternative to the Boyd's approach is to use a subcutaneous incision for the ulna and have a separate incision by the Kocher's approach for the radial head. The incision however is limited by the radial neck and as such is not very extensile.

Flowchart 13.1

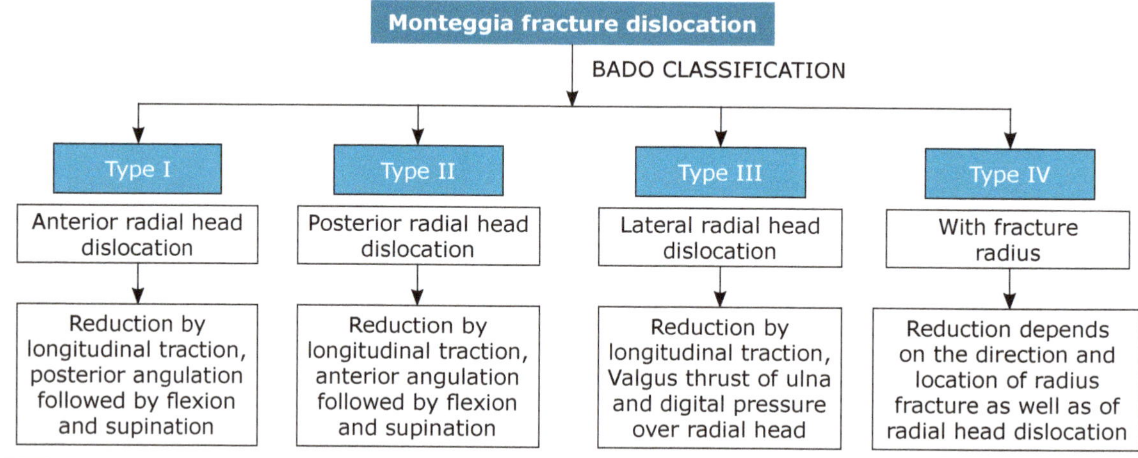

14 Miscellaneous Elbow Fractures

The fractures which we will be dealing with, in this chapter would be:

1) Medial condyle fractures
2) Medial Epicondyle fractures
3) Transphyseal injuries of distal humerus
4) Lateral epicondyle fractures
5) Olecranon fractures
6) Elbow dislocation
7) TRASH lesions

1) Medial Condyle Fractures

Introduction and Mechanism of Injury

- Medial condyle fractures are extremely uncommon fractures in children and account for only about 2% of all elbow fractures.
- These injuries occur by two means- either by a fall on outstretched hand or by a direct trauma to the olecranon which forces the medial condyle to fracture.

Classification

Killfoyle classification **(Fig. 14.1)**:

Type I: Undisplaced and incomplete- not extending to the articular surface

Type II: Undisplaced but complete- extending to the articular surface

Type III: Displaced and rotated fracture (similar to the lateral condyle fracture)

Clinical Features

- Pain, swelling and deformity over the medial aspect of the elbow.

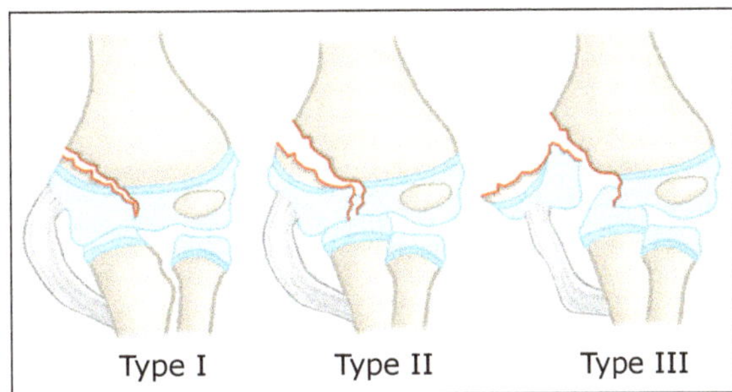

Fig. 14.1: *Killfoyle classification of medial condyle fractures*

- There is usually significant contusion over the medial side.
- Valgus instability is very common and always needs to be checked for.
- It is very rarely associated with ulnar nerve symptoms.

Imaging

- Plain X-rays are usually sufficient at least for the primary diagnosis of medial condylar fractures.
- A good quality AP, lateral and oblique elbow X-ray is important.
- Sometimes, a stress X-ray with mild valgus helps in getting an idea about the instability associated with the injury.
- It is important to note that the medial condyle is not ossified till 8 years of age, and hence any medial *epicondyle* fracture below 8 years of age is to be considered as medial *condyle* fractures unless proved otherwise.
- MRI is sometimes needed to exactly delineate the fracture as well as to

diagnose whether the fracture is intra-articular or stopping short of the articular surface.

Treatment

The treatment of medial condylar fractures depends on the type of injury.

- *Type I injury*: In-situ cast application for around 4 weeks
- *Type II injury*: Closed reduction and K-wire fixation with arthrogram confirmation.
- *Type III injury*: Open reduction and internal fixation with K-wires/ screws through the medial approach.

2) Medial Epicondyle Fractures

Introduction and Mechanism of Injury

- Medial epicondyle fractures are the third most common fractures around the elbow in children after supracondylar humerus fractures and lateral condyle fractures. The unique feature of medial epicondyle fractures is the attachment of the powerful common flexors to the epicondyle which causes displacement and which in turn helps in the reduction of the fragment.
- The mechanism of injury is usually an avulsion injury with a valgus force which creates this fracture due to the vigorous pull of the common flexors **(Fig. 14.2)**.
- It can be associated with elbow dislocations when it can be entrapped inside the joint along with the flexor mechanism.

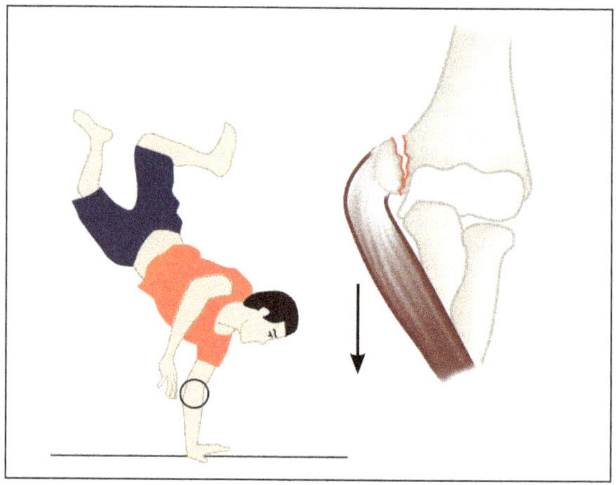

Fig. 14.2: *Mechanism of injury of medial epicondyle fractures- Fall on the outstretched hand with valgus thrust force.*

Classification

- Woods and Tully classification:

1) Undisplaced
2) Minimally displaced
3) Displaced- more than 5 mm.

- Elbow joint not dislocated
- Epicondyle not in joint
- Epicondyle in joint but elbow joint reduced
- Epicondyle in joint and elbow dislocated

Clinical Features

- The child presents with severe pain over the medial aspect of the elbow with significant swelling and contusion.
- The child usually has valgus instability in mid-flexion.
- In cases where the elbow is dislocated and the epicondyle is entrapped within the elbow joint, there may be symptoms of ulnar nerve palsy.

Imaging

- Usually plain X-rays are enough to diagnose medial epicondyle fractures. Standard good quality antero-posterior and lateral X-rays along with external rotation oblique X-rays give a good idea about the amount of displacement of the fracture.
- Gravity stress X-rays may be required to look for medial opening of the joint.

- In some cases, MRI may be needed to diagnose the exact amount of displacement of such fractures as well as to rule out the intra-articular extent of the fracture if any.

Treatment

- For the purposes of treatment, medial epicondyle fractures can be divided into three groups:
- Undisplaced and minimally displaced fractures (with less than 5mm displacement).
- Fractures with displacement more than 5 mm but the elbow reduced.
- Displaced fractures with elbow dislocated and the epicondyle incarcerated in the joint.

a) *Undisplaced and minimally displaced fractures* can be treated conservatively with long arm posterior slab/ cast for about 3 weeks. Usually the outcome of such fractures is excellent and with early range of motion, these kids get back to full function and power in a short time.

b) *Displaced fractures (more than 5mm) and elbow stable:* This is a relative indication for surgery. Even when the displacement is more than 5 mm, the child can be conservatively treated. However when there is significant instability, especially in the dominant hand of an athlete who requires full function and power of the elbow, fixation is indicated. The approach is medial, with a longitudinal incision, keeping the ulnar nerve away. Fixation is performed using a semi threaded 4 mm cannulated cancellous screw with a washer.

- Position: Supine with arm on arm board with tourniquet on upper arm. The limb is externally rotated so as to expose the medial side of the elbow. Supine position helps in ease of radiographic viewing. An alternative position is the lateral or prone position with arm over a radiolucent arm support (similar to the one used for the posterior approach to the humerus). The shoulder is then *internally* rotated in a Figure of 4 position in order to visualise the fragment and which gives a varus force and helps in the reduction **(Fig. 14.3)**.

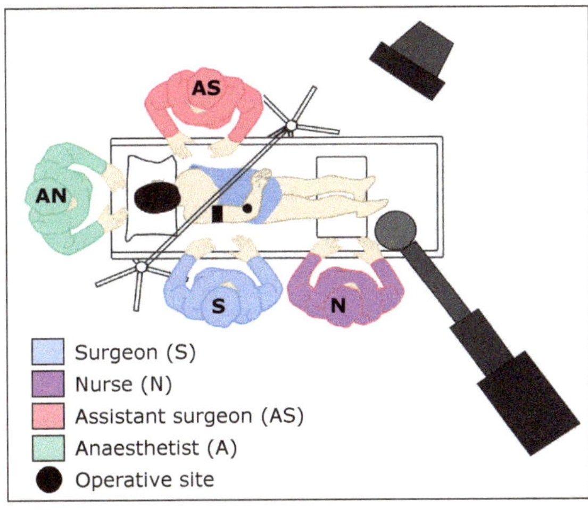

Fig. 14.3*: Position of the patient for fixation of medial epicondyle fractures with the patient in prone position and shoulder in full internal rotation so as to expose the medial aspect of the elbow.*

- After painting and draping and elevation of tourniquet, a 5 cm long incision is made over the medial supracondylar ridge extending upto and beyond the medial epicondyle.
- The ulnar nerve is exposed and retracted medially and posteriorly away from the fracture site **(Fig. 14.4)**.
- The medial epicondyle fragment along with the attached common flexor mass is identified (either intra or extra-articular). Care is taken to keep the soft tissue attachments of the medial epicondye intact. In case of incarcerated fragments, the ulnar nerve is usually entrapped or in close proximity to the

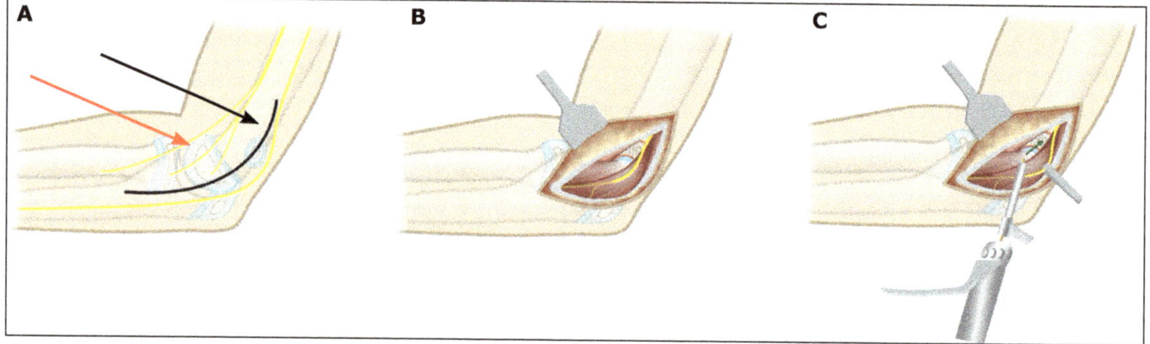

***Fig. 14.4**: (A) The exposure of the medial epicondyle through the medial approach (Black arrow) (keeping the antebrachial cutaneous nerve safe (Red arrow). (B) The ulnar nerve is retracted posteriorly and (C) The guide wire/K-wire is passed with a drill sleeve so as to protect the ulnar nerve.*

medial epicondyle and hence has to be carefully separated and retracted away **(Fig. 14.5)**.

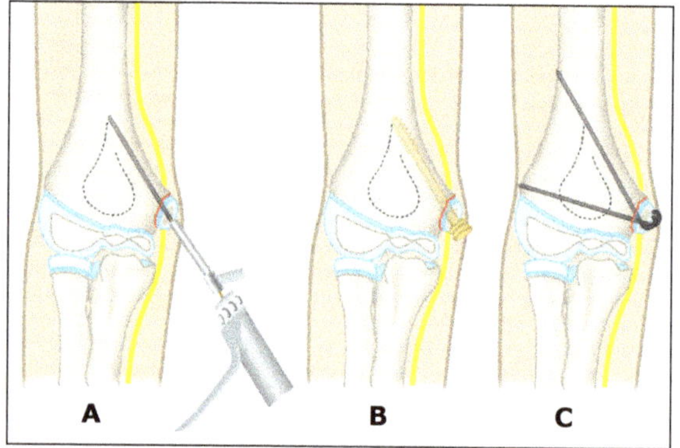

***Fig. 14.5**: Different methods of fixation of medial epicondyle fractures (A) Passing a guide wire (B) followed by fixation using a single cannulated cancellous screw or (C) by two divergent K-wires.*

- Reduction is performed either manually or with the help of small tenaculum clamps grasping the flexor-pronator mass (and not the fragment *per se*).
- Typically, the fragment gets reduced by flexion of the wrist and fingers so as to decrease the pull of the common flexor group.
- Once reduction is obtained, fixation is performed using a single 4-4.5mm cannulated cancellous screw. This screw may not be bicortical and can stop at the medial column in the dense cancellous bone. Usually a washer is used. Care should be taken that the fragment doesn't shatter or spin during drilling. Avoid over-tightening the screw. The author's preferred method of fixation is a 4.5 mm self-drilling/ self-tapping cannulated cancellous screw **(Figs. 14.6 and 14.7)**.
- Augmentation of fixation should be performed using thick non-absorbable sutures passed through the flexor-pronator mass and through the periosteum of the medial supracondylar ridge.
- Anatomical reduction of the joint as well as the fragment is confirmed on C-arm.
- Wound is closed and above elbow slab is applied.
- Mobilisation can be started early at around 2-3 weeks to prevent stiffness.

c) *Displaced fractures incarcerated in the joint with elbow dislocation:* This is an absolute indication for fixation of medial epicondyle fractures. The elbow has to be approached through the medial approach, ulnar nerve isolated

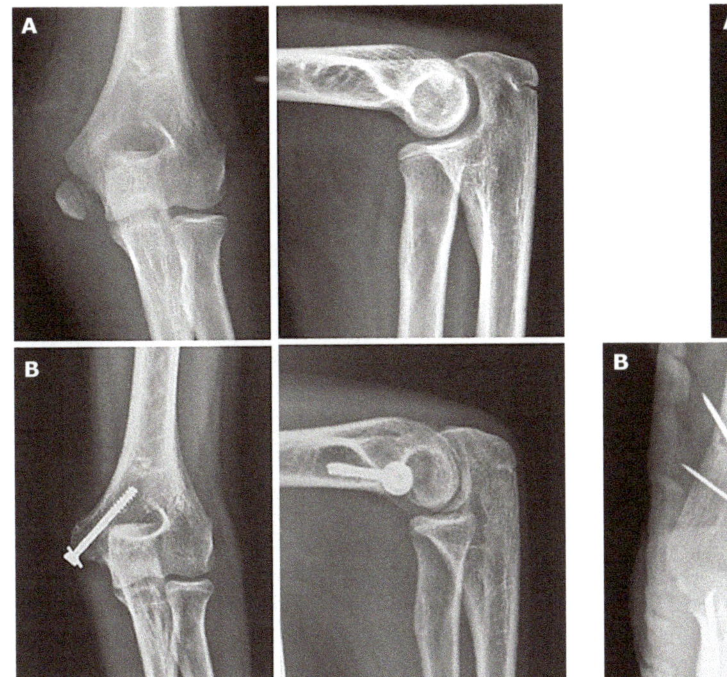

***Fig. 14.6**: (A) AP and lateral X-rays of the elbow in the dominant arm in a young gymnast showing a displaced medial epicondyle fracture (B) Treatment by open reduction and internal fixation using 4.5 mm CC screw showing excellent healing at 3 months post-operative.*

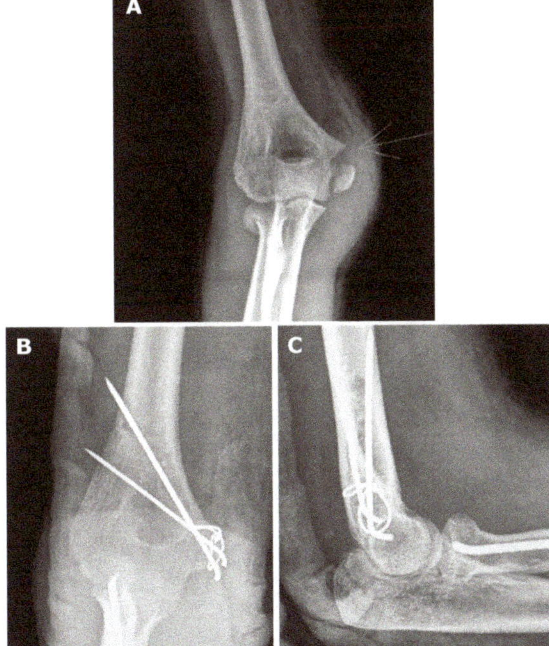

***Fig. 14.7**: Another method of fixation of displaced medial epicondyle fracture (A) using 2 divergent K-wires and TBW wire through flexor-pronator mass (B/C). The child incidentally also had a displaced radial neck fracture which was fixed with titanium elastic nail by the Metazieu technique.*

very carefully as it can be inside the elbow joint, medial epicondyle removed from the elbow joint with the common flexors and fixation done using semi threaded 4mm cannulated cancellous screws. Immobilisation has to be done for a slightly prolonged period to allow the soft tissues to heal **(Fig. 14.8)**.

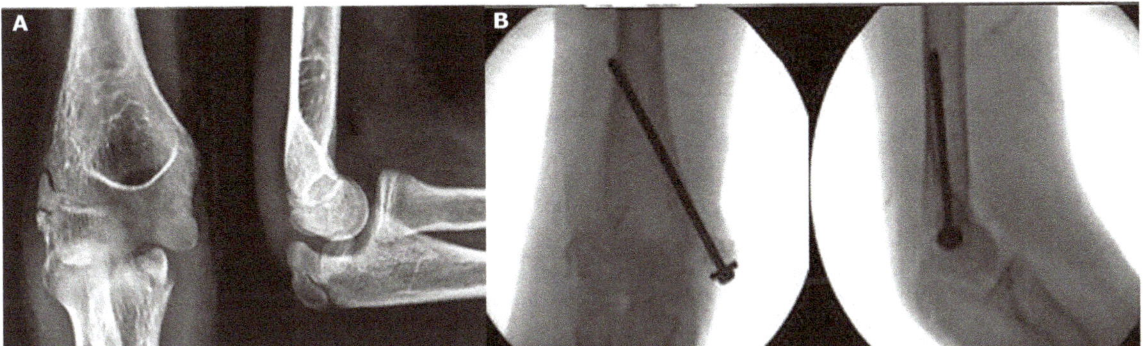

***Fig. 14.8**: (A) AP and lateral X-ray of elbow of a 10-year-old boy with elbow dislocation which was reduced but with an incarcerated medial epicondylar fragment (B) Post-operative C-arm picture of the same child after open reduction of the elbow dislocation and fixation of medial epicondyle with 4mm CC screw.*

Complications

A) *Late ulnar nerve dysfunction:* The incidence of this complication is about 10-15% when the fragment is outside the joint and is almost 50% when the fragment is incarcerated. The ulnar nerve dysfunction has been shown to be more in patients with incarcerated medial epicondyles in whom manipulative reduction is attempted before definitive fixation. The usual cause of this complication is a thick fascial band which develops between the ulnar nerve and the underlying muscle. This fascial band causes constriction and may require to be released.

B) *Symptomatic non-union and valgus instability:* Though radiological non-union of the medial epicondyle occurs in almost 40-50% of all fractures, only a small proportion of them lead to symptoms of pain and valgus instability. This is seen more in high level athletes who use the upper limb extensively like gymnasts and swimmers. The treatment of this condition is difficult and requires compression and fixation with / without bone grafting.

C) Hypertrophy of the medial epicondyle along with myositis ossificans.

3) Transphyseal Injuries of the Distal Humerus

Introduction and Mechanism of Injury

- Transphyseal injuries are extremely rare injuries occurring almost exclusively below 6 years of age.
- Transphyseal fractures occur in three instances:

1) Birth trauma: This is the commonest mechanism of injury especially when the arm gets entrapped during normal vaginal or caeserian section deliveries.
2) Non-accidental trauma: this is the second most common cause, especially when there is a twisting injury.
3) Trauma: This is quite uncommon but can occur when there is a posterior displacement with rotational movement.

Clinical Features

- The commonest presentation is that of a newborn child who has had a difficult delivery and then presents with painful pseudoparalysis of the upper limb.
- Initially it is many a time misdiagnosed as brachial plexus birth injury or an "elbow dislocation". However it can be easily differentiated from BPBI by the fact that there is significant amount of pain on movement and by the presence of swelling over the elbow. There may be some soft crepitus around the elbow.
- Older kids usually have severe swelling over the elbow with contusion on both sides of the elbow. A careful history is needed to rule out non-accidental trauma and appropriate social services references need to be done.

Imaging

- It is extremely difficult to diagnose transphyseal injuries since they occur in very young age and the entire distal humerus epiphysis is unossified. On plain X-rays, hence it is often diagnosed as an elbow dislocation. The diagnostic feature is that there is *posteromedial* displacement of the distal fragment as against *posterolateral* displacement seen in elbow dislocation **(Fig. 14.9)**.
- In most cases, a good quality AP and lateral plain X-ray is sufficient for diagnosis. In some, an arthrogram may be needed for the exact diagnosis.
- In older kids, MRI helps for documentation of the epiphyseal displacement and confirmation of diagnosis.

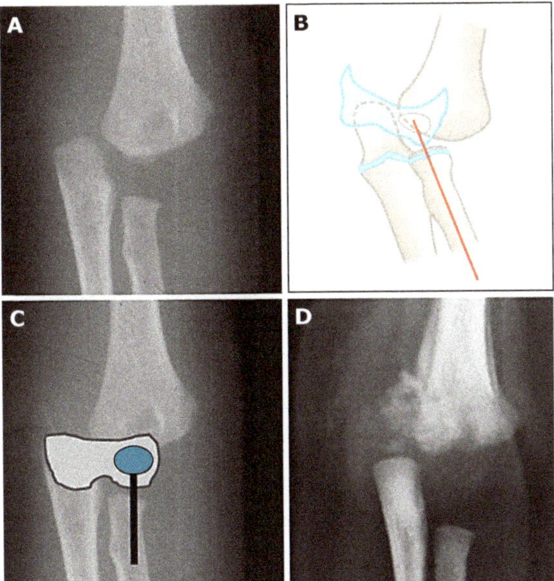

***Fig. 14.9**: (A) Pre-operative AP X-ray of a neonate with Transphyseal injury of elbow showing postero-medial displacement of the radio-ulnar complex. (B,C) Schematic diagram showing the radiocapitellar line which was lined up with the capitellar which denotes the injury proximal to the capitellum. (D) One month post-trauma radiograph showing good callus formation.*

Treatment

- The treatment of neonatal transphyseal injuries is dependent on the day of presentation to the orthopaedic surgeon.
- In case, the child is referred early (within two to three days) to the orthopaedic surgeon, an attempt can be made to reduce the fracture. Here the varus or the medial translation needs to be corrected and can be repositioned in a slab or a cast with a valgus mould. In rare cases, closed reduction under anaesthesia, arthrogram and K-wire fixation can be attempted. However performing a surgical procedure on a few-day old child is a challenge by itself.
- The usual presentation is at around 7 days post trauma at which time the fracture has already become a bit sticky. Here there is very little mobility and no attempt should be made at forceful reduction. A well moulded above elbow slab is enough for uneventful healing.
- In older kids, the treatment of choice is closed reduction and internal fixation with K-wires in a cross configuration.

Complications and Outcome

Transphyseal injuries of the distal humerus have a fairly good outcome in terms of healing. Kids may have some residual varus, which may or may not remodel. A call can be taken at around 2 years post trauma as to the need for corrective osteotomy and fixation.

4) Lateral Epicondylar Fractures

Lateral epicondylar fractures are extremely uncommon elbow injuries which are seen typically in older kids nearing adolescence.

Mecahnism of Injury

In children, the mechanism of injury is usually an avulsion injury of a part of the common extensor origin with extension of the elbow. In older children, adolescents or children very near skeletal maturity, the mechanism of injury can be a direct trauma to the lateral side of the elbow.

Clinical Features

The child presents with pain and swelling around the lateral aspect of the elbow. There is usually no deformity and very little contusion.

Imaging

Usually a plain radiograph of the elbow-AP, lateral and internal oblique view is sufficient for the diagnosis of this injury. This fracture is confused with the normal undulating physis of the distal humerus and vice versa. In this case, an opposite side elbow X-ray is of utmost importance to diagnose this fracture.

Treatment

The treatment of lateral epicondylar fractures (unless in rare circumstances when it is incarcerated) is conservative. An above elbow plaster cast in 90° flexion for about three weeks usually heals this fracture without any complications.

5) Olecranon Fractures

Introduction

Olecranon fractures are uncommon elbow injuries accounting for only about 2-3% of all elbow injuries in children. They usually occur in older children and around adolescence.

Mechanism of Injury

There are three mechanisms of injury:

1) Flexion type fractures- which have a failure of the *tension* side of the bone (posterior surface) followed by articular surface and then followed by complete avulsion.

2) Extension type injuries (Varus/ valgus): These injuries occur when the child falls on the outstretched hand with the elbow in extension. Usually when the elbow hyperextends, the olecranon hits against the supracondylar ridge leading to a supracondylar fracture. However, in the interim if there is a valgus or varus force, the olecranon fractures with a greenstick on the medial or lateral side respectively. The extension of this type of injury can carry the fracture line laterally and have a resultant fracture of the radial head or a type 3 Monteggia. The usual fracture line in this injury is at a level below the coronoid.

3) Direct trauma: This occurs when there is a direct trauma to the posterior aspect of the proximal ulna/olecranon and causes a shear injury. This is an extremely rare injury.

Classification

There are three types of olecranon fractures:

1) Fractures involving proximal apophysis of the olecranon
2) Metaphyseal fractures of the olecranon
3) Fractures of the coronoid process

Clinical Features

The child typically presents with pain on the posterior aspect of the elbow along with significant swelling. The child may also have restricted anti-gravity extension of the elbow in case of complete fractures.

Imaging

AP and lateral X-ray views of the elbow are sufficient to diagnose these injuries. In case of doubtful cases of apophyseal injuries, an opposite side X-ray may be necessary for confirmation.

Treatment

Non-operative management may be sufficient for most undisplaced or minimally displaced fractures with an above elbow cast in extension of the elbow.

Operative management is in the form of percutaneous or open reduction and K-wire/ screw fixation in case of displaced fractures with displacement of more than 4mm **(Fig. 14.10)**.

Complications

These fractures usually heal with very few complications like apophyseal arrest, delayed union, and restricted elbow extension.

6) Elbow Dislocation

Introduction

Elbow dislocations are uncommon elbow injuries and are usually associated with concomitant bony injuries in almost 50% of all cases.

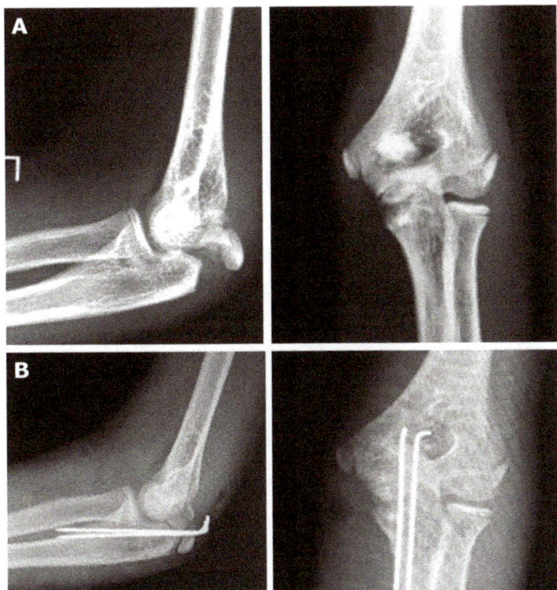

***Fig. 14.10**: (A) AP and lateral X-ray of the elbow in a 9-year-old child showing dispaced fracture of the olecranon (B) treated by open reduction and internal fixation with K-wire and trans-osseus suturing through the triceps by thick non-absorbable suture.*

Classification

1) Posterior elbow dislocation
2) Medial/ lateral elbow dislocation
3) Proximal radio-ulnar translocation

a) Posterior elbow dislocation:

   The typical mechanism of injury of posterior elbow dislocation in a child is a valgus force in an extended elbow which leads to a failure of the medial collateral ligament followed by posterior displacement of the proximal radius-ulna.

Clinical Features

The child usually has severe elbow pain and a grotesque deformity around the elbow. This leads to a prominence of the posterior aspect of the elbow with the olecranon jutting out posteriorly. There are common bony, soft tissue and neurovascular concomitant injuries:

- Concommitant bony injuries (Seen in almost 50%):

  Medial epicondyle, coronoid process and radial head and neck.

- Concomitant soft tissue injuries:

  Anterior capsule, Medial collateral ligament and annular ligament.

- Neurovascular concomitant injuries:

  Ulnar nerve (most common) associated with medial epicondylar fractures. The vascular injuries associated are injuries to the anterior recurrent ulnar artery and the inferior ulnar collateral artery.

Imaging

Plain X-rays of the elbow- AP and lateral views are sufficient for diagnosis and management in most cases. In some cases, MRI may be required for diagnosis of concomitant ligamentous injuries.

Treatment

The treatment of acute posterior dislocation of the elbow is usually non-operative and consists of closed reduction under sedation and short general anaesthetic.

There are two techniques for reduction of posterior elbow dislocation:

1) *Puller technique:* In this method, with the elbow flexed to 90°, the distal forearm is "pulled" with a counter-traction being given to distal aspect of the humerus by the assistant. Any medio-lateral force as necessary is applied depending on the direction of initial displacement.
2) *Pusher technique:* In this method, with the elbow again flexed 90°, the olecranon is "pushed" distally by the thumb of the surgeon while the entire hand gives counter-traction on the distal humerus by providing posteriorly directed force.

Operative Treatment

Operative treatment is indicated only in cases of neglected elbow dislocations, recurrent dislocation or associated bony or soft tissue injuries.

The operative treatment for neglected and recurrent elbow dislocations is beyond the purview of this book.

Elbow TRASH lesions

(The Radiographic Appearance Seemed Harmless)

There is a small group of elbow injuries which are easily missed on primary radiographs due to their benign appearance. But if treated incorrectly or insufficiently, they have the potential to cause long term issues in elbow function. They are primarily osteochondral injuries which occur in children below 10 years of age which follow elbow dislocations and spontaneous relocations. The conditions which are included in this group are:

1) Epiphyseal separations
2) Displaced intra-articular fractures of the medial condyles
3) Capitellar shear fractures
4) Radial head fractures with radiocapitellar subluxation
5) Osteochondral fractures of the olecranon, radial head and distal humerus with joint incongruity.
6) Lateral condylar avulsion shear fractures

The exact treatment of individual TRASH lesions may be beyond the purview of this book but the principles of management of these lesions are:

1) Any elbow injury with significant trauma, significant swelling and pain but with seemingly normal plain radiographs need to be considered as TRASH lesions unless proved otherwise.
2) MRI is the investigation of choice
3) Fixation is usually required and should be rigid to allow early range of motion.
4) Even with the best of treatment, it may be associated with significant long term elbow stiffness and a detailed informed consent needs to be taken regarding the same.

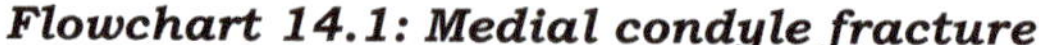

Flowchart 14.1: Medial condyle fracture

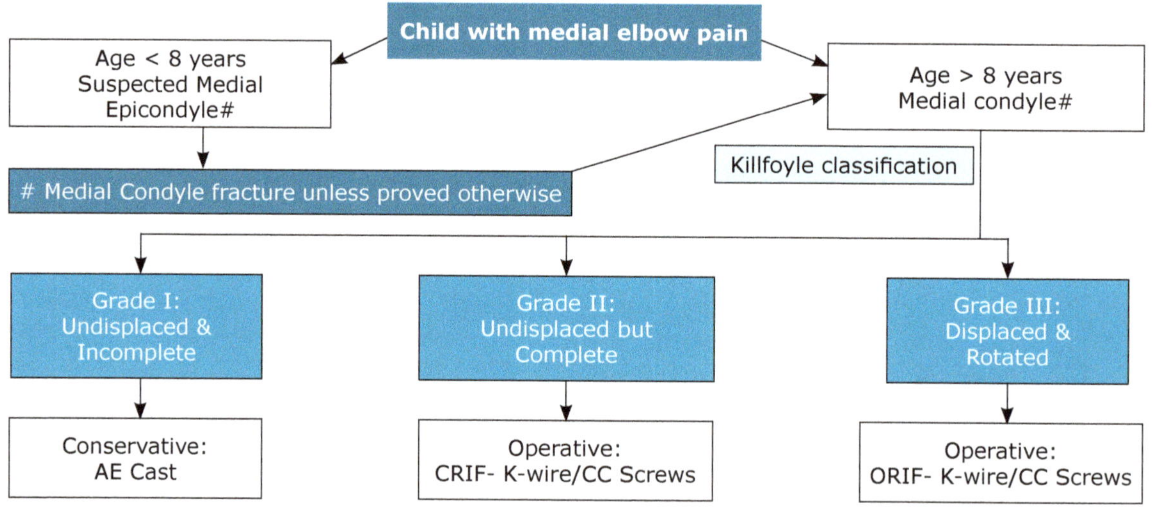

Flowchart 14.2: Medial Epicondyle fracture

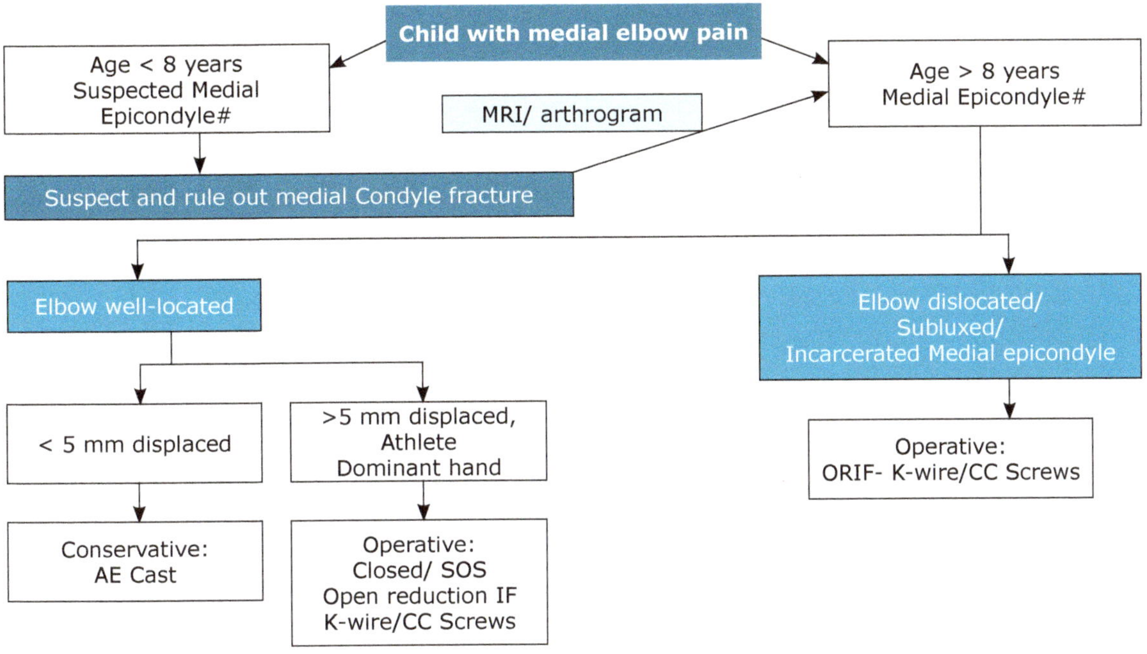

Flowchart 14.3: Trans-physeal injury distal humerus

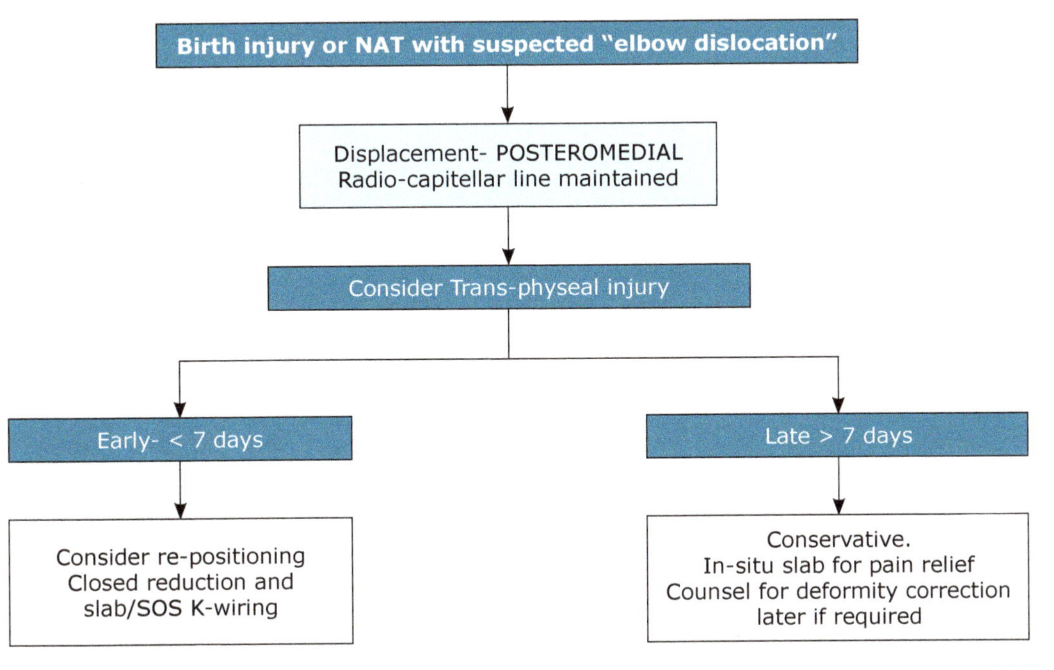

Flowchart 14.4: Elbow TRASH lesions

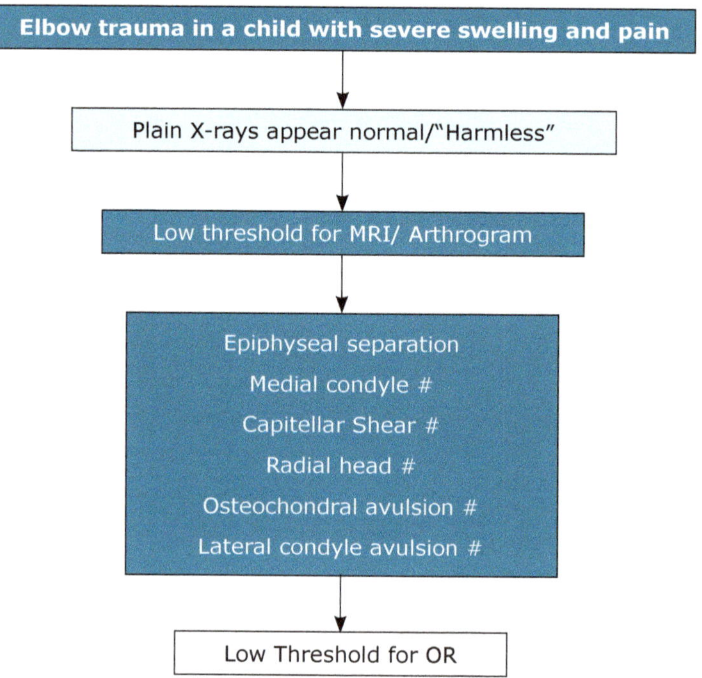

15 Radius and Ulna Shaft Fractures

Introduction

Fractures of the forearm bones are the commonest reason for children receiving orthopaedic treatment. Despite a high incidence, these fractures continue to challenge the clinician due to the wide variation in presentations, management options as well as complications. Though there has been a slightly increased rate of surgical fixation of these fractures in the last few years, the treatment of choice in most cases remains skillful conservative plaster casting, and it is imperative for all orthopaedic surgeons to master the art and science of good plastering, moulding, plaster care as well as re-manipulation of fractures.

Relevant Anatomy

Bony anatomy

The forearm anatomy is complex with the forearm bones articulating with each other through two joints (the distal radio-ulnar joint and the proximal radio-ulnar joint). The radius and ulna are also connected to each other through the tough interosseous membrane which runs from the ulna to the radius in a distal-ward manner and is the thickest in the middle third of the forearm. On the whole, the forearm can be described as a single non-synovial joint with an almost 180° arc of rotation.

The ulna is a relatively straight bone which has a very stable hinge articulation with the humerus at the elbow joint and is virtually subcutaneous through most of its length. It has a dorsal bow and ends in the ulnar styloid.

The radius on the other hand is a double-curved bone with a lateral bow of around 15° which peaks at around 60% of the length of the bone (commonly known as the *radial bow*) and a second smaller curve of around 10° which is apex medial near the upper third close to the bicipital tuberosity. The radial bow is an important factor for forearm rotations **(Fig. 15.1)**.

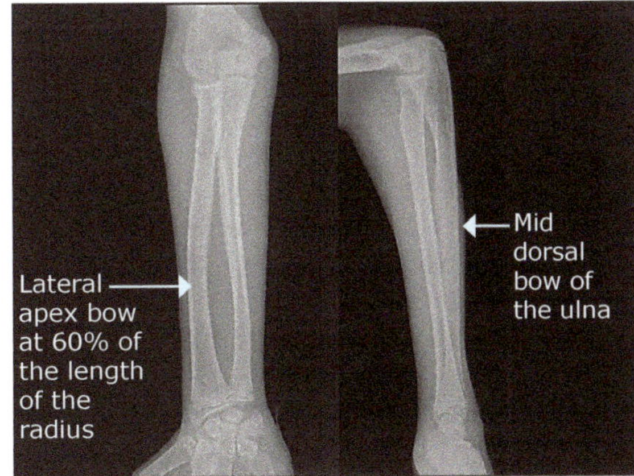

***Fig. 15.1**: Bony anatomy of radius and ulna.*

Muscular anatomy

The powerful supinators are attached to the proximal third of the forearm while the pronators are attached to the middle and distal third of the forearm **(Fig. 15.2)**.

Nerves and vessels of the forearm

- The radial nerve (terminating into the superficial radial and posterior interosseous nerves), the median nerve (terminating in the anterior interosseous nerve) and ulnar nerve are the three nerves of the forearm.

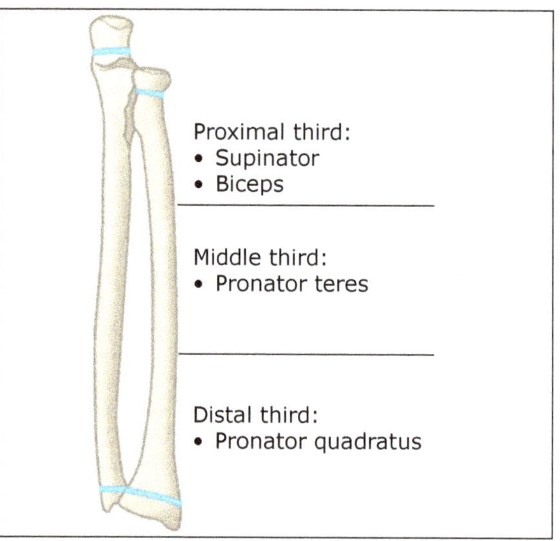

***Fig. 15.2**: Division of forearm into proximal, middle and distal thirds based on insertion of supinator and pronator muscles on the radius.*

- The brachial artery divides into the radial and the ulnar artery in the proximal third of the forearm. The radial artery is the predominant vessel of the forearm, but the ulnar artery can take over the radial vascular territory in case of any vascular trauma or surgical excision of the radial artery **(Fig. 15.3)**.

Classification

Mehlmann classified forearm fractures based on bones involved, levels and common types:

A) Based on number of bones involved:

- Single bone forearm fractures
- Both bone forearm fractures

B) Based on location:

- Upper third: Biceps and Supinator territory
- Middle third: Pronator teres territory
- Lower third: Pronator quadratus territory

C) Based on types:

- Torus fractures
- Greenstick fractures
- Plastic deformations
- Complete fractures

Clinical features

Forearm fractures usually occur following a fall on outstretched hand or a direct fall on the forearm.

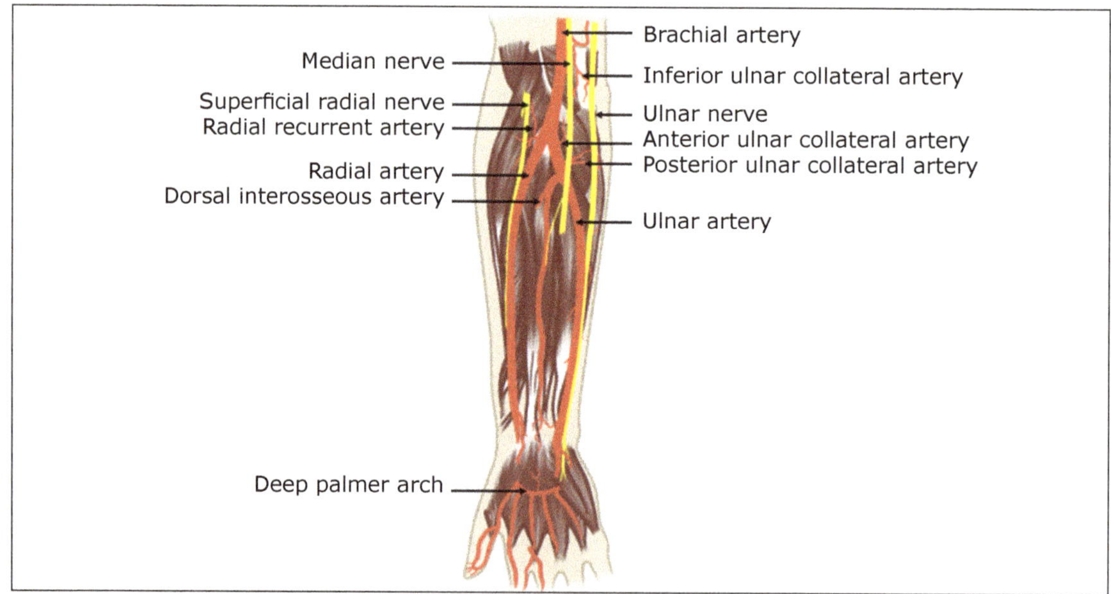

***Fig. 15.3**: Neuro-Vascular anatomy of the forearm*

Whereas pure bending forces without rotational component are responsible for forearm greenstick injuries with radius and ulna fractured at the same level, rotational deforming forces are implicated in the causation of injuries in which the radius and ulna are fractured at different levels. Pronation forces are responsible for fractures with apex dorsal angulation. On the other hand, fractures with apex volar angulation are caused due to supination forces **(Fig. 15.4)**. This information is vital in choosing closed reduction manoeuvre as described in the section on treatment.

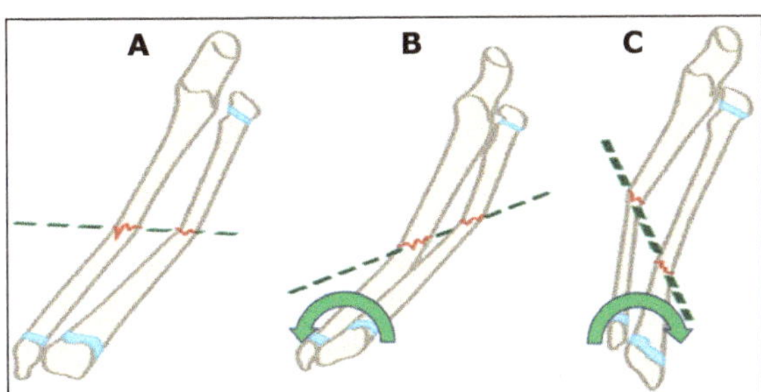

***Fig. 15.4**: Mechanism of injury in greenstick fractures of the radius and ulna: (A) When fractures of radius and ulna are at the same level, the mechanism of injury is pure bending force. On the other hand, (B) pronation rotatory force results in fracture with apex dorsal angulation, and (C) supination rotatory force results in fracture with apex volar angulation.*

Clinically, tenderness, swelling, deformity and restriction of range of forearm rotations may be observed. Clinical evaluation must include examination of neurovascular status and signs of impending or established compartment syndrome, especially in high velocity injuries and "floating elbow" injuries (fractures of radius and ulna with associated supracondylar humerus fracture). In incomplete fractures, the signs and symptoms can be very subtle and may be limited to just restriction of rotations especially supination, in minimally displaced greenstick fractures.

Imaging

AP and lateral plain X-rays are sufficient for diagnosis of radius-ulna fractures. The X-rays should include elbow and wrist joints to rule out associated elbow/wrist fractures and Monteggia/Galeazzi injuries.

In fracture radius ulna, the X-rays should be carefully evaluated to determine magnitude of radial bowing, angulation, rotation, translation and over-riding at the fracture site.

Radial bowing

As mentioned in the section of bony anatomy, radius has a lateral bow of about 15° which peaks at about 60% of its length. This bow should be restored during reduction for complete restoration of prono-supination movements.

Angulation

- It is relatively easy to assess the angulation on plain X-rays and can be measured with reasonable reliability. However, it should be borne in mind that if there is angulation in both antero-posterior and lateral radiographs, then it indicates an oblique plane deformity with the magnitude of deformity being greater than that seen in either AP or lateral views.
- As a general rule, angulation in the radius ulna fractures results in decreased range of prono-supination. The more proximal the fracture, the greater the restriction of forearm rotations.
- Since ulna is a subcutaneous bone, dorsal angulation at ulna fracture site results in poor cosmesis.

Rotation

- Malrotation in fracture radius-ulna needs proper analysis and if under-estimated can have serious consequences in terms of loss of prono-supination movements.

- One method of analyzing rotational alignment in forearm fracture is by assessing the positions of the bicipital and radial tuberosities on anteroposterior radiographs. If the rotational alignment is maintained, in a fully supinated forearm the bicipital tuberosity is seen to be pointing medially and the radial tuberosity laterally.
- Similarly, in the ulna, an anteriorly oriented coronoid process and posterior ulna styloid process in lateral radiograph of a fully supinated forearm indicates normal rotational alignment **(Fig. 15.5)**.
- *Radius cross-over sign* is a recently described radiological sign which is extremely useful to assess rotational alignment in forearm fractures. It is applied as follows:

• Full-length X-ray of the forearm from the elbow to the wrist is obtained, with the distal humerus seen in AP profile. In this X-ray, in a forearm with normal rotational alignment:

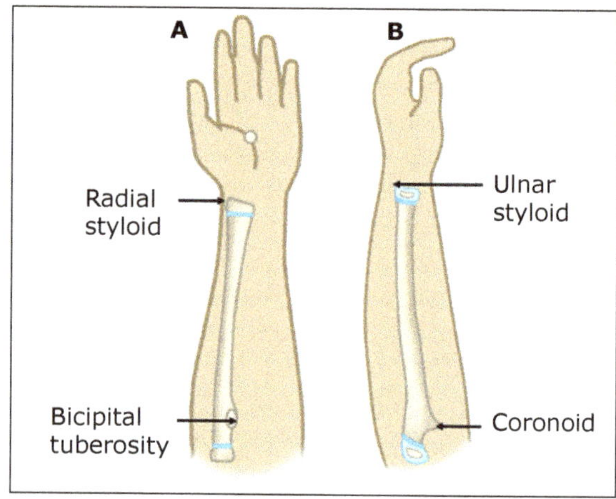

***Fig. 15.5**: (A) Medially pointing bicipital tuberosity and laterally pointing radial styloid process in anteroposterior radiograph of fully supinated forearm (B) Anteriorly pointing coronoid process and posteriorly pointing ulna styloid process in lateral radiograph of fully supinated forearm.*

(1) If the forearm is in full pronation, the radius crosses over the ulna in the upper third

(2) If the forearm is in neutral rotation, the radius crosses over the ulna in the lower third

(3) If the forearm is in full supination, the radius and ulna don't overlap **(Fig. 15.6)**.

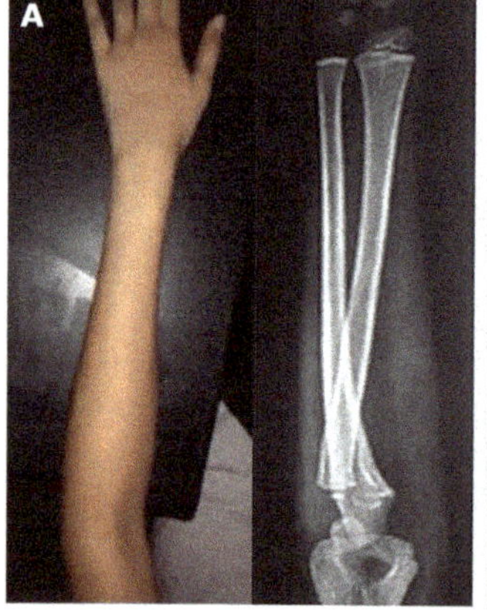

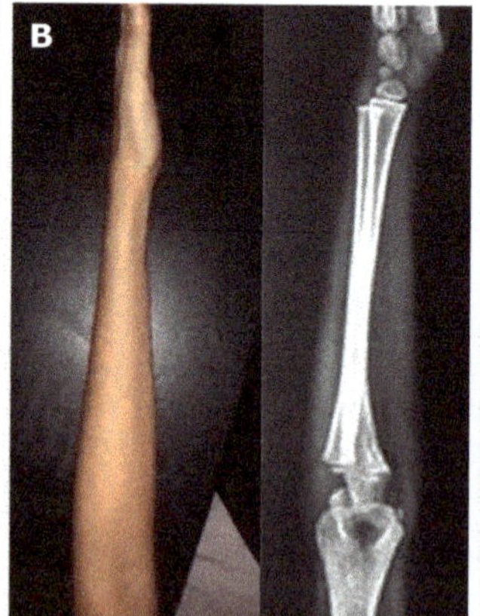

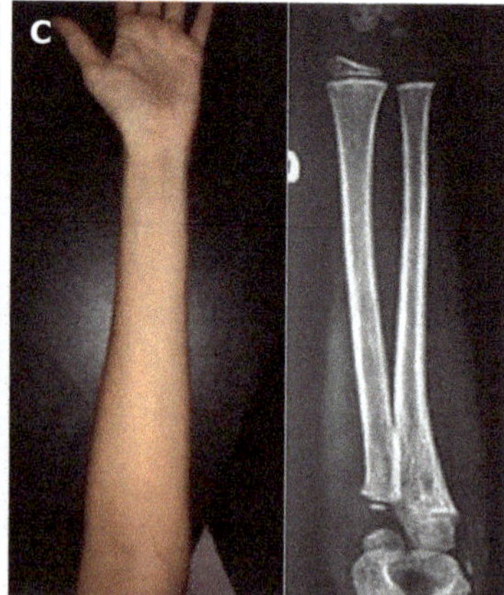

***Fig. 15.6**: AP X-rays of the forearm with the distal humerus seen in AP profile: (A) In full pronation, the radius crosses over the ulna in the proximal third (B) In neutral rotation, the radius crosses over the ulna in the distal third (C) In full supination, the radius does not cross over the ulna.*

Rotational malalignment at the level of the fracture can be identified if there is any mis-match between the alignment of the proximal and distal fragments. For example, **Figure 15.7A** is the AP X-ray of an 8 years old male child presenting with 3 months old fracture mid-shaft radius ulna treated with above-elbow cast application. Here the radius crosses over the ulna in the proximal third indicating that the proximal fragment is in full pronation. However, the position of the wrist indicates that the distal fragment is in mid-supination. This suggests that the distal fragment is in almost 120^{0} malrotation with respect to the proximal fragment. The child underwent a corrective osteotomy following which the rotational alignment of the proximal and distal fragments was restored **(Fig. 15.7B)**.

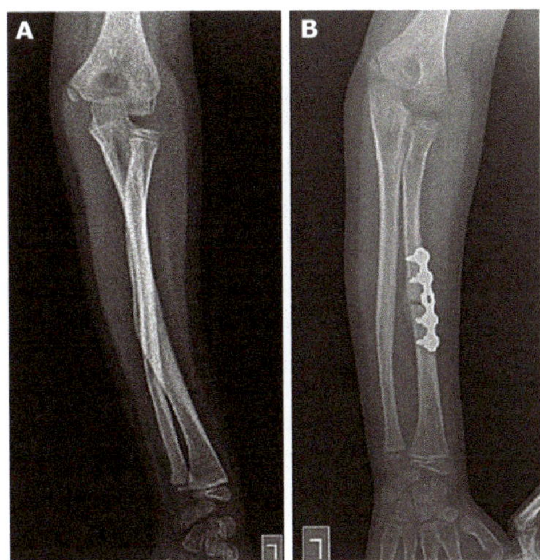

***Fig. 15.7**: Malunited fracture radius ulna (A) Proximal fragment in full pronation and distal fragment in mid-supination as assessed by the radius cross over sign (B) After corrective osteotomy, the rotational alignment is restored.*

Translation/over-riding

- Translation and over-riding are relatively better tolerated than angulation and rotation.
- 100% translated fractures of single or both bones, especially of the distal third are shown to completely and reliably remodel and have an excellent outcome.
- Over-riding of upto 1cm is well tolerated and is in fact supposed to be beneficial for restoration of range of motion through interosseous membrane relaxation.
- However, while accepting translation/ overlap in radius-ulna fracture, care should be taken to ensure that there is no encroachment of the interosseous space, which can result in restriction of prono-supination.
- Also, remodelling may not occur in the desired manner if less than 2 years of growth are left and hence adolescent fractures need to be treated with a much lower threshold for surgical treatment than younger children.

The acceptability criteria for radius-ulna fractures are summarised in **Table 15.1** below *(Price and Noonan criteria)*.

Treatment

Non-operative treatment

Majority of forearm fractures in children are treated non-operatively. Non-operative treatment consists of closed reduction and immobilisation in above-elbow cast. Closed reduction is not needed if

Table 15.1: Acceptability criteria for radius and ulna fractures

Age	Angulation	Malrotation	Displacement	Loss of radial bow
< 8 years	15^{0}	45^{0}	Complete	Yes
> 8 years	10^{0}	30^{0}	Complete	Partial

the fracture is in acceptable alignment at presentation. In such cases, above-elbow Cast may be applied in the Out-Patient Department without the need for sedation or anaesthesia. However, should closed reduction be needed, sedation or anaesthesia must be administered.

In case of forearm swelling at initial presentation, a non-circumferential above-elbow slab may be initially applied, which may be converted to a cast once the swelling subsides.

Closed reduction of radius-ulna fractures: Reduction in forearm fractures is achieved by three-point pressure, with the central pressure point being at the convexity of the apex of the deformity and the proximal and distal pressure points being on the concavity.

Closed reduction of specific fracture patterns:

- **Plastic deformation:**

  Closed reduction of plastic deformation of radius-ulna should be performed when the deformity exceeds 10° with restriction of range of forearm rotations, especially in children more than 8 years age. The reduction manoeuvre consists of application of a strong, sustained force at the convex apex of the bowing for a period of 5 to 10 minutes. A rolled towel or the surgeon's knee may serve as the fulcrum **(Fig. 15.8)**. Following correction, a well-moulded above-elbow cast with three-point pressure is applied.

- **Greenstick fractures:**

  As mentioned earlier, greenstick injuries of the forearm with radius and ulna being fractured at different levels, occur due to rotational forces, which need to be reversed during closed reduction. Supination forces cause radius-ulna greenstick fractures with apex volar angulation and should be reduced by forearm pronation. Similarly, pronation forces cause greenstick fractures with apex dorsal angulation and should be reduced by supination.

  On the other hand, greenstick fractures with radius and ulna fractured at the same level are caused by bending forces and can be reduced by application of three-point pressure with the central pressure point at the apex of the deformity on the convex side.

  There is a controversy whether a greenstick fracture should be completed before reduction and cast application. Proponents claim lower rates of redisplacement within cast and more solid healing with lower refracture rates if the fracture is completed prior to reduction. However, benefits of fracture completion have not been validated in multiple studies. We don't recommend completion of the fracture, but we do perform slight exaggeration of deformity to unlock the fragments before reduction and cast application.

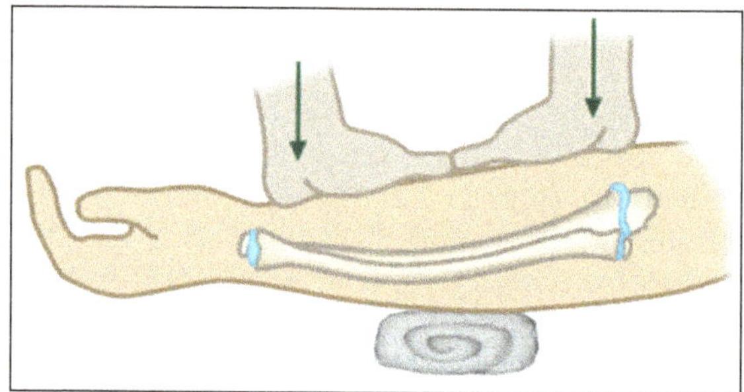

***Fig. 15.8**: Correction of plastic deformation of radius-ulna.*

- **Complete fractures:**

  Reduction of complete displaced fractures requires stretching of soft tissues which can be achieved by sustained manual traction. However despite sustained traction, reduction may not be achieved due to the thick, intact periosteum on the concave side of fracture. In these cases, reduction may be attempted by exaggeration of deformity at fracture site to relax the concave periosteum. Once reduction is achieved, the intact periosteum acts like a tension band and offers stability to prevent re-displacement **(Fig. 15.9)**.

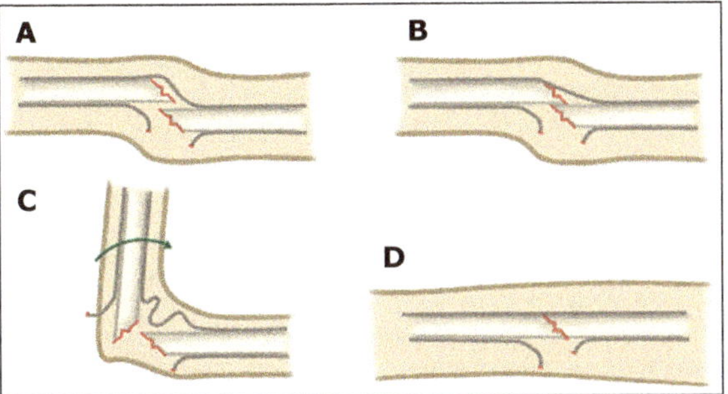

Fig. 15.9: *(A,B) Intact periosteum on the concave side of the fracture obstructs reduction in a completely displaced fracture (C) Hyper-exaggeration of deformity aids in relaxing the periosteum following which traction is applied (D) After reduction, tension band effect of the intact periosteum aids in maintaining reduction.*

Above Elbow Cast application in radius-ulna fractures:

Following reduction, an above-elbow cast should be applied, taking all precautions for safe cast application as mentioned in Chapter 3 on Casts and Splints. The steps of application above-elbow cast for forearm fractures are as follows:

(1) *Application of tubular bandage:* This is an optional step. The tubular bandage should extend from the axilla to beyond the MCP joints with a cut-out for the thumb.

(2) *Cast padding:* A single layer of cotton cast padding with overlap of half width should be applied from the axillary crease to the MCP joints. Extra padding should be applied at the olecranon bony prominence. There should be no crumpling of padding in the ante-cubital fossa.

(3) *Cast application:* A single layer of circumferential POP or fiberglass cast should be applied from the axilla to the distal palmar crease, with the elbow held in 90^0 flexion and forearm in appropriate rotation. The cast should be trimmed to allow free movements of the thumb and flexion of MCP joints. The cast material should be evenly distributed and the position of the limb should not be changed after application of first layer of cast material to avoid crumpling. The ends of the tubular bandage are then folded over the cast, following which another single layer of circumferential cast is applied. Care is taken that the edges of cast are smooth to avoid skin abrasions.

(4) *Moulding of cast:*

Moulding of the cast during cast setting is important to maintain the reduction achieved during closed reduction.

During cast setting, three-point pressure is applied to ensure adequate cast moulding. The central pressure point is at the convex apex of the fracture whereas the proximal and distal pressure points are on the concave side **(Fig. 15.10)**.

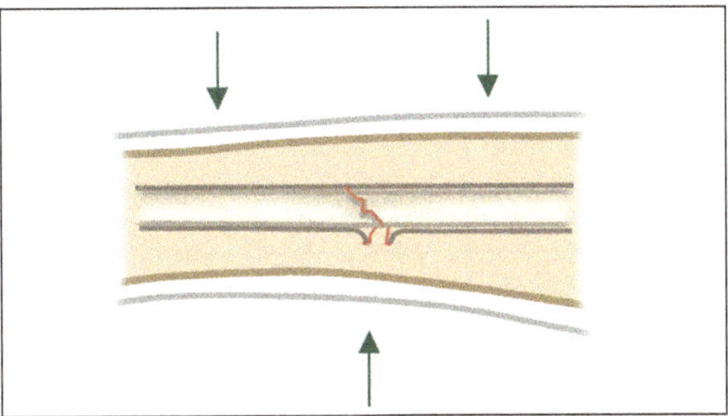

Fig. 15.10: *Three-point pressure moulding applied during cast setting with central pressure point at the convex apex of the fracture.*

Also, good interosseous mould is applied to achieve good spread of the interosseous membrane. The cast should be oval in cross-section with medial-lateral diameter more than anterior-posterior diameter **(Fig. 15.11).**

The cast index and various other indices such as padding index, three-point index, Canterbury index and gap index have been described to determine adequacy of cast moulding. These are described in greater detail in Chapter 16.

Additionally during cast setting, straight moulding of the dorsal border of ulna should be performed to avoid unsightly posterior angulation of the ulna.

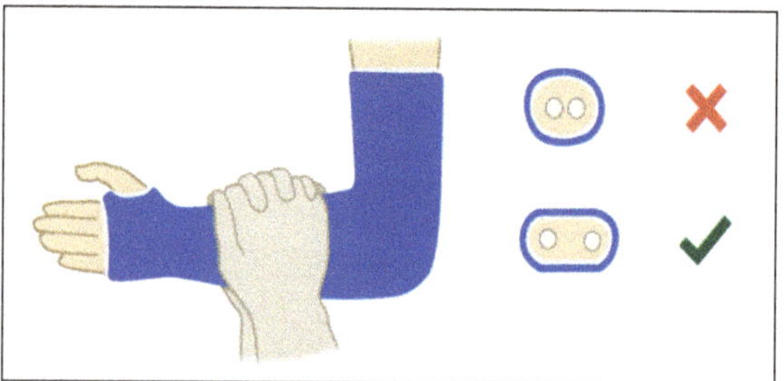

***Fig. 15.11**: Interosseous mould to achieve a good interosseous spread with oval cast.*

(5) *Position of forearm rotation* during immobilisation of complete forearm fractures is controversial. It is now accepted that the "rule of 3s", which recommends immobilisation of upper third fractures in supination, middle third in neutral and distal third in pronation is not valid. However we do prefer to immobilise proximal radius-ulna fractures in supination and fractures distal to pronator teres attachment in neutral.

(6) *Common pitfalls:*

Sometimes, radius ulna fractures of the proximal third angulate with a dorsal apex if the above elbow cast in applied in 90° elbow flexion. This occurs due to the deforming effect of the triceps on the proximal ulna fragment. In such cases, above-elbow casting in extension (elbow in 10 to 45° flexion) has been recommended for relaxing the triceps. Above-elbow cast in extension should have a good supracondylar mould and should incorporate the thumb in order to prevent cast slippage. Additionally, careful straight moulding of the dorsal border of ulna during cast setting is essential to avoid dorsal apex angulation at the ulna fracture site.

Follow-up

Following closed reduction and cast application, parents must be instructed to look for signs of compartment syndrome and to approach the hospital stat if any of these arise. Some surgeons perform bivalving of cast as a routine prophylactic measure against this rare but dreadful complication.

Weekly clinical and radiographic follow-up should be obtained for at least 3 weeks to watch for cast complications and re-displacement within cast.

In greenstick fractures, we prefer to continue cast immobilisation for at least 6 to 8 weeks to allow adequate fracture consolidation. Return to sports should be delayed for at least 3 months following trauma.

Operative treatment

Operative treatment in paediatric radius-ulna diaphyseal fractures is reserved for:

(a) Complete and displaced fractures in adolescents

(b) Open fractures

(c) Fractures associated with compartment syndrome

(d) Fractures associated with floating elbow injuries

(e) Unacceptable displacement following non-operative treatment

Surgical options:

The options for surgical management of radius-ulna shaft fractures include:

(1) Closed reduction and elastic nails fixation

(2) Open reduction and elastic nails fixation

(3) Open reduction and plate fixation

(4) External fixation (usually reserved for compound fractures)

Elastic nailing of radius-ulna shaft fractures

- Elastic nailing is a minimally invasive technique and can be performed closed or with minimal opening of fracture site. Hence, it is the ideal surgical procedure for fixation of radius ulna fractures in children.
- Various implants including K-wires, Rush nails, etc have been used, however Elastic Stable Intramedullary Nailing with Titanium Elastic Nails (TENS nails) is the most popular implant.

Principles:

- The ESIN technique for radius ulna fractures is based on achieving a stable three-point fixation in each bone. The proximal and distal fixation points are the proximal and distal metaphysis respectively. The central fixation point is at the convex apex of the pre-bent nail.
- The radius and ulna nails are inserted with their convexities facing laterally and medially respectively. This helps to achieve a "safety-pin" construct with spreading and stretching of the interosseous membrane which further increases fracture stability.

Implants and special requirements:

- TENS nail set with nails of all sizes, straight and curved awls, benders, T-handle with chuck, vice grips, slotted punch, hammer and nail cutter, periosteum elevators, Hohmann retractors, bone holding clamps (small) **(Fig. 15.12)**.
- Pneumatic tourniquet
- Image intensifier

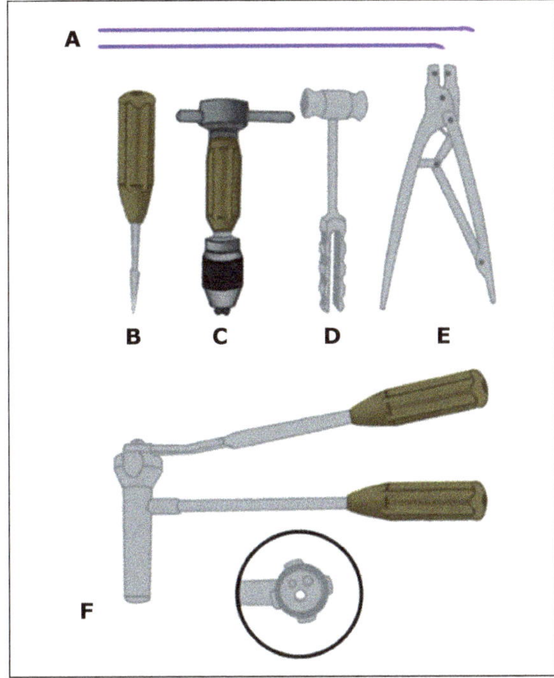

Fig. 15.12: *Instrument set for TENS nailing (A) TENS nails (2/2.5/3/3.5 and 4mm diameters, for radius-ulna usually 2 or 2.5mm nails are used (B) Bone awl (straight and curved) (C) T-handle with chuck (D) Mallet (E) Vice grip (F) Nail cutter.*

Patient positioning **(Fig. 15.13)**

- Supine with arm on radiolucent hand table
- Pneumatic tourniquet applied to upper arm
- A stirrup with folded towel placed at the level of the axilla gives counter-traction when traction is applied for fracture reduction

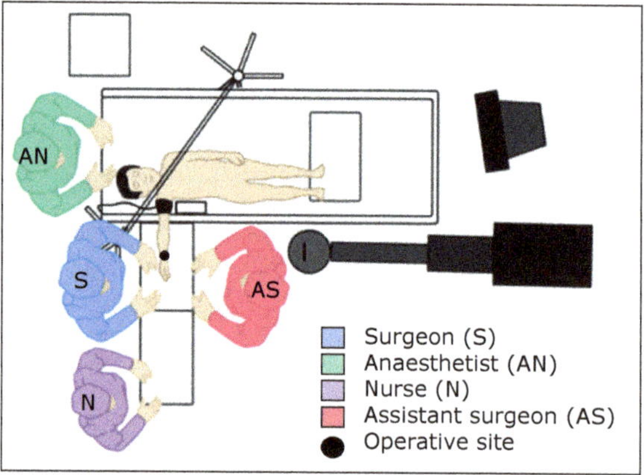

***Fig. 15.13**: Patient positioning for intramedullary nailing of radius-ulna fractures.*

Surgical technique:

In dual bone fixation, the radius nail is inserted first because manipulation of the elbow and reduction-nailing of the radius can be difficult after insertion of ulna nail.

Radius nail is always inserted retrograde and entry points for the same may be:

(1) Dorsal: This entry point is located just above the Lister's tubercle, about 2 cm proximal to the distal radius physis, between the 2nd (ECRL/ECRB) and 3rd (EPL) extensor compartments. The incision is about 2cm long extending from the entry point distally. The EPL tendon is identified and retracted during nail insertion **(Fig. 15.14a)**.

(2) Lateral: This entry point is located on the lateral aspect, proximal to the radius styloid process, just volar to the tendons of Extensor Pollicis Brevis (EPB) and Abductor Pollicis Longus (APL) (1st extensor compartment). The superficial radial nerve is at risk of injury in this approach **(Fig. 15.14b)**.

Ulna nail may be inserted either antegrade or retrograde and options for entry points may be

(1) Proximal metaphysis: The usually preferred entry point in the ulna is the proximal ulna metaphysis lateral aspect and is used for antegrade insertion of ulna nail **(Fig. 15.14c)**.

(2) Distal metaphysis: Distal ulna metaphyseal entry point is used for retrograde insertion of ulna nail and is located on the ulnar border about 1.5 cm above the distal ulna physis **(Fig. 15.14d)**.

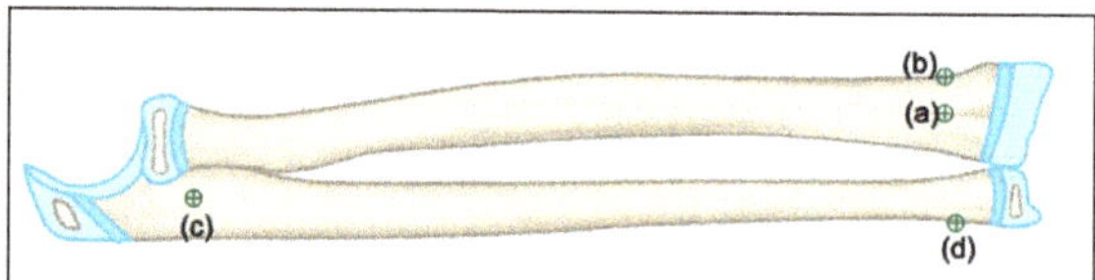

***Fig. 15.14**: Entry points for TENS nail in the radius and ulna (a) Radius dorsal entry point (b) Radius lateral entry point (c) Ulna proximal metaphyseal entry point (d) Ulna distal metaphyseal entry point.*

- A straight awl is inserted perpendicular to the bone to create the intial entry point. The awl is then inserted at 45° to the long axis of the bone to create tract for the elastic nail. Care should be taken to avoid perforation of the contralateral cortex.
- TENS nail of diameter equal to 60 to 70% of the narrowest diameter of the radius medullary canal is chosen. Typically radius isthmus is located in its mid portion. Usually TENS nails of 2 to 2.5 mm diameter are appropriate for fixation of paediatric radius ulna diaphyseal fractures.
- The nail is pre-bent such that the diameter of the bend is equal to three times the diameter of the bone. Also the apex of the bend should coincide with the level of the fracture.
- The nail is mounted on the T-handle with chuck and is introduced into the entry point, at an angle of 45° to long axis of shaft with the hockey-stick tip

pointing distally. Once the tip hits the opposite cortex, the nail is rotated through 180° so that the tip points towards the medullary canal. The convex side of the curved tip is then used to negotiate the contra-lateral cortex. If tip is impacted in contra-lateral cortex, nail is removed and tip is further bent to facilitate nail insertion **(Fig. 15.15).**

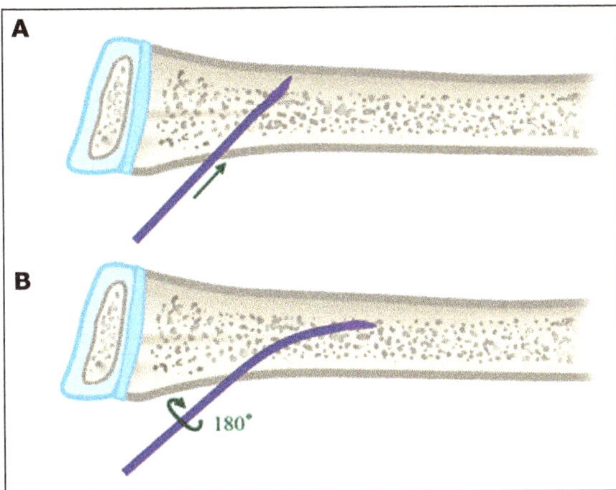

***Fig. 15.15**: Initial insertion of radius TENS nail (A) the nail is initially inserted with the hockey-stick tip pointing distally (B) after the nail tip hits the contra-lateral cortex, the nail is rotated so that the nail tip points towards the medullary canal.*

- Once in the medullary canal, the nail is advanced with rotatory movements till the nail tip reaches the fracture site **(Fig. 15.16).**

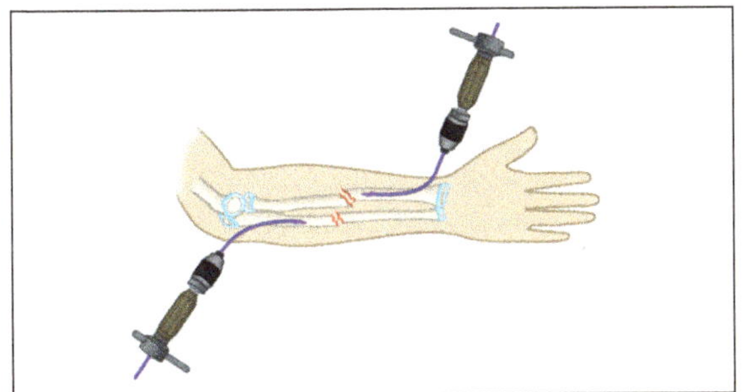

***Fig. 15.16**: Advancement of nail tip till fracture site.*

- In case of impaction in the medullary canal, the nail is withdrawn about 1cm, rotated by 90° and then re-advanced. Hammering of nail should be avoided to prevent shattering of cortex.
- Once the nail tip has reached the fracture site, closed reduction of the fracture is attempted by traction-counter traction and correction of angulation- translation **(Fig. 15.17).**

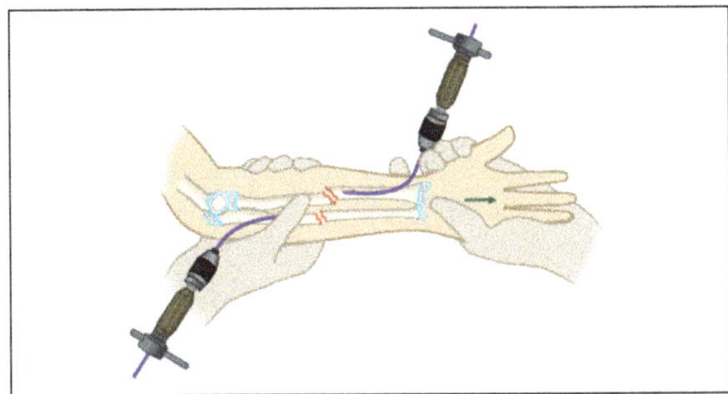

***Fig. 15.17**: Once the nail tip reaches the fracture site, the fracture is close reduced by traction-counter traction and digital pressure.*

- The F tool may be used to aid in reduction. In case of completely translated fractures, a K-wire introduced into the fracture site percutaneously may be used to lever the fragments into alignment.
- The nail may be rotated under image intensifier control so that the J shaped nail tip engages the medullary canal of the proximal fragment. The nail is then derotated to reduce the fracture **(Fig. 15.18).**
- If alignment is achieved with above closed reduction techniques, the nail is advanced across the fracture site and the nail tip is perched about 2cm beyond the fracture. Multiple failed attempts at passage of nail across the fracture site should be avoided as it damages the soft tissues of the forearm compartments thereby increasing the risk of compartment syndrome.

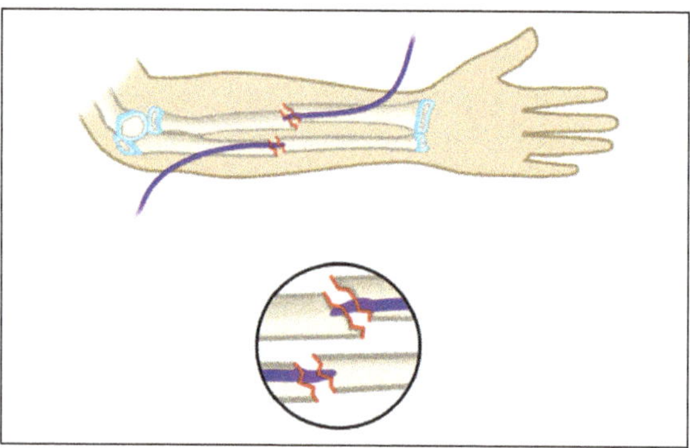

***Fig. 15.18**: Image intensifier guided rotation of nail tip for fracture reduction.*

- In case of failure of closed reduction, attempt may be made to insert the ulna nail first if closed reduction of ulna fracture looks feasible.
- Or else, minimal opening of the fracture site should be performed through a 3 to 4 cm incision using the volar Henry's approach (described in detail in section on plating). An assistant holds the fracture fragments with bone holding clamps while the surgeon advances the nail across the fracture site **(Fig. 15.19)**.

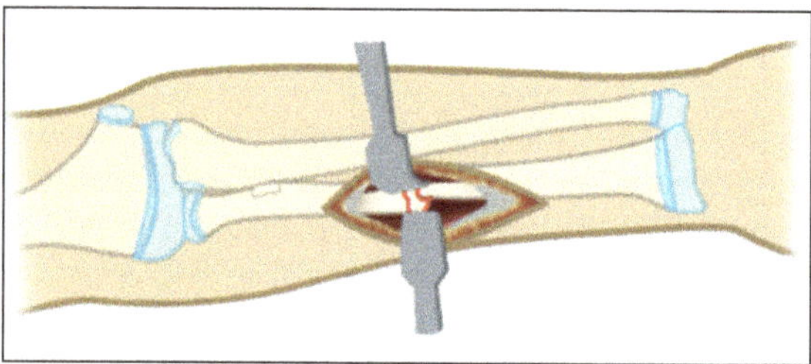

***Fig. 15.19**: Minimal opening of fracture site following failed closed reduction.*

- The radius nail is advanced only about 2 cm across the fracture site. Further insertion of radius nail is avoided at this stage, to facilitate easy manipulation of the ulna fracture site. The ulna nail is then advanced across the fracture site.
- Both radius and ulna nails are then advanced till their nail tips reach the bicipital tuberosity of the radius and distal metaphysis of ulna respectively. With the forearm supinated, the nails are then rotated such that convexity of the radius nail faces laterally and convexity of ulna nail faces dorso-medially. In this position, the normal radial bow of the radius and dorsal bow of ulna are restored and the interosseous membrane is spread. The nails are then withdrawn by 1cm, and cut 2cm distal to the nail entry point in the bone. The nails are then hammered back to their final positions, so that 1cm of the nail is left protruding beyond the nail entry points. If dorsal entry point of radius is used, the cut end of the nail is bent dorsally by 90^{0} so that it comes to lie between the tendons of EPL and ECRB. This is done to prevent attrition rupture of the EPL tendon due to chronic rubbing against the sharp cut end of the nail **(Fig. 15.20)**.
- Surgical wounds are then closed and above-elbow slab is applied.
- Some authors recommend single bone nail fixation, and fixation of the other bone only if reduction is deemed to be unsatisfactory after nailing of the first bone. Ulna is usually the more preferred bone for single bone nailing due to easier entry site and easier approach for open reduction, should it be needed.

Post-operative

- Post-surgery, an above-elbow slab is applied and maintained for a period of 10 days.
- If the fracture fixation is stable, slab is removed at 10 days and mobilisation is commenced.
- In comminuted fractures, rigid immobilisation in cast is continued for a period of 4 weeks.

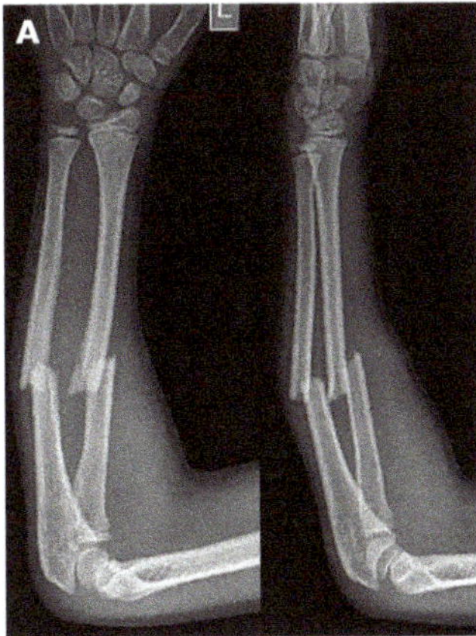

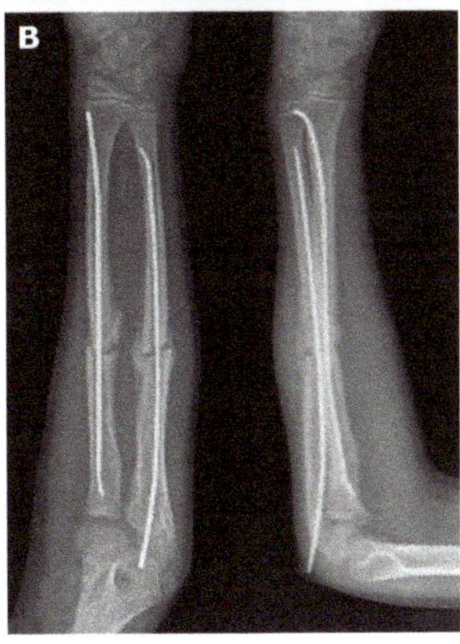

Fig. 15.20: *(A) Completely displaced fracture of radius ulna shaft in a 11 years old boy (B) Closed reduction- internal fixation performed with Titanium Elastic (TENS) Nails. Note the bent tip of the radius nail at the dorsal entry point. This ensures that the nail lies between the extensor tendons and attrition rupture of EPL is avoided.*

- Return to sports is permitted once fracture consolidation is seen on X-rays, usually at 10 to 12 weeks. It may be further delayed in cases where open reduction has been performed and consolidation is delayed.
- Implant removal should be performed at one year post-surgery.

Open Reduction and Plate Fixation of Radius-ulna Shaft Fractures

- Although the functional results of plating and TENS nails are similar, the need for larger incisions, soft tissue stripping and unsightly scar make plating a less popular option in paediatric radius-ulna shaft fractures.
- Plating is usually preferred in late presenting maluniting fractures or re-fractures where callus at the fracture site or obliteration of medullary cavity may preclude closed intra-medullary nailing.
- Plating may also be preferred in fractures at the metaphyseal-diaphyseal junction which are too proximal for K-wire fixation, and, too distal for intra-medullary nail fixation.

Implants and special requirements:

- 3.5mm DCP/tubular plate and screws
- 2.7mm plates and screws
- 3.5mm set with 2.5 mm drill-bit/tap/screw-driver, periosteum elevators, Hohmann retractors, bone holding clamps, plate holding clamps
- Power drill
- Pneumatic tourniquet
- Image intensifier

Patient positioning:

- Same as for intramedullary nailing **(Fig. 15.13)**.
- Pneumatic tourniquet applied to upper arm.

Surgical technique:

- The order of plate fixation in radius-ulna fractures is a matter of surgeon preference. But as a convention, usually radius followed by ulna are exposed first and then the two bones are fixed in the same order.
- Radius is most commonly approached through the volar Henry's approach,

which can be used to exposed the entire radius.

- The incision is along a straight line extending from the medial border of the biceps tendon to the radial styloid process. The length of the incision depends on the extent of exposure desired **(Fig. 15.21)**.

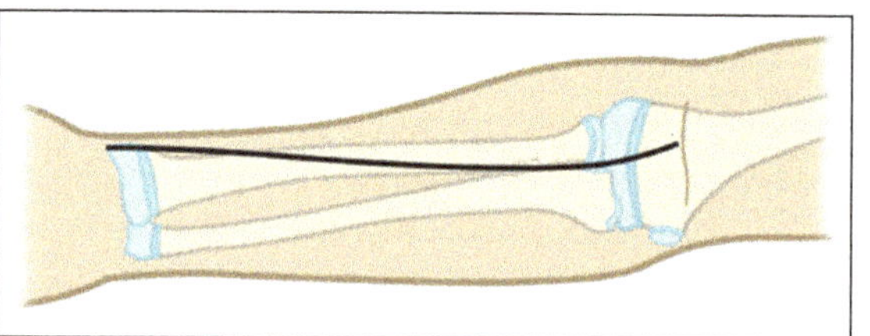

***Fig. 15.21**: Incision for volar Henry's approach to the radius lies along a line extending from medial border of the biceps tendon to the radial styloid process*

- The superficial plane lies between the brachio-radialis (mobile wad) laterally and flexor carpi radialis medially. The radial artery lies underneath the medial border of brachioradialis in the proximal and mid-shaft, and is retracted medially after ligation of muscular branches to the mobile wad of Henry. In the distal third, the radial artery lies between the brachioradialis and flexor carpi radialis. The superficial radial nerve lies lateral to the radial artery in the proximal two-thirds and is retracted laterally. In the proximal third, the posterior interosseous nerve (PIN) is at risk for injury and should be protected **(Fig. 15.22).**
- In the deep plane, the supinator covers the lateral aspect of proximal third of radius. The posterior interosseous nerve lies within its substance. The forearm is supinated to visualise the medial extent of its attachment on the radius which lies just lateral to the biceps tendon insertion and its bursa. The muscle is detached off its insertion

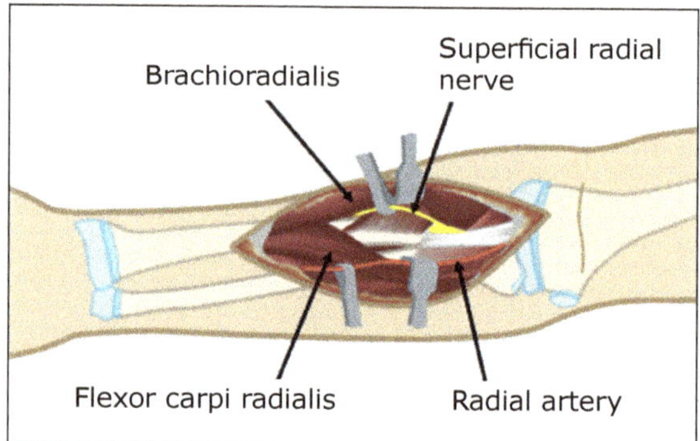

***Fig. 15.22**: Superficial dissection in volar approach to forearm lies between the mobile wad of Henry and flexor carpi radialis tendons.*

on the radius and is sub-periosteally elevated laterally just enough to achieve sufficient exposure so as to avoid injury to the PIN.

- In the middle thirds, the forearm is pronated to identify the insertion of pronator teres which is disinserted and sub-periosteally elevated medially. Similarly, in the distal thirds, the forearm is pronated and muscles are elevated: the flexor pollicis longus proximally and the pronator quadratus distally **(Fig. 15.23)**.
- The ulna is exposed through a dorsal incision along a line joining the tip of the olecranon process and the ulnar styloid process. The intermuscular plane lies between the flexor carpi ulnaris and extensor carpi ulnaris muscles **(Fig. 15.24).**
- Once the fracture site is exposed, the fracture ends are gently freshened and the medullary canals are opened at either end. The fracture is then reduced with reduction clamps.
- 3.5 mm plates or one-third tubular plates or 2.7 mm plates may be chosen depending on bone diameter. The plate may be contoured so as to conform to the contours of the underlying bone.

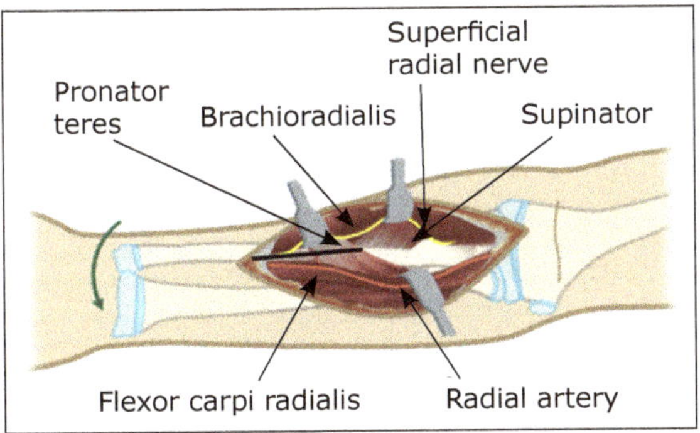

***Fig. 15.23**: Deep dissection in volar Henry's approach to the radius. (a) In the proximal thirds, the forearm is supinated and supinator is elevated laterally off its insertion (b) In the middle thirds, the forearm is pronated and the pronator teres is elevated medially (c) In the distal thirds, the forearm is pronated and the flexor pollicis longus in the proximal extent of the incision and the pronator quadratus distally is disinserted and elevated medially.*

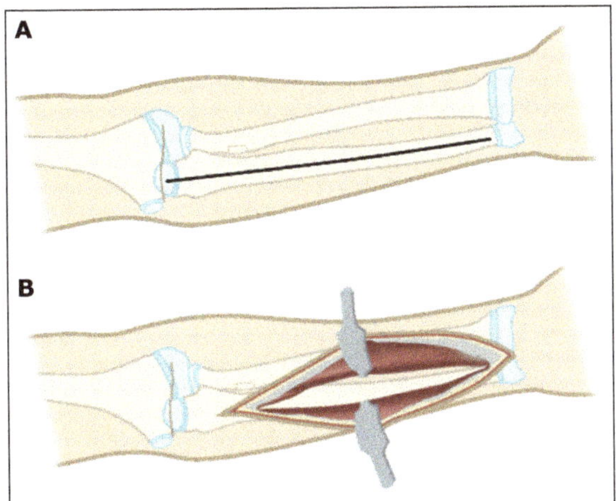

***Fig. 15.24**: Dorsal approach to the ulna (A) incision along a line joining the tip of the olecranon and the ulna styloid process (B) the inter-muscular plane lies between the flexor carpi ulnaris and extensor carpi ulnaris muscles.*

- If Dynamic Compression Plates are used, in order to achieve uniform compression across the width of the bone, before insertion of the screws, the plate is pre-bent so that its centre stands 1 to 2 mm from the anatomically reduced fracture surface. Compression at the fracture site can be achieved by inserting a centric screw through a hole on one side of the fracture, and then an eccentric screw on the other side of the fracture. As the eccentric screw is tightened, compression is achieved at the fracture site.
- Remainder screws may be inserted in neutral mode if no more compression is needed. Four cortex fixation on either side of the fracture is adequate for fixation of paediatric radius-ulna shaft fractures **(Fig. 15.25)**.
- At the end of fixation, unrestricted range of motion of elbow joint and forearm rotations is confirmed.
- Few authors have described single bone plate fixation, either the radius or ulna, instead of dual bone plate fixation and have reported similar functional results with lower complication rates. Plating of the other bone may be performed in the event of unsatisfactory alignment after fixation of the first bone.
- Suction drain is inserted before wound closure. The muscles fall back to their anatomical position and need not be reattached. The fascia should not be closed due to risk of compartment syndrome. The subcutaneous tissue and skin are closed with absorbable sutures to spare the child distress during removal of non-absorbable sutures.
- An above-elbow slab is applied after wound closure. In the post-operative period, the limb is elevated on pillow and child is observed for signs of compartment syndrome. The drain is usually removed on 2nd post-operative day, and slab is discarded after two weeks. X-ray is repeated after 4 weeks. Return to sports is allowed after radiographic healing, usually after 2 to 3 months. Implant removal may be planned after 6 months.

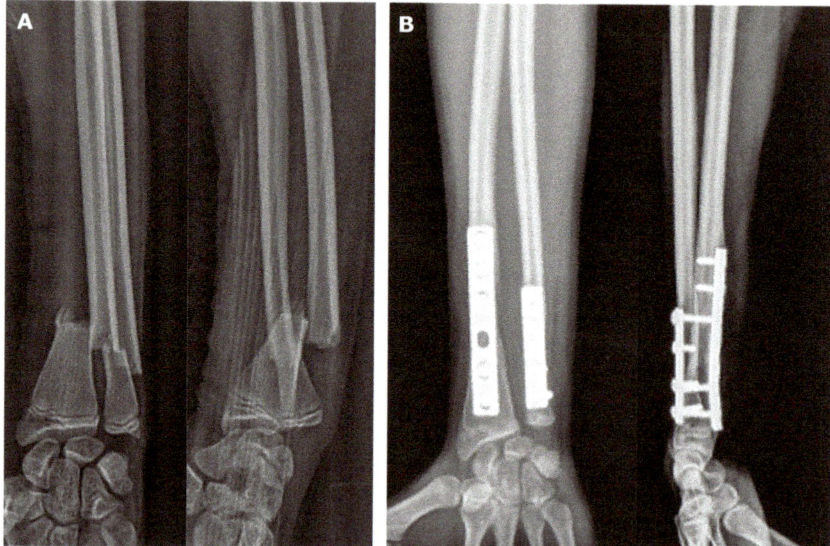

Fig. 15.25: *(A) AP and lateral X-rays of the Right forearm in a 12 years old girl reveals fracture radius-ulna distal third completely displaced (B) Post-operative X-rays following Open Reduction and internal fixation with 3.5 mm Dynamic Compression Plates and Screws.*

Compound radius-ulna fractures

- Even innocuous appearing Grade 1 compound radius-ulna fractures may be complicated by serious infections due to contamination of medullary cavity **(Fig. 15.26)**.
- For this reason, exploration of medullary cavity, debridement and prophylactic antibiotics is recommended even for Grade 1 compound fractures.
- Need for fixation after debridement of compound fractures depends on nature of wound and fracture characteristics.
- It is not necessary to fix every Grade 1 compound fracture after debridement, and these can be safely managed by cast immobilisation with regular review of wound through cast window till wound healing.
- Fixation of Grade 1 compound fractures after debridement, with TENS nails or plates has also been shown to be safe.
- However in larger and contaminated wounds, external fixation may be warranted in view of risk of infection and to facilitate wound management.

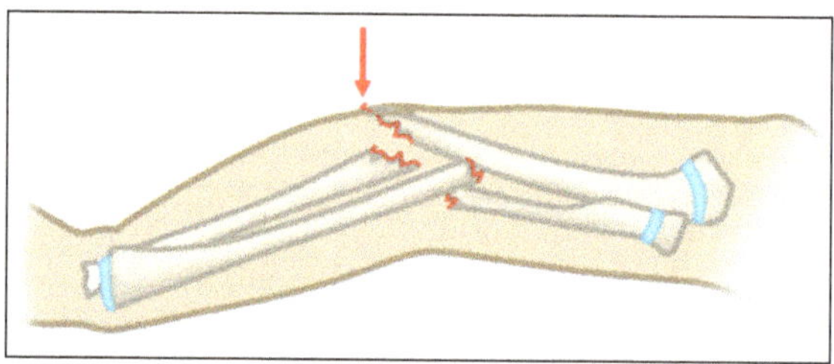

Fig. 15.26: *In compound fracture, the bone fragment protrudes through the skin laceration leading to contamination. Reduction of the fracture carries the contamination into the medullary cavity which may lead to frank osteomyelitis.*

Complications of Radius Ulna Shaft Fractures

Re-displacement within Cast:

Re-displacement within cast is one of the commonest complication following closed reduction and casting for radius-ulna shaft fractures. It is especially common after proximal shaft fractures, and, as has been already mentioned, cast for proximal shaft fractures should be applied in elbow extension with good moulding of the subcutaneous border of ulna. Lack of adequate moulding during cast setting is the commonest surgeon-related cause of fracture re-displacement within cast. Re-displacement tends to occur most commonly in the first two weeks after cast application, when the soft tissue swelling subsides leading to loosening of the cast. For this reason, weekly radiographs is recommended for the first two weeks after cast application.

Once re-displacement within cast is identified, options include acceptance of the deformity if within acceptable limits for the child's age, cast wedging, re-manipulation and application of new cast, or surgical intervention in the form of closed/ open reduction and elastic stable intra-medullary nailing or plating.

Malunion:

Malunion following fracture of shaft of radius and ulna have functional and cosmetic implications. Loss of range of forearm rotations is more severe following malunion of proximal third forearm fractures. Also malunions of ulna with dorsal apex angulation cause cosmetically displeasing bump. Whereas malunions in the coronal and sagittal planes are easily visualised on antero-posterior and lateral radiographs, rotational malunions are assessed by analysing the relative orientations of the radius bicipital tuberosity and styloid process on antero-posterior view, and, ulna coronoid process and styloid process on lateral view. The radius cross-over sign described earlier also helps to assess rotational malunion.

Remodelling following radius-ulna malunion occurs more effectively in younger children, sagittal plane malunions and distal forearm fractures. Rotational malunions don't remodel. Also, extent of loss of forearm rotations may not correlate with radiological malunion and functional deficit may be minimal even in radiologically significant malunions.

Radius-ulna malunions presenting in the first 3 weeks following trauma may be managed by closed osteoclasis. Osteoclasis of callus which is not yet consolidated may be performed with percutaneous drilling with K-wires followed by deformity correction and casting. Internal fixation may not be mandatory especially in younger children. Later presenting malunions with consolidated callus need formal open osteotomy and internal fixation. Plates are usually preferred as the medullary canal may be obliterated by the healed fracture. Open osteotomy if needed should preferably be performed if functional limitation of forearm rotations persists at the end of 6 months following trauma. Osteotomy performed later than this may not restore full rotations due to contractures of interosseous membrane and soft tissues. Level of osteotomy, and, single versus both bone osteotomy are decided after careful deformity analysis on radiographs. Recently, CT scans and 3D printed bone models have been used for accurate planning of deformity correction in complex cases.

Re-fractures:

Radius ulna fractures are the commonest bones to undergo re-fracture with a reported incidence of 4 to 8%. Re-fractures are commoner in adolescent boys with proximal and middle third forearm fractures and occur at average interval of 6 months following the original injury. Greenstick fractures are more likely to refracture than complete fractures. In children undergoing surgical treatment, re-fractures have been reported to occur following implant removal.

Re-fractures can be managed successfully by closed reduction and cast application with surgical treatment being recommended in case of failure of closed reduction or in complete displaced fractures in older children.

In cases with re-fractures with intra-medullary nails in-situ, straightening out the bent nails and closed reduction may be attempted, but if that fails, open reduction with implant removal and re-fixation with intramedullary nails or plate-screws may be needed.

Flowchart 15.1: Algorithm for the management of radius and ulna shaft fractures in children

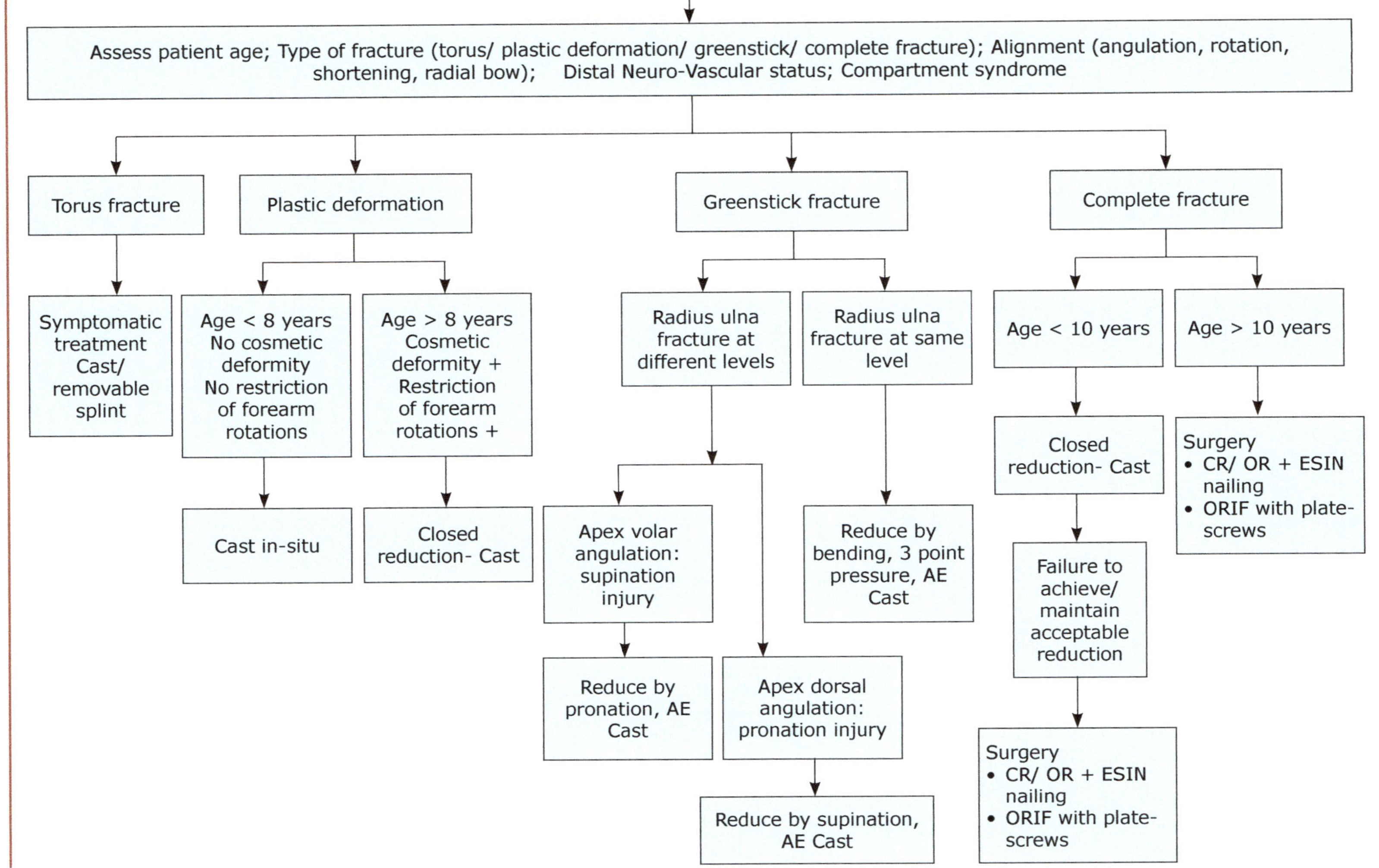

16 Fractures of the Distal Radius and Ulna

Introduction

Forearm fractures are the commonest long bone fractures in children and comprise 40% of all paediatric fractures. In forearm fractures, fractures of distal radius and ulna are the commonest. In distal radius, metaphyseal fractures are commonest followed by physeal. Fractures may be incomplete (torus/greenstick) or complete with bayonet apposition and shortening. The peak age of incidence of these fractures is during the pre-adolescent growth spurt.

Classification

- *Metaphyseal fractures:*
- Incomplete fractures:
1. Torus
2. Greenstick
- Complete fractures:
1. Undisplaced
2. Dorsal displacement
3. Volar displacement
- *Physeal fractures*
- Salter Harris Type 1 and 2
- Salter Harris Type 3 and 4 (extremely rare)
- *Paediatric Galeazzi fractures*
- With distal ulna Salter Harris Type 1 physeal fracture (paediatric Galeazzi equivalent)
- With soft tissue DRUJ disruption (extremely rare)

Associated injuries

50% of distal radius fractures are associated with ulna fractures. The ulna fracture may be physeal fracture or metaphyseal greenstick/complete fracture.

Distal radius fractures with concomitant elbow fractures are called "floating elbow" injuries and are at high risk for compartment syndrome/neurovascular compromise.

Severely displaced distal radius fractures can cause median nerve compression and carpal tunnel syndrome.

Clinical features

Children with distal radius ulna fractures present with history of fall on the outstretched hand. Whereas falls with the wrist extended lead to fractures with dorsal displacement, falls with flexed wrist lead to volar displacement of distal fragment.

On clinical examination, pain, swelling and deformity is seen at the distal radius fracture site. In torus fractures, the clinical signs may not be evident due to intact periosteum and inherent fracture stability. Additionally, torus fractures typically occur in the toddler age group. Consequently, these fractures often have a delayed presentation.

Imaging

Plain antero-posterior and lateral radiographs are sufficient to confirm diagnosis of distal radius ulna fractures. Undisplaced distal radius Salter Harris

Type 1 fractures may not be identified on plain radiographs. A mild widening of the physis or an elevated pronator quadratus fat pad may provide a clue to diagnosis in these cases.

Treatment

(1) DISTAL RADIUS METAPHYSEAL FRACTURES

(a) Torus fractures:

- Torus fractures are unicortical buckle fractures in compression, and hence are inherently stable **(Fig. 16.1)**.
- Hence the sole aim of immobilisation in torus fractures is to relieve pain and avoid repeat trauma.
- Various studies have compared rigid casts, removable splints and soft bandages in the management of torus fractures and no difference in outcome is observed. However, before opting for non-rigid immobilisation, careful evaluation of X-rays should be done to differentiate torus fractures from bi-cortical undisplaced fractures. Failure to do so can result in late displacement and sub-optimal outcome.

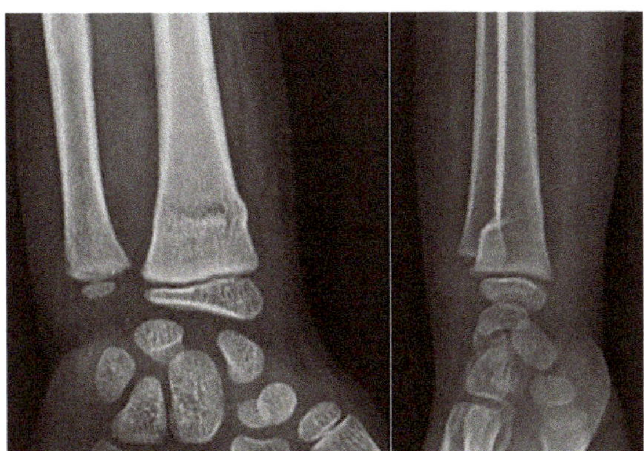

***Fig. 16.1**: Distal radius torus fracture.*

(b) Greenstick fractures:

- Greenstick fractures of the distal radius may occur with or without ulna fracture.
- These fractures should be treated with closed reduction and cast immobilisation.
- Greenstick injuries in which radius and ulna are fractured at different levels occur due to rotatory deforming forces.
- Thus, greenstick fractures with apex volar angulation are caused by supination rotatory force. These fractures are reduced by pronation of forearm and application of dorsal to volar force.
- On the other hand, fractures with apex dorsal angulation are caused by pronation rotatory force. These are reduced by forearm supination and volar to dorsal force.
- The fracture is then immobilised in a well moulded cast. A well moulded cast should consist of appropriate 3-point moulds to counteract the bending forces at the fracture site **(Fig. 16.2)**.

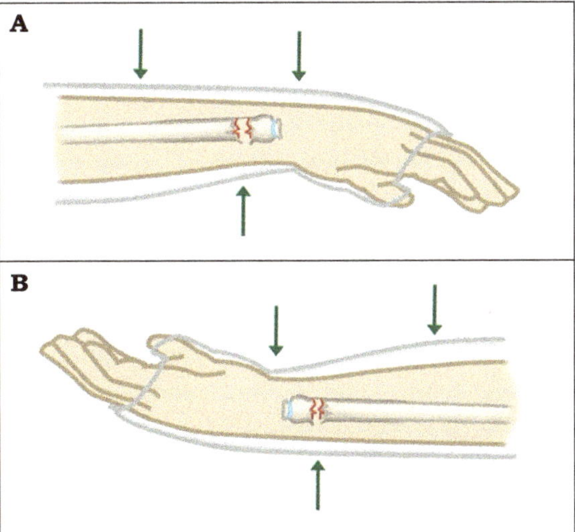

***Fig. 16.2**: Features of a well-moulded cast: (A) 3-point moulding in a fracture with apex volar angulation, with proximal and distal pressure points on the dorsal aspect and middle pressure point on the volar aspect at the apex of the fracture (B) 3-point moulding in a fracture with apex dorsal angulation, with proximal and distal pressure points on the volar aspect and middle pressure point on the dorsal aspect at the apex of the fracture*

- Additionally, on cross-section, well moulded casts should be oval rather than spherical with the medial-lateral diameter being greater than antero-posterior diameter. This ensures adequate stretch of the interosseous membrane.
- Various radiographic indices have been described to provide an objective measure of adequacy of cast moulding. Cast index which is a ratio of the antero-posterior diameter to the medial-lateral diameter is the most commonly used quantitative measure of cast moulding. A cast index less than 0.7 indicates an adequately moulded cast **(Fig. 16.3)**.
- Since prevention of forearm rotations is important in greenstick fractures, above elbow casts should be preferred over below elbow casts.
- Other radiographic indices described are the padding index, three-point index and Canterbury index **(Table 16.1)**.

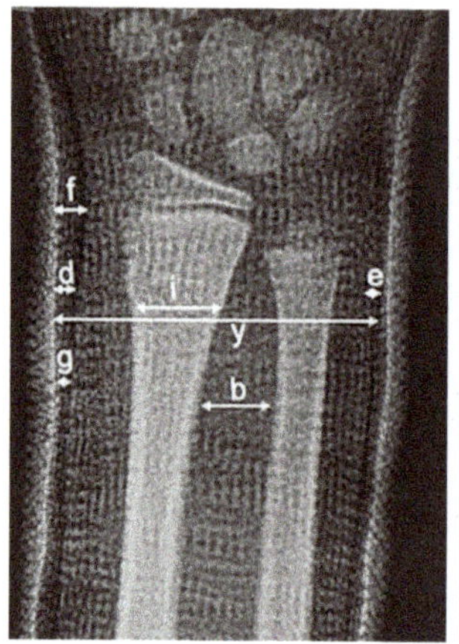

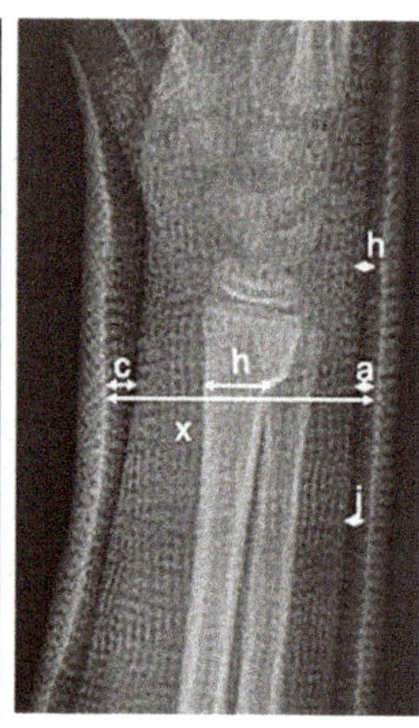

***Fig. 16.3**: Radiographic indices for assessing adequacy of cast moulding (Refer Table 16.1).*

COMPLETE METAPHYSEAL FRACTURES

(a) Undisplaced or minimally displaced fractures:

- Bicortical distal radius metaphyseal fractures which are undisplaced or which are angulated within acceptable limits may be effectively managed non-operatively by application of plaster cast in situ.
- Provided the cast is well moulded with cast index less than 0.7, a below-elbow and above-elbow cast have been shown to be equally effective in maintaining reduction in distal radius metaphyseal fractures.
- However, there is a risk of late displacement and check radiographs should be obtained weekly for 2 to 3 weeks to look for late displacement.

Table 16.1: Radiographic indices to assess adequacy of cast moulding in forearm fractures

Cast index	Inner cast diameter lateral view (x)/Inner cast diameter AP view at fracture site (y)	< 0.7
Padding index	Dorsal gap lateral view at fracture site (a)/maximum interosseous distance (b)	< 0.3
Canterbury index	Cast index + Padding index	< 1.1
Gap index	[Radial gap (d) + Ulnar gap (e) at fracture site /inner diameter of cast AP view (y)] + [Dorsal gap (a) + Volar gap (c) at fracture site / inner diameter of cast lateral view (x)]	<0.15
Three point index	[Distal radial gap (f) + Ulnar gap at fracture site (e) + Proximal radial gap AP view (g)/Diameter of radius bony contact AP view (i)] + [Distal dorsal gap (h) + Volar gap at fracture site (c) + Proximal dorsal gap lateral view (j)/Diameter of radius bony contact lateral view (h)]	<0.8

(b) Displaced fractures:

- Being close to the rapidly growing distal radius physis, distal radius metaphyseal fractures have a tremendous remodelling potential and this has a strong influence on their management.
- Remodelling depends on age of the child (more in younger children) and plane of angulation (sagittal angulation in plane of motion of wrist joint remodels more).
- Acceptability criteria for distal radius metaphyseal fractures are as described in the table 16.2.

Table 16.2: Acceptability criteria in distal radius fracture

	Age < 10 years	Age > 10 years
Dorsal-volar angulation	25°	20°
Radio-ulnar angulation	15°	15°
Shortening/Bayonet apposition	1 cm	0

- The radial inclination on anteroposterior view averages 22° and may be lower in younger children, whereas volar tilt averages 11° on lateral view. This information is helpful in quantifying angulation in distal radius fractures.
- Bayonet apposition with complete over-riding of fracture fragments has been shown to remodel completely in children less than 10 years. Application of plaster cast with correction of angulation in sagittal and coronal planes is an option in these fractures and may be performed without need for anaesthesia.

Non-operative treatment

Indications

- Metaphyseal fractures with displacement within acceptable limits
- Metaphyseal fractures which are amenable to closed reduction and maintenance of acceptable alignment with cast immobilisation.

Technique of closed reduction

- Closed reduction of metaphyseal fractures with dorsal over-riding of distal fragment:

• Due to the stout intact dorsal periosteum, closed reduction of these fractures by simple longitudinal traction is almost never possible **(Fig. 16.4)**.

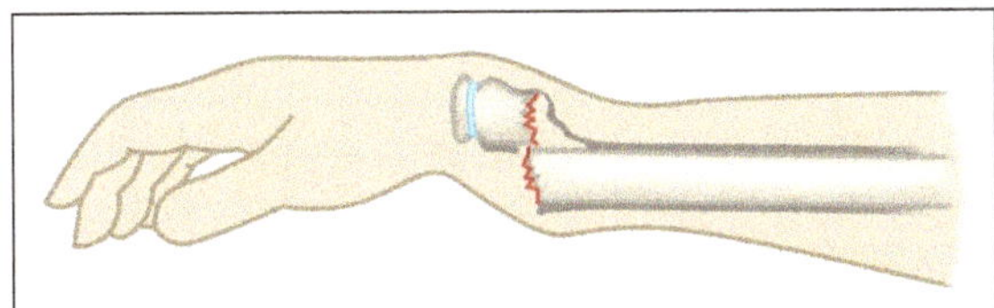

***Fig. 16.4**: Intact dorsal periosteum in distal radius metaphyseal fractures with dorsal displacement of distal fragment.*

• The reduction manoeuvre recommended for these fractures consists of initial dorsiflexion and exaggeration of the deformity at fracture site. This relaxes the dorsal periosteum.

• Longitudinal traction is then applied to the distal fragment.

• Once the distal fragment is pulled beyond the distal end of the proximal fragment, the distal fragment is flexed and translated volarly to reduce the fracture **(Fig. 16.5)**.

• Well-moulded cast is then applied to maintain the reduction. As mentioned earlier, if the casts are well-moulded, below elbow casts are as effective as above elbow casts in maintaining reduction in distal radius fractures.

• Additionally, three point pressure should be applied during cast setting with proximal and distal pressure points on the dorsal aspect and middle

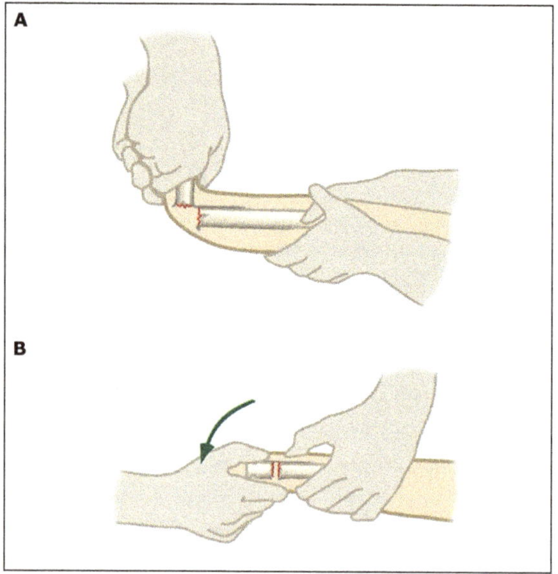

***Fig. 16.5**: Reduction manoeuvre for dorsally displaced distal radius metaphyseal fractures. (A) Initial dorsiflexion and exaggeration of deformity (B) Longitudinal traction followed by flexion and volar displacement of distal fragment.*

pressure point on volar aspect at the level of the fracture.

- Some surgeons prefer to bivalve casts as a preventive measure against the rare but dreaded complication of compartment syndrome.
- Once the oedema decreases in the initial few days after cast application, the cast tends to loosen which may result in fracture re-displacement. For this reason, it is essential to perform weekly check radiographs after cast application.

- Closed reduction for metaphyseal fractures with volar displacement of distal fragment:

- In metaphyseal fractures with volar displacement of distal fragment, the fracture is reduced by traction and direct volar pressure on the distal fragment with wrist dorsiflexion. Well moulded cast is then applied with three-point pressure during cast setting, with proximal and distal pressure points on the volar aspect and middle pressure point on dorsal aspect at the fracture level **(Fig. 16.6)**.

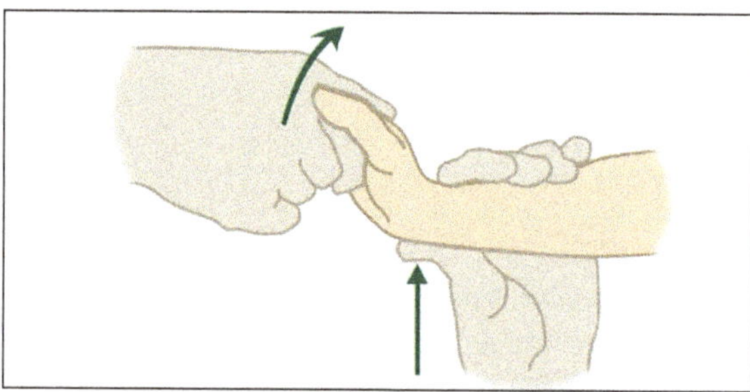

***Fig. 16.6**: Reduction manoeuvre for distal radius fractures with volar displacement of the distal fragment: longitudinal traction is applied, wrist if dorsiflexed and thumb pressure is applied on the volar aspect of the distal fragment.*

Operative treatment

Indications

- Unstable fractures: If closed reduction manoeuvres described above are successful, manual pressure is released and stability of reduction is checked. If unstable, surgical fixation may be considered.
- Irreducible fractures
- Fractures associated with compartment syndrome/neurovascular compromise/ median neuropathy
- Associated elbow fractures (floating elbow injuries)
- Compound fractures
- The threshold for surgical management is lower in adolescents closer to skeletal maturity.

Closed Reduction and K-wire Fixation

- If closed reduction is successful, but fracture is unstable, fixation is performed with cross K-wires. In high metaphyseal fractures, this can be achieved without breaching the physis **(Fig. 16.7)**.

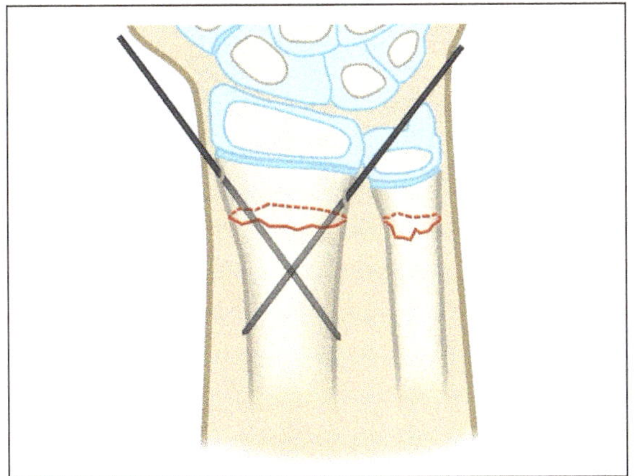

Fig. 16.7: *Cross K-wire fixation for distal radius metaphyseal fracture.*

- However, if the fracture line is more distal, K-wire fixation may cross the physis. Preacautions to be taken while inserting trans-physeal wires to avoid physeal damage are described in the section on physeal injuries **(Fig. 16.8)**.

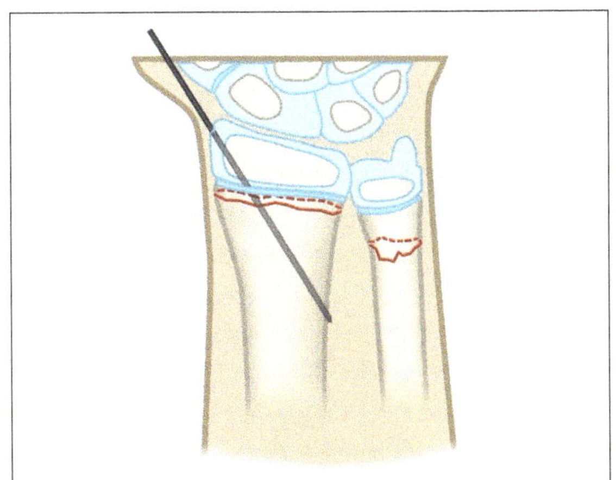

Fig. 16.8: *Transphyseal K-wire fixation for distal radius metaphyseal fracture.*

- If there is associated ulna fracture, it usually reduces and stabilises once the radius fracture is reduced and fixed. Fixation of distal ulna fracture is almost never needed and should be avoided. However, if at all ulna fixation is needed, it should avoid the physis **(Fig. 16.9)**.

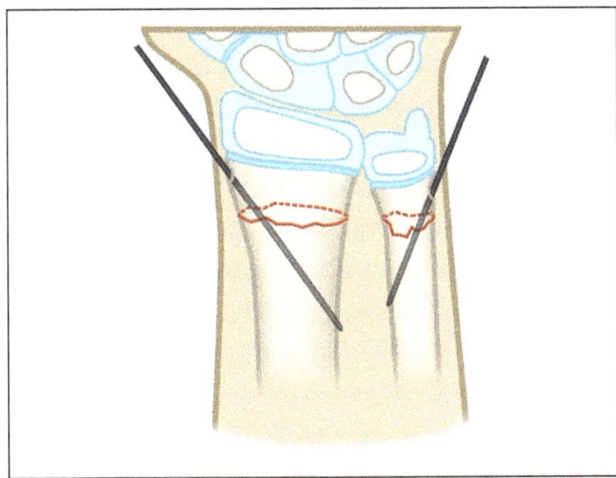

Fig. 16.9: *Fixation of distal ulna fracture. The K-wire should avoid the physis.*

- Closed reduction and fixation by intra-focal K-wire leverage (Kapandji technique) for fractures with dorsal displacement of distal fragment:

  Occasionally, distal radius fractures with dorsal displacement cannot be close reduced by the manoeuvres described above. The intra-focal K-wire leverage technique is an extremely effective technique for closed reduction and fixation of these fractures.

Technique

- Patient position: Supine on radiolucent hand table **(Fig. 16.10)**

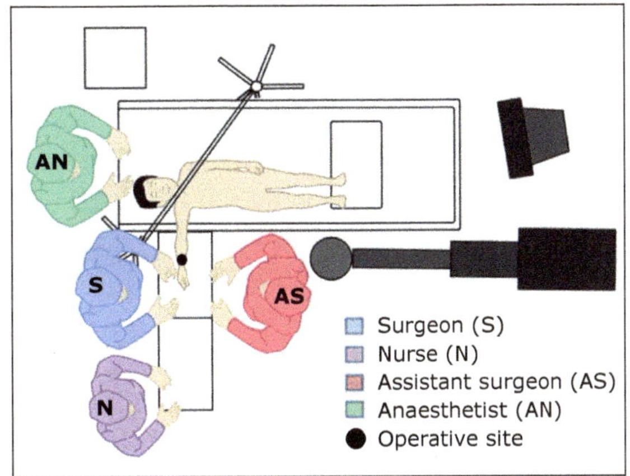

Fig. 16.10: *Patient positioning.*

- Requirements:
  - o Image intensifier
  - o Power drill
  - o K-wires 2.5mm
- Technique **(Fig. 16.11)**:
  - o A thick 2.5mm K-wire is inserted percutaneously under image-intensifier control from dorsal aspect into the fracture site.
  - o The K-wire tip is then hitched on the distal end of proximal fragment.
  - o The K-wire is then used like a lever and and is rotated distally to reduce the fracture fragment.
  - o Once reduced, the same wire is advanced across the volar cortex of the proximal fragment to provide intra-focal fixation.
  - o Well moulded cast is then applied. Cast

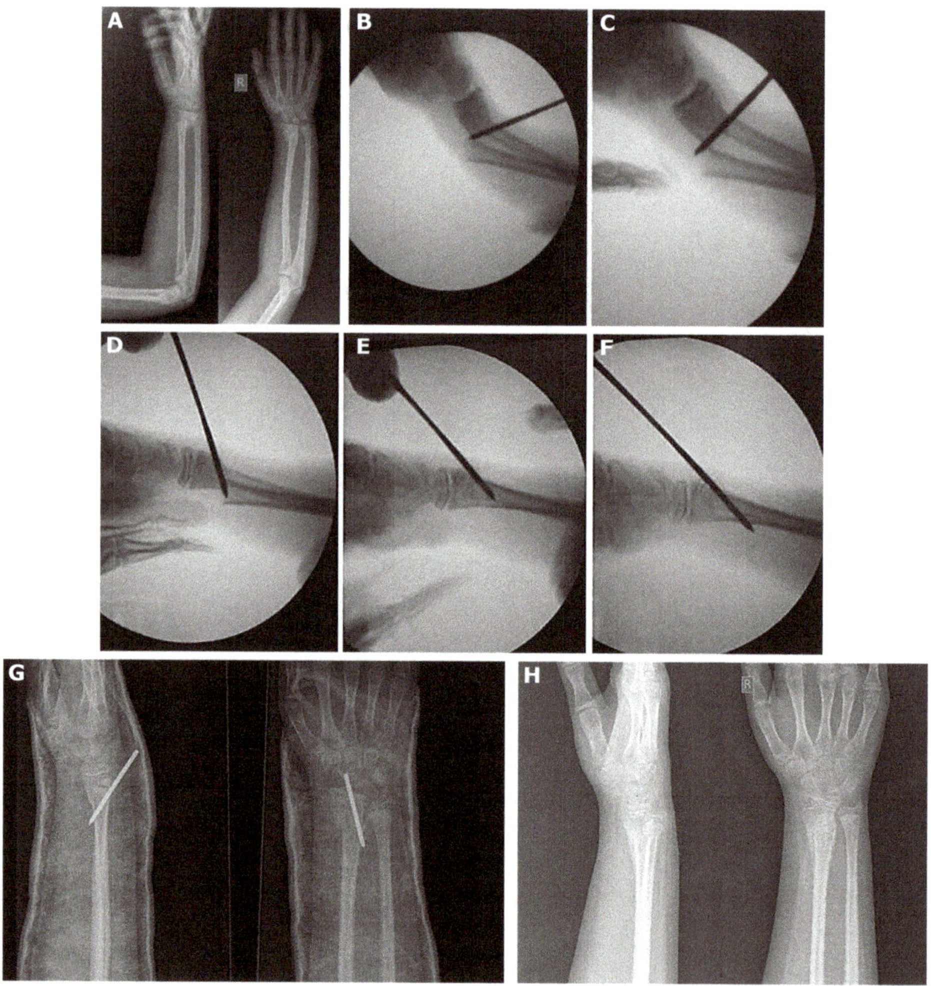

***Fig. 16.11**: Intrafocal K-wire for leverage and fixation of distal radius metaphyseal fractures with complete over-riding of the distal fragment. (A) Distal radius metaphyseal fracture with complete over-riding of distal fragment (B) 2.5mm K-wire is inserted percutaneously into fracture site from dorsal side (C) K-wire used to lever and reduce fracture fragment (D,E) same K-wire advanced across volar cortex of distal fragment to provide intra-focal fixation (F) post-operative radiographs, immediate and at 6 weeks after removal of cast and K-wire (G,H).*

and wires are maintained for 6 weeks till fracture union is seen on X-rays.

- **Open reduction and plate fixation:**

- In patients close to skeletal maturity where rigid fixation is desired, open reduction and fixation with plate and screws is an option for treatment of distal radius fractures.
- Also fractures at the metaphyseo-diaphyseal junction are too proximal and unsuitable for intra-focal K-wire fixation. At the same time, they are too distal for TENS nail fixation. Open reduction and plate fixation may be appropriate for such fractures which lie in the "grey zone".
- The distal radius is exposed by volar approach, which is a distal extension of Henry's volar approach to the radius, described in greater detail in the chapter on radius-ulna shaft fractures.
- The superficial dissection is between the brachioradialis laterally and the flexor carpi radialis with the radial artery medially.
- This exposes the pronator quadratus attachment on distal radius which is detached by a sharp incision on the periosteum along its lateral border.
- The fracture surface is exposed, cleared and reduced. Fixation is then performed with 3.5 mm or 2.5 mm plate and screws. Straight plates or distal radius plates are used depending on size of distal fragment. The distal tip of the plate must stop short of the distal radius physis. The plate may be slightly contoured to accommodate the anatomical volar tilt of distal radius **(Fig. 16.12)**.
- After fixation of radius, the reduction and stability of distal ulna is assessed. If reduced and stable, ulna may be left alone. Options for ulna stabilisation include Closed/Open reduction and TENS nail fixation (inserted from the olecranon), or Open reduction and plate fixation.

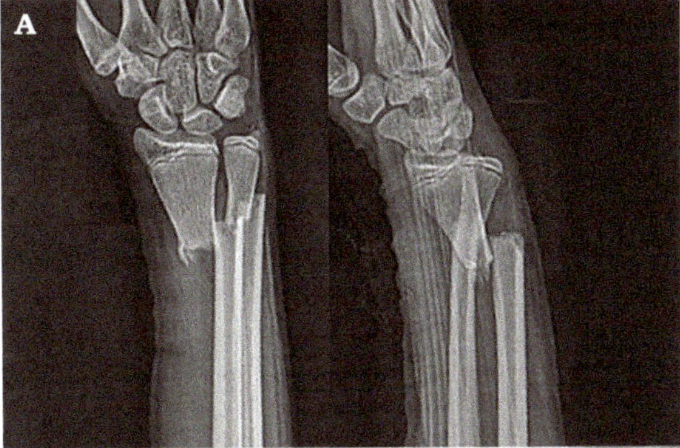

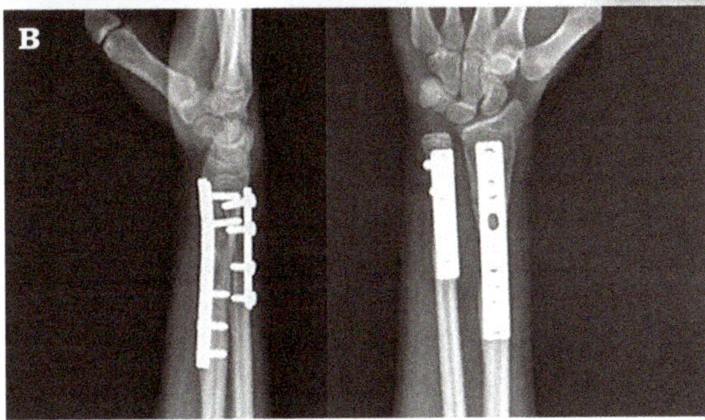

***Fig. 16.12**: (A) Distal radius ulna metaphyseal-diaphyseal junction fracture in a 13 years old girl (B) Open reduction internal fixation with plate and screws.*

- Technique of fixation of ulna fractures is described in chapter on radius-ulna fractures. The implant should not breach the distal ulna physis as it has a high propensity for growth arrest.

(2) DISTAL RADIUS PHYSEAL FRACTURES

- Salter Harris Type 1 and Type 2 physeal fractures of the distal radius may present with either a dorsal (commoner) or volar (rarer) displacement of the distal fragment.
- Undisplaced Salter Harris Type 1 fractures may be difficult to diagnose acutely. A displaced volar pronator quadratus fat pad due to sub-periosteal

haemorrhage may provide a clue to diagnosis.

- Careful evaluation is needed to differentiate this injury from an undisplaced scaphoid fracture which presents with tenderness overlying the scaphoid fossa and displaced scaphoid fat pad.

Non-operative treatment

Closed reduction of distal radius physeal injuries

- Physeal fractures of the distal radius are usually treated with closed reduction and cast application.
- The reduction manoeuvre consists of longitudinal traction and disimpaction of the fracture fragments followed by flexion (for dorsally displaced fractures) or extension (for volar displaced fractures). Initial traction for disimpaction is of great importance to prevent grating of the physis by the sharp metaphyseal corner of the proximal fragment **(Fig. 16.13)**

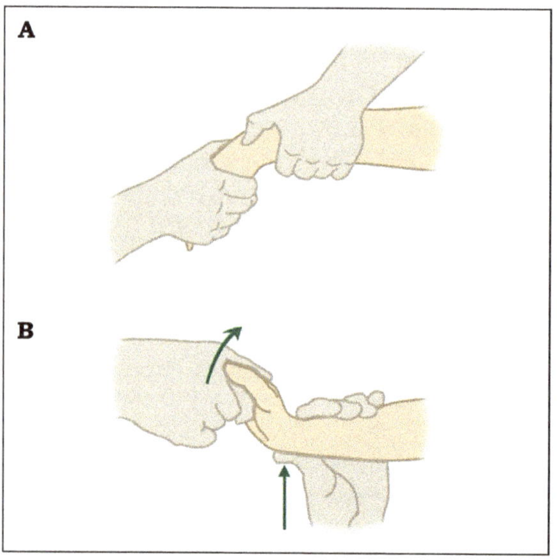

***Fig. 16.13**: Reduction manoeuvre for distal radius physeal fractures with (A) dorsal displacement and (B) volar displacement.*

- These fractures are usually stable after closed reduction due to the splintage offered by the thick intact periosteum on the side of fracture displacement.
- If after closed reduction, the fracture is found to be unstable, that is, it re-displaces on release of manual pressure, K-wire fixation may be considered.
- However if the fracture is stable, well-moulded cast may be applied. Principles of cast application in distal radius physeal fractures are the same as for distal radius metaphyseal fractures mentioned earlier.

Operative treatment

Closed reduction and K-wire pinning for distal radius physeal fractures:

- As mentioned earlier, K-wire pinning for distal radius physeal injuries may be considered in case of fracture instability.
- Cross K-wire configuration is usually used for fixation of distal radius physeal fractures.
- First K-wire is inserted from the tip of styloid process retrogradely towards the medial cortex of proximal fragment.
- Second wire is inserted from the dorso-medial corner of the epiphysis towards the volar and lateral cortex of the proximal fragment. In case of Salter Harris Type 2 fracture, wire may pass through the metaphyseal Thurston Holland fragment rather than the physis **(Fig. 16.14)**.
- Passage of K-wires across the distal radius physis is reasonably safe and not associated with growth arrest provided a few basic rules are followed:

o Use smooth, thin K-wires (1 mm for younger children, 1.5 for older children).

o Use one or maximum two K-wires.

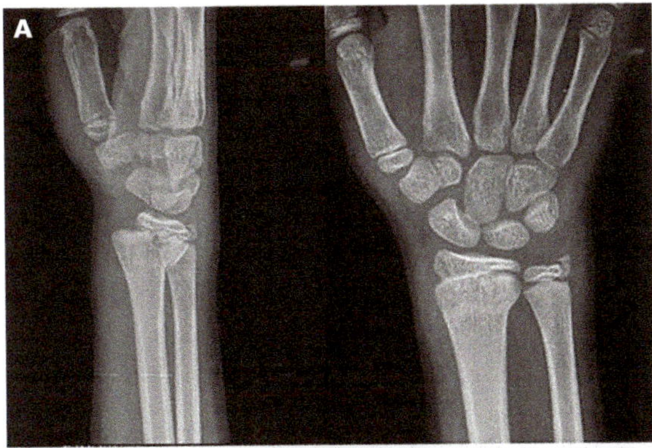

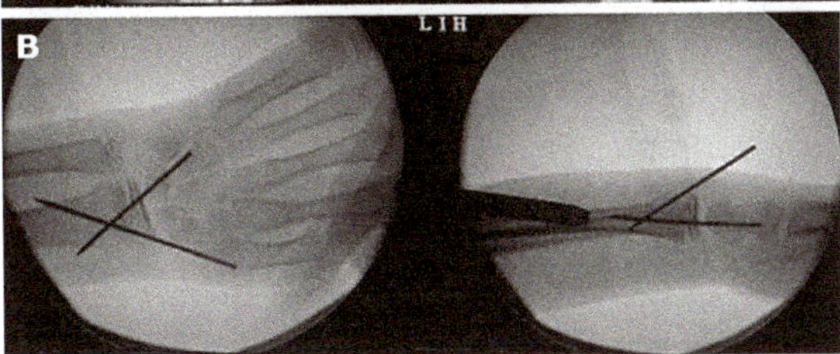

Fig. 16.14: *(A) AP and lateral X-ray of the wrist showing distal radius Salter Harris Type 2 physeal injury (B) K-wire configuration for fixation of distal radius physeal fracture.*

- o Avoid multiple attempts at insertion of K-wires across the physis. Before actual insertion, confirm accurate trajectory of the K-wire on both antero-posterior and lateral views under image intensifier.
- o Avoid insertion of K-wires across the periphery of the physis, as this region is more vulnerable to growth arrest.
- o Use low torque drill with stop-and-start mode to avoid thermal necrosis as the wire is advanced across the physis.
- o K-wires should be removed within 4 weeks. Early removal is safe as physeal fractures heal faster than bony fractures.

Late presenting distal radius physeal injuries:

Reduction should not be attempted in distal radius physeal fractures presenting more than one week post injury. Manipulation of these late presenting fractures is associated with a risk of growth arrest, the consequences of which can be severe in young children and needs complex surgical reconstructions. On the other hand, remodelling potential of these fractures is tremendous if there is growth remaining and the displacement is in the plane of motion of wrist joint.

(3) PAEDIATRIC GALEAZZI FRACTURE-DISLOCATION

- Distal radius fractures in association with disruption of the Distal Radius-Ulna Joint (DRUJ) is called Galeazzi fracture dislocation.
- In children, DRUJ disruption may either be in the form of:
  - Distal ulna physeal frature (Galeazzi equivalent injuries, commoner) ,or,
  - True ligamentous disruption (rarer)
- This injury occurs due to axial loading in association with rotational forces.
  - Supination forces lead to distal radius fractures with apex volar angulation and volar displacement of the distal ulna.
  - Pronation forces lead to distal radius fractures with apex dorsal angulation and dorsal displacement of the distal ulna.

Clinical examination

- Ulna head may be prominent on clinical examination. DRUJ tenderness and instability may be elicited on palpation (piano key sign).

Treatment

- Unlike adult Galeazzi injuries which are "fractures of necessity" and need surgical treatment, most paediatric Galeazzi fracture- dislocations can be managed non-operatively by closed reduction and casting.

- For radius fractures with apex volar angulation and volar displacement of ulna head, reduction can be achieved by pronation and volar to dorsal three point pressure on the radius at the level of fracture.
- Conversely, for radius fractures with apex dorsal angulation and dorsal displacement of ulna head, reduction can be achieved by supination and dorsal to volar three point pressure on the radius at the level of fracture.
- Fracture immobilisation is achieved by above elbow cast in pronation or supination in apex volar and apex dorsal angulations respectively.
- Ulna physeal injuries in Galeazzi equivalent injuries usually reduce after closed reduction of the radius fracture and do not need separate management, provided the DRUJ is well-aligned and ulna malalignment is less than 10°. However open reduction and K-wire fixation may be considered in irreducible fractures in adolescents close to skeletal maturity. K-wire fixation across the distal ulna physis should be avoided in younger children as there is a high risk of growth arrest.

(4) RADIAL PHYSEAL STRESS INJURIES

- o Repeated axial loading of the distal radius can lead to radial physeal stress injuries.
- o These are typically seen in gymnasts following a prolonged period of excessive training.
- o These injuries typically present with chronic soreness aggravated by wrist flexion/extension and tenderness localised to the distal radius physis.
- o Radiologically, these injuries are identified by widening and haziness of the distal radius physis, metaphyseal sclerosis and cysts, epiphyseal beaking and reactive new bone formation.
- o MRI will reveal peri-physeal oedema. Bone scan will show increased physeal uptake but is non-specific.
- o These injuries resolve with a limited period of rest. This may be achieved by application of a removable splint and abstinence from sports but in cases where compliance may be doubtful, rest may be enforced by application of a below-elbow plaster cast for several weeks. The immobilisation should be continued till the child is symptom free. Gradual return to sports should be allowed over a period of 3 to 6 months.
- o Radial physeal stress injuries may lead to premature distal radius physeal closure and this should be monitored by periodic radiographs. If this happens, it can lead to positive ulna variance with resultant ulno-carpal impingement and TFCC tears.

Complications

Re-displacement within cast:

Re-displacement within cast is known to occur in 20 to 30% cases. The risk factors for re-displacement include:

- Severe initial displacement
- Bayonet apposition
- Age > 10 years
- Translation > 50%
- Apex volar angulation > 30°
- Isolated radius fractures
- Associated ulna fracture at the same level
- Inadequate cast moulding with cast index less than 0.7.

  Fixation with K-wires may be considered in fractures with these risk factors

Prevention and management

- In fractures with the above risk factors

for re-displacement, K-wire fixation may be primarily considered.

- Re-displacement is most likely to occur in the first two weeks following cast application, as the oedema resolves. Hence weekly radiographs for the first three weeks should be performed to look for re-displacement.
- In case of physeal injuries, displacement noted more than one week following injury should not be re-manipulated, due to risk of iatrogenic growth arrest. These fractures should be allowed to malunite and corrective metaphyseal osteotomy may be performed if unacceptable deformity persists after one to two years of remodelling.
- In case of metaphyseal fractures, re-manipulation may be considered in case of deformities outside the limits of acceptability. Osteoclasis and closed reduction may be successful in the early stages, but in presentations later than two weeks a K-wire inserted percutaneously in the fracture site may be used for breaking the callus. The same wire may then be used for intra-focal leverage and fixation by the Kapandji method as previously described. This technique is usually successful for up to four weeks following the initial trauma.

Malunion:

Malunited distal radius fractures have excellent remodelling potential due to the following factors:

- The deformity is in proximity to distal radius physis.
- The malunion generally occurs in the sagittal plane which is the plane of motion of the wrist.
- The distal radius physis accounts for 60 to 80% increase in length of the radius.
- The remodelling potential is even higher in the younger child than in adolescents.

Malunited distal radius fractures may lead to the following sequelae:

- Limitation of range of motion, especially forearm rotations. The loss of forearm rotations is even greater in malunited Galeazzi fracture-dislocations which lead to incongruity of the distal radius-ulna joint.
- Significant extension malunion can lead to carpal instability and degenerative arthritis at long term follow-up.
- Malunited Galeazzi fracture-dislocations can lead to Triangular Fibrocartilage Ligament Complex (TFCC) tears. Hence, MRI evaluation is recommended for malunited distal radius fractures presenting with ulnar sided wrist pain.

Treatment:

- Malunited distal radius fracture should be observed for 6 to 12 months for remodelling. Failure to remodel to acceptable limits is an indication for surgery. Surgery consists of open-wedge osteotomy with trapezoidal bone graft harvested from the iliac crest inserted in the osteotomy site to restore radius-ulna variance and congruity of the distal radius-ulna joint. Osteotomy is stabilised with plate-screws or external fixator.
- In case of TFCC tears, in addition to correction of bony malunion, arthroscopy for repair or debridement of the tear is indicated. If distal radius-ulna joint instability persists after TFCC repair, reconstruction with local tendon graft of extensor retinaculum is rarely needed.

Distal radius growth arrest:

This is usually an iatrogenic complication, may occur in the following situations:

- K-wire insertion across the distal radius physis: This can be avoided if proper technique is followed. The precautions to be taken for K-wire insertion across the physis include:

- Multiple insertions and withdrawal of wires should be avoided. Wires should be inserted in one or at the most two attempts.
- Use smooth wires of 1 or 1.5 mm diameter.
- Wires should be inserted with low-torque drill to minimise heat generation during insertion.
- Wires should be removed within four weeks.

- Distal radius growth arrest may also occur if attempts are made to manipulate physeal fracture presenting more than 7 days following injury.
- This may also occur if during closed reduction of physeal fractures, initial dis-impaction of fragments by application of traction is not done. In that case, the sharp metaphyseal spike grates against the physis and causes physeal damage.

The consequences of growth arrest to distal radius include:

- positive ulna variance with ulno-carpal impingement and wrist pain
- angulation of distal radius articular with abnormal radial tilt and inclination

Distal radius growth arrest may be treated by:

- Growth restoration by physeal bar resection: can be tried in a younger child with localised bony physeal bar. However, attempts at restoration of growth at distal radius by physeal bar resection usually fail
- Completion of distal radius epiphysiodesis and radius osteotomy: for correction of radius deformity
- Ulna shortening and distal ulna epiphysiodesis: for correction of ulna variance
- Radius lengthening: for correction of ulna variance.

Flowchart 16.1: Algorithm for management of distal radius and ulna fractures in children

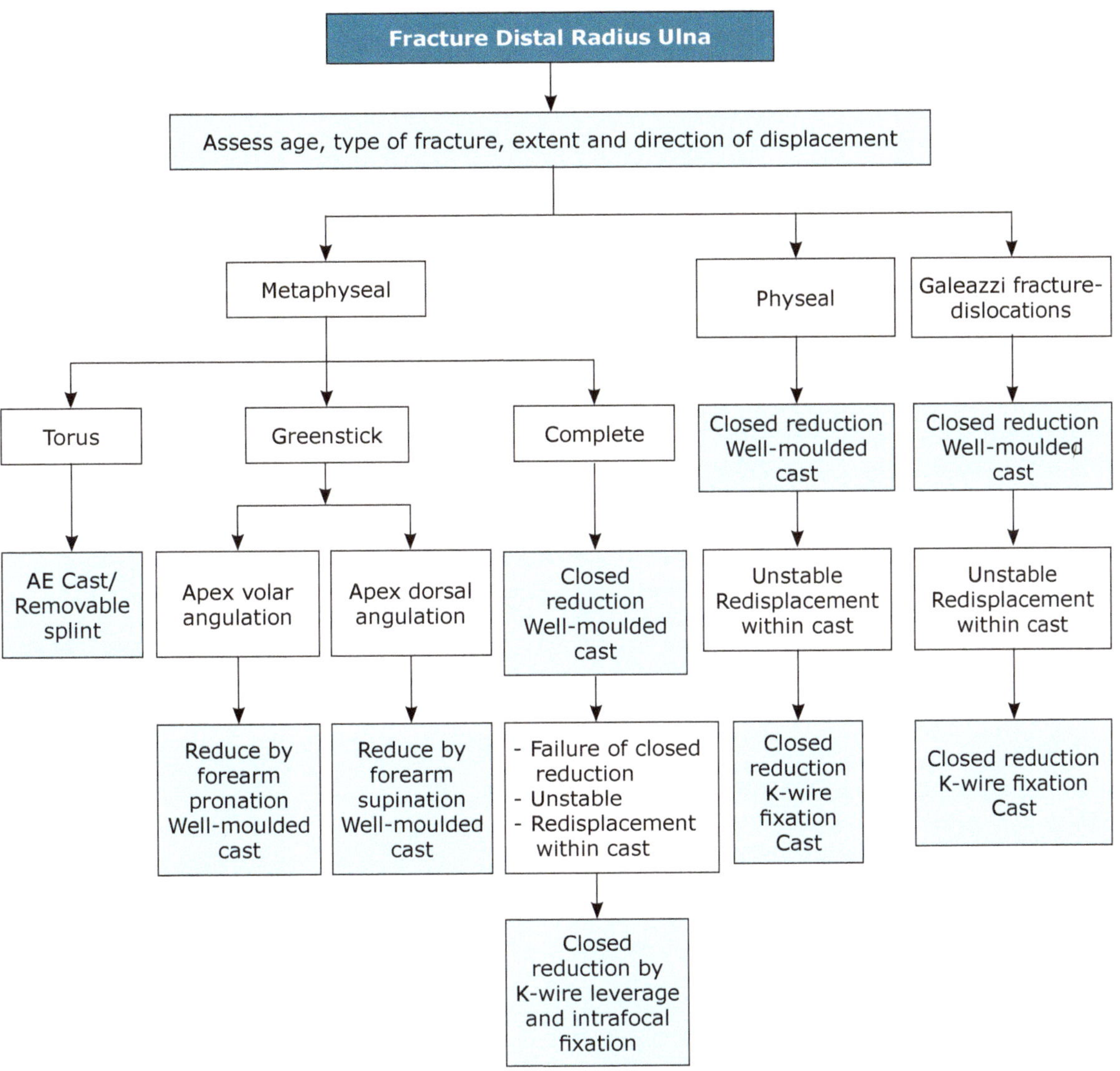

17 Fractures and Dislocations of the Hand and Carpus

Introduction

Finger injuries in children are mainly of two types: crush injuries (distal phalanx most commonly involved); and, physeal injuries (proximal phalanx most common). Finger injuries in children show a biphasic age distribution: Toddlers (crush injuries common) and adolescents (twisting injuries, contact sports common).

The border digits (thumb and little finger) are most commonly injured.

Amongst carpal bones, scaphoid fracture is the commonest.

Relevant anatomy of hand and carpus

Secondary ossification centres are seen at proximal ends of all phalanges.

Secondary ossification centres are seen at distal ends of 2nd/3rd/4th and 5th metacarpals, and at proximal end of 1st metacarpal.

The scaphoid ossifies in the fifth year of life in a distal to proximal direction. The differential ossification of the scaphoid leads to increased space between the scaphoid and lunate and can be mis-diagnosed for a ligamentous disruption *(pseudo-Terry Thomas sign)*. Comparison X-ray of the contralateral hand can resolve the confusion.

DISTAL PHALANX FRACTURES

Classification

Distal phalanx fractures in children are classified as:

1) According to location:
- Extraphyseal
  - Transverse diaphyseal
  - Longitudinal
  - Comminuted
  - FDP avulsion injuries
- Physeal
  - Salter Harris 1 and 2 including Seymour fracture
  - Salter Harris 3 and 4 including extensor tendon avulsions (Paediatric mallet) and FDP avulsion (Jersey finger)

2) According to mechanism of injury:
- Crush
- Hyperflexion
- Hyperextension

3) Closed or compound. A compound fracture is associated with nail bed laceration. In the presence of an intact nail plate, a subungual haematoma greater than 50% is assumed to indicate underlying nail bed laceration and compound fracture.

Clinical Features

Distal phalanx fractures usually occur following crush injuries, with door trap injuries being a common mechanism.

Malrotation in these fractures is diagnosed by noting digital scissoring during active grasp. If the child is unable to do active finger flexion, passive wrist extension will cause finger flexion by flexor tendon tenodesis and helps to look for digital scissoring.

Tendon injuries are assessed by noting finger position during rest and active grasp.

Neurovascular injuries are difficult to assess and a high index of suspicion is essential for their diagnosis. Digital artery lies just dorsal to the digital nerve. Pulsatile bleeding from a digital injury is indicative of a digital artery injury. In presence of digital artery injury, digital nerve is assumed to be injured.

Imaging

- Plain radiographs

- Anteroposterior, lateral and oblique views are recommended.
- Lateral finger cascade view gives simultaneous lateral visualisation of all digits. **(Fig. 17.1A)**
- Where single digit is involved, dedicated anteroposterior and lateral views of the affected digit may be obtained. **(Fig. 17.1B)**

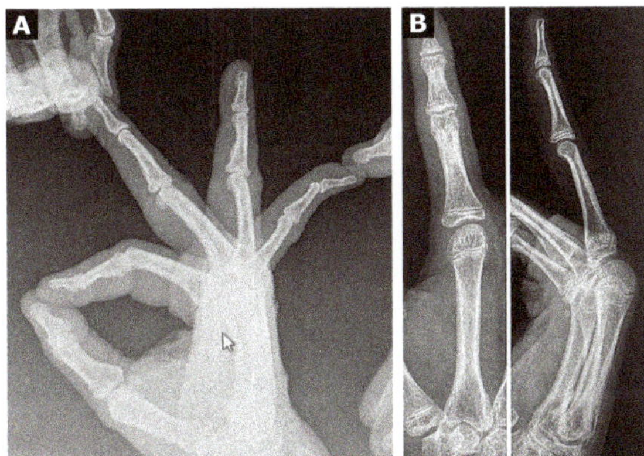

***Fig. 17.1**: (A) X-ray Lateral finger cascade view allows simultaneous lateral visualisation of all digits; (B) X-ray anteroposterior and lateral views of index finger.*

- Phalangeal line test: In a normal finger, line drawn along centre of phalangeal neck through centre of physis should pass through centre of preceding phalangeal or metacarpal head irrespective of flexion of the joint.

Salter Harris Type 1 and 2 physeal injuries

- In Salter Harris Type 1 and 2 physeal injuries of the distal phalanx, the terminal tendon of the extensor apparatus inserts into the dorsal aspect of the proximal epiphyseal fragment and pulls the proximal fragment dorsally.
- On the other hand, the Flexor Digitorum Profundus tendon which inserts on the volar aspect at the meta-diaphyseal region pulls the distal fragment into flexion. **(Fig. 17.2A)**
- *Seymour fracture:* In case of overlying nail bed laceration, the nail bed matrix may invaginate and get entrapped in the fracture gap. This pattern is called "Seymour fracture". If undetected, reduction of fracture will be obstructed and the fracture being compound, is prone to infection and osteomyelitis. Seymour fracture and its treatment is described in detail in a later section of this chapter.

Salter Harris Type 3 and 4 physeal injuries

- Salter Harris Type 3 and 4 fractures of the dorsal aspect of distal phalanx occur following hyperflexion injury. They are actually bony avulsions of the extensor tendon and result in bony mallet finger. **(Fig. 17.2B)**
- On the other hand, hyperextension injuries can cause bony avulsion of the metaphyseal insertion of FDP resulting in SH 4 injuries of the volar aspect of distal phalanx *(Jersey finger)*. **(Fig. 17.3)**

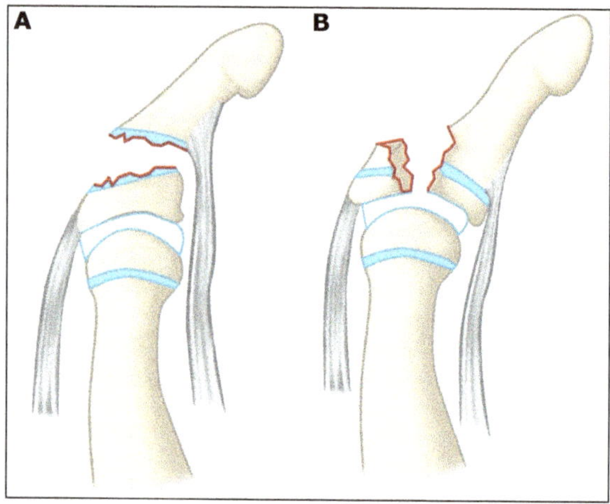

***Fig. 17.2**: (A) Salter Harris Type 1 fracture of the distal phalanx; (B) Dorsal Salter Harris Type 4 fracture of distal phalanx.*

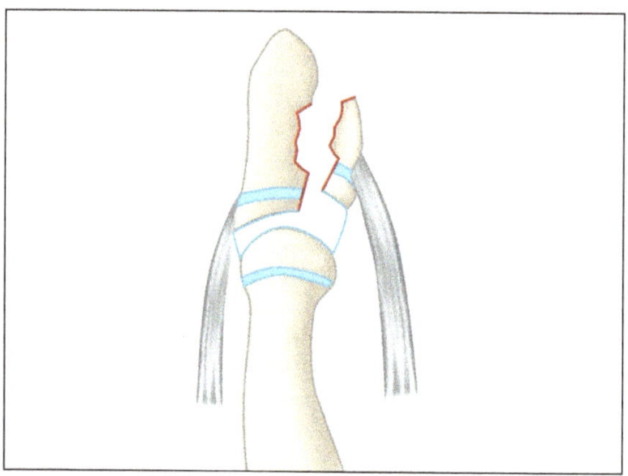

***Fig. 17.3**: Volar bony avulsion of metaphyseal insertion of FDP tendon (Jersey finger).*

Treatment

Non-operative treatment:

- Non-operative treatment of paediatric distal phalanx fractures is indicated in fractures which are closed, stable and with low risk of nail deformity and growth plate arrest.
- In case of extraphyseal injuries, immobilisation in simple volar or dorsal splint for few weeks suffices. **(Fig. 17.4)**
- In case of mallet finger deformity, finger splinting in extension is performed.

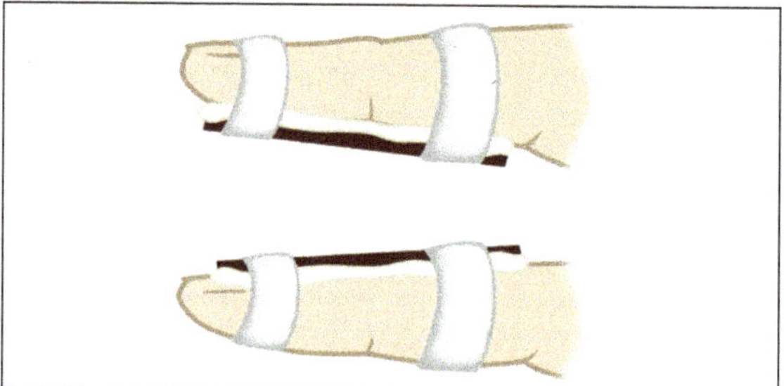

***Fig. 17.4**: Volar and dorsal splints for immobilisation of distal phalanx fractures.*

Surgical treatment

(1) *Subungual haematoma evacuation*

- Evacuation of subungual haematoma is recommended if in the presence of an intact nail plate, the haematoma exceeds 50% area of nail bed with severe pain.
- Nail plate trephination is performed with a sterile hypodermic needle **(Fig. 17.5)**.

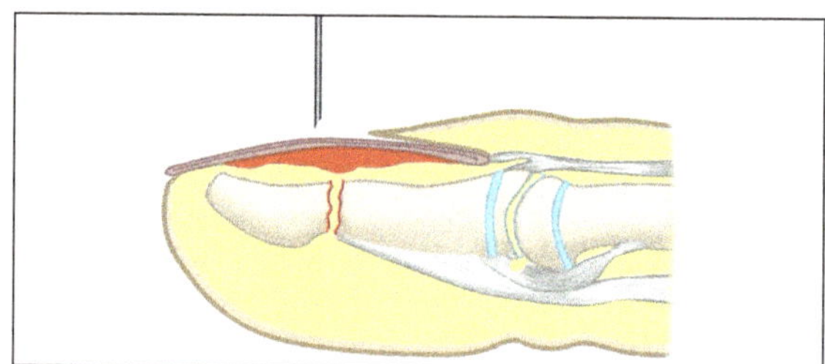

***Fig. 17.5**: Nail plate trephination for drainage of subungual haematoma.*

- Haematoma drainage has no benefits in injuries presenting after 12 to 24 hours due to haematoma coagulation.

(2) Nail bed laceration repair

- Nail bed repair is indicated for obvious lacerations and subungual haematomas with irreducible fractures indicating possible entrapment of the nail matrix in fracture gap.

Technique **(Figs. 17.6 and 17.7)**

- In children, nail bed repair is usually done in operating room under appropriate anaesthesia.

- Digital tourniquet is used.
- If overlying nail plate is still intact, it is removed by gently inserting a Freer elevator between the nail plate and nail bed. Avoid using artery forceps to remove the nail plate, as it may cause further damage to the underlying germinal matrix. Curved incisions may be made on the eponychial folds for proximal exposure of the germinal matrix.
- Haematoma is evacuated with saline irrigation.
- Nail matrix if entrapped in fracture gap, is gently extracted.
- Nail bed laceration should be sutured as precisely as possible. Interrupted sutures with 6-0 absorbable material are placed **(Fig. 17.6A)**.
- During placement of sutures, eversion or inversion of matrix should be carefully avoided to prevent permanent nail deformation.
- Dorsal nail fold is kept open by reinserting previously removed nail plate. This is done in order to:
  • Prevent scarring between the eponychium and matrix.
  • Nail provides splintage to underlying fracture.
  • Nail plate serves as template for future nail growth.
- If the nail plate is not available, cut foil of suture pack may be used for the same purpose.
- Nail plate reinsertion may be performed by passing a 5-0 non absorbable suture from the dorsal aspect of eponychium to the base of the nail plate and back from the nail plate to the eponychium **(Fig. 17.7)**. The nail plate is gently reinserted into the dorsal nail fold. The two ends of the suture are tied over a small cotton piece. **(Fig. 17.6B)**.
- Remember to remove the digital tourniquet at the end of the procedure.
- Volar splint is then applied as mentioned in section on non-operative management.
- Dressing is discontinued in 2 weeks. The replaced nail plate adheres to the underlying matrix but falls off in 4 to 6 weeks with growth of new nail plate.
- Splinting may be discontinued in 4 weeks.

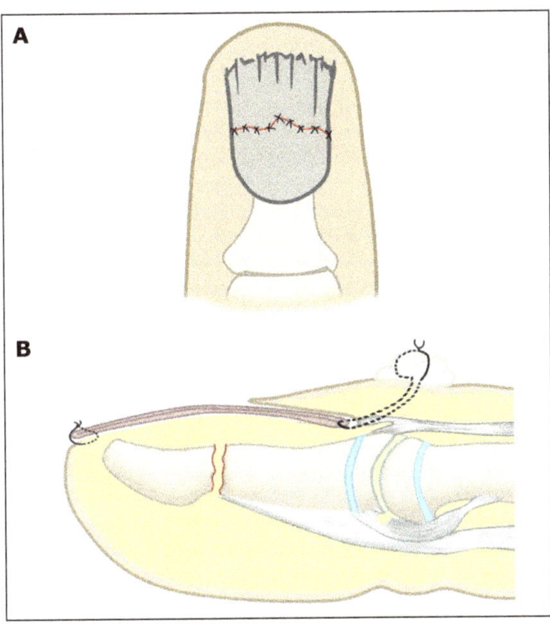

***Fig. 17.6**: Repair of nail bed laceration: (A) Nail bed laceration sutured with interrupted sutures, (B) Replacement of nail plate to keep dorsal nail fold open.*

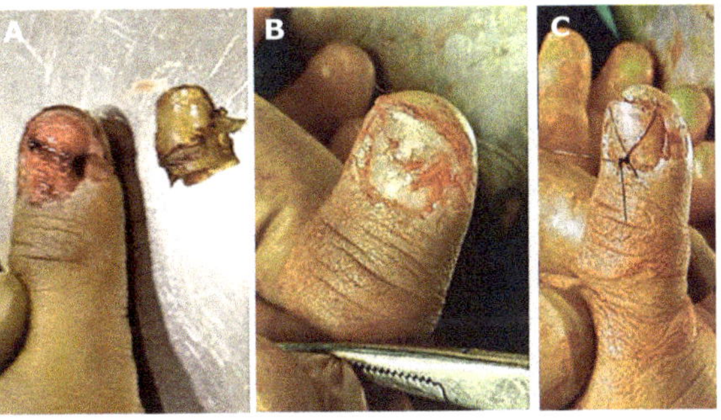

***Fig. 17.7**: (A) Nail bed laceration of the thumb with avulsion of nail plate. (B) After repair of nail bed laceration. (C) Repositioning of nail plate and fixation with suture.*

(3) Fingertip amputation

- Fingertip amputations are often compound fractures of underlying distal phalanx.
- Fingertip amputations with minimal loss of tissue usually heal by secondary intention. Even if minimal bone is exposed, these wounds may heal with repeated dressing.
- Options for raw area coverage in dorsal oblique and large volar oblique finger amputations include:

(a) Primary closure

(b) Bone shortening and closure **(Fig. 17.8)**

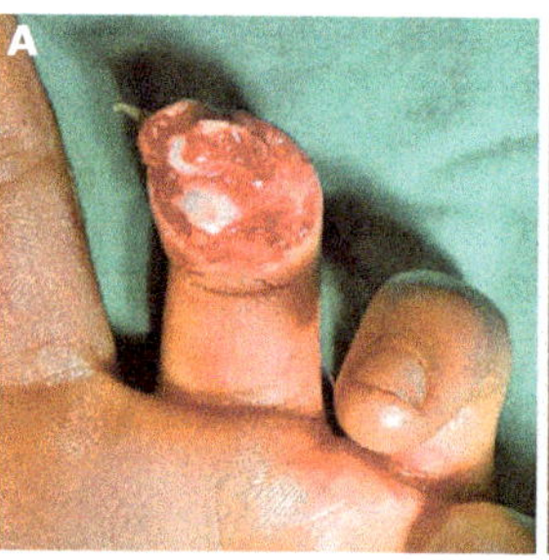

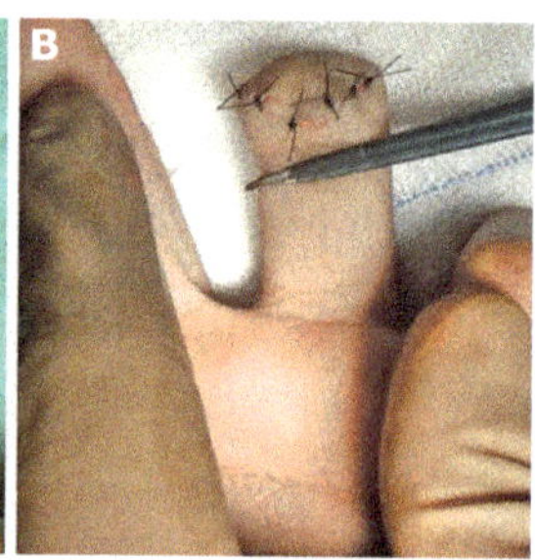

***Fig. 17.8**: (A) Finger amputation at the level of middle phalanx of ring finger. (B) It was treated by bone shortening and closure with skin flap mobilised from the dorsum.*

(c) Full-thickness skin grafts: may be obtained from amputated part or from remote site like medial arm.

(d) Local Flap closure: options include V-Y advancement flap, oblique flap, thenar flap, cross-finger flap **(Figs. 17.9 and 17.10)**

(e) Remote flap: options include abdominal flap, groin flap.

- If nail bed loss is more than 50%, primary nail ablation should be performed.
- Plastic surgery team should be involved for reconstruction of complex finger tip defects.

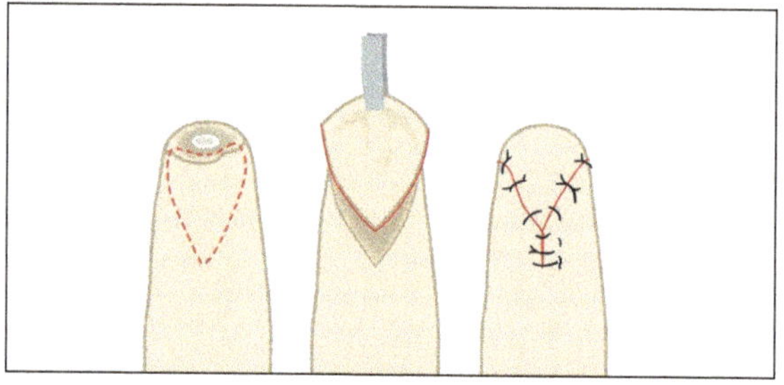

***Fig. 17.9**: V-Y flap for coverage of finger-tip injury. These flaps are used for coverage of transverse or dorsal oblique finger-tip avulsions. The distal edge of the wound forms the base of the flap. The apex of the flap is at the distal interphalangeal joint crease. The skin, subcutaneous tissue and septae anchoring the pulp tissue to bone are released and the flap is mobilised distally. Upto 1cm flap mobilisation can be achieved. The flap is sutured in the shape of Y.*

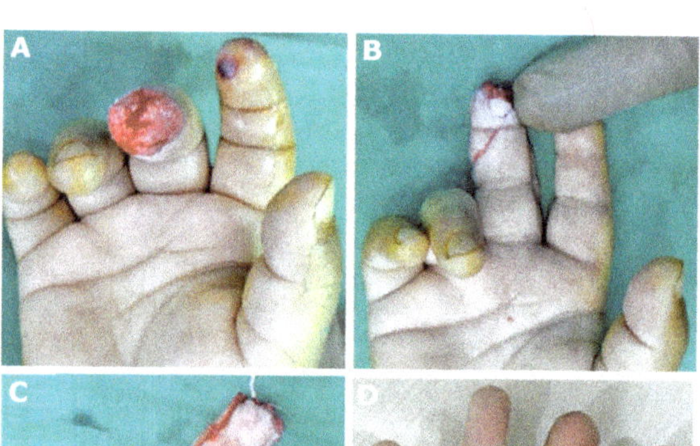

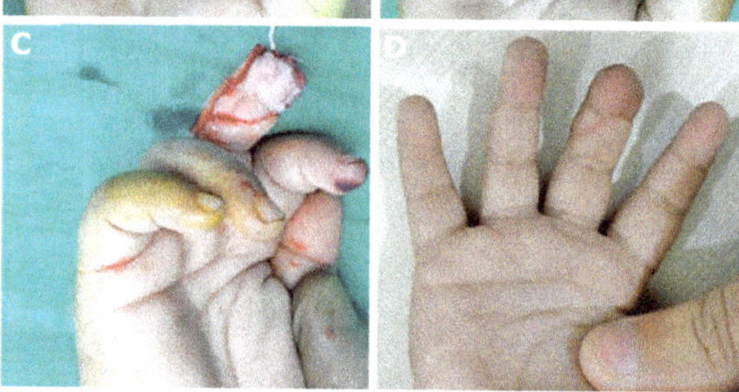

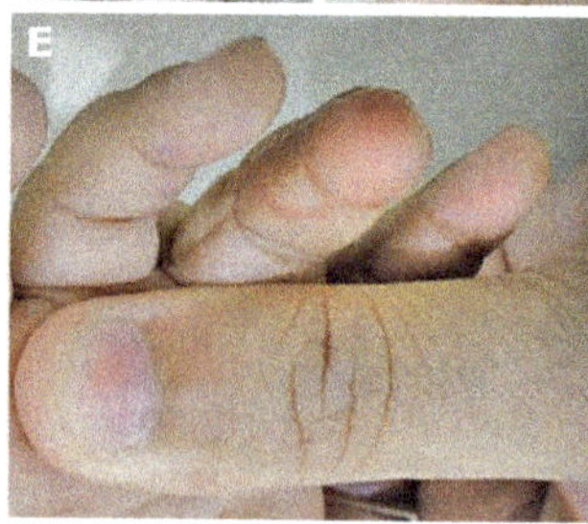

***Fig. 17.10**: (A) Fingertip amputation of the middle finger. (B,C) The raw area was closed by raising a V-Y advancement flap with the apex based on the ulnar side of the finger. (D,E) Healing at one month post-operation.*

- Post-operative immobilisation is performed with a splint applied in safe (functional/ Edinburgh) position with wrist in slight dorsiflexion, MCP joints in 70-90^{0} flexion and IP joints extended. The safe position is maintained for a period of 3 weeks. **(Fig. 17.11)**

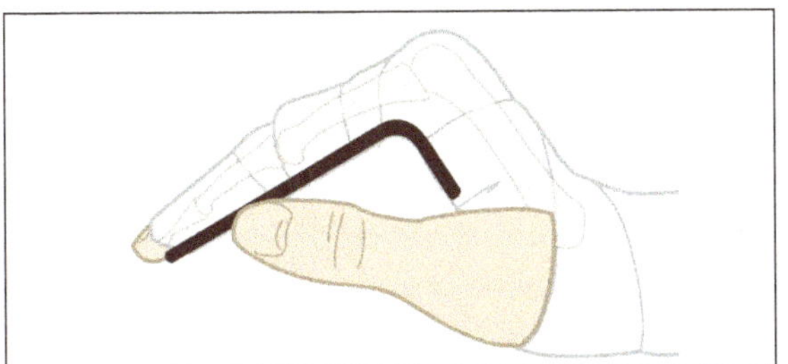

Fig. 17.11: *Safe position for hand immobilisation.*

(4) Extra-physeal fractures

- It is important to repair nail bed lacerations in association with these fractures. These lacerations may be difficult to recognise in the presence of intact nail plate. In many cases, retraction of the interposed nail bed and replacement of nail plate is sufficient to achieve reduction and stability in these fractures.
- Most of these fractures are treated conservatively by splint application. However if displaced or malrotated, closed reduction and fixation with K-wire inserted from phalanx tip may be performed **(Fig. 17.12)**
- In case of open fractures, the K-wire may be inserted retrograde through the fracture surface by inside out technique.

(5) Physeal fractures

Seymour's fracture

- Seymour's fractures which are compound Salter Harris Type 1 injuries with entrapment of nail matrix should be open reduced. Overlying nail bed laceration is repaired. After nail bed repair and nail plate replacement, fracture alignment and stability is usually restored and fracture fixation is not required. **(Fig. 17.13)**

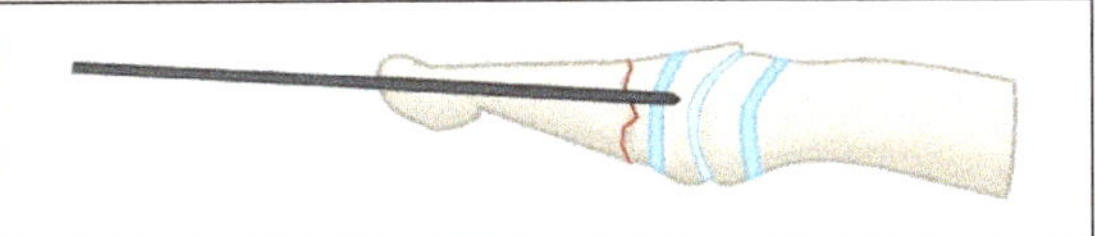

Fig. 17.12: *Fixation of distal phalanx with K-wire inserted from phalanx tip.*

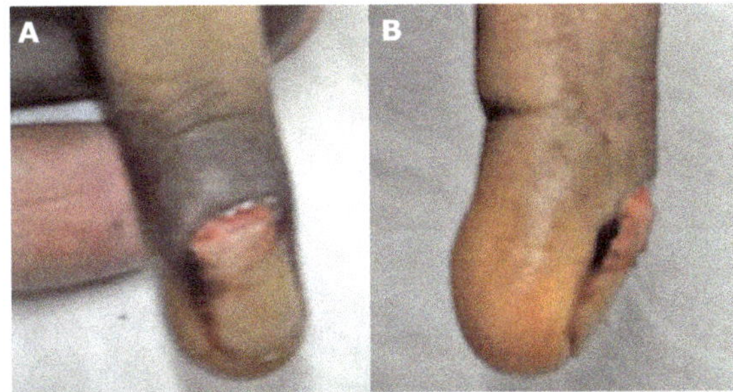

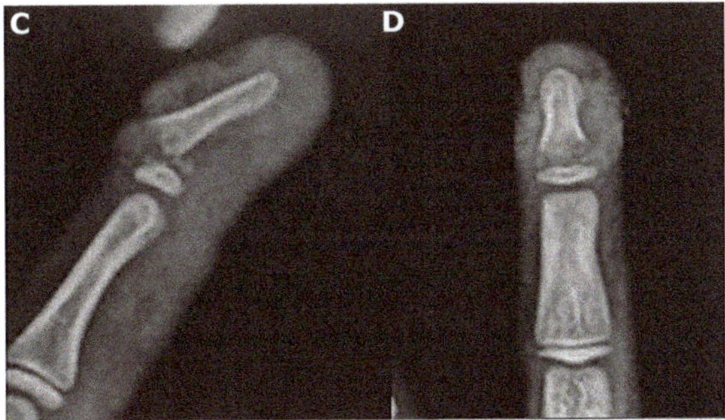

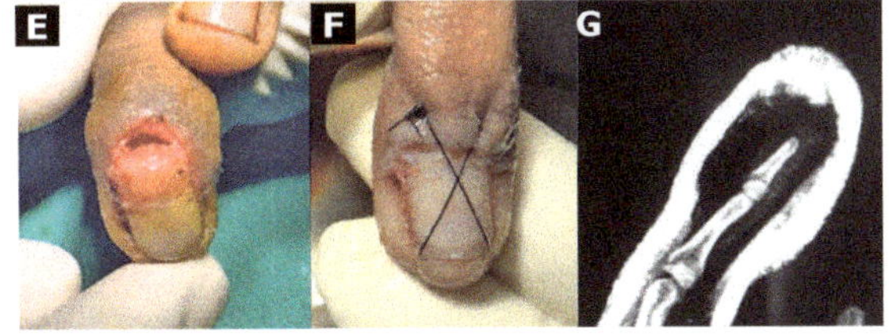

Fig. 17.13: *(A,B) Seymour fracture of index finger. 7 years old child presented with door-trap injury to the index finger. (C,D) X-rays index finger AP and lateral views showing Salter Harris Type 1 fracture of the distal phalanx with physeal widening due to entapment of nail bed germinal matrix. (E,F) Child was operated, entrapped germinal matrix was removed, fracture was reduced, nail bed laceration repaired and nail plate replaced (G) Post-operative X-ray shows normalisation of physeal width.*

- However if fracture continues to be unstable, it may be fixed with single K-wire from phalanx tip to epiphysis.
- Post-operative splint is applied.
- K-wire is removed at 4 weeks.

(6) Paediatric mallet finger

- Majority of these injuries are treated by closed reduction and volar splint application with DIP joint held in slight extension.
- However fixation may be needed for fractures which are severely displaced and irreducible, involve more than 50% articular surface and those with associated subluxation of DIP joint
- Fixation options include K-wire fixation of the DIP joint in extension or extension block pinning with splint application **(Fig. 17.14)**.

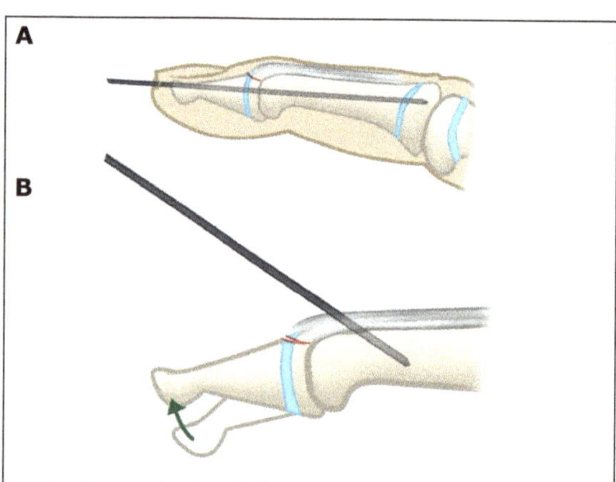

Fig. 17.14: *Fixation of paediatric bony mallet finger (A) with K-wire inserted from the phalanx tip, and, (B) with extension block pinning.*

- Rarely if fracture is irreducible, open reduction and fixation with mini-fragment screws or transosseous pull through sutures is needed.
- Post-operative extension splint is discontinued and K-wire is removed after 4 weeks.

(7) Jersey finger

- These are rare S-H type 3 or 4 volar fractures of distal phalanx occurring due to volar plate or FDP avulsion and should be open reduced and fixed.
- They are treated by volar approach, fixed with K-wire or transosseous pull-through suture.

MIDDLE AND PROXIMAL PHALANX FRACTURES

Classification

- Middle and proximal phalanx fractures can be classified as
- • Physeal (S-H 1/2/3/4)
- • Extraphyseal
  - o diaphyseal
  - o neck
  - o condyles

Clinical Features

- Unlike distal phalanx fractures, proximal and middle phalanx fractures are mostly caused by rotatory or angular forces rather than crush injuries.
- As in distal phalanx fractures, malrotation should be assessed by observing for digital scissoring on finger flexion **(Fig. 17.15)**.

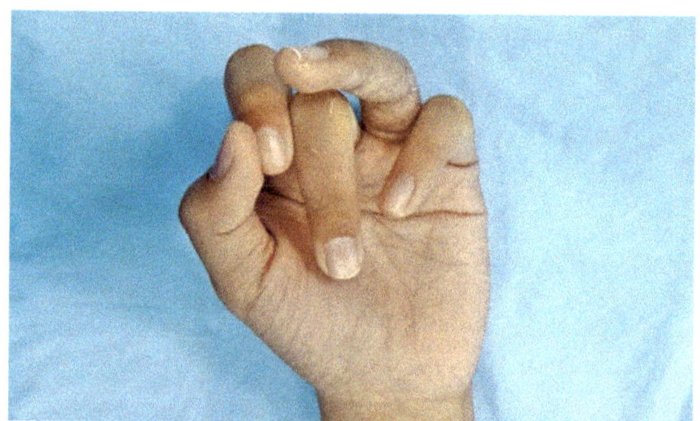

Fig. 17.15: *Digital scissoring in a child with mal-rotated fracture of the proximal phalanx of the ring finger.*

Imaging

- AP, lateral, oblique views should be ordered for evaluation of these injuries. Additionally, finger cascade and isolated finger AP/ lateral views may be requested.
- A S-H type 2 fracture of the base of proximal phalanx of little finger with ulnar deviation is denoted by the eponym *"extra-octave fracture"* because malunion in this position is of benefit to a pianist by virtue of increase of digital span. **(Fig. 17.16)**

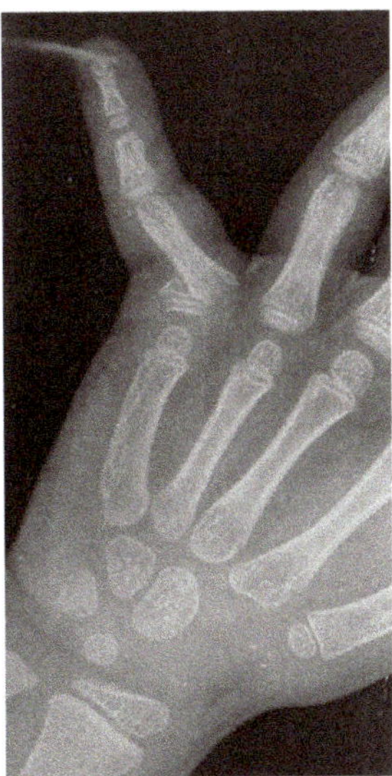

***Fig. 17.16**: Extra-octave fracture (Salter Harris type 2 fracture of base of little finger with ulnar deviation).*

- Dorsal S-H type 3 and 4 fractures of the middle phalanx occur due to hyperflexion injury with avulsion of central slip of extensor tendon (paediatric Boutonniere injury).
- On the other hand, hyperextension results in volar S-H 3 or 4 fractures due to volar plate avulsion.
- Medial S-H type 3 injury of thumb base occurs due to lateral deviation injury and avulsion of Ulnar Collateral Ligament (UCL) attachment. This is analogous to the adult "gamekeeper injury". The UCL with attached fragment may herniate out of the adductor pollicis aponeurosis *(Stener's lesion)*. Failure to treat these injuries leads to grip weakness. Open reduction of these fractures is indicated in the presence of Stener's lesion or MCP instability.
- Neck fractures are often hyper-extended. These may be irreducible due to interposition of volar plate in the fracture gap. Malunion of these fractures results in flexion block of the corresponding inter-phalangeal joint.

Treatment

Non-operative treatment

- Most of the proximal and middle phalanx physeal and diaphyseal fractures can be successfully treated with non-operative management. On the other hand, many neck fractures need operative treatment.
- An extra-octave injury with ulnar displacement can be reduced by placing a gauze ball in the 4th web space to serve as a fulcrum over which the little and ring fingers are approximated. Immobilisation is then achieved by buddy taping the little and ring fingers with/without application of splint in safe position.
- Non-operative treatment may be considerered in Salter Harris Type 3 and 4 injuries if the fracture fragment is less than 25% of the articular surface area and there is no instability of the adjacent joint. A dorsal injury is immobilised in extension and volar injury is immobilised in flexion.

Operative treatment

- In Salter Harris Type 1 and 2 injuries, closed reduction and cross K-wire fixation may be considered for irreducible or unstable fractures.

- In Salter Harris Type 3 and 4 injuries involving more than 25% of articular surface or with instability of the adjacent joint, closed reduction and K-wire fixation may be attempted. If irreducible by closed means, open reduction and fixation with K-wires or mini-fragment screws or pull-through sutures is performed. Approach depends on location of fracture fragment.
- In gamekeeper's thumb with Stener's lesion, fracture exposure can be achieved with incision of adductor fascia. After reduction and fixation, the fascia should be closed.
- In shaft fractures, an angulation of upto 30° in children < 10 years age and 20° in adolescents is acceptable. If this is not achieved with non-operative methods, closed reduction and K-wire fixation may be performed with longitudinal or transverse K-wire depending on fracture configuration.
- In phalangeal neck fractures, closed reduction is performed by distraction, volar directed pressure on the dorsally displaced distal fragment, with flexion of the interphalangeal joint. In few cases, an interposed volar plate may block reduction. In these cases, closed reduction may be attempted by using an intra-focal K-wire technqiue. Fixation is performed with K-wires inserted from the lateral aspect of the distal fragment into the contralateral cortex of the proximal fragment. Alternatively wire may be inserted retrogradely from the tip of distal phalanx.

Complications

Malunion:

Malrotation is often underestimated and missed on X-rays and leads to grip disturbances. Malunion of phalangeal neck fractures leads to functional block. Despite being away from physis, neck malunions show good remodelling in younger children. However osteotomy is needed in older children for restoration of flexion

Non union:

It can occur in neck fractures due to volar plate interposition.

METACARPAL FRACTURES

Classification

- Metacarpal fractures in children can be:
- Physeal fractures
- Neck fractures
- Diaphyseal fractures
- Base fractures

Clinical Features

- Metacarpal fractures are usually caused by fall of heavy object on hand. Metacarpal neck fractures may be caused due to trauma to closed fist as in boxing.
- Clinical evaluation for malrotation is essential.
- Multiple metacarpal fractures may be associated with compartment syndrome of hand

Imaging

Antero-posterior, lateral and oblique views.

Metacarpal neck fractures

- Metacarpal neck is the commonest site of metacarpal fractures as the cortex is thinnest in this part.
- These are analogous to adult boxer's fractures.
- They are commonest in the peripheral two digits. i.e. small and ring fingers.

Diaphyseal fractures

- They are relatively common.
- Central ray fractures are usually stable due to attachments of inter-metacarpal ligaments, whereas peripheral ray fractures are more unstable and prone to displacement and shortening.

Base fractures

- Metacarpal base fractures are rare in children.
- In first metacarpal base fractures (Bennet's fracture), the abductor pollicis longus which inserts into the first metacarpal base is the main deforming force.
- In fifth metacarpal base fractures, proximal pull of the extensor carpi ulnaris can cause fracture-dislocation of the little finger carpo-metacarpal joint (reverse Bennet's fracture).

Treatment

Non-operative treatment

- Majority of metacarpal fractures in children are treated non-operatively
- In metacarpal neck fractures, reduction is performed by Jahss manoeuvre. It consists of flexion of the MCP joint to 90°, longitudinal pressure along the long axis of the finger so as to push the metacarpal head dorsally into anatomical alignment with simultaneous push on the dorsal aspect of metacarpal neck to provide counter-pressure. **(Fig. 17.17)**
- Fractures of 2nd to 5th metacarpals are immobilised by application of splint in safe position (MCP joints in 70-90° flexion, interphalangeal joints extended).
- Fractures of 1st metacarpal are immobilised with thumb spica cast.

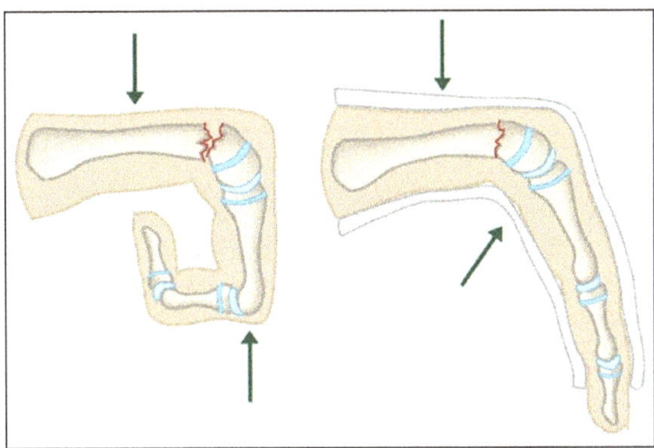

***Fig. 17.17**: Jahss manoeuvre: The metacarpo-phalangeal joint is flexed to 90°, longitudinal compression is applied along the long axis of the finger, followed by application of a well-moulded splint.*

Operative treatment

- Surgical treatment is reserved for
  - Multiple fractures
  - Extensive soft tissue injury
  - Malrotated fractures
  - Intra-articular fractures
  - Irreducible fractures
  - Unstable fractures
- Surgical treatment consists of closed reduction or open reduction and fixation. Fixation options include crossed K-wires or intramedullary antegrade K-wires introduced from metacarpal base or inter-fragmentary screws or plate and screws depending on the fracture configuration.
- *Bennet's fracture:* These are intra-articular fractures and are treated surgically. Reduction is effected by digital pressure on lateral aspect of the displaced metacarpal. K-wire fixation may be performed percutaneously traversing the physis and CMC joint. Alternatively, the shaft fragment may be fixed transversely to the 2nd metacarpal. **(Fig. 17.18)**

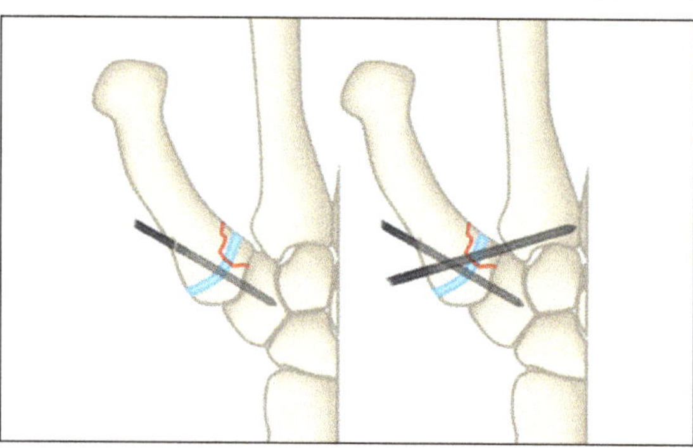

***Fig. 17.18**: Fixation of Bennet's fracture.*

Complications

Malunion:

In extra-articular fractures, malunion is well tolerated. Malunion in intra-articular fractures can lead to arthrosis and pain in the long run.

FRACTURES OF SCAPHOID

Introduction

- Fractures of scaphoid are rare in children due to the predominant cartilaginous component of the scaphoid. Due to differential ossification from distal to proximal, avulsion fractures of distal pole are commoner in younger children, whereas scaphoid waist fractures and proximal pole fractures are commoner in older children and adolescents engaged in contact sports.
- Differential ossification of the scaphoid also leads to increased radiographic clear space between the scaphoid and lunate, which may be mis-interpreted as a sign of carpal instability (pseudo-Terry Thomas sign).

Classification

- Type A: Distal pole fractures
    - A1: Distal pole extra-articular
    - A2: Distal pole intra-articular
- Type B: Middle third (waist) fractures
- Type C: Proximal pole fractures

Clinical features

- Scaphoid fractures usually occur following fall on outstretched hand with extended wrist.
- Clinical evaluation reveals tenderness and oedema overlying the anatomical snuff box. Tenderness is aggravated on ulnar deviation of the wrist.

Imaging

- AP/ lateral/ oblique views
- *Scaphoid view:* is obtained by placing the palm down on the X-ray receptor with maximal ulnar deviation of the wrist. This projection places the long axis of scaphoid parallel to the X-ray film and provides full profile view of the scaphoid. **(Fig. 17.19)**

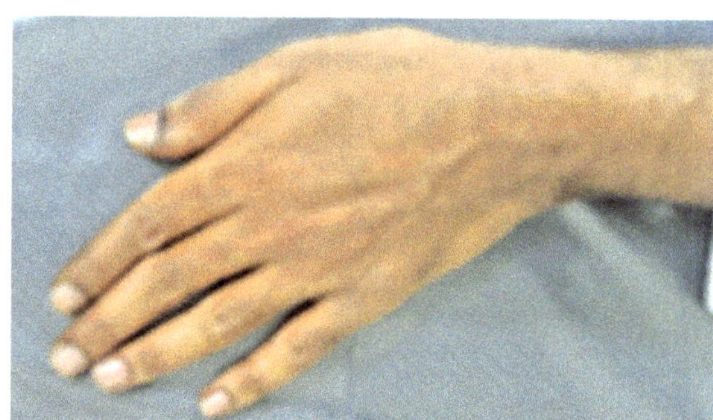

***Fig. 17.19**: Positioning for obtaining scaphoid view X-ray.*

- MRI: is useful in assessment of clinically suspected scaphoid fractures with plain radiographs being normal.
- CT scan: CT scan is useful for diagnosing scaphoid fractures and assessing union. CT cuts along longitudinal axis of scaphoid should be specifically requested for.

Treatment

Non-operative treatment

- Undisplaced fractures can be effectively

managed with thumb spica cast application.

- The cast is applied with slight extension and radial deviation of the wrist joint. The thumb is in glass-holding position. Most surgeons allow free movement of the thumb interphalangeal joint within the cast.
- Below elbow cast is adequate for adolescents, however in younger children, cast should be extended above the elbow to prevent cast slippage.
- Cast should be continued for a period of 8 weeks. However for proximal pole fractures, immobilisation is continued for 12 weeks.
- In the event of normal post-injury radiographs, in the presence of positive clinical findings of scaphoid fracture, cast should be applied for a period of two weeks. At the end two weeks, the cast should be removed, child should be clinically assessed and radiographs should be repeated.
- If two weeks radiographs confirm fracture, cast immobilisation should be continued for 8 weeks.
- If at the end of two weeks, clinical signs are positive, but radiographs still don't reveal any fracture, MRI is performed to detect occult fractures.

Operative treatment

- Closed reduction-internal fixation may be attempted in minimally displaced fractures. If satisfactory closed reduction is achieved, percutaneous screw fixation is performed.
- Open reduction and internal fixation is indicated for fractures with more than 1mm displacement or more than 10° intra-scaphoid angulation. Approach for open reduction may be volar or dorsal. Compression screws are mainly used for internal fixation, though K-wires may occasionally be used.

Complications

Non union:

Rarer than in adults.

Avascular necrosis:

AVN is more common after proximal pole fractures of the scaphoid.

Inter-carpal instability:

It can occur as a consequence of long standing non-union.

FRACTURES OF OTHER CARPAL BONES

- These are extremely rare.
- They occur following high energy trauma and are usually a component of a larger injury like a peri-lunate or lunate dislocation.
- They may be complicated by compartment syndrome of hand.
- Hamate fractures may involve the hook or body. CT scan may be needed for diagnosing these fractures.
- Trapezium fractures can occur in association with injuries to the thumb carpo-metacarpal joint.

Treatment

- Fractures of most of the other carpal bones are treated conservatively if undisplaced and by open reduction-internal fixation if displaced. Other associated peri-lunate injuries are simultaneously repaired.
- Hook of hamate fractures are treated with excision of the fracture fragment if small.

Dislocations of Inter-phalangeal and Metacarpo-phalangeal Joints

Introduction

- Dislocations of IP and MCP joints are rare in children as ligaments are stronger than physes, and hence, physeal fractures are commoner than joint disruptions.

Classification

- *Depending on direction:*
• Dorsal
• Volar
• Lateral
- *Depending on severity:*
• Simple: easily reducible by closed means
• Complex: irreducible due to interposition of volar plate with/ without FDP tendon

The two can be differentiated by the fact that in simple dislocation, the dislocated bone is at right angles to the preceding bone. On the other hand, in complex dislocations the two bones are parallel to each other.

Clinical Features

Dislocations are diagnosed by history of trauma followed by pain, swelling, shortening and deviation of the involved digit in the direction of dislocation.

Imaging

- AP and lateral view of the involved digit.
- MCP joint dislocations may not be obvious and careful evaluation of oblique radiographs is needed to diagnose these.

Treatment

- Closed reduction:
• Possible in simple dislocations
• The closed reduction manoeuvre consists of traction, exaggeration of the deforming force followed by translation of the dislocated bone over the preceding bone.
• K-wire if unstable, splint in stable position for 3 weeks
- Open reduction:
• For irreducible dislocations
• Dorsal or volar approach
• SOS K-wire, splint in stable position

Complications

- Digital nerve injury:

  Iatrogenic injury following volar approach, especially in MCP joint dislocations.
- Redislocation
- Stiffness

Flowchart 17.1

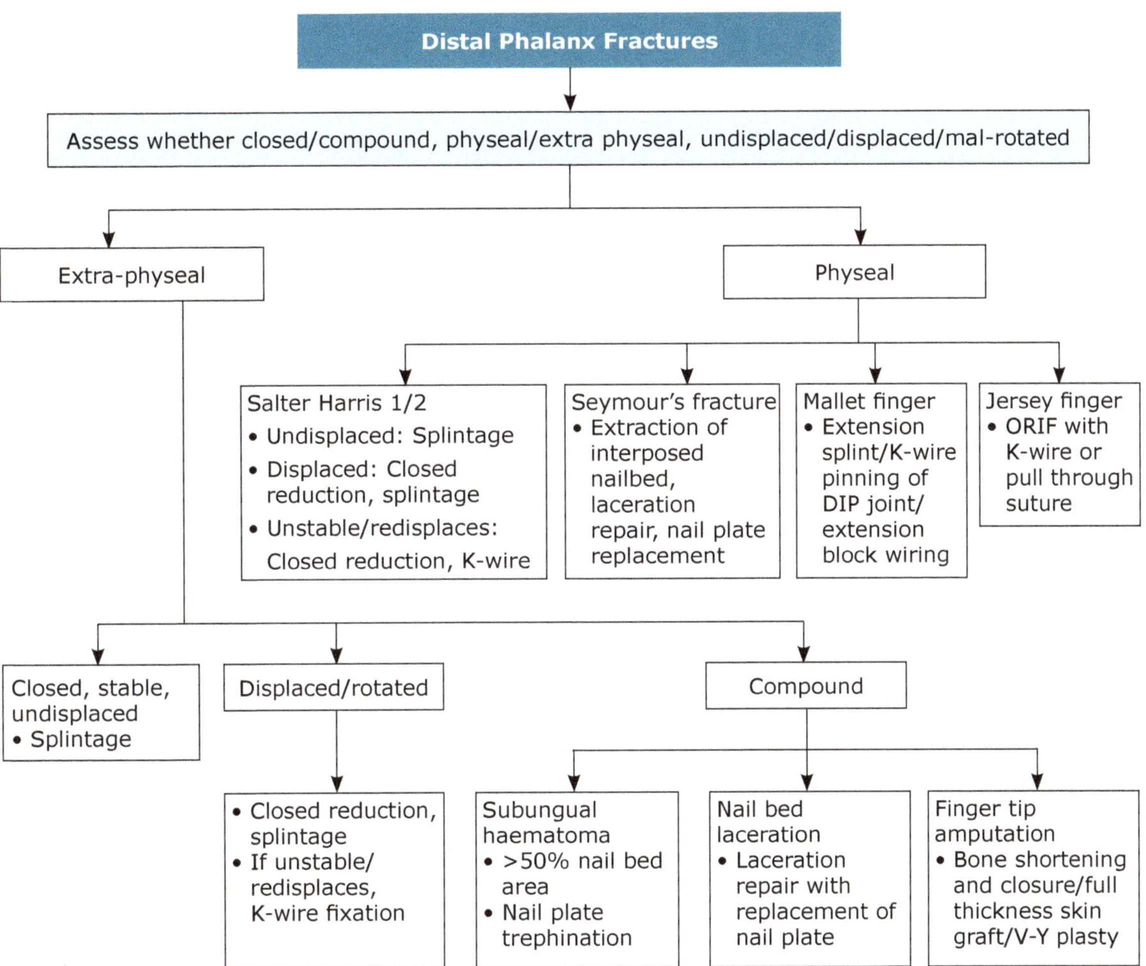

Flowchart 17.2

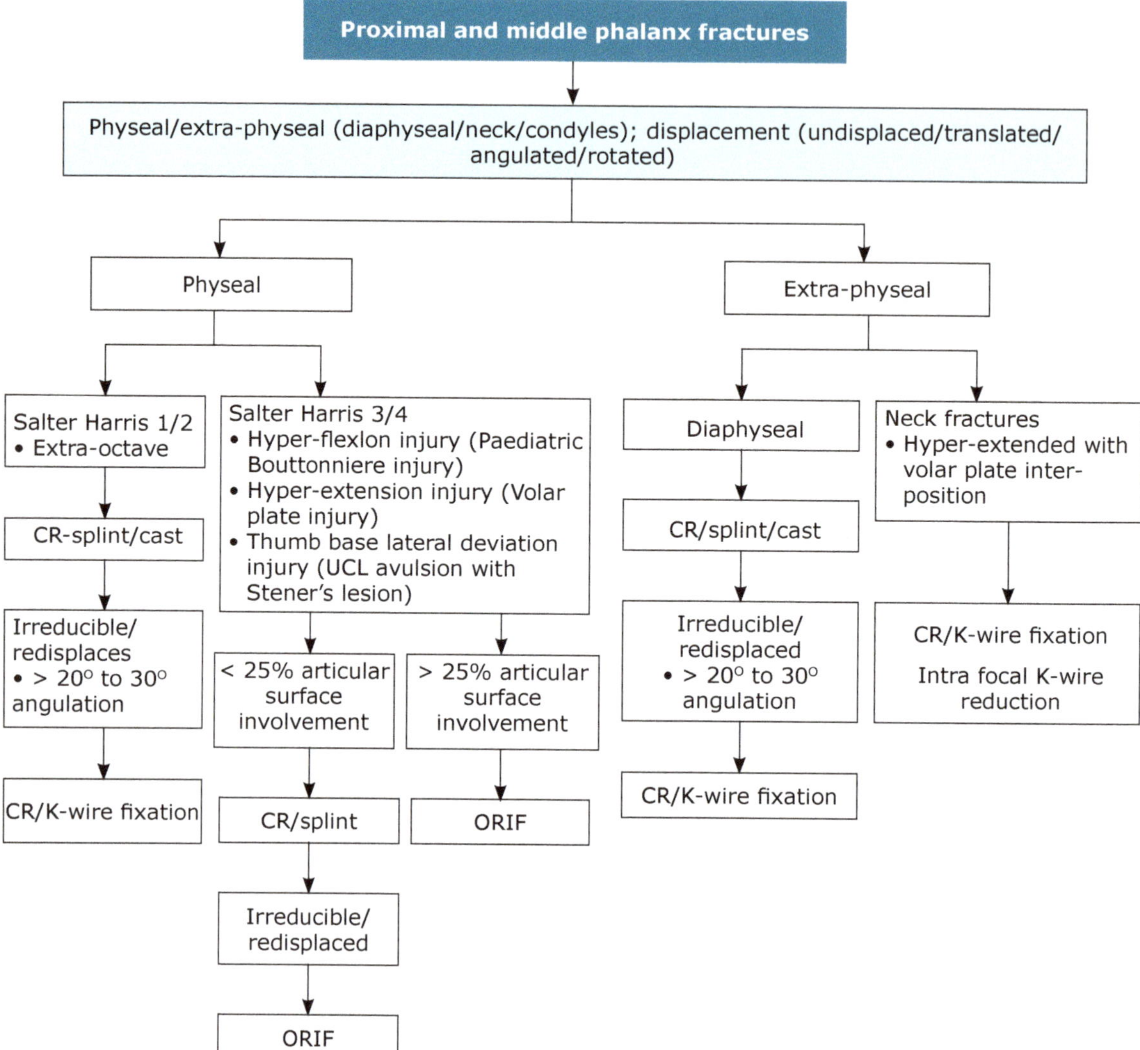

Flowchart 17.3

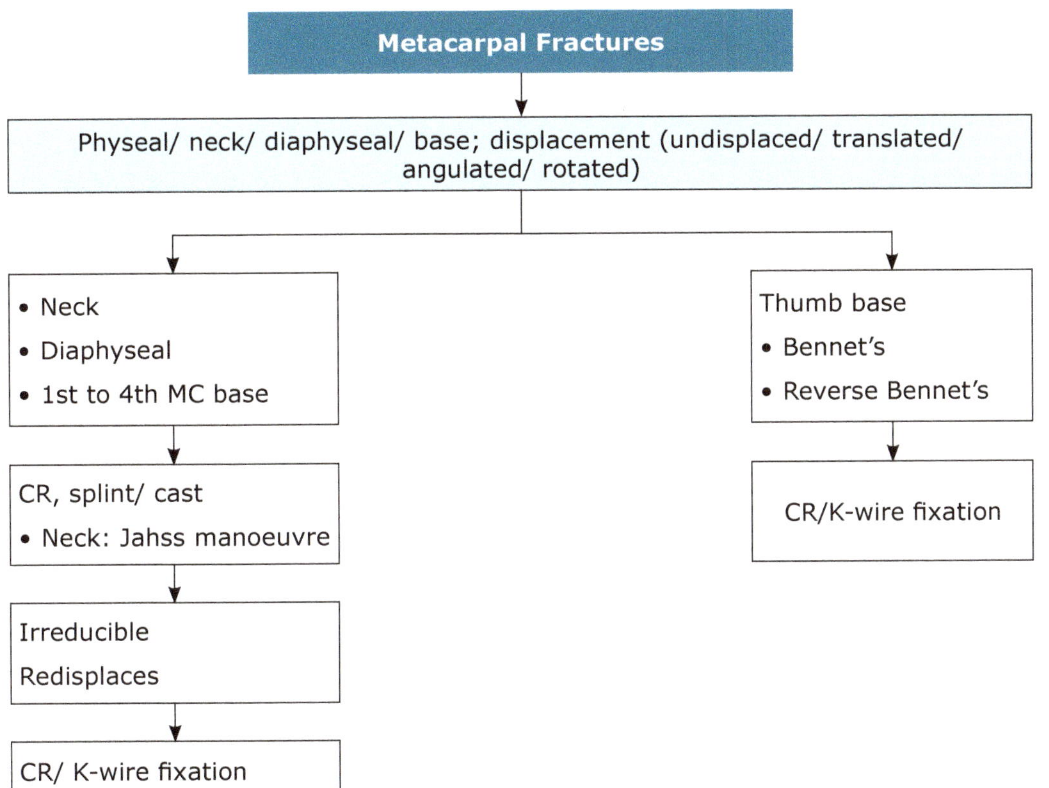

18 Acetabular and Pelvic Fractures

Introduction

Pelvis and acetabulum fractures are uncommon, accounting for <1% of all paediatric fractures. These fractures represent high energy injuries like motor vehicle accidents or fall from height and present with many associated injuries. Due to the presence of triradiate cartilage in children, these fractures are prone for growth arrest if not managed properly.

Children sustain more of lateral compression injury as opposed to antero-posterior force in adults, hence it does not result in expansion of pelvic ring or disruption of sacroiliac (SI) joint, thereby having less intra pelvic haemorrhage. Also, increased contractility of a child's smaller arterial vessels leads to greater vasoconstriction after injury and less haemorrhage following pelvic injury as compared to adults. Hence mortality rate solely from pelvic injury is lower in children.

Pathoanatomy

- Sacrotuberous, sacrospinous and anterior and posterior sacroiliac ligaments, in addition to iliolumbar and lumbosacral ligaments provide stability to the pelvis. **(Fig. 18.1)**
- Nervous, genitourinary and vascular systems lie adjacent to the pelvis. Lumbosacral Coccygeal plexus ,sciatic nerve and common iliac vessels are in close proximity.
- Bladder and urethra are the structures of the urinary system that are most commonly injured after a pelvic fracture.

Associated Injuries

- Intra-abdominal injuries (15%), like

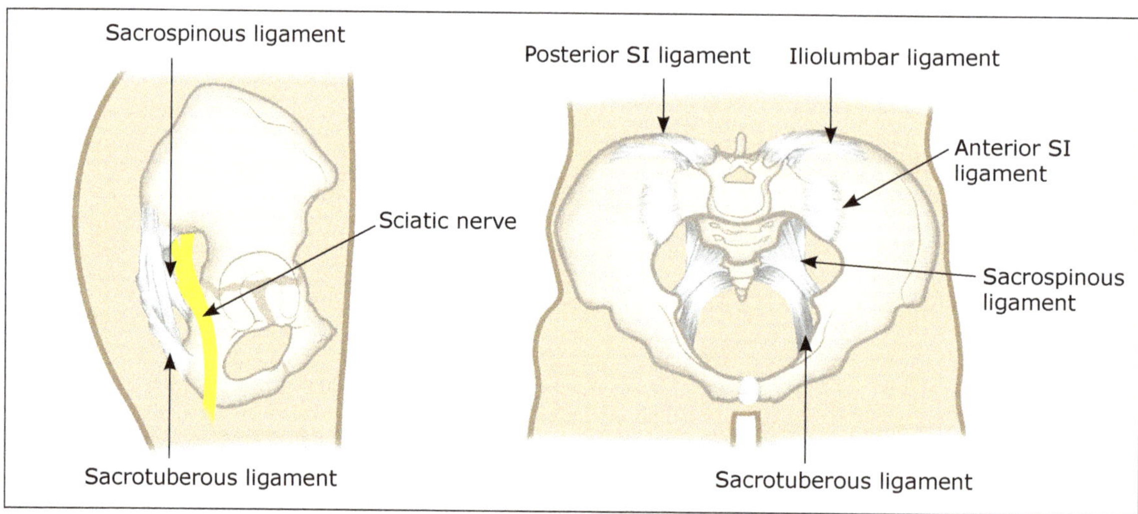

***Fig. 18.1**: Ligaments around the Pelvic ring.*

contusion/laceration of the spleen, liver or kidney, large intestine or small intestine

- Neurological injuries (50%)
- Musculoskeletal injuries (50%)
- Genito urinary injuries(10-20%)

Clinical Features

- In case of pelvic and acetabular fractures, the clinical evaluation should begin with ABC (Airway, Breathing, Circulation) of polytrauma and complete neurovascular examination. After haemodynamic stabilisation of the child, secondary survey and evaluation specific to pelvic injuries can be carried out. Gentle palpation of different sites of the pelvis like symphysis pubis, anterior superior iliac spine (ASIS), iliac crest and SI joint and gentle pelvic compression-distraction test will help in identification of specific fracture. **(Fig. 18.2)**

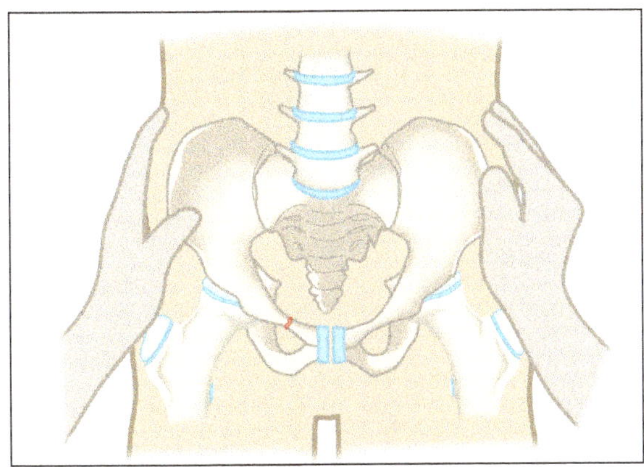

***Fig. 18.2**: Pelvic compression-distraction test.*

- Sporting activities mainly result in avulsion fracture of the secondary ossification centre of growing pelvis, especially in 11-17 years old children. These avulsion injuries are a result of forceful contraction of large muscles, typically those that traverse both hip and knee with origins on pelvic apophyses. These apophyses need to be palpated for tenderness. For example, violent pull of hamstrings can result in acute ischial tuberosity avulsion fracture in gymnasts. ASIS avulsion fracture due to pull of sartorius and anterior inferior iliac spine (AIIS) avulsion fracture due to pull of rectus femoris are seen in soccer players and long distance running can result in iliac apophysitis due to pull of external oblique muscles of abdomen.
- Pelvis and perineum need to be evaluated for lacerations and ecchymosis.
- Gentle log-rolling of the child allows complete inspection for Morel-Lavallee lesion which is a degloving injury where skin and subcutaneous fat is sheared from the underlying muscle, creating a large space where haematoma can form.
- Genitourinary and rectal examination need to be done for evaluation of rectal laceration, urethral tears, bladder disruption and haematuria.
- It is essential to do complete spine examination and lower limb evaluation for associated fractures.
- Head injury needs to be ruled out in all the children with high energy injury, before definite management of pelvic and acetabular fractures.

Imaging

Pelvis AP, Inlet (60° caudal), Outlet (45° cephalad) and Judet views are essential for diagnosis of fracture.

Inlet view helps to assess antero-posterior displacement of the pelvic ring whereas outlet view helps to define superior to inferior displacement of the pelvic ring. **(Figs. 18.3 and 18.4)**

Iliac oblique view shows the posterior

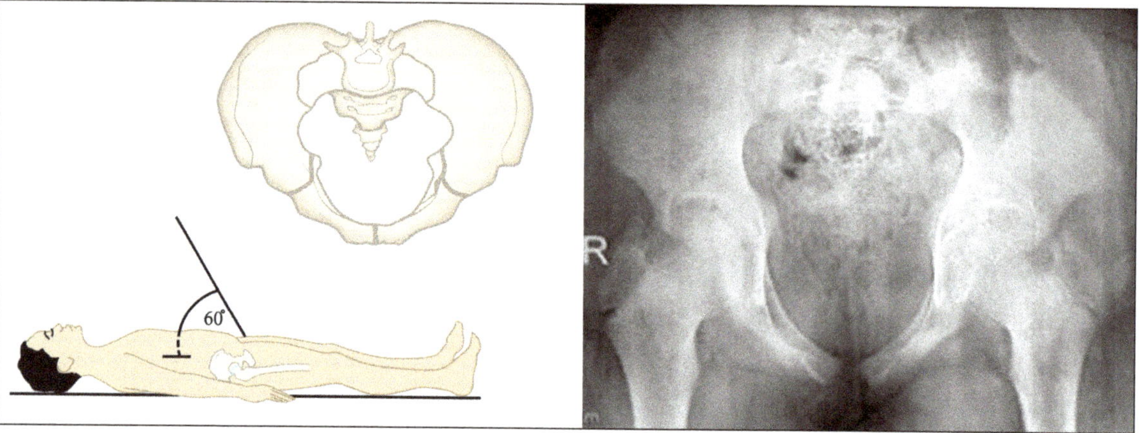

***Fig. 18.3**: Pelvic inlet view.*

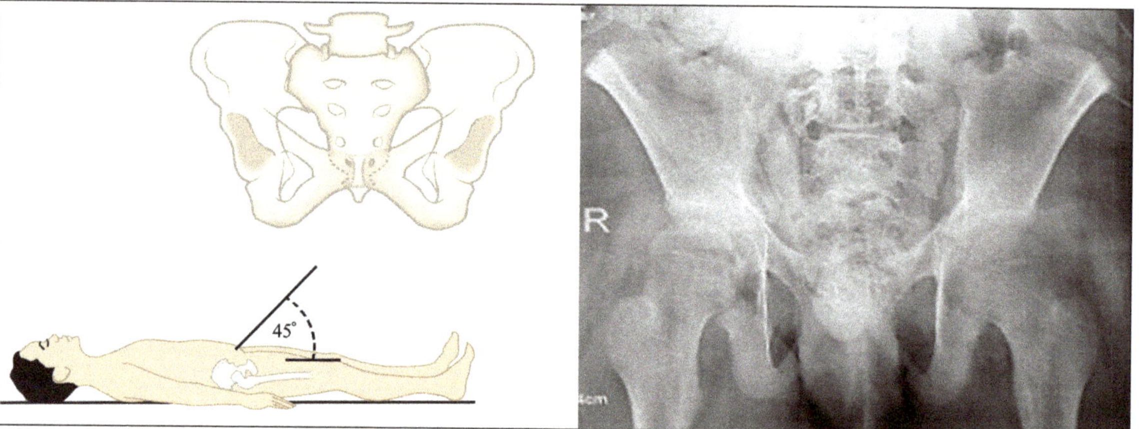

***Fig. 18.4**: Pelvic outlet view.*

column and the anterior wall whereas the obturator oblique view shows the anterior column and the posterior wall. **(Figs. 18.5 and 18.6)**

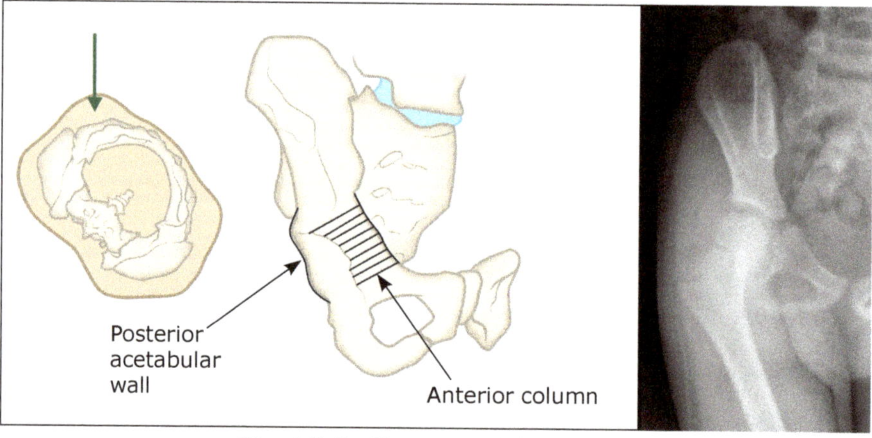

***Fig. 18.5**: Obturator oblique view.*

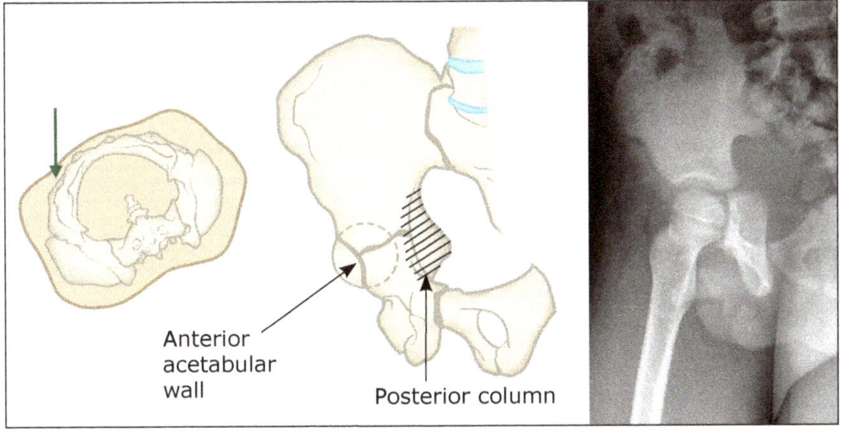

Fig. 18.6: *Iliac oblique view.*

Comparison views of the opposite side is required in c/o avulsion injuries.

CT scan with 3-D reconstruction is the best modality for evaluation of bony pelvis. **(Fig. 18.7)**

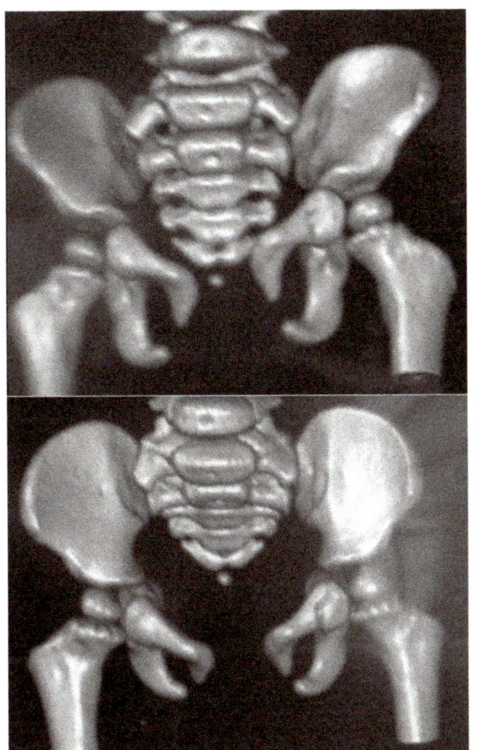

Fig. 18.7: *3-D CT Pelvis showing pubic symphysis diastasis.*

MRI may be required for occult stress fracture, avulsion fracture, acetabular fracture and soft tissue injuries.

At the time of fusion of ischium to pubis, a lucent area is noted on the X-ray, it is asymptomatic and represents ischiopubic synchondrosis. It is often bilateral and should not be confused with acute/stress fracture.

Classification

Pelvic fracture classification

Modified Torode and Zieg classification **(Fig. 18.8)**

I. Avulsion fractures

II. Iliac wing fractures

a. Separation of the iliac apophysis

b. Fracture of the bony iliac wing

III. Simple ring fractures

a. Anterior only ring fracture

b. Stable Anterior and Posterior ring fracture

IV. Unstable ring disruption

a. Double anterior ring disruption:

- Straddle fracture

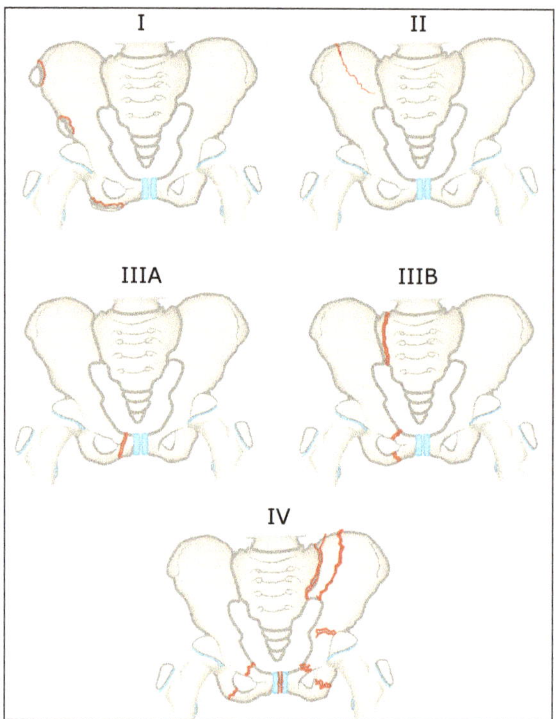

Fig. 18.8: Modified Torode and Zieg classification of Pelvic fractures.

(Bilateral superior and inferior pubic rami fractures)

b. Anterior and posterior pelvic ring (Double ring) disruption:

Fractures involving anterior pubic rami or pubic symphysis and the posterior elements (SI joint or sacral ala)

c. Multiple crushing injury:

Fractures that produce at least two severely comminuted fractures located at any site in the pelvic ring or create an unstable segment between the anterior ring of pelvis and acetabulum.

Pelvis is considered 'unstable' if there is

- Break in anterior and posterior pelvic ring
- Displaced posterior ring fracture
- Displaced triradiate fracture
- Extremely misshapen pelvis

Acetabular Fracture Classification:

Acetabular fracture is very rare, comprising ~ 5-10 % of all pelvic injuries in children.

Type I: Small fragment fracture that occurs with dislocation of the hip

Type II: Linear fractures that result in one or more large, stable fragments

Type III: Linear fractures that result in hip instability

Type IV: Fractures that are secondary to central dislocation of the hip

Isolated triradiate cartilage injuries are difficult to recognise primarily on X-ray, may require thin section (2-3 mm) CT cuts and are prone for premature physeal closure and shallow acetabulum.

Treatment

Torode and Zieg Type I (Avulsion fracture)

- The common avulsion injuries in the pelvis are at
- Ischial tuberosity (attachment of hamstring and hip adductor)
- ASIS (attachment of sartorius)
- AIIS (attachment of direct head of rectus femoris)
- Iliac crest (attachment of iliopsoas)
- Majority are due to athletic injury, occurring mostly in boys of age 12-14 years, due to sudden strenuous activities like kicking a ball or making a quick turn.
- Majority avulsion fractures are treated conservatively with rest, with extremity position in such a way to minimise muscle stretch and partial-weight bearing on axillary crutches for around 2 weeks. Normal activities are usually resumed after 6-8 weeks.
- For ischial tuberosity avulsion

fractures, there is some controversy. Non union rate is quite high, upto 68%. Open reduction and internal fixation is recommended by some for:

- > 1-2 cm displacement and painful non union
- Bony prominence interfering with sitting

Some recommend excision of ischial apophysis if chronic pain and disability persists after displaced fracture.

Surgical steps for open reduction of ischial tuberosity fracture:

- In a prone position, take 7-10 cm incision along the gluteal crease.
- Develop a plane between gluteus maximus and hamstrings.
- With the hip extended and knee slightly flexed, fracture fragments can be easily reduced.
- Fix with a cancellous screw with/ without washer and additional fixation with suture anchors/cables or wires, if needed.

Post-operative protocol:

- Initial period of non-weight bearing and gradual resumption to full-weight bearing over 3-6 weeks.
- Sitting is permitted with hips and knees slightly flexed to reduce stress on hamstrings.
- Resumption of full activities are usually permitted by 12 weeks once adequate strength of the muscles is restored.

Torode and Zieg type II (Isolated iliac wing fracture)

- These are relatively rare injuries (~15 % of all pelvic fractures).
- Mechanism is usually an external force exerted on the iliac wing or a lateral compression type force. The iliac wing is tethered by the abdominal muscles and hip abductors, hence severe displacement is rare and usually occurs laterally. But spasm of hip abductor muscles leads to painful Trendelenburg gait.
- Majority are treated symptomatically for pain and with Partial-weight bearing on axillary crutches till pain persists. Some injuries may have significant blood loss and may require blood transfusion. Ileus may develop after an iliac wing fracture and may require general surgeon consultation. Rarely, large fragments with severe displacement require open reduction and fixation with screws or plates. **(Fig. 18.9)**

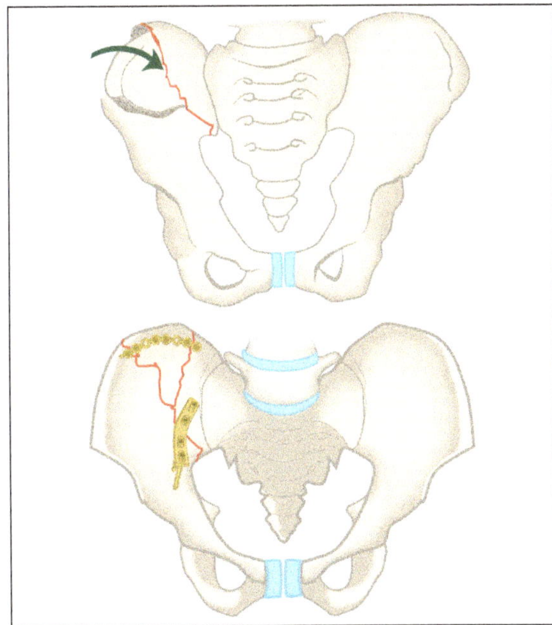

Fig. 18.9: *Internal fixation of large, displaced iliac wing fracture with reconstruction plates.*

Other stable fractures

Fracture of Sacrum

- Sacral fractures are of 2 types:
- Spinal-type injury: Crush injury with

vertical foreshortening or horizontal fracture

It is a significant injury and may damage sacral nerve with loss of bladder, bowel function

- Alar–type injury: Vertical fracture through sacral ala or foramina

  It may represent the posterior break of double ring fracture.

- Clinically, sacral fracture presents with localised pain and tenderness.
- On X-ray, it may be difficult to identify, but one must closely look for minimal offset of the foramen or offset of the lateral edge of the body of the sacrum. 35° caudal view of pelvis may be sometimes helpful for detecting fracture of body of sacrum. CT scan or MRI is best for diagnosis of sacral fracture.
- Treatment is mainly symptomatic. But in rare cases, if there is sacral nerve root impingement, decompression is necessary.

Fracture of Coccyx

- Fracture of coccyx presents with severe localised pain, pain on defecation and severe pain with abnormal mobility on per-rectal examination.
- Lateral X-ray of coccyx should be taken with hips flexed maximally, for better visualisation.
- Apex posterior angulation of coccyx is a normal variant and should not be mistaken for fracture. CT scan/MRI may be useful in differentiating between fracture and physeal plate.
- Majority coccyx fractures are treated symptomatically with activity restriction and pressure relieving cushion for sitting. Symptoms usually resolve in 4-6 weeks. Rarely, local injection or sometimes coccygectomy may be required in adolescents for intractable pain.

Torode and Zeig type III A and B: Simple ring fracture

- Most common fracture type, accounting for upto 55% of all pelvic fractures.
- Unlike in adults in whom a pelvic fracture in one part of the ring may be associated with fracture in another part, children can have fracture in a single aspect of pelvic ring without an associated fracture.

1. Superior pubic ramus fracture

- Clinically, this fracture presents as pain and tenderness at pubic ramus. Child may be unable to walk due to guarding of muscles around the hip. Pelvic ring is grossly stable to rocking and compression.
- Diagnosis can be confirmed on PBH X-ray, Pelvic inlet-outlet views or sometimes with the help of a CT scan.
- Treatment is symptomatic. The child is kept Non-weight bearing for 1-2 weeks. Gradual weight bearing and full activities are restored by 6-8 weeks.

2. Unilateral Superior and Inferior Pubic ramus fracture

These fractures present similar to above mentioned fracture, they are usually stable fractures, but may be associated with injury to abdominal viscera, especially genito-urinary system like bladder or urethral rupture. Special investigations like cystourethrogram may be required in suspected injuries.

Treatment is conservative, as mentioned in the previous fracture.

3. Widening of symphysis pubis

- The child presents with severe pain anteriorly at the pubic symphysis. There may be an external rotation attitude of lower limb and FABER (Flexion, Abduction, External Rotation) sign is positive.

- X-ray PBH/CT scan: >2.5 cm diastasis or rotational deformity >15° suggests significant instability and is an indication for reduction.

  It is also important to look for SI joint disruption and triradiate cartilage fracture.

- Treatment is symptomatic if there is an isolated injury of the pubic symphysis with diastasis < 2 cm. If diastasis is wider, closed reduction and external fixator or open reduction and plating are recommended.

4. *Isolated fracture near or through SI joint*

- Unlike in adults, anterior SI ligaments rarely tear through the entire ligament complex. Hence SI joint injury is usually in the form of physeal separation of ilium adjacent to the joint.
- Clinically, there is pain and tenderness at SI joint, FABER test may be positive.It is important to check distal neurovascular status, as lumbosacral nerve root avulsion can be associated with this injury.
- Radiological diagnosis can be made by pelvic inlet/outlet views or CT scan. Offset of distal SI articular surface is an indication of SI joint disruption.
- Treatment is symptomatic with limited weight bearing with axillary crutches.

  In some cases, open reduction and plate fixation may be required.

Torode and Zeig type IV: Unstable fracture patterns-Ring disruption

Type IV fractures have the highest incidence of associated genito-urinary, neurological and musculoskeletal injuries and also a high mortality rate (~13%)

Bilateral fractures of the Superior and Inferior Pubic Rami (Straddle or floating injuries)

- This type of injury occurs due to lateral compression of pelvis or sudden impact while riding a motorised cycle or fall while straddling a hard object.
- Bilateral superior and inferior pubic rami fracture or disruption of pubic symphysis and unilateral fracture of rami, both these fracture patterns result in a floating anterior segment of pelvic ring, that can displace superiorly, pulled in the direction of rectus abdominis muscle.
- Bladder and urethral disruptions are commonly associated injuries. (~20%)
- Pelvic inlet view/CT scan is helpful in accurate assessment of true displacement.
- Treatment is rest with the hip slightly flexed to relax the abdominal muscles and analgesics. Skeletal traction is not required and pelvic binder is contraindicated as further lateral compression may cause medial displacement of ilium. Fractures take 6-8 weeks to heal. In case of significant displacement, especially in adolescents, surgical treatment with screw/plate fixation may be necessary.

Anterior and Posterior ring disruptions

- This type of injury occurring as a result of antero-posterior or lateral compression, is a serious injury, as it is associated with retroperitoneal and intraperitoneal bleed and can lead to severe, life threatening haemorrhage. This injury results in an unstable pelvis.
- Clinically, there is local pain, tenderness and also limb length discrepancy and asymmetry of pelvis.
- X-ray pelvis inlet and outlet views and sometimes CT scan helps in the diagnosis of this fracture. **(Fig. 18.10)**

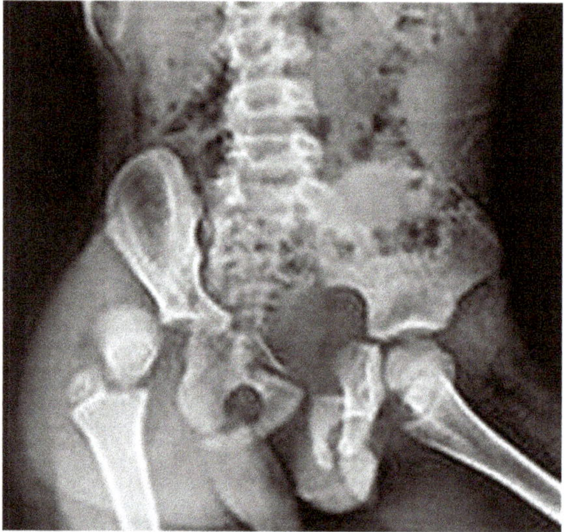

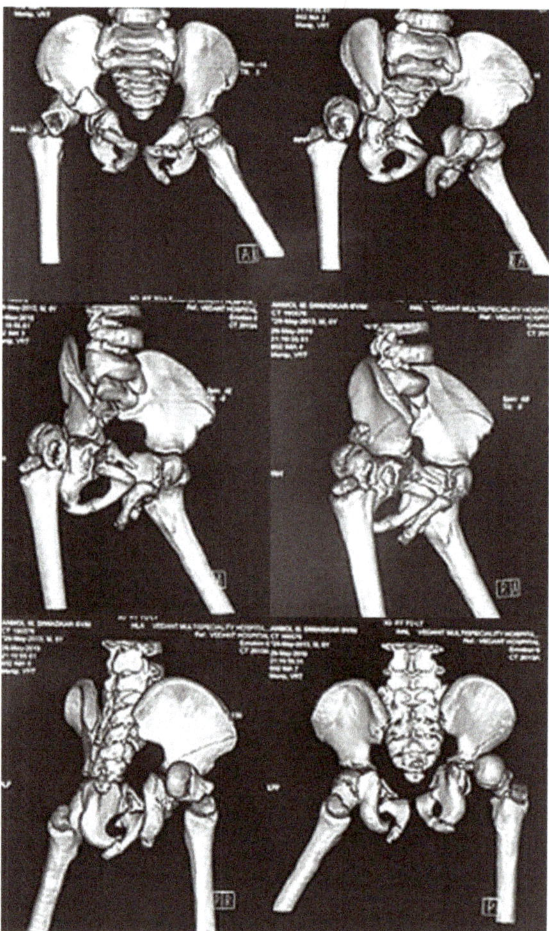

Fig. 18.10: *X-ray Pelvis and 3-D CT scan showing anterior and posterior pelvic ring disruption and transcervical neck femur fracture*

- Initial treatment should be like a polytrauma case taking care of ABC. In anteroposterior compression injury in older children/adolescents, binders/ sheets can be placed circumferentially across greater trochanter to prevent further expansion of pelvic ring and severe haemorrhage. Occasionally, embolisation of arterial vessels is required to control bleeding.

Minimally displaced fractures

- In minimally displaced fractures, treatment comprises analgesics, restricted weight bearing and close radiological follow up.
- Spica cast immobilisation is recommended in small children (< 8 years).
- In some older children and adolescents, fracture fixation is done occasionally to relieve pain and facilitate early mobilisation.

Displaced fractures

- Pelvic asymmetry does not completely remodel even in young children. Hence surgical treatment is recommended for fractures displaced >2 cm and pelvic asymmetry >1.1 cm. With surgical treatment, early mobilisation can be started, anatomic or near anatomic alignment of fracture can be restored and long term poor outcomes like SI arthrosis,limb length discrepancy, back pain can be avoided.
- In case of associated injuries like genitourinary injuries, teamwork/ multidisciplinary approach is needed. Timing of surgery depends on the needs of the individual patient. Emergency external/internal fixation may be required to control haemorrhage in open book injury, whereas sometimes delayed surgery 7-10 days after the initial injury is recommended as per concept of Damage control orthopaedics.

- Surgical options for anterior ring stabilisation are
- External fixator
- Symphyseal and/or rami plate fixation
- Screw fixation of rami and anterior column
- Surgical options for posterior stabilisation are
- SI screw fixation
- Plate fixation

Technique of External fixation

- Indications

1. To control haemorrhage in case of haemodynamic instability that is refractory to blood and fluid resuscitation.
2. Anterior pelvic ring displacement associated with posterior instability in a rotationally and vertically unstable fracture.

- Position

Supine on a radiolucent table **(Fig. 18.11)**

- Steps

- Attempt manual reduction. If required, longitudinal traction can be applied through a supracondylar femoral traction pin. Confirm reduction under fluoroscopy.

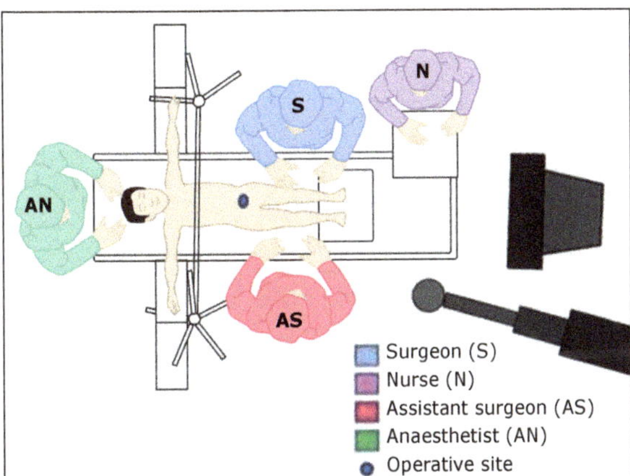

***Fig. 18.11**: Supine position on a radiolucent table for surgical treatment of pelvic fractures.*

- One to three half pins need to be inserted into each iliac crest. 4 to 4.5 mm diameter pins are required for small children and 5 mm pins for children > 8 years and adolescents.
- Iliac apophysis is split, stab incisions are made perpendicular to the crest on the ilium, approximately 2 cm posterior to ASIS.
- For supra-acetabular pins, incisions are made 2 cm superior to joint and medial to an imaginary line connecting ASIS and AIIS.
- It is important to direct the drill bit and pins from lateral to medial in approximately 30° angle to avoid perforating the medial or lateral cortex. The threaded aspect of the pin should be completely buried in the thickened aspect of the bone.
- Alternatively, the drill may be used only to create the entry point for the Schanz pin and thereafter the pin may be inserted with the T-handle. This helps to avoid perforation of the cortex.
- Confirm pin placements under fluoroscopy.
- Attach a small rod to each pin cluster.
- Connect the two small rods via two larger rods that extend medially and obliquely across the middle of abdomen. **(Fig. 18.12)**
- Stability of construct is confirmed by manual stressing under fluoroscopy.
- The frame should be adjusted to allow adequate room for the abdomen and should be positioned such that the patient can sit in a reclining chair.
- Post-operatively, daily pin tract care has to be taken. Weight bearing is limited for 4-6 weeks. Frame is usually removed after 6-10 weeks.

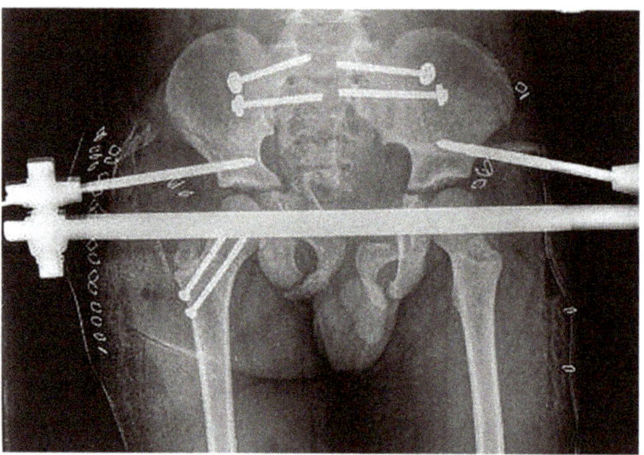

Fig. 18.12: *X-ray PBH showing external fixator and bilateral SI screw fixation for unstable pelvic fracture involving both the anterior and posterior ring. The transcervical neck femur fracture is fixed with two cancellous screws.*

Symphyseal plating

3.5 mm reconstruction plates are normally used for symphyseal plating. The advantage of plate over external fixator is that the plate is less bulky and surgery can be performed at the time of other procedures done for associated genitourinary or abdominal injuries.

Technique of open reduction of the symphysis pubis

Indications: Similar to those for external fixation

1. Fracture with > 2.5-3 cm symphyseal displacement
2. Unstable, open book type fracture with posterior ring disruption

This technique should not be used when haemodynamic instability is present, where an external fixator is a better option as it can be done quickly, without much blood loss.

Foley's catheter is a must before surgery, in order to decompress the bladder.

Position

Supine **(Fig. 18.11)**

Incision **(Fig. 18.13)**

Standard transverse Pfannenstiel incision, approximately one finger breadth above the pubic tubercle.

Steps

- Spermatic cord is identified and retracted.
- Anterior rectus sheath is incised transversely, leaving a small attachment to the symphysis pubis for later reattachment.
- Fatty tissue anterior to the bladder is bluntly dissected off the symphysis

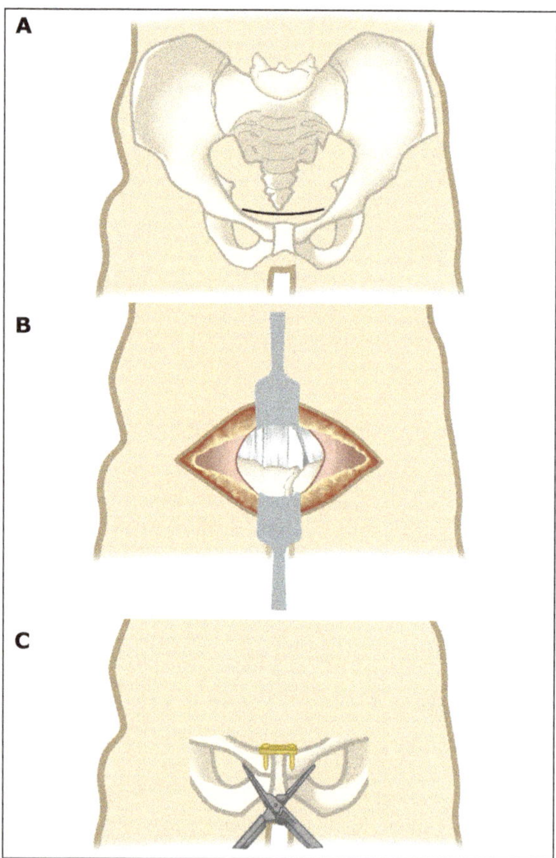

Fig. 18.13: *Technique of open reduction and plating for symphysis pubis diastasis:*
A. Pfannenstiel incision
B. Exposure of rectus femoris sheath
C. Reduction and plating

pubis where a sponge is packed to protect the bladder.

- Subperiosteal dissection is carried out laterally to get enough exposure for plate fixation.
- 4 hole 3.5 mm DCP or reconstruction plate for older children or 2 hole 1/3rd or semitubular plate for younger child (< 8 years) is recommended.
- Reduction is achieved by spanning the bone reduction forceps across the obturator foramina.
- Anatomical reduction is confirmed under direct vision.

SI screw fixation

This should be undertaken after stabilisation of the anterior ring. In children, there is a narrow corridor for safe screw placement, hence careful pre-operative CT scan evaluation is essential to understand the fracture pattern, displacement, comminution and ideal entry position and safe trajectory.

- Child is placed in a supine position, such that it allows intra-operative AP/ inlet/outlet/lateral views. **(Fig. 18.14)**

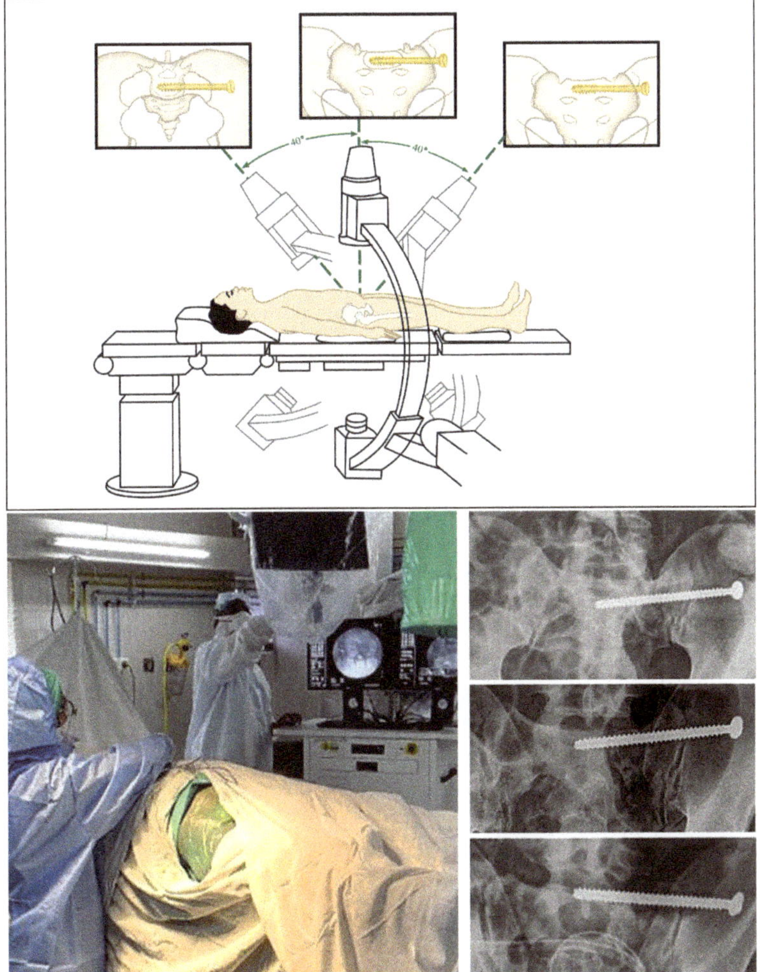

***Fig. 18.14**: Supine position of the child on a radiolucent table such that it allows intra-operative Inlet, AP and Outlet views and Insertion of Sacroiliac screws under fluoroscopy guidance.*

- Distal femur pin may be inserted for intra-operative traction.
- With longitudinal traction and compression, the sacral fracture or SI joint separation is manually reduced. The reduction is confirmed under fluoroscopy with AP, inlet and outlet views.
- 4.5/6.5 mm screws are used for younger children and 7.3 mm for adolescents, based on pre-operative CT evaluation.
- Screw entry point is determined based on inlet, outlet and lateral views. In a true lateral view, greater sciatic notches should overlap completely.
- Entry point laterally is at the intersection of the long axis of femur and a vertical line drawn posteriorly from ASIS.
- On AP outlet view, the entry point is just lateral to S1 neural foramen. Guide pin is directed towards the safe zone, the area between alar cortex supero anteriorly and sacral neural foramen posteriorly.
- Guide pin placement is confirmed under fluoroscopy on inlet, outlet and lateral views. Inlet view shows the screw placement in the axial projection, whether it is anterior or posterior. Outlet view shows the screw in cephalo-caudal orientation whether the screw is between the neural foramina. **(Fig. 18.15)**
- After advancing pin to the middle of the sacrum, length is reconfirmed under fluoroscopy and appropriate size screw with washer is inserted after drilling. Second screw may be added if rotational instability is still present after first screw. **(Fig. 18.16)**
- Post-operative spica cast immobilisation is required in young children and in case of unstable fixation, weight bearing is restricted for 6 weeks. Once the fracture unites, the screws are removed.

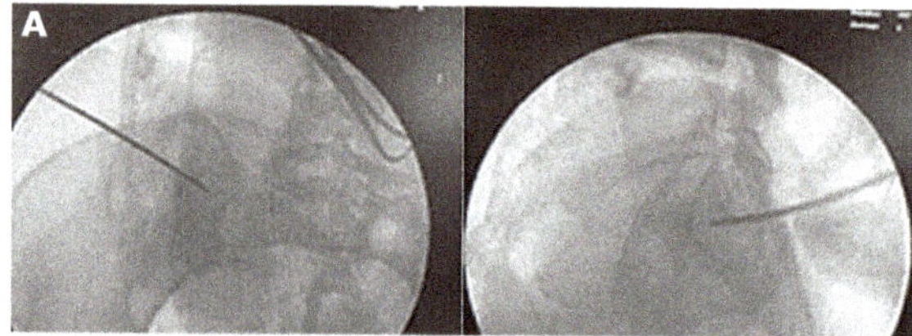

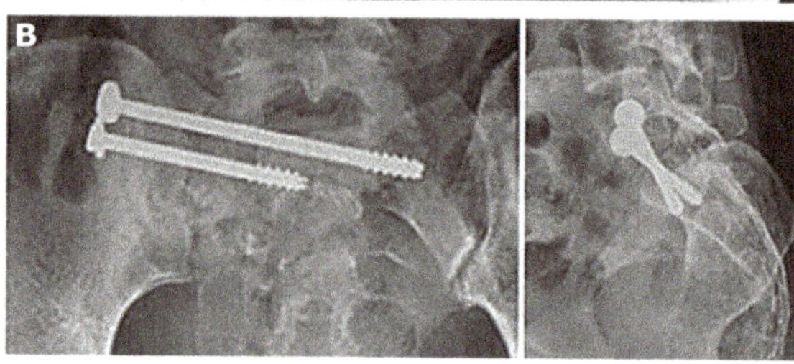

***Fig. 18.15**: A. Fluoroscopic images of the guide pin placement B. Screw insertion over the guide pins.*

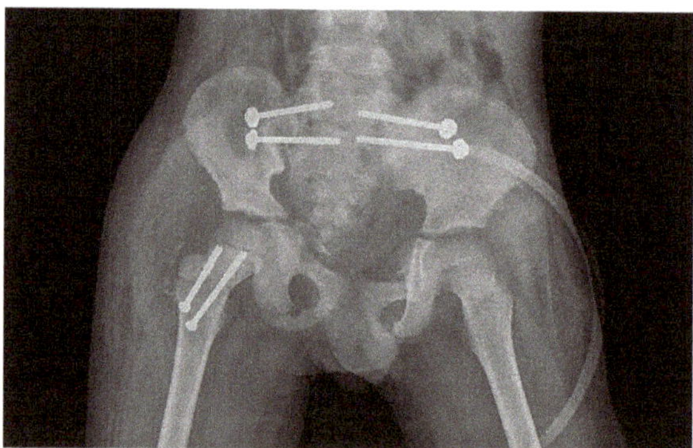

***Fig. 18.16**: Bilateral percutaneous sacroiliac screw fixation for unstable anterior and posterior ring disruption.*

SI plate fixation

Open reduction and 3.5 mm plate fixation via retroperitoneal/ posterior approach is indicated for large vertical displacement of hemipelvis where closed reduction can't be achieved.

Posterior approach for SI plating

Position:

Prone

Incision**:**

Vertical 2 cm lateral to posterior superior iliac crest

Steps:

- Reflect the gluteal muscles off the iliac wing subperiosteally.
- Origin of the gluteal maximus is reflected off the sacrum and the greater sciatic notch is exposed to fully visualise the fracture reduction.

- For sacral fracture, dissection is carried down to the sacral notch by reflecting gluteus maximus, erector spinae and multifidus muscles.
- Internal fixation is done with single or double screws or 3.5 mm reconstruction plate.

Treatment of Acetabular Fracture

Conservative

Majority can be treated conservatively. All type I and most type II and some type IV fractures with < 2 mm displacement following hip joint reduction can be treated with bed rest/skin or skeletal traction for a short period until comfortable and then Non-weight bearing walking with axillary crutches.

Follow up CT scan/X-ray should be done to reconfirm no further displacement. Progressive weight bearing can be started after 8-10 weeks.

Surgical: ~ 25 %

- The approach depends on the type of fracture.
- Posterior column and posterior acetabulum wall fracture can be fixed through Kocher Langenbeck approach. **(Fig. 18.17)**

Position:

Prone on a radiolucent table

Incision:

Lateral to PSIS extending to the posterior aspect of greater trochanter and down along the lateral aspect of femoral shaft.

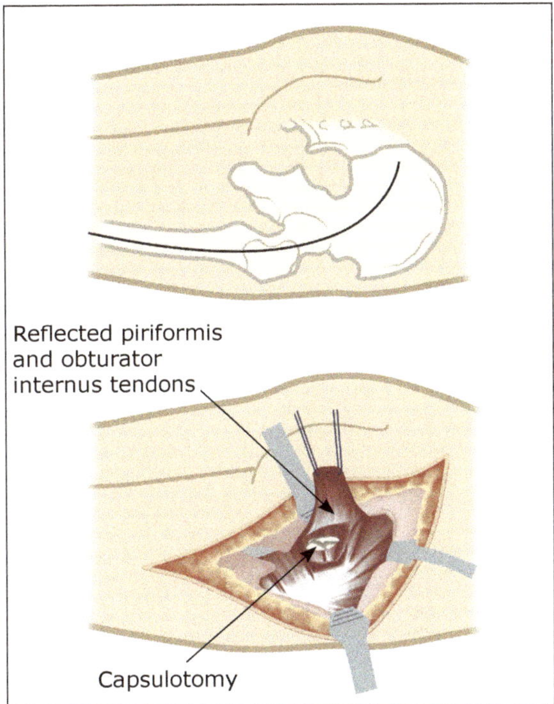

***Fig. 18.17**: Kocher Langenbeck posterior approach to the acetabulum.*

Steps:

- Fascia lata is split in line with femur.
- Gluteus maximus insertion is released from femur.
- Sciatic nerve is identified superficial to quadratus femoris.
- Piriformis and obturator internus tendon are taken off the trochanter and greater and lesser sciatic notches are exposed.
- The inferior aspect of the iliac wing is exposed by subperiosteal dissection.
- Capsulotomy is performed to expose the posterior aspect of the acetabulum and femoral head.

- Anterior column and inner innominate bone fracture is fixed through

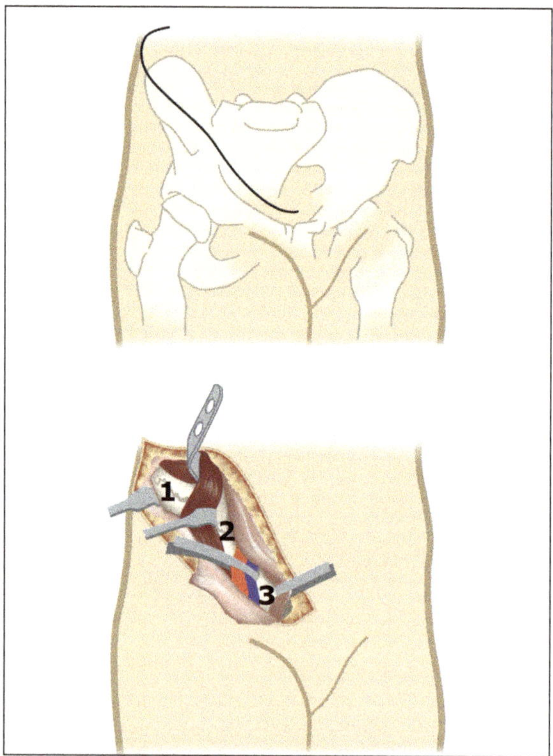

***Fig. 18.18**: Ilioinguinal approach to the acetabulum with creation of 3 windows.*

ilioinguinal approach (described by Letournel) **(Fig. 18.18)**

Position:

Supine

Incision:

3-4 cm above the pubis, continuing to the ASIS and along the iliac crest

Steps:

- Subperiosteal dissection is done along the iliac crest to expose the anterior SI joint and internal iliac fossa.
- External oblique aponeurosis is incised to expose the inguinal canal.
- Following structures are identified and rubber catheters are placed around them

1. Spermatic cord
2. Psoas tendon and lateral cutaneous nerve of thigh
3. External iliac vessels and lymphatics

- 3 windows are created

- First window is between iliac fossa and the psoas muscle and gives access to the internal iliac fossa, anterior SI joint and upper portion of the anterior column
- Second window is between the psoas muscle and the iliac vessels and provides access to the pelvic brim from the anterior SI joint to the lateral extremity of the superior pubic ramus
- Third window is medial to the iliac vessels and provides access to the symphysis pubis and the retropubic space of Retzius

Complications

Mortality associated with pelvic fracture in children is ~ 2-11%

Non orthopaedic complications:

- Neurogenic and genitourinary system injury
- Haemorrhage
- Laceration of vagina and rectum
- Urinary tract infection
- Pulmonary complications

Orthopaedic complications:

- Non union
- Delayed union
- Malunion
- Sacroiliac pain
- Premature triradiate fusion
- Heterotopic ossification

Flowchart 18.1

Pelvic Fractures
Torode and Zieg classification
Type I (Avulsion fractures)
Type II (Isolated iliac wing fractures)
Majority
> 1-2 cm displaced ischial tuberosity fracture interfering with sitting
Conservative treatment
• Rest
• Partial weight bearing on axillary crutches for 2 weeks
Open reduction and internal fixation with screws
Majority
Large fragment with signifcant displacement
• Symptomatic treatment
• Partial weight bearing on axillary crutches
Open reduction and internal fixation with screws or plates

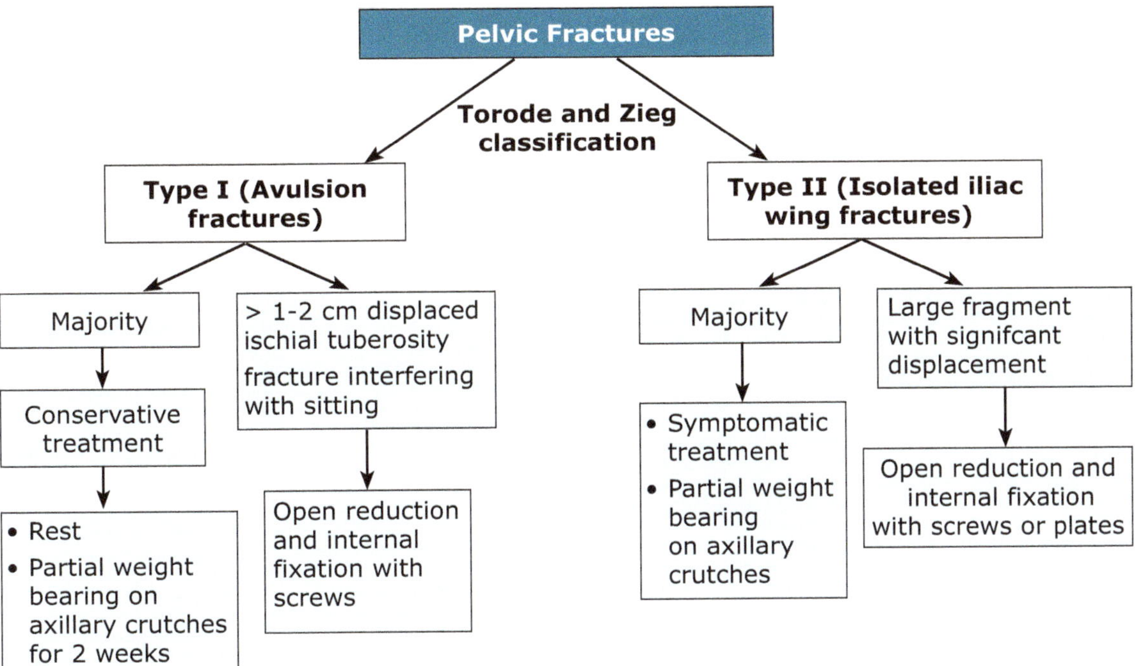

Flowchart 18.2

Pelvic Fractures
Torode and Zieg classification
Type III (Simple pelvic ring fractures)
1. Superior pubic ramus fracture
2. Unilateral superior and inferior pubic ramus fracture
3. Widening of symphysis pubis
4. Isolated fracture near or through SI joint
• Symptomatic treatment
• Non weight bearing walking for 1-2 weeks
Additional management for any associated bladder, genitourinary and abdominal injuries
< 2 cm
> 2 cm
Closed reduction and external fixator
Open reduction and plating
Rarely
Symptomatic treatment as in 1
Open reduction and internal fixation

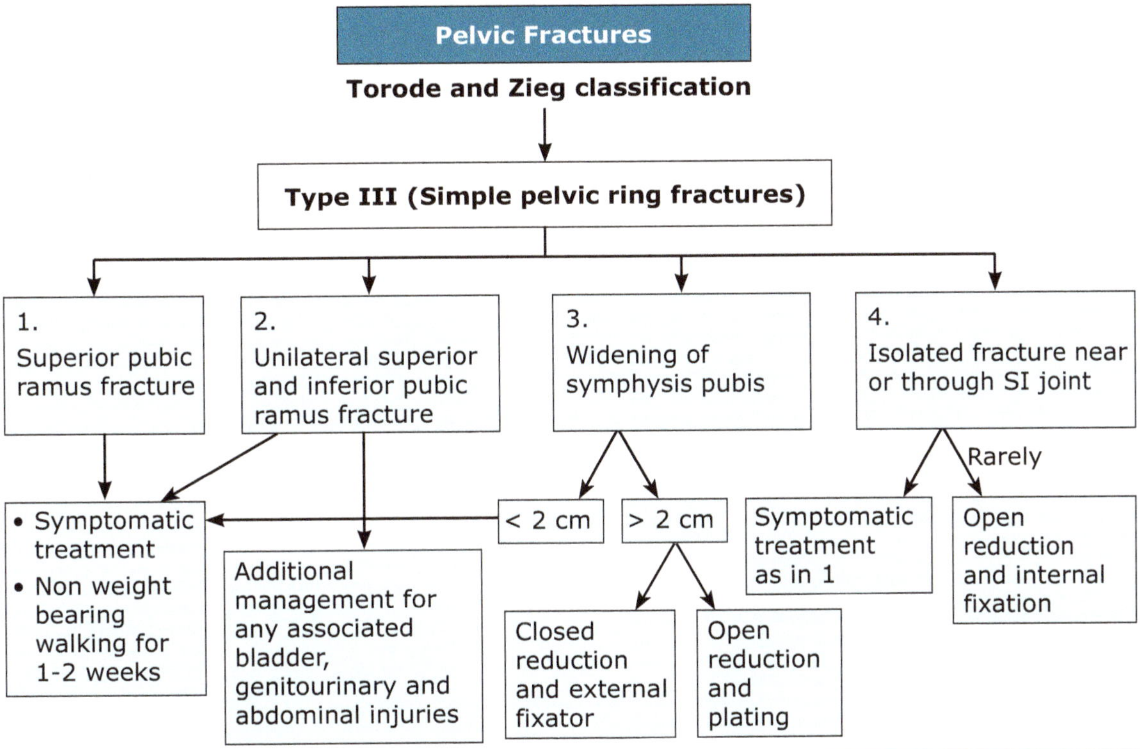

Flowchart 18.3

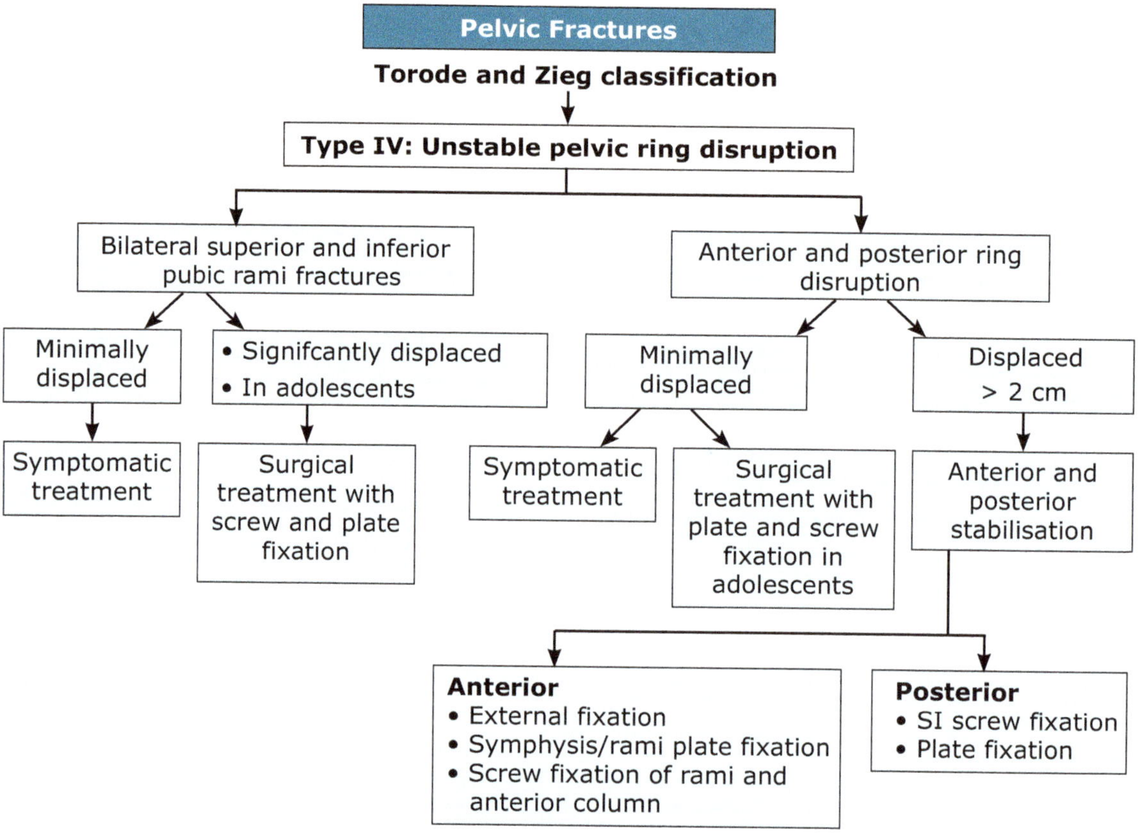

Pelvic Fractures

Torode and Zieg classification

Type IV: Unstable pelvic ring disruption

- Bilateral superior and inferior pubic rami fractures
  - Minimally displaced → Symptomatic treatment
  - • Signifcantly displaced • In adolescents → Surgical treatment with screw and plate fixation
- Anterior and posterior ring disruption
  - Minimally displaced
    - Symptomatic treatment
    - Surgical treatment with plate and screw fixation in adolescents
  - Displaced > 2 cm → Anterior and posterior stabilisation
    - **Anterior**
      - External fixation
      - Symphysis/rami plate fixation
      - Screw fixation of rami and anterior column
    - **Posterior**
      - SI screw fixation
      - Plate fixation

Flowchart 18.4

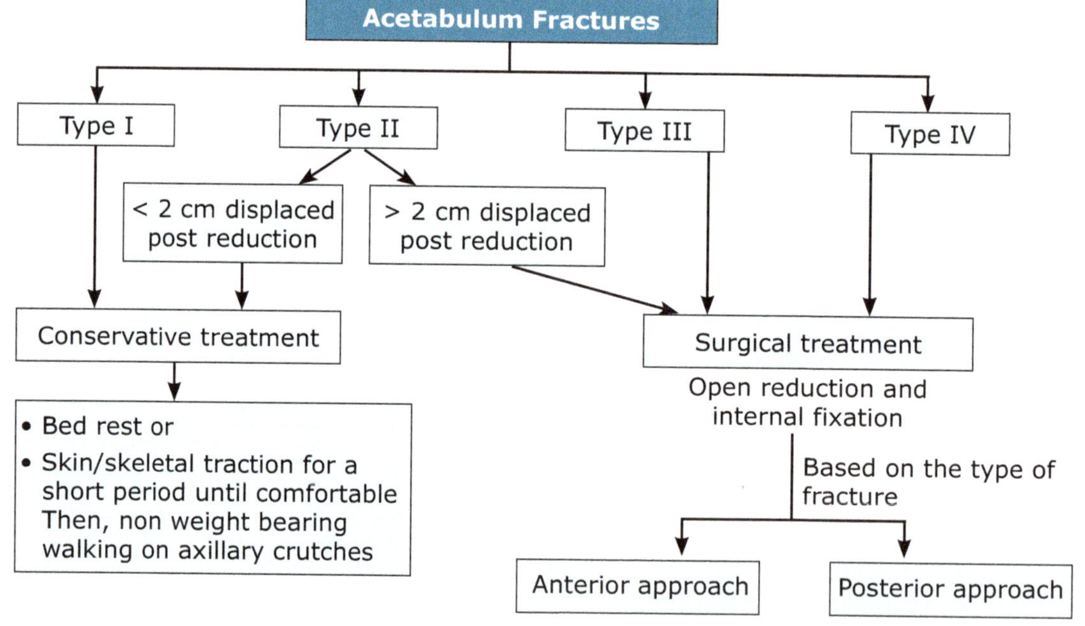

19 Fractures of the Femoral Neck and Hip Dislocation

FRACTURE NECK FEMUR

Introduction

Though paediatric neck of femur fractures are extremely rare injuries (less than 1% of all paediatric fractures), they are very important due to the highly increased chance of complications. The low incidence is attributed to the thick and strong periosteal cover and to the tough strong bones of children. Most of these injuries (80% to 90%) are due to high-velocity trauma and associated with other injuries in about 30-40%.

The anatomy of the paediatric hip differs from the anatomy of adult hips and this accounts for differences in treatment and complications. A thorough understanding of anatomy is important to ensure proper treatment and to understand associated complications to prevent high morbidity rates.

Relevant Anatomy

The proximal femoral physis is the growing physis of the proximal femur though only about 30% of the femoral growth takes place in the proximal end. As against that, the greater trochanteric physis is a traction *apophysis* and is thus not a growing physis and does not contribute to the growth of the limb as such.

The vascular anatomy of the proximal femur is extremely important and is derived from two main arterial trees: the main supply coming from the medial circumflex femoral artery and its branches while the lateral circumflex femoral artery and its branches supply the smaller part of the proximal femur. Extra capsular arterial ring located at the base of the femoral neck, the ascending cervical branches of the arterial ring at the surface of the femoral neck, and the arteries of the ligamentum teres contribute a minor percentage of the blood supply **(Fig. 19.1)**.

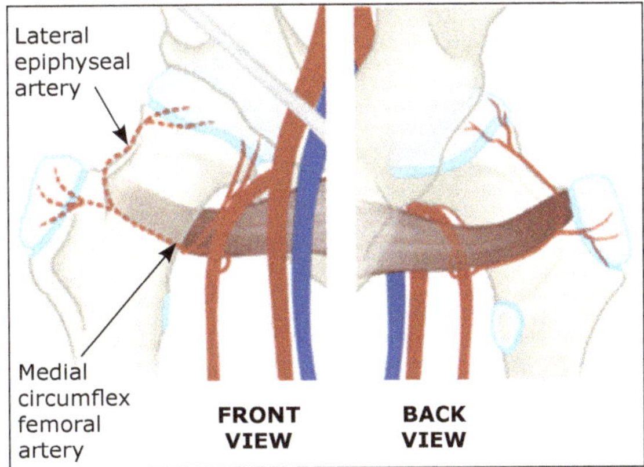

***Fig. 19.1**: Relevant vascular anatomy of the proximal femur showing the importance of the piriformis in the vascular supply of the neck and head of femur.*

Classification

The Delbet (modified by Colonna) classification is most commonly used for paediatric neck of femur fractures. This classification (though initially based on just six cases) has been backed by literature to have excellent correlation with the rates of complications, especially AVN with type I having an AVN rate of as much as 80 to 100% while type IV has an AVN rate of as less as 1 to 2%. **(Table 19.1 and Fig. 19.2)**

Clinical Features

The mechanism of injury is usually a

Table 19.1: Delbet classification

Type	*Description*	*Incidence*	*Chance of AVN*	*Chance of Nonunion*
Type I	Transphyseal IA - without dislocation of epiphysis from acetabulum IB - with dislocation of epiphysis	<10%	40-100% (AVN 100% in type IB)	Not defined
Type II	Trans-cervical	40-50%	28%	15%
Type III	Cervico-trochanteric (or basi-cervical)	30-35%	18%	15-20%
Type IV	Intertrochanteric	10-20%	5%	5%

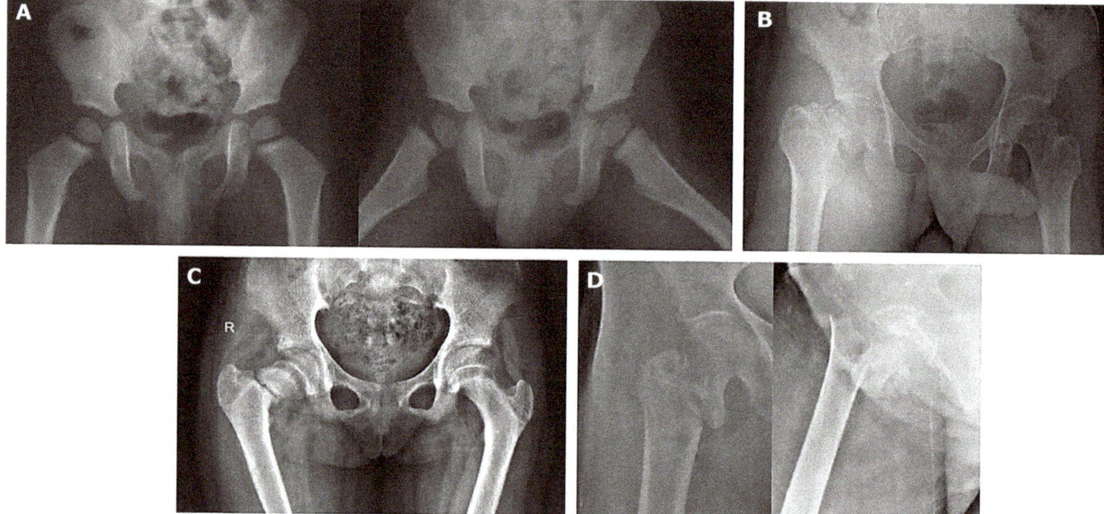

Fig. 19.2: *Plain radiographs denoting fractures according to the Delbet classification. (A) Type I fractures which are trans-epiphyseal, (B) Type II fractures which are trans-cervical, (C) Type III fractures- Cervico-trochanteric and (D) Type IV- Inter- or Transtrochanteric fractures.*

high velocity trauma in the form of fall from height or a motor vehicle accident. The child is unable to bear weight on the affected extremity which is shortened and externally rotated. These fractures can be associated with other systemic and skeletal injuries in the setting of polytrauma and a close lookout should be kept for other significant injuries (head injuries, abdominal injuries, etc).

Imaging

Plain radiographs are usually adequate for the primary diagnosis and classification of femoral neck fractures in children. Care should be taken while taking a cross table lateral or frog leg lateral view to ensure that there is minimal movement of the affected limb so that the fracture doesn't displace more. CT scan or MRI may be required for the diagnosis of subtle undisplaced fractures or when there is a suspicion of pathological or stress fractures.

Treatment

Non-operative treatment:

Non-operative management can be used only in very young kids less than one year of age who can be treated with either a Pavlik harness or a Hip spica cast.

In older children, undisplaced fractures can be treated with a Hip spica cast provided a close watch is kept for any further displacement and fixation is performed for re-displacement.

Non-operative and spica cast treatment alone is not optimal in older children due to very high incidence of non-union as well as coxa vara in non-operatively managed paediatric proximal femoral fractures.

Operative treatment:

There are various modalities of operative treatment of paediatric femoral neck fractures. In all the treatment modalities, certain principles need to be taken care of, which are:

1) Operative treatment should be undertaken as early as possible preferably as soon as basic preoperative investigations as well as imaging is done.
2) Especially in cases done early with a high velocity trauma, a capsulotomy should be done in order to decrease the tamponade effect of the intracapsular haematoma. This has been proved to decrease the rate of AVN in these injuries.
3) Stability of fixation is more important than the integrity of the proximal femoral physis especially in older kids as the contribution of the proximal femoral physis to the composite growth of the limb is comparatively less and it is more important to achieve good stable fixation with compression at the fracture site.
4) A supplemental spica cast (single leg) may be needed for most of the fractures even after fixation especially in younger kids.

The treatment also depends on the Delbet types as well as the age of the child. According as a general rule, Delbet I-III fractures below around 3 years of age, can be treated with K-wires, those between 4-10 years can be treated by K-wires or 4- 6.5mm CC screws while those above 10 years should be treated with 6.5 mm or 7 mm CC screws. Delbet type IV fracture is a unique fracture type which require good stable fixation and usually is fixed with a screw and side-plate construct. The other alternative is a 3 CC screw construct. Usually in this case, the screws can stop short of the physis **(Fig. 19.3)**.

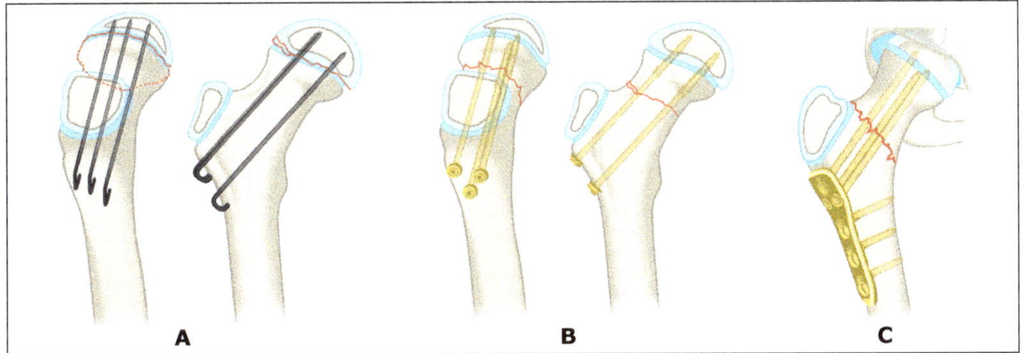

Fig. 19.3*: Treatment of femoral neck fractures according to the Delbet classification. (A) Type I transepiphyseal fracture treated with smooth K-wires. (B) Type II trans-cervical fractures treated with multiple cannulated cancellous screws and (C) Type III (cervico-trochanteric) or Type IV inter-trochanteric fractures treated with screw-and-side plate device like a proximal femoral locking plate or a paediatric DHS screw-plate.*

The treatment modalities are as follows:

1) Closed reduction and internal fixation with CC screws (CCS) with capsulotomy.
2) Closed reduction and internal fixation with DHS/ Proximal femoral locking plate (PF LCP).
3) Open reduction and internal fixation with CCS/ DHS/ PF LCP
4) Fixation with DHS with sub-trochanteric valgus osteotomy (for delayed presentations or non-unions)
5) Fixation with DHS with sub-trochanteric osteotomy with non-vascularised fibula grafting.

1) Closed reduction and percutaneous pinning/internal fixation (CRPP) with CC screws with capsulotomy

a) OR table: Fracture table or radiolucent table with a small bump under the ipsilateral buttock.

b) Position/positioning aids: supine with a "bump" under the thoracolumbar spine to the posterior-superior iliac spine to access the greater trochanter for screw insertion or placing the patient on a Fracture table.

c) Fluoroscopy location: between the legs in case of a fracture table or on the opposite side of the surgeon in radiolucent table.

d) Closed reduction of fracture by traction in flexion, internal rotation followed by extension and adduction. The foot should remain neutral or internally rotated at the end of the manoeuvre and not externally rotated.

e) Reduction is confirmed on AP and lateral views

f) Before draping, it is essential to check whether good-quality AP and lateral C-arm pictures are easily obtained with the femoral head and the physis is clearly visible.

g) The prominent bony markings such as anterior superior iliac spine (ASIS), greater trochanter, and the lateral femoral condyle are marked with a sterile marking pen.

h) Position of the guidewires is marked on the skin on both views.

i) Stab incisions are made and guide wires are inserted. An inverted triangle of fixation (2 superior- 1 each superolateral and superomedial, and one inferior screw) is the preferred mode of fixation.

j) Smooth pins if used can cross the physis at any age. If CC screws are used, then preferably stop short of the physis especially if age is less than 10 years. However, as mentioned earlier, if stability is compromised with the screws stopping short of the physis, it is better to extend fixation beyond the physis and achieve a better stability.

k) Insert smooth pins and cross physis (do not penetrate articular surface of femoral head).

l) Depending on the age of the child and type of fracture, the choice of implant can be chosen. In younger children 2-2.5 mm smooth pins should be used crossing the physis. In children older than 3 years, 4 mm cannulated cancellous screws can be applied in standard configuration keeping in mind not to cross the physis. In older children and adolescents 6.5mm or 7.3 mm cannulated cancellous screws can be used in standard configuration.

In fresh fractures, especially in Delbet I/II fractures, a capsulotomy is advisable. The surgical steps of the capsulotomy are as follows:

Capsulotomy

Emergent reduction and capsulotomy (<24hours) may diminish risk of AVN by restoring blood flow through kinked vessels. As a preliminary step, aspiration with wide bore needle through sub-adductor approach or anterior hip approach can be done to reduce the tamponade effect and reduce the risk of AVN.

Open capsulotomy also can be done by performing a hip arthrotomy through the anterior approach using the Smith Peterson interval.

Surgical Steps (Capsulotomy)

- OR table: Fracture table/ Simple radiolucent table.
- Fluoroscopy location: Standard position, between the legs (in fracture table) or opposite the surgeon in simple table.
- A small incision is made in the hip crease about 2 cm medial and 2 cm distal to the ASIS (centered on the AIIS). This incision is a skin crease incision and is very cosmetic. Alternatively a Smith Peterson incision can be used.
- Perform sharp dissection through the skin and subcutaneous tissue and identify the plane between the Sartorius and the Tensor Fascia lata taking care of the lateral cutaneous nerve of the thigh.
- The straight head of rectus femoris is identified and retracted medially so as to expose the glistening white capsule underneath. The capsule is cleared of all the peri-capsular fat with the help of a blunt periosteal elevator .
- A small incision is made in the capsule to perform the capsulotomy. In fresh fractures, one will find a gush of haemorrhagic fluid bursting out of the capsule.
- The capsule is usually not closed to prevent tamponade effect.
- The joint is thoroughly irrigated and the wound is closed in layers under a negative suction drain.

2) Closed reduction and fixation with DHS and CC screws/ 130° proximal femur locking plate (Figs. 19.4 and 19.5)

- OR table: Fracture table. (simple radiolucent table if the patient is very small)
- Gentle closed reduction is performed.
- Lateral approach to the hip is used and dissection is done in layers.
- Once reduction is obtained, the guidewire for the Dynamic Hip screw is placed in the inferior quadrant on the AP view and central on the lateral view. This will allow one more screw above the DHS.
- Triple reaming and tapping (especially in adolescent bones) is performed and the DHS is inserted.

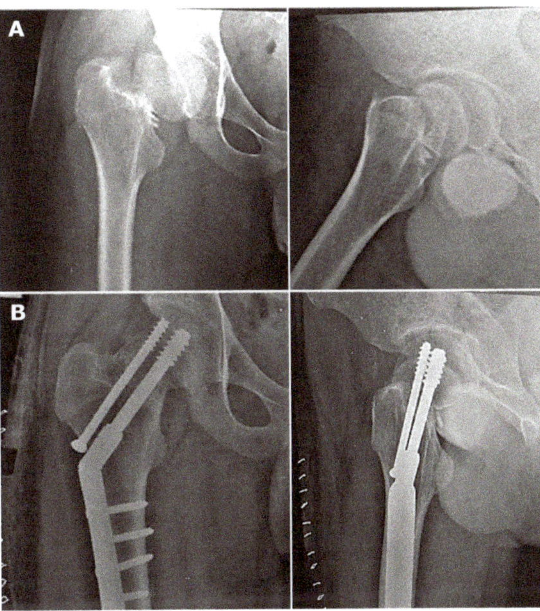

***Fig. 19.4**: (A) AP and lateral X-rays of hip showing a transcervical fracture neck of femur (Delbet type II) in a 11-year-old girl (B) Treated with closed reduction and internal fixation with paediatric DHS and single derotation CC screw.*

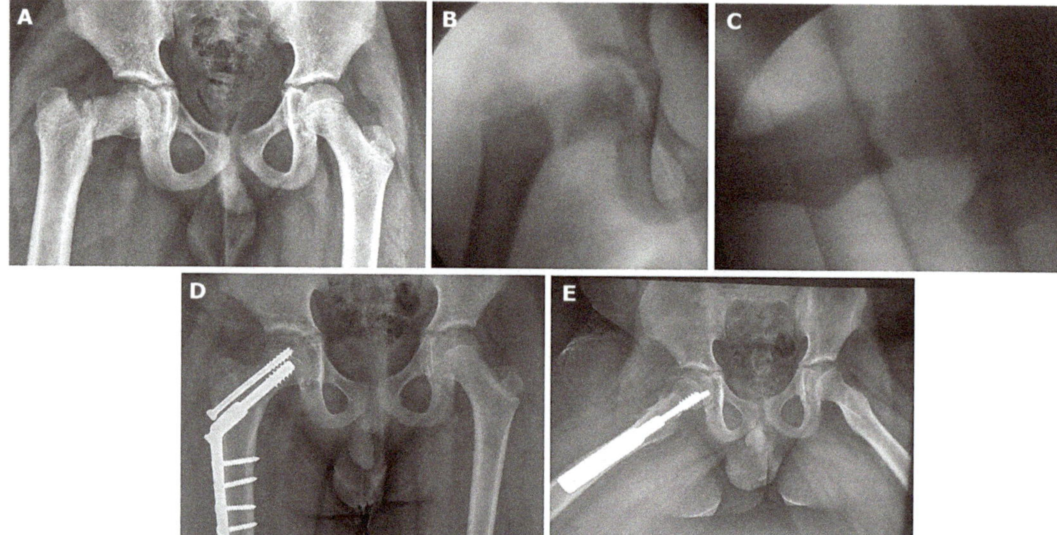

***Fig. 19.5**: (A) AP and lateral X-rays of hip showing Delbet type III fracture neck of femur (Cervico-trochanteric) (B and C). Intra-operative C-arm picture showing perfect reduction (D and E) Post-operative AP and frog-leg lateral view of the same patient at 3 months after paediatric DHS/CC screw fixation showing excellent healing, alignment and no changes of AVN.*

- Cannulated cancellous (CC) screw is inserted just superior and parallel to the central screw for added stability and compression.
- Paediatric DHS is applied in standard fashion.
- Final compression is done with the Top screw insertion after inserting 2 distal cortical screws.
- AP and lateral views are checked so as to detect spinning of the head during final tightening.
- Similarly after reduction, guide wire for 130° proximal femur locking plate is inserted.
- 130° proximal femur locking plate is inserted in standard manner.

3) Open reduction and internal fixation (Fig. 19.6)

- There should be a very low threshold for open reduction and internal fixation for these fractures as primary anatomical reduction is the key in obtaining good result.
- There are multiple approaches to open reduction of femoral neck fractures, like Watson-Jones approach, Smith-Peterson approach, Sommerville approach and the safe surgical dislocation (Ganz approach). The authors' preference is using a Watson-Jones approach as it is a versatile approach giving good exposure to the fracture site and also can be extended for definitive fixation with a DHS/PFLCP or CC screws.
- Position: Supine on a fracture table or on a simple radiolucent table with a bump under the ipsilateral buttock.
- A lateral incision is made centred over the greater trochanter starting about 8-10 cm proximally in a slightly anteriorly curving manner and then extending distally along the mid-lateral line of the thigh till about 10 cm distal to the trochanter.

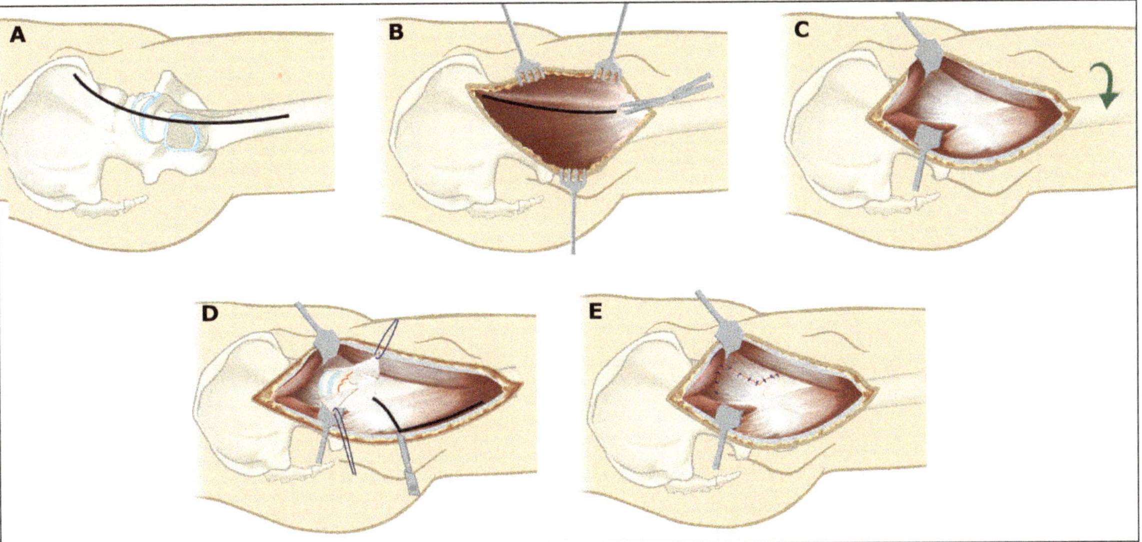

***Fig. 19.6**: Surgical steps of open reduction of femoral neck fractures using a lateral Watson-Jones approach. (A) Skin incision centred on GT and curving slightly anteriorly towards the ASIS. (B) Fascia cut in line with the incision. (C) Limb externally rotated and anterior surface of the joint capsule exposed through the interval between the TFL and the gluteus maximus. (D) Hip capsule opened using a Z-or T-shaped incision exposing the fracture site, draining the haematoma and allowing reduction of the fracture. If required, laterally the Vastus lateralis cut in a L-shaped manner for placement of the screws and plate. (E) Capsulotomy closed if required by loose sutures.*

- The fascia lata is incised longitudinally. Care is taken to save the superior gluteal nerve which is about 5 cm proximal to the greater trochanter. The internervous plane between the TFL and gluteus medius is developed and the TFL is retracted anteriorly. If necessary, the anterior-most fibers of the gluteus medius tendon can be detached from the trochanter for wider exposure.
- The hip capsule is seen anteriorly and a transverse capsulotomy is performed. The fracture haematoma is drained and the fracture site is exposed.
- A 2 mm K-wire is passed into the proximal fragment and used as a joystick to reduce the fracture.
- Once the reduction is obtained and confirmed on C-arm, fixation is performed using CC screws or Side plate in a routine manner.
- The capsule is closed by only a couple of loose sutures taking care that the closure is not too tight.

Post-operative care

- Supplementary spica casting should be considered for the majority of patients with proximal femoral fractures. Casting is indicated in all type I fractures in younger children. For type II and III fractures, it is recommend to use a hip spica cast for at least 6 weeks, especially in patients whose implants do not cross the femoral physis.
- Children older than 12 years can be treated with transphyseal fixation that is stable enough to avoid cast application. But the use of a postoperative cast depends on the stability of fracture fixation and the patient's compliance.

- Fractures treated with a hip screw and side plate do not require cast immobilisation.
- Formal physiotherapy usually is not required unless persistent limp or stiffness is seen, which is rare.

Complications

The two most important and most dreaded complications of paediatric femoral neck fractures are avascular necrosis and non-union.

1) Avascular necrosis: Avascular necrosis is related more to the initial injury rather than the treatment and is directly correlated to the Delbet type of fracture. The treatment of AVN post femoral neck fractures is related to the amount of femoral head involved and the symptoms of the child. The exact details of the treatment are beyond the purview of the book.

2) Non-union:

- The important causes of non-unions in femoral neck fractures in children and adolescents are related to the mode and severity of the injury, obliquity of fracture as well as the primary treatment provided for the fracture.

a) Mode and severity of injury: These fractures are usually high energy injuries (unlike in elderly) which cause severe shearing of the vasculature as well as significant capsular tamponade.

b) Obliquity of the fracture: The obliquity of the fracture plays a very important role in causing femoral neck non-unions. More vertical fractures are more prone to non-union due to significant shearing forces at the fracture site. The verticality of the fracture is one of the major modifiable factors in femoral neck non-unions and the treatment is based on this principle.

c) Method of reduction: Another cause of delayed/ non-union of femoral neck fractures is related to the local vascularity which is altered or damaged during reduction manoeuvres. Forceful or vigorous closed reduction methods are strictly not advisable in neck femur fractures in children though they are mainly responsible for the complication of avascular necrosis rather than non-union.

d) Method of fixation: The stability of fixation and the method of fixation are important factors in causation of non-union of femoral neck fractures. Implants like K-wires or threaded pins may not provide the adequate stability especially in older children or in vertically oriented fractures.

Classification

It is important to classify femoral neck non-unions by the *Sandhu's classification* as this classification accurately predicts the chances of success of osteosynthesis as well as the methodology required to treat it. This is a radiological classification based on X-rays and MRI (CT scans, if MRI is not available). The classification works on the principle that the changes that occur in the region of the fracture line such as smoothening of the fracture margins, absorption of neck of the femur, increase in the gap between the fragments, decrease in the size of the proximal fragment and appearance of avascularity of the proximal fragment have a definite bearing on the outcome of any procedure aimed at osteosynthesis. Though this classification is not limited to femoral neck non-unions in children, it can be utilised in children also as the principles of management remain the same.

The classification divides femoral neck non-unions into three groups **(Table 19.2)**:

Table 19.2: Classification of femoral neck non-union

Group	Fracture surface	Size of proximal fragment	Size of fracture gap	Changes of avascularity
I	Irregular	>2.5 cm	<1 cm	None
II	Smoothened	>2.5cm	>1cm but <2.5cm	None
III	Smoothened	<2.5cm	>2.5cm	Yes

This classification has a prognostic as well as therapeutic value as group I has 100% chance of union (in their series), group II has 88 % chance of union while group III has only about 30% chance of union.

Imaging

Plain radiographs of the pelvis with both hips –Anteroposterior and lateral views form the cornerstone of investigations for diagnosis of femoral neck femur non-unions in children. It is always useful to first classify a femoral neck fracture by the standard Pauwel or Garden's classification in order to get an idea about the obliquity of the fracture line. However these classifications would not be very useful in diagnosis of non-unions following femoral neck fractures.

In some cases, advanced imaging may be necessary to diagnose and plan management for femoral neck non-unions. CT scans may be used to see the bony appearance of the stipled area and bony sclerosis, trabecular resorption, microfracture and subchondral collapse. Some changes of AVN may also be seen on CT scans. CT scans also are very useful in diagnosis of femoral neck non-unions following fixation since it is very difficult to get an MRI done in presence of metal implants.

MRI may be used in some cases to diagnose if there is concomitant avascularity. It is also a very sensitive tool for accurate diagnosis of non-unions. The Sandhu et al classification, in fact, is based on MRI scans for better delineation of the fracture lines as well as more accurate measurement of the fracture fragments.

Preoperative planning/surgical options

The goals of treatment in femoral neck non-unions in children and adolescents are:

1) To obtain a painless, mobile and stable hip
2) To cause the least possible amount of physeal damage
3) To prevent secondary changes such as greater trochanteric over-riding.
4) To cause the least limb length discrepancy at skeletal maturity.

The treatment depends on age, physical status of the child, the duration of symptoms, amount of resorption of the femoral neck, the Pauwel angle and, most importantly the Sandhu et al grade of the fracture. The options for management are:

1) Osteosynthesis with or without vascularised or non-vascularised single or dual fibula grafting
2) Osteosynthesis along with osteotomy (displacement or angulation type)
3) Osteosynthesis using muscle pedicle bone grafting (Refer to standard textbooks of techniques)

The author's preferred mode of treatment is osteosynthesis using a side plate-and-screw construct with a Valgus angulation osteotomy with or without a single non-vascularised fibula grafting. Sandhu et al grade I fractures require only osteosynthesis with valgus osteotomy while grade II/III fractures require fixation/osteotomy along with fibula grafting.

Pre-operative planning and operative steps in detail of the above-mentioned procedure are described below.

- Preoperative planning is performed from the radiograph of the normal hip to study various anatomical landmarks like the location of the normal physis, to select the appropriate implant for osteosynthesis as well as to better define the surgical steps.
- The tracing of the pre-operative X-ray is drawn in the anteroposterior view. The Pauwel angle is drawn.
- The aim of the surgical procedure of osteotomy is to convert a very high Pauwel angle to a low one preferably around 25°.
- The entry of the proximal screw/s is drawn which is parallel to the femoral neck and a subtrochanteric/ intertrochanteric wedge is drawn. The angle of the wedge is equal to the difference between the actual and the intended Pauwel angle. For example, if the current Pauwel angle is 45 degrees and the intended angle is 25°, then the angle of the wedge will be 45-25 which is 20°.
- A lateral closing wedge osteotomy is planned which helps to convert a vertical fracture line with shear forces across the fracture fragments to a horizontal fracture line with compressive forces across the fracture line. The osteotomy is drawn and completed and fixation is done using a side plate device. In case fibula grafting is to be performed in addition, then the entry point of the proximal screw is made slightly distally and fibula is inserted proximal to it. The detailed pre-operative planning is shown in **Fig. 19.7.**

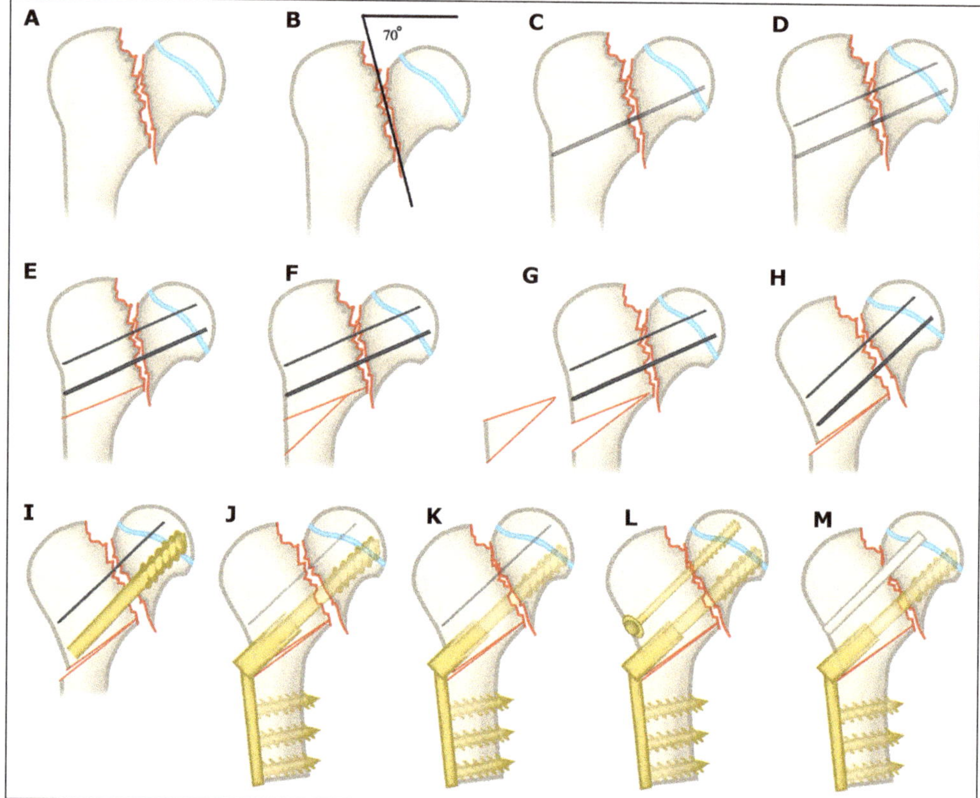

Fig. 19.7*: Sub-trochanteric valgus osteotomy by lateral closed wedge resection and fixation with DHS and CC screw (Figure 7L) or DHS and single fibula (Figure 7M).*

Surgical procedure

- The procedure is performed in supine position on a radiolucent table with a small radiolucent bump under the ipsilateral buttock. Before draping, it is essential to check whether good quality anteroposterior and frog-lateral C-arm pictures are easily obtained. The entire leg is draped free.
- The prominent bony markings such as ASIS, greater trochanter and the lateral femoral condyle are marked with a sterile marking pen. Closed reduction, if possible is obtained using traction and internal rotation and provisionally fixed using two thick K-wires. The femur is exposed using the lateral approach, cutting the fascia lata widely and elevating the vastus lateralis sub-periosteally. In case, closed reduction is not possible, open reduction is performed by extending the same incision proximally by the Watson-Jones approach between the tensor fascia lata and the gluteus medius.
- The authors' preferred implant of choice is either a paediatric DHS screw and plate device or a locking proximal femoral hip osteotomy plate. Once reduction is obtained, the guide wire for the proximal screw is placed in the inferior quadrant on the AP view and central on the lateral view. This will allow either one more screw or fibula just above the first screw. Once this guidewire is accepted, the screw is predrilled and kept slightly loose and not completely seated in the bone.
- The subtrochanteric osteotomy is then planned just below the lesser trochanter. A wedge equal to the angle of correction is osteotomised and lateral based wedge is closed. The distal fragment is then lateralised and the side plate or locking plate (as appropriate) is placed and fixed with cortical screws **(Fig. 19.8)**.
- In case of group II/III fractures, fibular osteosynthesis is performed.
- About 6-8 cm of fibular graft is harvested from the middle third. The graft width and length is measured. The size of the expected fibular graft is exactly measured and it is cut to that

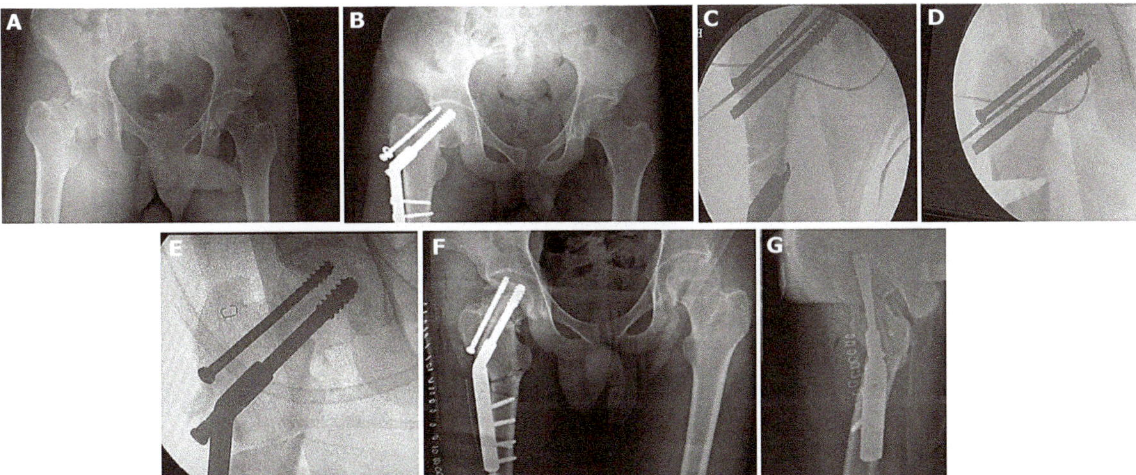

***Fig. 19.8**: (A) Pre-operative radiograph of a trans-cervical fracture neck of femur (B) treated initially with DHS and CC screw fixation which had cut through. (C) Intra-operative images of the revision surgery with a subtrochanteric wedge marked, (D) excised and (E) closed and translated. (F, G) Post-operative AP and lateral radiographs after definitive fixation after valgus osteotomy.*

size. The width (diameter) of the graft is usually 6-7 mm and if thicker than that, the graft is shingled to that size.

- In order to prepare the tract at the superior border of the femoral neck, sequential reaming is performed using cannulated drill bits and finally by a triple reamer so as to make the canal of adequate size. It is very important to see to it that the canal is dilated adequately so as to not shatter the fibular graft. The fibula is passed over the guide wire and gently tapped using a bone punch. The seating of the graft is ensured till about 5mm of the subchondral surface.
- Once the seating is confirmed on AP and lateral views on C-Arm, the extra portion of the fibular graft is cut using a sharp bone cutter. In case of some Group III fractures, when the gap between the fracture fragments is too large, it is sometimes necessary to fill the graft using iliac crest cancellous bone grafts. However, it is very rare for this to be required especially in children.

The final position is confirmed on antero-posterior and frog leg lateral view on C-Arm. The wound is thoroughly irrigated and closed in layers under negative suction drain.

- Another method of valgus osteotomy is by performing a transverse osteotomy at the sub-trochanteric level and abducting the proximal segment along with lateral translation of the distal fragment so as to achieve an *end-to-side* apposition of the fragments. The advantage of this method is that alignment of the mechanical axis is better with good lateral translation of the distal fragment **(Fig. 19.9).**

Methods of Fixation and Implant Choice

Various methods of fixation have been described and used. The commonest method of fixation is an angled plate and screw device which helps to provide adequate compression at the fracture site as well as adequate stability to the osteotomy site. As described previously, the authors' preferred method is a

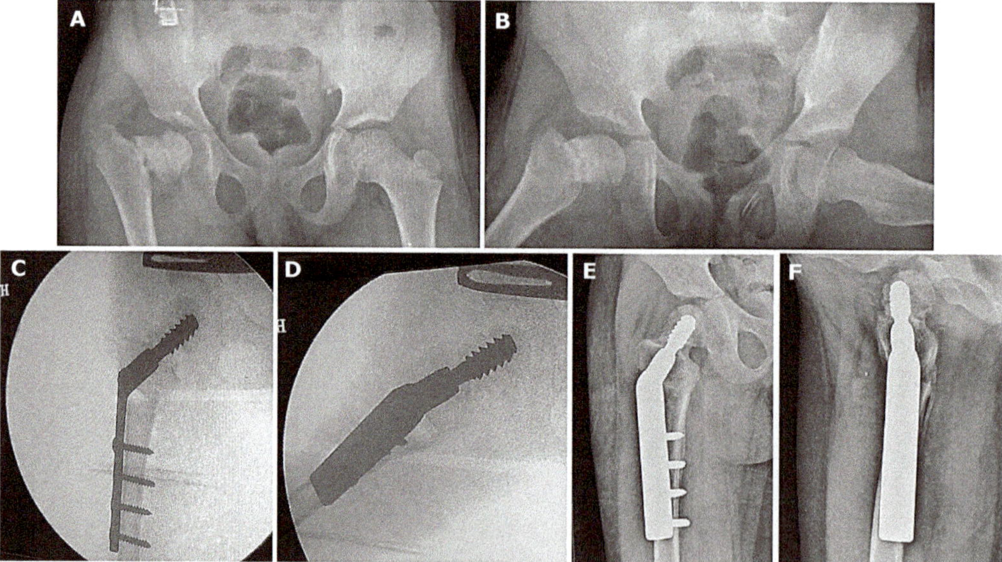

***Fig. 19.9**: (A/B) Pre-operative radiographs of a neglected non-union of the neck of femur (C/D) Treatment with Sub-trochanteric valgus osteotomy (without wedge resection). (E/F) 6 months post-operative radiographs show excellent healing of both the fracture and the osteotomy.*

paediatric DHS, the other implants which can be used are the angled blade plate and the proximal femoral osteotomy locking plate. Another implant which can be used is a reconstruction or a 1/3rd tubular plate which can be bent at an angle and hammered in. This relatively older and less technologically intensive method is quite modular and works quite well in experienced hands. Simple cannulated cancellous screws can also be used in case only fixation of the non-union site is to be performed without osteotomy.

Post-operative Care

The patient is to be kept non-weight bearing for at least six weeks. Drains are removed after 48 hours. In very young children, it is better to put the child in a single leg hip spica for a few weeks to maintain the fixation. After six weeks, depending on the status of union (both of the fracture and osteotomy site), hip range of motion and partial weight bearing is started. As a general guideline, full weightbearing is permitted only after full radiological union, which is usually after about eight to twelve weeks. The patient is kept under follow-up for a long period to look for signs of avascularity.

HIP DISLOCATION

Introduction

Hip dislocation is an uncommon injury in children, constituting < 5% of all paediatric dislocations.

Mechanism of Injury

- Posterior dislocation is the most common and occurs when a force is applied to the leg with the hip flexed and adducted.
- Anterior dislocation constitutes <10% of hip dislocations, anterosuperior dislocation occurs when the hip is extended while undergoing forced abduction and external rotation. Anteroinferior dislocation occurs when the hip is flexed while in abduction and external rotation.
- Luxatio erecta femoris or infracotyloid dislocation occurs extremely rarely where the femoral head dislocates directly inferiorly.
- In younger children (<6 years), dislocation occurs due to high energy injuries like MVA/sports injuries, but with predisposing factors like coxa valga, hyperlaxity and acetabular dysplasia.

Associated injuries

- Posterior hip dislocation is associated with sciatic nerve injury in ~ 5 %
- Anterior hip dislocation may be associated with femoral neurovascular injury.
- Tears of the capsule and acetabular labrum are common and prevent concentric reduction of the hip. Hence post reduction confirmatory imaging is important.
- Ipsilateral knee injury is common in high energy trauma.

Clinical Features

Child with hip dislocation presents with severe acute pain following trauma and inability to bear weight. The characteristic attitude of the limb (depending on the direction of dislocation) is as follows:

- Posterior dislocation:
  - Flexed, adducted and internally rotated.
  - The limb appears shorter than the other side.
  - The femoral head can be palpated posteriorly.
- Anterior dislocation-

  Abducted, flexed and externally rotated **(Fig. 19.10)**

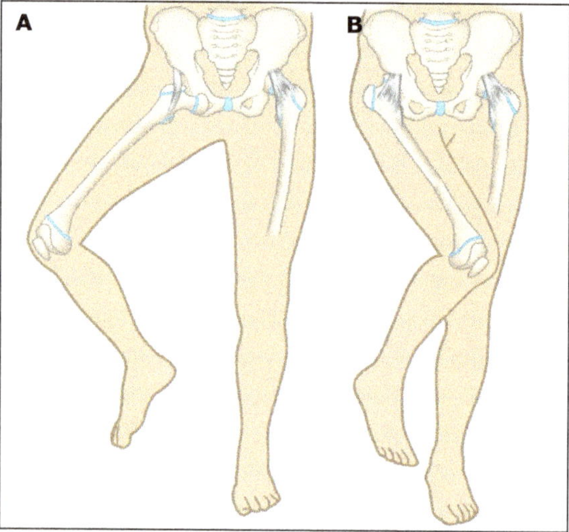

Fig. 19.10: Position of the limb in anterior dislocation of the hip (A) and posterior dislocation of the hip (B).

- Antero-inferior and inferior dislocations:

  Severely flexed, abducted and externally rotated.

- The limb appears longer than the other side
- The femoral head may be palpated anteriorly.

- Central dislocation:

- There may be some narrowing of the pelvic width but no characteristic attitude of the limb.
- The leg length is similar to the opposite side.

- Sometimes pain may be referred to the knee.
- Clinical assessment of distal neurovascular deficit is important.

Imaging

- Plain X-ray -

  Sometimes it is difficult to differentiate between posterior and anterosuperior hip dislocation on AP view. The following two features help to differentiate between the two types.

1. In posterior hip dislocation, the femoral head is internally rotated and hence the lesser trochanter is often obscured on AP view.

   In anterosuperior hip dislocation, the femoral head in externally rotated and hence the lesser trochanter is more visible on AP view.

2. In posterior hip dislocation, the femoral head appears smaller then the contralateral side whereas in anterosuperior hip dislocation, the femoral head appears larger than the contralateral side on a well centred AP view, on account of geometric magnification.

- MRI is helpful to rule out dislocation and spontaneous relocation with interposed soft tissue.
- CT scan can be helpful for confirmation of concentric reduction and presence of interposed bony fragment/s.

Classification

1. Depending on the direction of displacement: **(Fig. 19.11)**

   Posterior/ Anterosuperior/ Anteroinferior / Infracotyloid

   Posterior dislocations are further classified as per the location of the femoral head into Iliac, Ischial, Obturator and Pubic.

2. Based on associated fracture: Stewart-Milford classification **(Fig. 19.12)**

   Grade I : Dislocation without an associated fracture/ small bony avulsion of acetabulum

   Grade II : Posterior rim fracture associated with stable hip after reduction

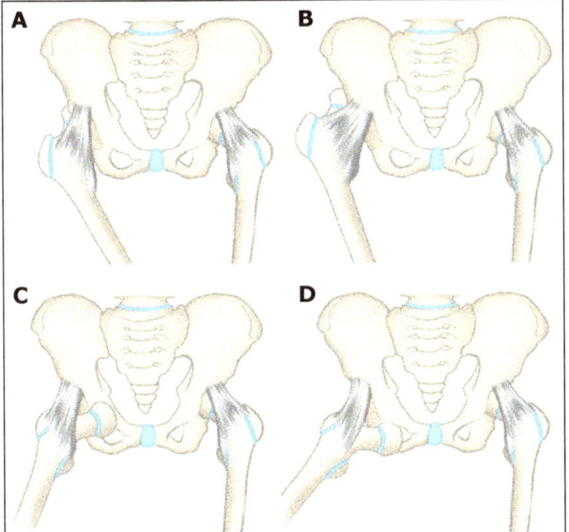

Fig. 19.11: *Classification of dislocations of the hip based on the direction of displacement. (A) Iliac (B) Ischial (C) Obturator (D) Pubic.*

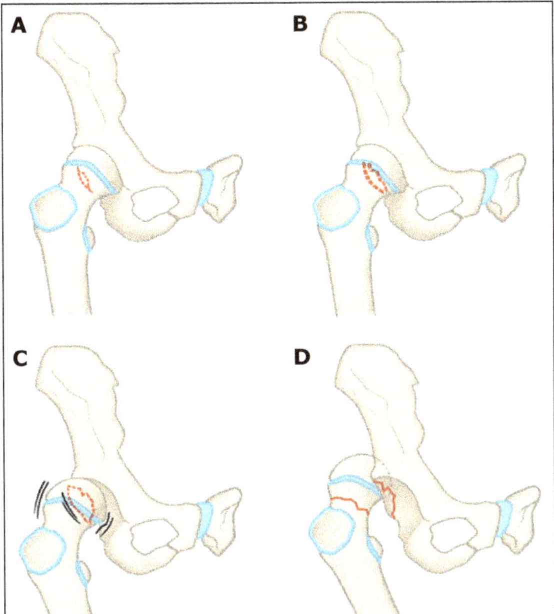

Fig. 19.12: *Stewart- Miford classification of hip dislocations. (A) Grade I (B) Grade II (C) Grade III (D) Grade IV.*

Grade III : Posterior rim fracture with unstable hip

Grade IV : Dislocation with associated head/neck fracture

3. Pipkin classification:

- Type 1: Associated with femur head fracture caudal to the fovea with a resultant small fragment
- Type 2: Associated with femur head fracture cranial to the fovea with a resultant large fragment
- Type 3: Combined femoral head and neck fracture
- Type 4: Any femoral neck fracture with an acetabulum fracture

Treatment

The goal of treatment in hip dislocation is to achieve a prompt, stable and concentric reduction . Care is to be taken to do a gentle manipulation and closed reduction under anaesthesia , in order to prevent rupture of Y ligament, damage to the sciatic nerve and prevent iatrogenic fracture.

Posterior dislocation of hip:

Closed reduction should be attempted by any of the following methods

1. ***Allis manoeuvre:*** Easiest, most common and most effective method

Steps **(Fig. 19.13):**

- Child is under GA and in supine position
- The assistant stabilises the pelvis by applying direct pressure over the ASIS.
- The hip and knee are flexed to 90°, thigh is in slight adduction and internal rotation.
- The surgeon keeps the forearm behind the child's knee and leg and applies an anteriorly directed force, in order to release the femoral head from behind the posterior lip of the acetabulum and closed reduction is performed.
- Further adduction and internal rotation of the hip may be required to relax the hip joint capsule if there is soft tissue

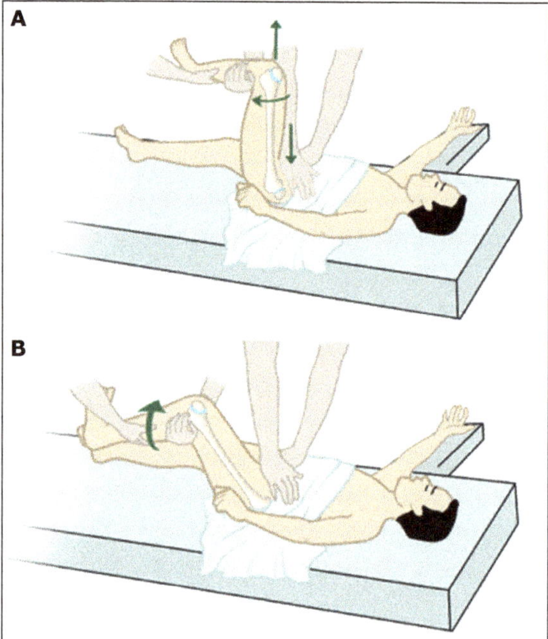

***Fig. 19.13**: Steps of the Allis method for reduction of posterior hip dislocation.*

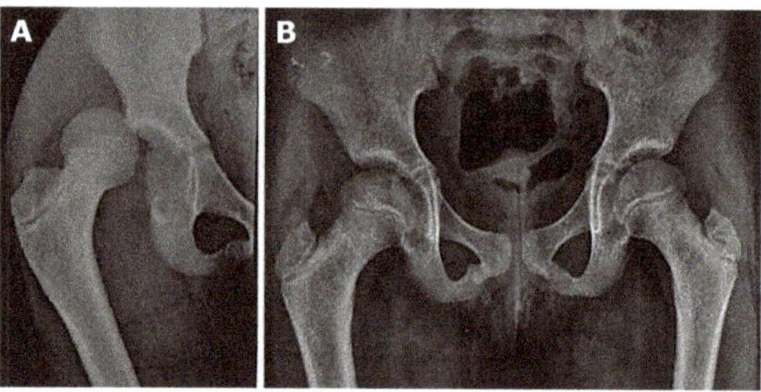

***Fig. 19.14**: (A) X-ray of the hip in a 14-year-old boy showing posterior dislocation (B) Treatment with Allis method showing concentric reduction.*

resistance. The assistant can help in the reduction by applying anteriorly directed pressure on the femoral head.

2. ***Bigelow's manoeuvre* (Fig. 19.15)**:

   Child is under GA and in supine position

- The assistant applies counter traction on the ASIS.
- The surgeon holds the affected limb at the ankle with one hand and places the opposite forearm around the patient's knee.

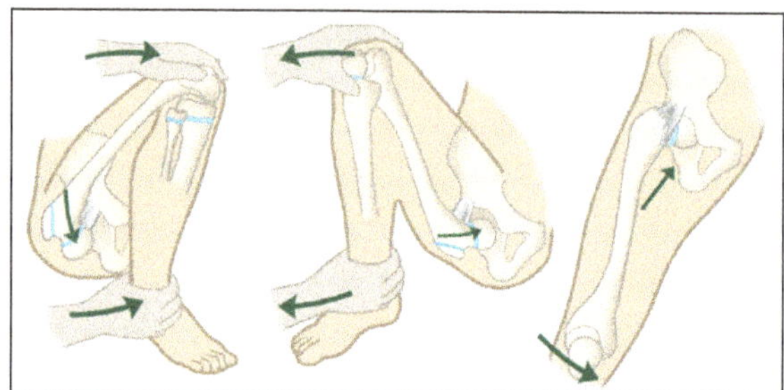

***Fig. 19.15**: Bigelow method for closed reduction of posterior hip dislocation.*

- The hip is flexed to 90° with the thigh adducted and internally rotated and longitudinal traction is applied in order to relax the Y ligament. The femoral head is then freed from the rotator muscles by gently rotating the thigh back and forth. Finally, by gentle abduction, lateral rotation and hip extension, the femoral head is levered back into the acetabulum.

3. ***Stimson manoeuvre* (Fig. 19.16)**:

- It may be used in younger patients
- Child is under GA and in prone position
- Child is kept at the edge of the table with hip and knee flexed to 90°
- Gravity along with downward push on

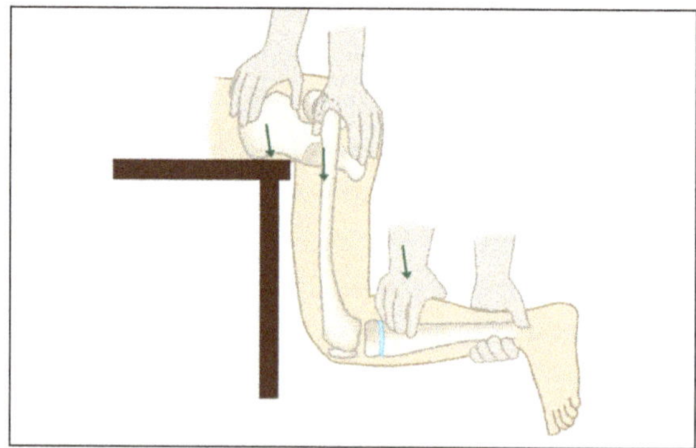

***Fig. 19.16**: Schematic representation of the Stimson's method for reduction of posterior hip dislocation.*

the lower leg while using the ankle to apply internal and external rotation helps to achieve the reduction.

Anterior dislocation of hip

Modification of Allis technique

- Supine position
- With hip in full abduction, the hip and knee are flexed to 90^{0} **(Fig.19.17A)**
- Traction is applied directly in line with the long axis of the femur, while the assistant applies posterior pressure on the anteriorly dislocated femoral head **(Fig.19.17B)**.
- Then the surgeon adducts the hip and reduces the head into the acetabulum by using the patient's thigh as the lever **(Fig.19.17C)**.

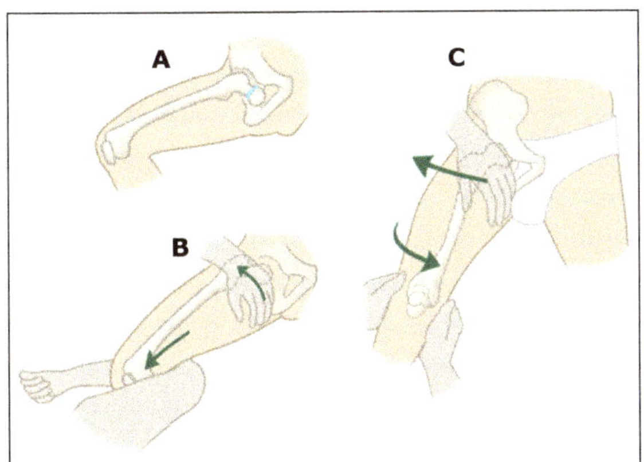

Fig. 19.17: *Modified Allis method for closed reduction of anterior hip dislocation.*

Central Dislocation of Hip

Central dislocation of hip is usually associated with acetabular fracture, hence reduction is achieved using skeletal traction. Distal femur traction, along with skeletal traction pin in the greater trochanter for lateral traction is used. The traction can be kept for 3-4 weeks. Some active ROM of the hip is allowed to promote moulding of the acetabulum.

Open Reduction:

Indication:

- Failed closed reduction
- Non concentric closed reduction
- Dislocation associated with displaced femur head, neck or acetabulum fracture

Approach:

Depends on the direction of hip dislocation

Goal:

- To clear obstacles to concentric reduction (piriformis tendon, hip capsule, inverted limbus, osteocartilaginous loose bodies)
- Anatomical fixation of acetabulum/ femur head fracture
- Repair of soft tissue envelope

Posterior approach for posterior dislocation:

- Lateral position
- Skin incision is made from the PSIS to the GT and down the lateral aspect of the thigh
- The sciatic nerve is identified and protected. The short external rotators are divide 1 cm. from the insertion.
- The partially torn posterior capsule is incised to allow visualisation of the acetabulum.
- The femoral head can be distracted using a Schanz screw placed into the GT for better visualisation.
- The joint is irrigated, any osteocartilaginous debris is removed.
- Any associated acetabular rim fracture should be internally fixed with screws in the young child and 3.5 mm. reconstruction plate in adolescents.

- Repair of the capsule and labral tears is performed.

Anterior/Anterolateral approach for anterior dislocation: (Smith-Peterson or Watson Jones)

- Rarely required as majority anterior dislocations are treated by closed reduction.
- Principles same as in posterior approach.

Post reduction protocol:

- Post reduction confirmation with a CT scan is a must.
- Young children < 6-7 years: Spica cast with hip in neutral extension and mild abduction or skin traction for 4-6 weeks
- Older children: Non weight bearing walking with axillary crutches for 6 weeks
- In c/o fracture –dislocation:
  - Young child: 6-8 weeks immobilisation
  - Older child: 12 weeks immobilisation

Gradual Partial weight bearing and then Full weight bearing is allowed.

Complications

- Avascular necrosis:
  - Most common complication in posterior hip dislocation ~8-18%
  - More common in older age (>8 years),

    Delayed treatment (>24 hours post injury), severe trauma
  - Changes of AVN evident at 3 months-2 years
- Sciatic nerve injury:
  - Rare
  - Upto 5 % of posterior dislocation
  - Usually seen in older children with high energy trauma
  - Commonly partial nerve injury
  - Exploration recommended if no recovery beyond 3 months
- Recurrent hip dislocation:
  - In children <10 years
  - Due to inadequate healing / attenuation of posterior capsule
  - Treatment by open surgical repair/ immobilisation of hip in 45° flexion and 20° abduction for 4-6 weeks
- Degenerative arthritis:
  - Rare
  - Due to AVN
- Vascular injury:
  - In anterior dislocation
  - Surgical emergency
  - Needs prompt reduction followed by vascular repair
- Injury to triradiate cartilage:
  - Can result in shallow acetabulum and hip subluxation.

Flowchart 19.1

Fracture Neck Femur

DELBET CLASSIFICATION

- **Type I**
  - Type Ia
    - Trans-epiphyseal WITHOUT hip dislocation
    - Fixation with smooth K-wires
    - High chance of AVN (around 40-50%)
  - Type Ib
    - Trans-epiphsyeal WITH hip dislocation
    - Fixation with smooth K-wires
    - Very High chance of AVN (almost 100%)
- **Type II**
  - Trans-cervical fracture
  - 20% chance of AVN
  - Fixation with DHS/ CC Screw
- **Type III**
  - Cervico-trochanteric fracture
  - Low chance of AVN
  - Fixation with DHS/ CC Screw
- **Type IV**
  - Intertrochanteric fracture
  - Almost no chance of AVN
  - Fixation with DHS/CC Screw

Flowchart 19.2

Non-union Fracture Neck Femur

SANDHU et al CLASSIFICATION

- **Type I**
  - Fracture surface irregular with >2.5cm proximal segment and <1cm fracture gap.
  - Treatment- Fixation with DHS with/without valgus osteotomy
  - Low chance of non-union
- **Type II**
  - Fracture surface smooth with Proximal segment >2.5cm, gap >1cm and <2.5cm, changes of AVN +
  - Treatment- Fixation with valgus osteotomy with fibula grafting
  - Moderate chance of non-union
- **Type III**
  - Fracture surface smooth with proximal segment <2.5cm, fracture gap >2.5 cm with changes of AVN
  - Treatment – Fixation with valgus osteotomy with fibula and pure cancellous bone grafting
  - High chance of non-union

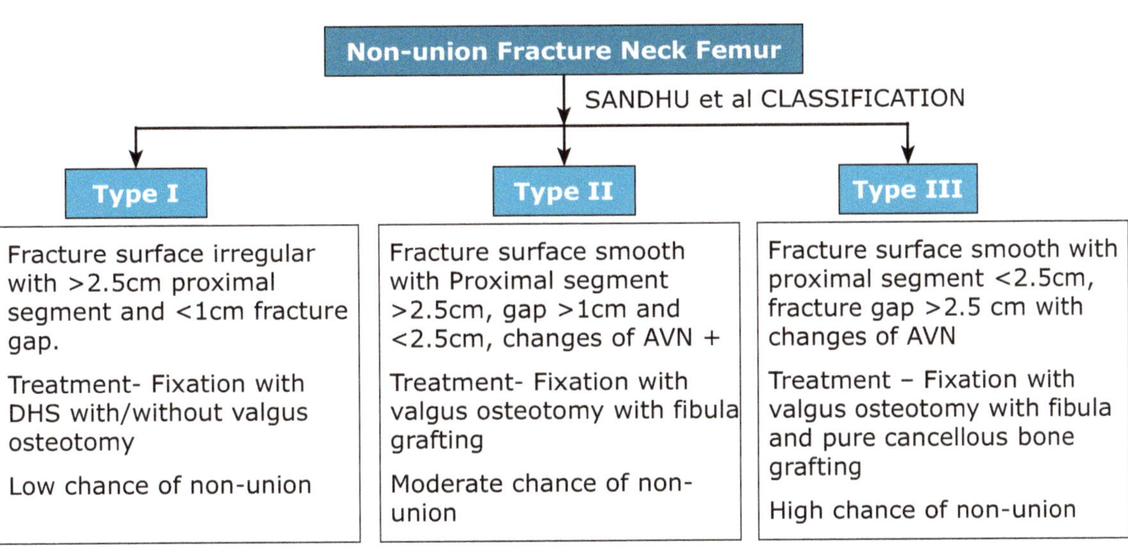

Flowchart 19.3

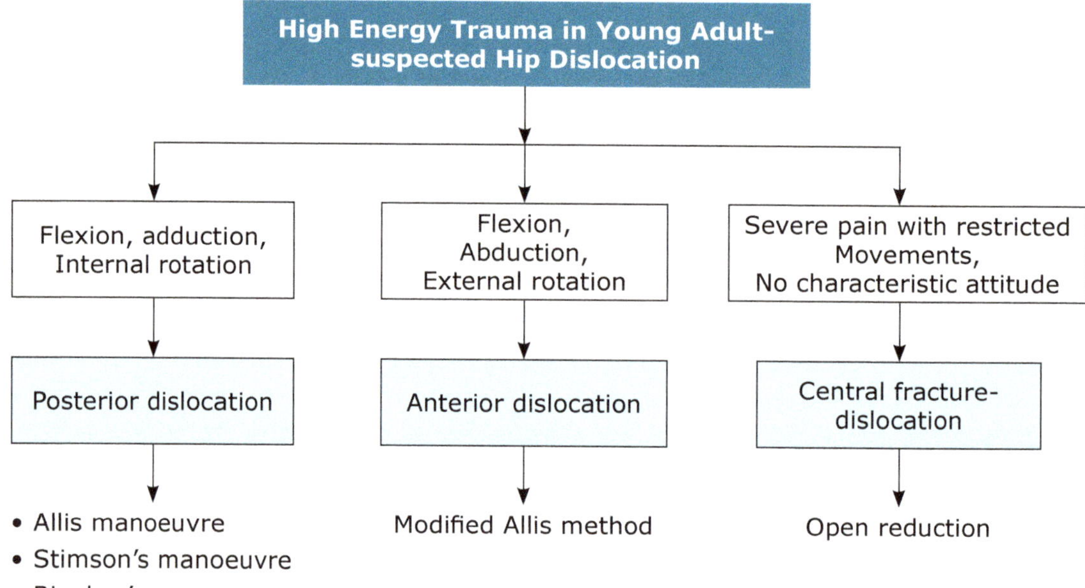

20 Slipped Capital Femoral Epiphysis

Introduction

Slipped capital femoral epiphysis is one of the commonest adolescent hip disorders, which is associated with significant morbidity and is associated with significantly increased risk of early degenerative joint disease and avascular necrosis. Early diagnosis and prompt and proper treatment is essential to prevent or minimise these issues.

Relevant anatomy

The proximal femoral physis is the growing physis of the proximal femur, though only about 30% of the femoral growth takes place in the proximal end. As against that, the greater trochanteric physis is a traction *apophysis* and is thus not a growing physis and does not contribute to the growth of the limb as such.

The vascular anatomy of the proximal femur is extremely important for the treatment of slipped capital femoral epiphysis and is derived from two main arterial trees: the main supply coming from the medial circumflex femoral artery and its branches while the lateral circumflex femoral artery and its branches supply the smaller part of the proximal femur. Extra capsular arterial ring located at the base of the femoral neck, the ascending cervical branches of the arterial ring at the surface of the femoral neck, and the arteries of the ligamentum teres contribute a minor percentage of the blood supply.

The importance of this anatomy lies in the fact that the proximal femoral epiphysis slips posteriorly leading to kinking of the posterior vasculature. Any forcible attempt to reduce a slip from its posteriorly displaced position will lead to stretching on the blood supply with resultant vascular compromise and avascular necrosis. Also the callus which is formed posteromedially abuts against the posterior vasculature and hence removal of the callus has to be performed in an extremely careful manner without disturbing the blood supply **(Fig. 20.1)**.

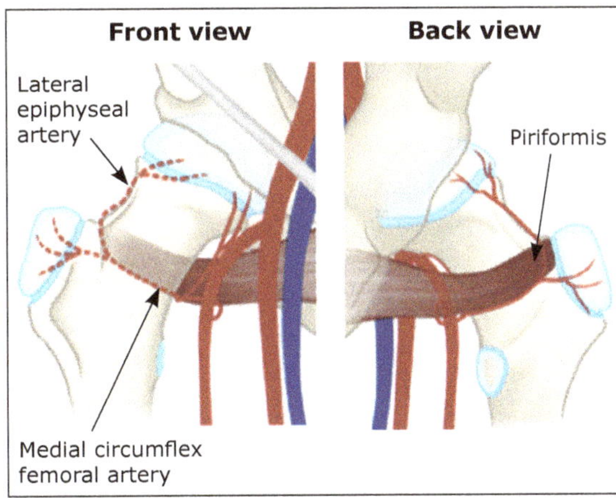

Fig. 20.1*: Front and back view of the proximal femoral vascular anatomy relevant to SCFE.*

Classification

Classification of SCFE helps in deciding the treatment modality of the patient and also helps in the prognostication. There are various classification systems of Slips based on the chronological acuity, the stability of the physis, the degree of the slip angle as an indicator for future mechanical damage to the hip joint and other anatomical factors like acetabular and femoral retroversion, anatomical depth, etc.

1) ***Chronological classification***

- One of the oldest classifications.
- Least useful in determining the eventual outcome of this condition

Acute slip :

Symptoms less than 3 weeks with or without a period of prodromal symptoms. 10-15% of all slips present in this manner

Chronic slip :

Commonest type of slip.

Symptoms more than 3 weeks.

Acute-on-chronic slip :

Acute-on-chronic SCFE occurs when a child who has had hip pain and symptoms since the past few weeks to months, suddenly has severe exacerbation of the pain due to a trivial fall or trauma.

This classification is however less commonly used nowadays, with some clinicians suggesting discarding this schema, which has little correlation with the pathomechanics found in SCFE.

2) ***Stability classification***

- Most frequently used classification and one which is most important for prognosis.
- This classification described by Randall Loder, describes the mechanical stability of the slip and classifies it into stable and unstable.
- *Stable:* The child is able to bear weight on the limb with or without support (AVN rate 1%)
- *Unstable:* The child is unable to bear weight with or without support (AVN rate – 60-80%).

3) ***Morphological classification***

Based on the displacement of the epiphysis on AP and lateral views with the accurate assessment of the deformity being made on the lateral view.

It depends on 2 factors: the percentage of displacement of the head on the neck and the Southwick angle (defined as the angle between a line perpendicular to a line that connects the anterior and posterior margins of the physis and a line along the axis of the femoral shaft). The classification is as follows **(Fig. 20.2)**:

1) *Pre-slip:* Just widening of the physis, no displacement
2) *Mild slip:* Less than 30% of displacement and 0-30° of Southwick angle
3) *Moderate slip:* Between 30-50% of displacement and 30-60° of Southwick angle
4) *Severe slip:* More than 50% of displacement and more than 60° of Southwick angle.

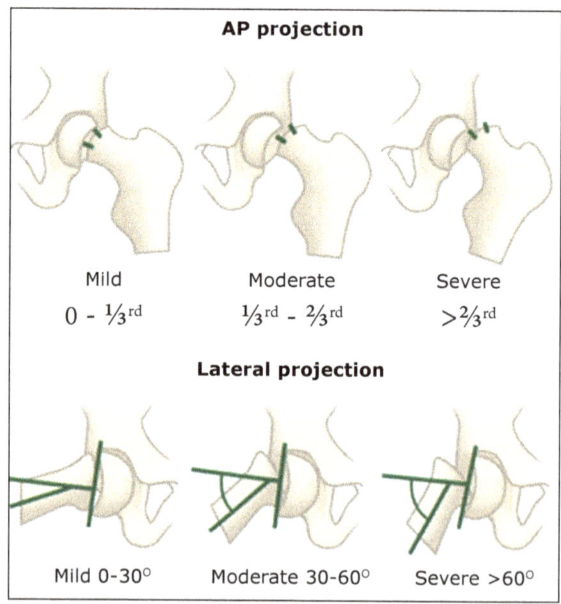

***Fig. 20.2**: Severity classification of SCFE as seen from the AP and lateral projection.*

Clinical Features

The clinical presentation of SCFE is very variable and depends on four features:

1) Temporal acuteness
2) Physical stability of the physis which is slipping
3) Degree of actual displacement
4) Amount of deformity which the protruding anterior metaphysis causes to the anterior acetabular rim during extreme hip range especially flexion.

- SCFE is a typically adolescent hip pathology with the common age being between 13-16 years in boys and 11-14 years in girls. It is much more common in boys as compared to girls with the male: female ratio being 1.5-2:1. It is bilateral in almost 10-20% of cases though there is a wide variabilility in the bilaterality in various studies.
- Obesity is the most important risk factor and is associated with endocrinopathies in about 20% in the form of hypothyroidism, Juvenile diabetes, Down's syndrome, etc.
- The typical presenting feature of a chronic stable slip is pain in the distal thigh or hip which is dull aching and associated with mild restriction of activities.
- The child has a typical out-toeing gait with mild antalgia and is able to sit cross legged. In late cases, and with severe deformities, there can be associated restricted flexion which prevents the child in squatting or even sitting on a chair.
- On examination, the typical feature is an external rotation deformity. The pathognomonic feature is *Drehmann sign*, which is described as movement of the knee towards the ipsilateral shoulder on hip flexion. There may be some shortening and may be associated with restricted flexion.
- In case of unstable, acute or acute-on-chronic slips, the child is unable to bear weight. The limb is in severe external rotation and is extremely painful on any movement.

Imaging

- The pelvis with both hips-anteroposterior and frog leg lateral view are the two basic X-rays to be done in all cases of suspected SCFE. The radiographs demonstrate the typical postero-inferior displacement of the epiphysis relative to the metaphysis, which is often only seen on the frog leg lateral view. Frog leg lateral view may be difficult to perform in a child with severe pain. In this case, a cross table view may be useful to decrease the patient discomfort during positioning.

There are a few signs which can be seen on the anteroposterior view which helps in proving the diagnosis of SCFE in the early stages **(Fig. 20.3)**.

1) Widening and irregularities of the physis as compared to the opposite side
2) The anterior aspect of the femoral neck loses its anterior concavity
3) Cystic change in the metaphysis, remodelling and periosteal reactions in cases of chronic SCFE.
4) A relative loss of height of the epiphysis on AP projection
5) *Metaphyseal blanch sign of Steel:* The metaphyseal blanch sign of Steel is a radiographic double density created by the posteriorly displaced epiphysis overlapping the medial metaphysis, as seen on the AP radiograph. This is a very early sign and can be easily missed if not looked for, carefully.

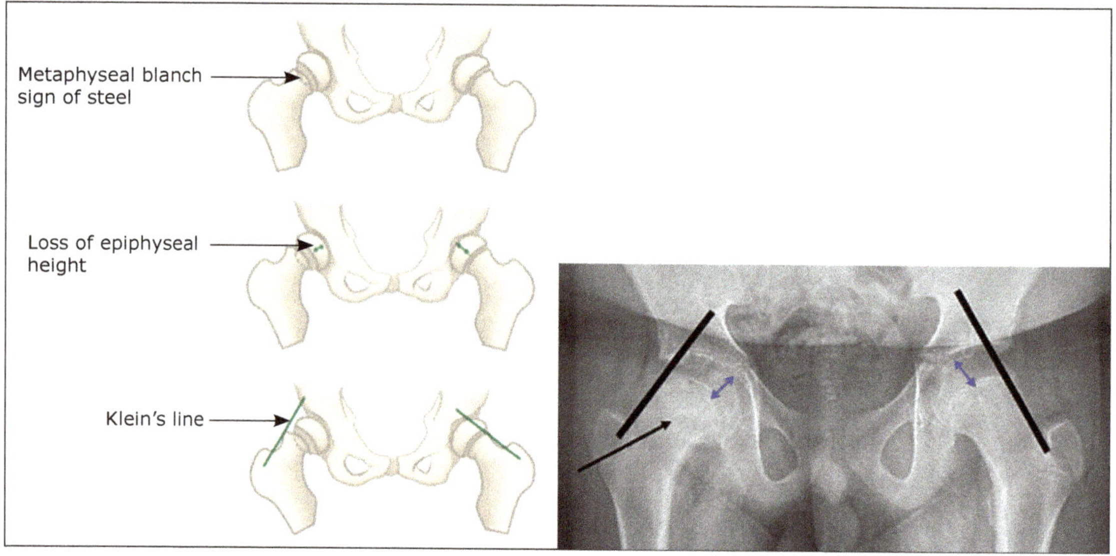

Fig. 20.3: *Schematic and X-ray of a mild SCFE showing various signs. Metaphyseal sign of Steel is shown by the faint white line of the metaphysis denoted by the thin black arrow, Klein's line is denoted by the bold black line which is not intersecting the epiphysis on the left and the loss of epiphyseal height on the left is denoted by the blue arrows.*

6) *Klein's line:* Klein's line is a line drawn along the superior border of the femoral neck on the AP radiograph. In a normal hip, this line should intersect the epiphysis (ie some part of the epiphysis should lie superior to the metaphysis). On the other hand, in a chronic slip, the epiphysis lies flush with or below this line. This denotes a subtle inferior displacement of the epiphysis as compared to the metaphysis.

As the slip becomes more and more chronic, more changes start becoming apparent on the X-rays There is metaphyseal remodelling and retroversion of the femoral neck in long standing cases of SCFE. There is metaphyseal rounding at the anterosuperior portion of the neck and callus formation on the postero-inferior aspect of the femoral neck on the frog leg lateral view.

The X-ray findings in acute and acute-on-chronic slips are much more apparent. Usually only an AP radiograph can be obtained due to severe discomfort of the patient. This shows an abrupt displacement of the epiphysis with respect to the metaphysis. If it is an acute on chronic slip, then there will be a variable amount of remodelling seen on the anterior metaphysis. As against that, in case of an acute slip (which is in fact very rare), these changes are not seen.

Other imaging

Further imaging in form of CT scan or MRI are needed in specific circumstances.

MRI is indicated in very early cases of suspected SCFE especially in the so-called "Pre-slip" or imminent slip. MRI in this stage shows widening of the physis, bone marrow oedema, joint effusion and synovitis.

CT scan is typically needed in case of suspected mild SCFE which is not picked on the standard AP and frog lateral radiographs. This is also useful in mild to moderate slips in order to exactly quantify the amount of displacement and further plan the management vis a vis in-situ fixation versus reduction and fixation.

Treatment

The treatment of SCFE is controversial and in a state of constant flux over the years. The main goals of treatment of SCFE are:

1) Prevention of slip progression by obliteration of physis
2) Prevention of Femoro-Acetabular Impingement (FAI) by correcting the slip angle and improving the lateral Alpha angle
3) At the same time, maintaining (in some cases, restoring) the vascularity of the femoral head.

With these goals in mind, the main modalities of treatment are as follows:

1) In-situ pin/Screw fixation
2) Closed/incidental/Serendipitous reduction and screw fixation
3) Anterior mini-open "reduction" and screw fixation (Parsch) method
4) Anterior open reduction with Cuneiform osteotomy
5) Safe surgical dislocation with modified Dunn osteotomy

The full surgical details of all the procedures is outside the purview of this textbook. We will be discussing in-situ pinning and Safe surgical dislocation/Modified Dunn osteotomy in detail.

1) ***In-situ Fixation***

   In-situ fixation has been the oldest and most widely used method of treating SCFE. In fact in a landmark study by Carney et al, a 41 year followup of SCFE treated with in-situ pinning showed 70% good to excellent results and very low conversion to THR.

The indications for in-situ pinning are:

1) All mild slips
2) Moderate slips with good/fair internal rotation
3) Severe stable slips- in conjunction with proximal femoral derotation osteotomy
4) Severe unstable slips- (relative indication)

Procedure:

- Position: Supine on a fracture table (unstable slips), or on a simple radiolucent table with a small bump below the ipsilateral buttock (stable slips)
- It is extremely important especially in case of slips, to be able to visualise the complete femoral head including the articular surface on both AP and lateral views. On the fracture table, one needs to get a complete shoot through lateral view, while when the patient is on a simple table, lateral view is to be obtained by flexing the hip to 30° and turning the C-arm by 30°, so as to obtain a frog lateral view of the hip.
- After sterile painting and draping, marking of the screw trajectory is very important . This is performed by placing guidewires on the AP and lateral view on the skin. The screw trajectory should be such that the screw is central on the femoral epiphysis on the AP and lateral view. Traditionally the direction of the screw was described to be perpendicular to the physis, with its entry point being on the anterior aspect of the proximal femur with the direction from anterior to posterior.
- However this anterior starting point of the screw is in a less dense bone and can lead to an inadequate fixation inspite of good position. The other difficulty in placing this screw is the close proximity to the anterior neurovascular bundle.

As against that, the newer concept is passing an oblique screw with an entry point on the lateral aspect of the femur, with the trajectory passing posteriorly in the neck but ending centrally in the femoral capital epiphysis **(Fig. 20.4)**.

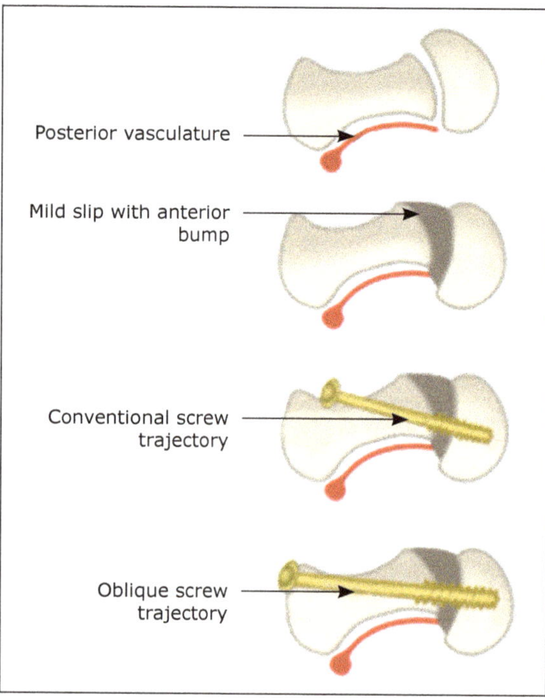

***Fig. 20.4**: Traditional (conventional) trajectory of the screw for in-situ fixation in mild SCFE.*

- Once the screw trajectories are marked on the AP and lateral views, the point on the skin where they intersect is the point where the incision is centred.
- The typical incision is a small 5 cm incision , with a fascia lata underneath being cut widely from proximal to distal. This step is extremely important as the fascia lata usually prevents accurate placement of the guidewire.
- The trajectory of the oblique screw starts on the anterolateral edge of the femur, just lateral to the inter-trochanteric line and proximal to the lesser trochanter. The usual screw which is used is a 7.0mm fully threaded or 32 mm threaded cannulated cancellous self drilling self tapping screw. This screw should pass in the posterior quadrant of the neck and hold the femoral epiphysis in the central third. It is important to note that this screw is *not* perpendicular to the physis (as conventionally described).
- Once the guidewire trajectory and screw size is confirmed, the screw is passed. This screw should end within about 5 mm of the sub-chondral surface and should have at least 3-5 screw threads crossing the physis. It is of utmost importance to confirm on multiple C-arm views as well as fluoro shots that the screw threads are not intra-articular as that can lead to severe chondrolysis.
- In stable slips, one central 6.5-7.0 mm screw is enough while in unstable slips, two screws may be necessary **(Fig. 20.5)**.
- In moderate slips, this can be combined with an anterior approach mini-open osteoplasty with the help of a burr, in order to remove the anterior bump and decrease the chance of FAI.
- Wound closure is performed in a usual manner.
- In chronic stable slips, weightbearing is started immediately as per pain tolerance. As against that, in unstable slips, weight bearing is withheld till radiological signs of union/fusion of physis are seen.

2) ***Closed/Incidental reduction and screw fixation:***

Closed/incidental reduction, by definition, is the reduction which takes place as soon as the patient is placed on the operation table or the fracture table after anaesthesia, *without any extra force or manipulation*. It is paramount to remember that the posterior vasculature

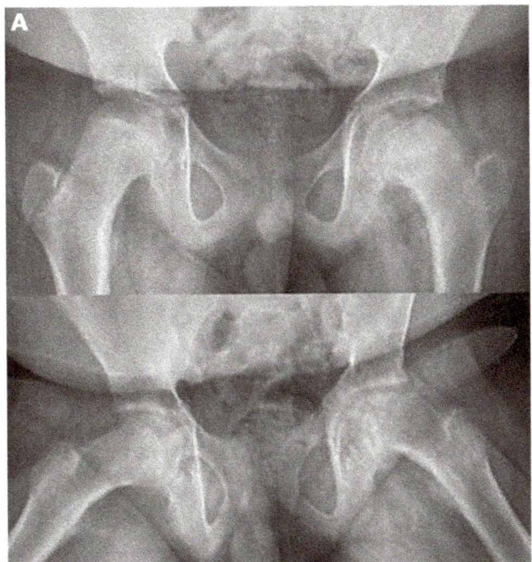

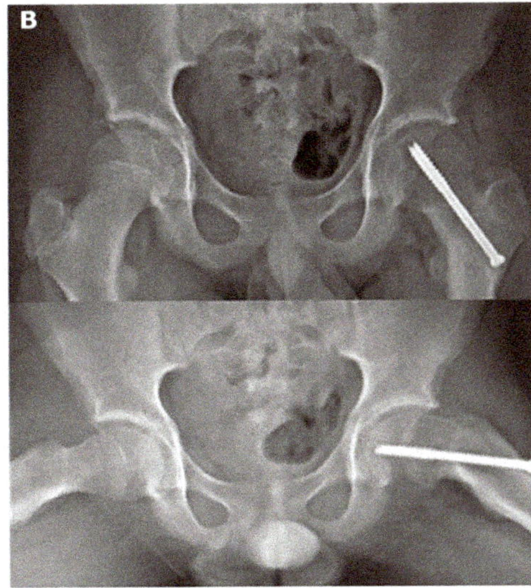

Fig. 20.5: *(A) Pre-operative AP and frog-leg lateral X-rays of a 15 year old boy with left sided mild, chronic stable SCFE treated with in-situ screw (oblique) fixation using a single 7.0 mm cannulated cancellous screw. (B) One year post-operative X-ray showing excellent healing and remodelling of the deformity.*

in slipped capital femoral epiphysis is shortened and kinked and any attempt to internally rotate the hip even while positioning the child on the fracture table can lead to vascular compromise of the femoral head. The exact amount of this "gentle" manipulation which is tolerated by the femoral head is extremely variable and hence this method of "gentle" closed reduction has the highest rates of avascular necrosis. On the whole, "gentle", "serendipitous" and "incidental" reduction should be avoided as much as possible unless the reduction is obtained without any manipulation at all during positioning.

3) ***Anterior mini-open partial "reduction" and screw fixation (Parsch method)***:

This unique method of treatment of acute-on-chronic SCFE has found favour in a few centres. The principle here is to convert a severe acute on chronic slip to its "pre-acute" slip levels and convert it to a mild slip and then fix it in a routine manner. The steps of the Parsch method in brief are as follows:

- Position: The child is usually taken on a fracture table and positioned without any manipulation of the lower limb.
- The hip is exposed using the anterior Smith-Peterson approach.
- Anterior capsulotomy is performed and the haemarthrosis (which is usually present in an acute-on-chronic, unstable slip) is drained.
- A small flat instrument such as a large periosteal elevator is then inserted through the rent in the capsule on the anterior surface of the proximal femur and gentle force is applied so as to decrease the severity of the slip. Care should be taken to be extremely gentle in this step and stop after even the slight amount of resistance keeping a check on the C-arm.
- Once partial reduction is obtained, screw fixation is performed with either one or two screws from the lateral/ anterolateral aspect in the routine manner.

- In smaller patients, instead of a periosteal elevator or an instrument, the surgeon can use the digital force with the help of the thumb in order to partially reduce the slip and then fix it from the lateral side.
- The capsule is usually not closed as that can lead to tamponade with vascular compromise of the head of the femur.
- Wound is closed in a routine fashion and usually no immobilisation is required.
- The child is kept non-weight bearing for about 6 weeks till radiological signs of physeal closure appear.

4) ***Anterior open reduction and Dunn osteotomy***:

Anterior open reduction and Dunn osteotomy was described in the early 1960's and was popular in the United Kingdom for a few decades. The principle of the surgery is correction of the deformity at the level of the deformity so as to achieve maximum correction. The steps of procedure include exposing the hip through the anterior Smith-Peterson approach, doing an anterior capsulotomy and removing a cuneiform wedge, shortening the femoral neck and fixing the slip in a standard manner. This procedure usually leads to a robust correction of the deformity albeit at the expense of significant neck shortening. Initial results especially in some British centres had very good results in terms of correction as well as very low rates of AVN. However over the years, a number of series emerged which showed significantly high rates of AVN. The probable reason was that there was no access to the blood supply of the femoral head as the approach was anterior which resulted in inadvertent damage and kinking of the blood vessels. This procedure is very rarely performed in today's age and is almost of historical interest. Further details of this procedure can be obtained in older editions of standard textbooks and is beyond the purview of this book.

5) ***Safe surgical dislocation with Modified Dunn procedure:***

The "modified" Dunn osteotomy is nothing but the Dunn cuneiform osteotomy performed through the "Ganz" safe surgical dislocation approach. It combines the efficacy of the Dunn procedure (in which the deformity is corrected as close to the CORA as possible) with the safety of the Ganz method in terms of maintaining vascularity. Over the last decade or so, the "Ganz" modified Dunn osteotomy has emerged as the treatment of choice for moderate to severe slips and its efficacy and safety has been seen in a number of series at many centres throughout the world.

However it should be noted that it is an extremely technically demanding procedure and needs to be performed by a surgeon well versed with the surgical dislocation method along with a well-trained team.

Indications:

- Severe unstable slips
- Moderate slips (relative indication)
- Severe chronic slips (relative indication)
- Chronic healed slips with severe head-neck deformities.

Procedure:

- The patient is placed in a lateral position with the affected hip up, a bump placed anteriorly in such a way as to allow the hip to be flexed up to 90° intra-operatively.
- While draping, a pouch is fashioned anteriorly, which could hold the limb during dislocation in a sterile manner.

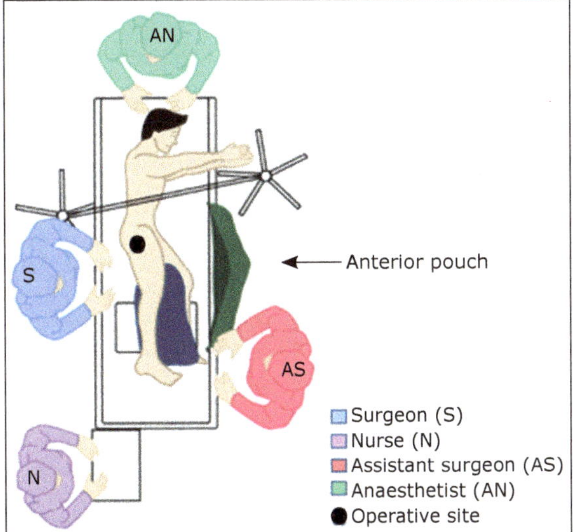

***Fig. 20.6**: Intra-operative positioning of the child with right sided severe SCFE planned for modified Dunn osteotomy. Note the sterile pouch made of the drapes anteriorly in order to hold the leg during dislocation.*

- The incision is centered over the greater trochanter, extending 5 cm proximally towards the iliac crest, and 8 cm distally along the mid-lateral line The deep fascia is cut distally in line with the incision, and proximally between the gluteus maximus and tensor fascia lata.
- The digastric osteotomy is started with an oscillating saw, from the posterior margin of the origin of the vastus lateralis, to the tip of the greater trochanter. This ensures that the thickness of the trochanteric flap is around 1 to 1.5 cm, and also that the majority of the fibers of the gluteus medius are attached to the mobile trochanter, with only a small part remaining on the stable trochanter.
- However, to accommodate for the external rotation deformity of the limb in SCFE, the cut is completed with a curved, broad osteotome directed laterally.
- The hip is then flexed, abducted and externally rotated to allow visualisation of the anterior hip joint surface. The hip capsule is exposed anteriorly by raising from its surface, the gluteus minimus proximally, and the vastus intermedius and iliocapsularis distally, from the acetabular labrum to the intertrochanteric line.
- The Z shaped capsulotomy is then made, the central limb along the femoral neck, inferior limb along the intertrochanteric line, and the superior limb along the acetabular margin. The capsule is first sharply entered using the bovie or knife. A gush of haemorrhagic fluid when the capsular rent is widened with a blunt hemostat proved the presence of an unstable slip.
- Next, the hip is flexed, adducted and externally rotated, and the leg is placed anteriorly in the sterile pouch. The anterior surface of the femoral neck is exposed and the anterior periosteal flaps are fashioned.
- Before dislocating the hip fully, it is necessary to temporarily fix the femoral epiphysis in the slipped position with two thick K-wires, particularly in unstable slips. The hip is then further rotated externally to dislocate it fully by cutting the ligamentum teres with stout scissors. At this stage, the vascularity of the epiphysis is checked by drilling a small hole using a Kirschner wire and checking for active pulsatile bleeding.
- The hip is then reduced again so as to further prepare the retinacular flaps, starting from the posterior aspect of the stable trochanter, by removing all of the cancellous bone from the supra-apophyseal part of the trochanter. The entire metaphysis of the femoral neck is thus denuded of the retinacular flaps.
- The hip is then dislocated again. Before removal of the provisional fixation pins,

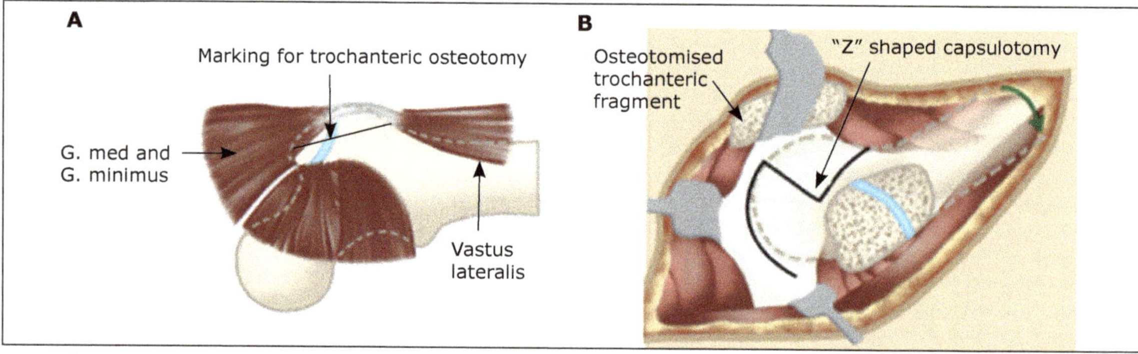

***Fig. 20.7A and B**: (A) Schematic diagram of the proximal femur showing the marking for the digastric trochanteric osteotomy extending from the tip of the trochanter to just below the vastus ridge, lined proximally by the Gluteus medius and minimus and distally by the Vastus lateralis. (B) Schematic diagram for the anterior Z-shaped capsulotomy.*

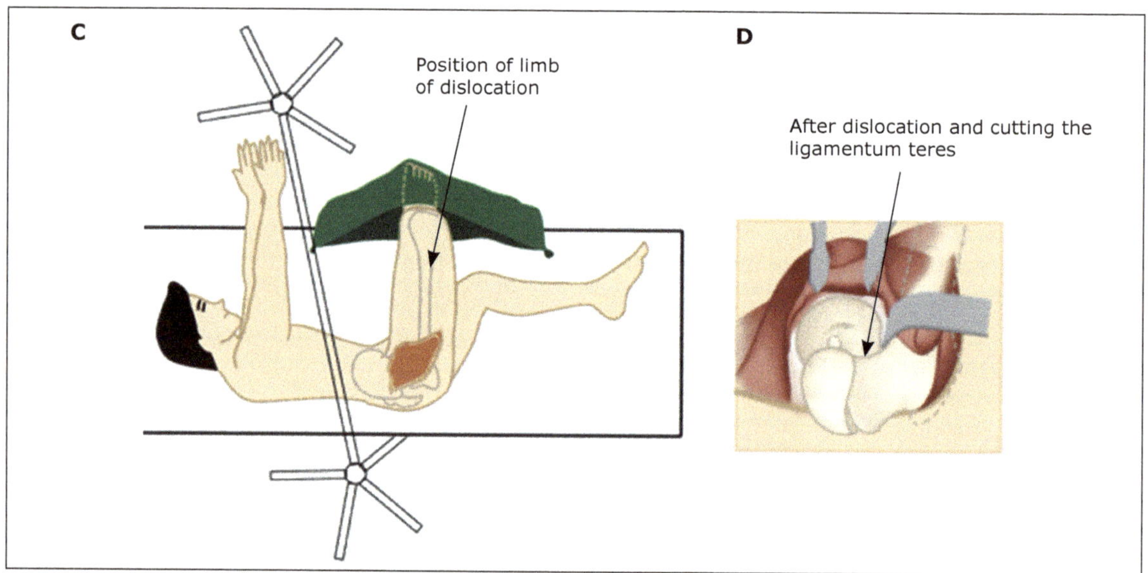

***Fig. 20.7C and D**: (C) Position of the limb during dislocation with the leg being placed in the sterile bag. (D) Corresponding view of the wound after sectioning of the ligamentum teres.*

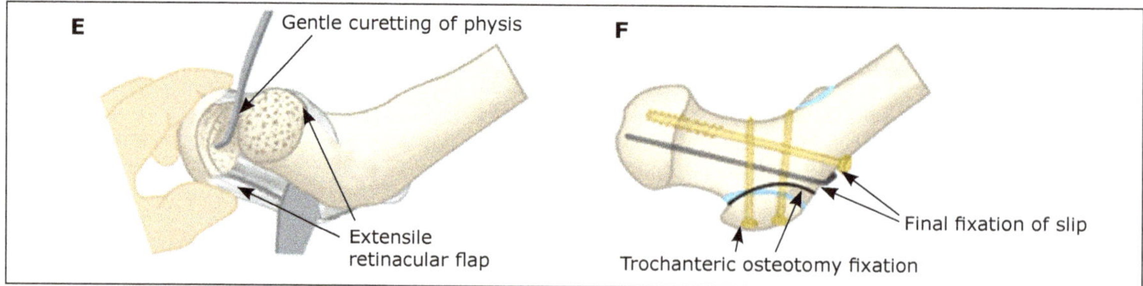

***Fig. 20.7E and F**: (E) Schematic diagram showing the curetting of the physis keeping the extensile retinacular flap intact. (F) Final fixation using one 6.5 mm cannulated cancellous screw and one K-wire for fixation of the slip and two 3.5 mm cortical screws for fixation of the trochanteric osteotomy.*

the acetabular cavity is packed with roller gauze to prevent inadvertent slippage of the epiphysis back into the acetabulum.

- The epiphysis is now carefully separated from the metaphysis. In true unstable slips, this occurs easily. In acute on chronic slips, the epiphysis often does not separate so easily and requires careful separation using osteotomes.
- Once the entire neck is exposed, the posteromedial callus and anterior metaphyseal bump are removed using rongeurs, curettes and scoops. This important step allows realignment of the head to its anatomic location without stretching the retinacular vessels and embarrassing the capital femoral blood supply.
- The femoral physis is curetted carefully to remove all the physeal cartilage. The femoral head is then reduced and fixed provisionally with K-wires passed retrogradely. At this stage, vascularity of the head is re-checked. If there is no bleeding, the fixation has to be removed immediately and the neck checked again for any residual callus or bump.
- Final fixation is done from the lateral cortex of the femur; our preference is to use one 6.5 or 7 mm cannulated cancellous screw supplemented with one or two K-wires.
- The hip joint is reduced, and the trochanter is fixed slightly distally using 3.5 mm self-tapping cortical screws. The image intensifier is used to assess the alignment of the femoral head as well as trochanteric fixation.
- The wound is closed in the routine manner over a negative suction drain.
- Post-operatively, the limb is immobilised in a knee immobiliser to prevent hip flexion in bed, and in some abduction to reduce stress on the trochanteric fixation. The child is allowed in bed skateboard exercises as tolerated, after which bedside sitting and knee range of motion exercises are begun.
- An X-ray is obtained prior to discharge, and then at 6 weeks post op. Once

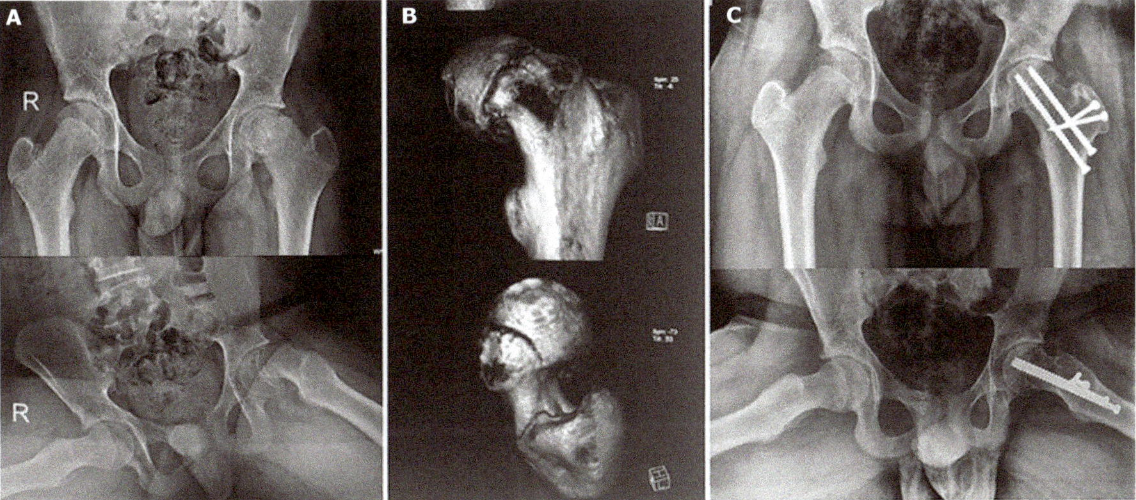

***Fig. 20.8**: (A) Pre-operative AP and lateral views of a 14 year old boy with left sided chronic, severe slip. (B) Pre-operative CT scan of the same patient showing a severe deformity with a large anterior metaphyseal bump. (C) Two years post-operative X-ray showing excellent correction of the deformity with no AVN.*

union at the trochanteric osteotomy is confirmed, the child is allowed unrestricted weight-bearing. Further follow-up is at 6 monthly intervals.

Complications

1) Avascular necrosis of the femoral head

AVN of the femoral head is one of the most dreaded complications of SCFE- which is both due to the actual injury itself as well as due to the treatment given. The commonest cause of AVN in SCFE is an unstable slip with reported rates being as much as 10-60% in various series. The usual causative event is a severe shearing off of all the vasculature from the metaphysis related to the sudden instability of the condition. Even after performing a safe surgical dislocation in these hips, it is found that the femoral head doesn't bleed after placing a small drill hole in the periphery and that is an indicator of the imminent avascularity of the femoral head.

The other cause for AVN in SCFE is iatrogenic with sudden forceful closed reduction as the main factor. As discussed before, in some severe, acute or acute on chronic slips, even positioning of the child and "gentle" traction can be deleterious to the femoral head vascularity and as such, no manipulation should be allowed.

2) Femoro-acetabular impingement and increased chance of early Hip Arthritis

This is seen more often in moderate and severe slips which have been pinned in-situ. However long term follow-up has shown increased incidence of FAI, with significant labral damage even in mild slips managed with in-situ pinning. The typical variety of FAI which is seen in SCFE is the cam type with a pistol-grip deformity due to the metaphyseal bump caused by the slippage. This is a pre-arthritic condition and is one of the commonest causes of total hip arthroplasty in younger age.

3) Intra-articular screw penetration and chondrolysis

This occurs more commonly in slips which have been fixed in-situ rather than through the modified Dunn procedure. The trajectory of the screw in case of a mild to moderate slip is from anterolateral side to posterior with a very oblique course. This results in an inadvertent under-estimation of the tip to surface distance of the screw with resultant intra-articular penetration of a few threads of the screw. This can cause severe chondrolysis and stiffness and once set in, is very difficult to reverse.

A key point to be remembered during in–situ fixation of a slip is the "fluoro-shot" which is nothing but a continuous shoot of the hip on C-arm in all range of motion so as to ensure that the screw tips are not inside the joint. At the end of the procedure, none of the screws should be less than 5mm from the surface of the joint.

Flowchart 20.1

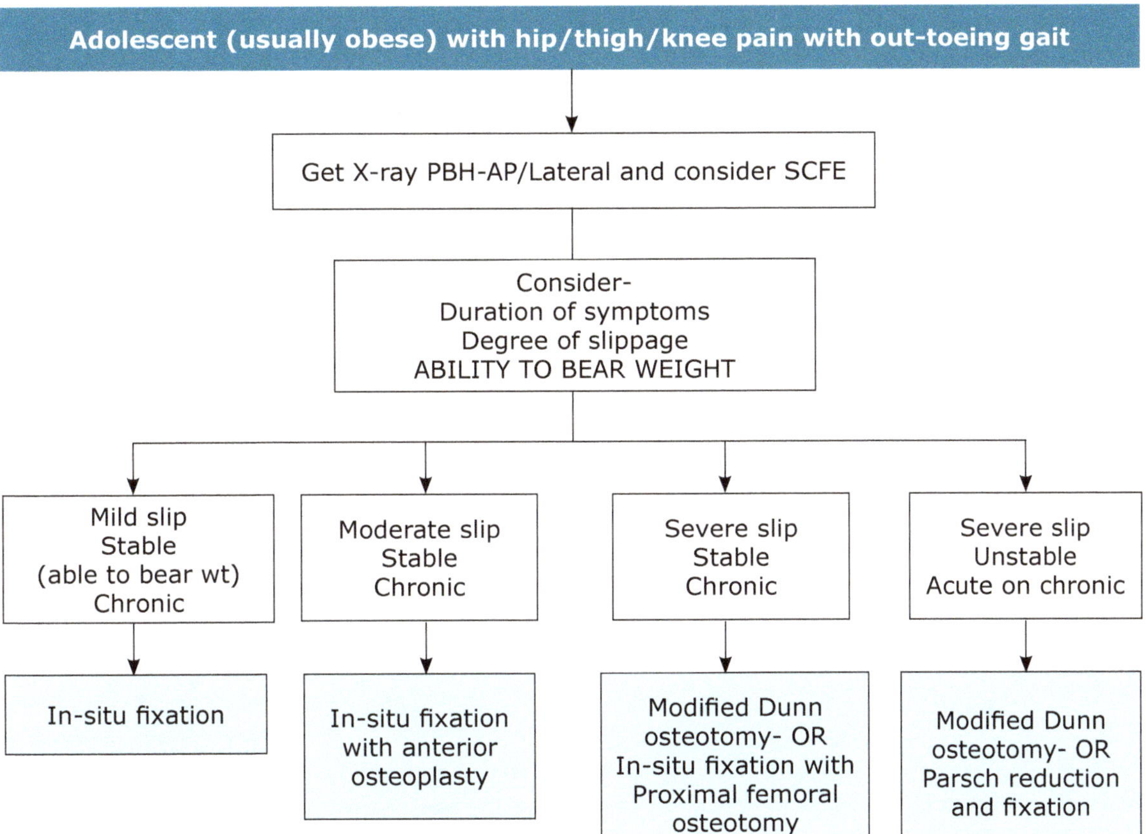

21 Fractures of the Femoral Shaft

Introduction

Femoral shaft fractures are common, representing about 1.6 % of all bony injuries in children. There is bimodal distribution of femoral shaft fractures between 1–4 years and between 11-16 years. In early toddler years, the femur is relatively weak and breaks usually from simple falls whereas with progressive increase in bone strength, high velocity trauma is required to fracture the femur in adolescent age. Before walking age, about 80% of femoral fractures are caused by abuse. Stress fractures may occur at any location in the adolescent femoral shaft from extreme overuse and sports. Also, pathological fractures may occur in femur in patients with osteogenesis imperfecta, neurological conditions like cerebral palsy or meningomyelocele, metabolic disorders or neoplasms, mostly benign lesions like Non ossifying fibroma, Aneurysmal bone cyst, Unicameral bone cyst, Fibrous dysplasia and Eosinophilic granuloma **(Fig. 21.1)**.

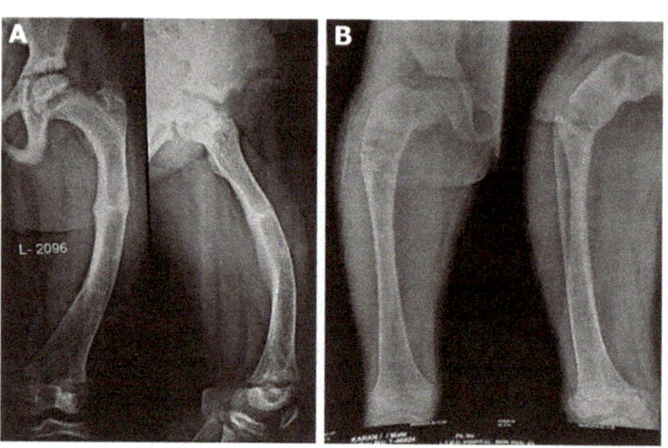

Fig. 21.1: *Pathological femur fracture in a child with A. Hypophosphatemic rickets; B. Fibrous dysplasia.*

The strong pull of muscles of the thigh at various levels account for the typical displacement and deformity seen in femur shaft fractures **(Fig. 21.2)**.

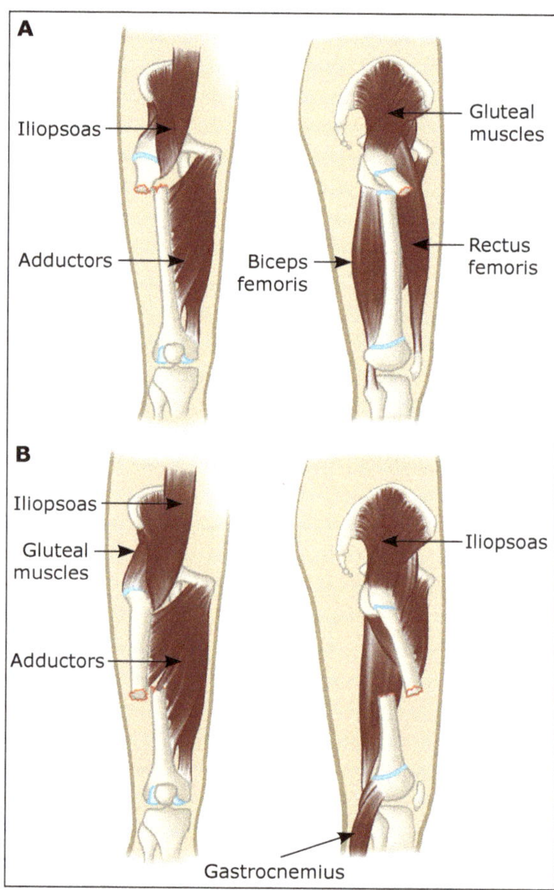

Fig. 21.2: *Characteristic displacement patterns in femur shaft fractures: A. Proximal fracture: Flexion (iliopsoas), abduction (abductor muscle group) and external rotation (short external rotators); B. Midshaft fracture: Less marked flexion, abduction, external rotation due to balancing effect of adductors and extensors attachment on the proximal fragment*

Clinical Features

Clinical diagnosis of femoral shaft fracture is obvious with a clear mechanism of injury, localised pain, swelling of the thigh and deformity. A comprehensive physical examination is necessary to look for other associated injuries like head injuries and intra-thoracic or intra-abdominal injuries. In case of polytrauma, rapid stabilisation of femur fracture is essential for overall care and to achieve haemodynamic stability. Hypotension rarely results from isolated closed femur shaft fracture and other sources of blood loss should be carefully evaluated. Presence of any associated neurovascular injury should be documented.

Imaging

Anteroposterior (AP) and lateral X-rays of the entire femur, including hip and knee should be done for diagnosis of femur shaft fracture and any associated fracture. X-rays should be carefully evaluated for comminution, classification (transverse/spiral/oblique) or presence of any non displaced 'butterfly' fragment, as this helps in planning of treatment.

Treatment

Treatment of femoral shaft fractures in children depends on two primary considerations: age and fracture pattern. Some other secondary considerations, especially for surgical treatment, include the child's weight, mechanism of injury, associated injuries and economic concerns.

Infants

Due to the presence of thick periosteum, femoral shaft fractures in infants are usually stable. Once any metabolic abnormality and abuse is ruled out, most proximal and mid shaft femoral fractures are successfully treated with Pavlik harness, just to provide comfort and some stability and to improve the resting position of the fracture. Pavlik harness can be applied with the hip in moderate flexion and abduction, in order to align the distal fragment with the flexed proximal fragment. **(Fig. 21.3)** Excessive hip flexion in the presence of a swollen thigh may lead to femoral nerve palsy and weekly evaluation of quadriceps function must be performed during treatment.

With thick periosteum and tremendous remodelling potential **(Fig. 21.4)**, newborns rarely need a manipulative reduction or rigid external immobilisation. But if there

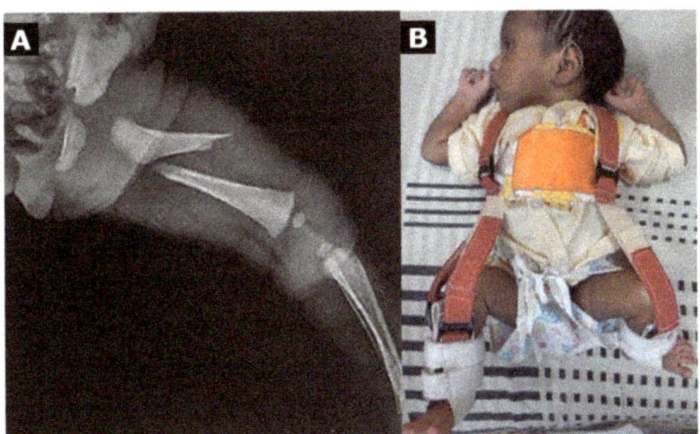

Fig. 21.3: *(A) Mid shaft femur fracture in a 2-month-old child (B) Treatment with Pavlik harness.*

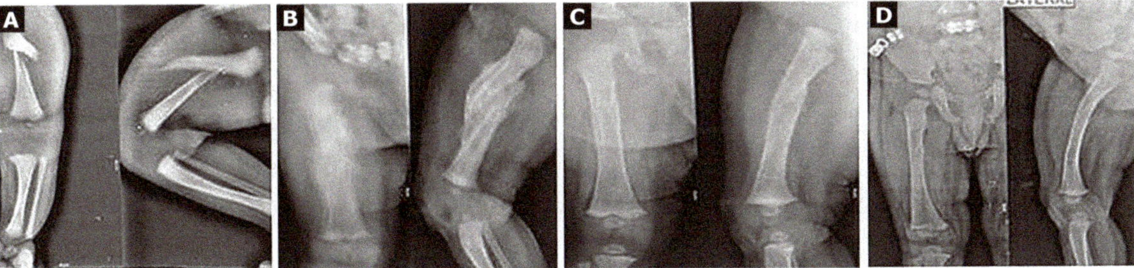

Fig. 21.4: *Remodelling in neonatal femur shaft fracture (A) At birth (B) At 4 weeks (C) At 3 months (D) At 6 months.*

is excessive shortening (> 1-2 cm) or angulation > 30°, spica cast may be used.

Pre-School Children: (6 months–6 years)

- For children with fractures without much swelling and < 2 cm of initial shortening, early spica casting is the treatment of choice. In low-energy fractures, even " walking spica" can be given.

Advantages of a spica cast:

- Low cost
- Good results with acceptable leg length equality, healing time and motion
- Safe, with minimal complications.

"Telescope Test" (described by Thompson et. al.)

Children are examined with fluoroscopy at the time of reduction and casting. If > 3 cm of shortening is demonstrated with gentle axial compression, 3-10 days of skin or distal femur skeletal traction is advised rather than immediate spica casting. **(Fig. 21.5)**

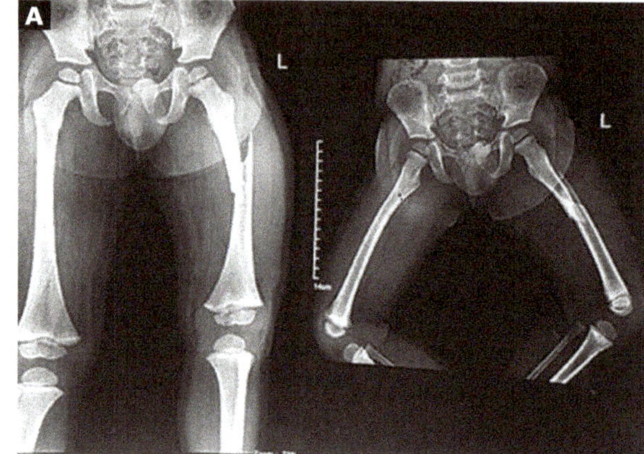

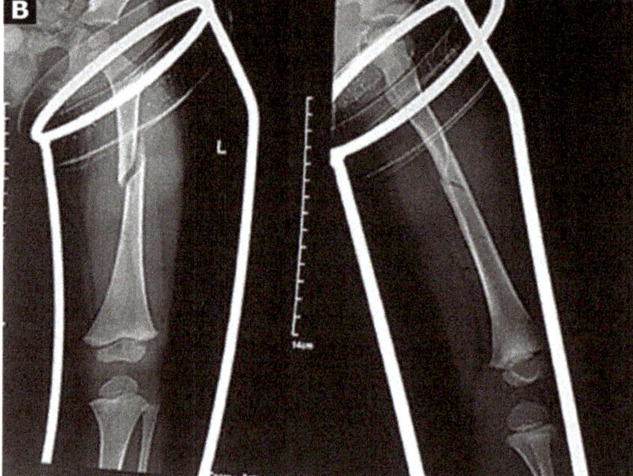

***Fig. 21.5**: (A) Midshaft femur fracture in a 4-year- old child with > 2 cm. shortening; (B) Initial treatment with skin traction in Thomas splint*

Spica cast application technique

The trolley is prepared with all the materials required for the spica cast application. **(Fig. 21.6)**

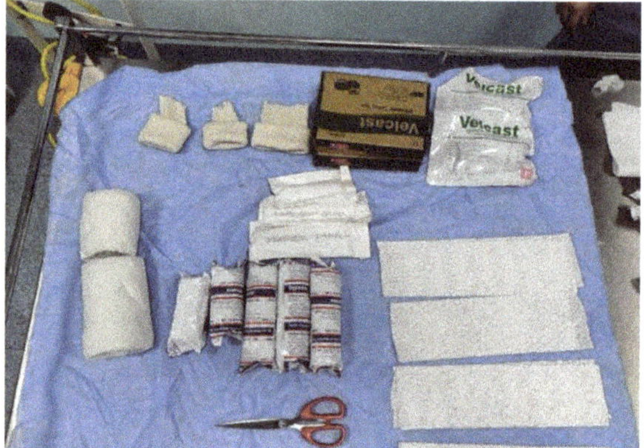

***Fig. 21.6**: Materials required for spica cast application.*

- Cast should be applied in the operation theatre or emergency room under anaesthesia.
- Child is placed on a spica table. Adequate padding is applied from abdomen above umbilicus to foot on the affected side and above knee on the normal side. Extra padding should be applied in the popliteal area.
- It is important to avoid excessive traction as risk of compartment syndrome and skin sloughs are high.
- *Position of the limb:* The position of the hip and knee in the spica cast is controversial. The more proximal the

fracture, the more hip should be flexed. The usual position is hip in 60°-90° flexion, 30° abduction and 15° external rotation, knee in 45-60° flexion and ankle in neutral.

- Strengthen the cast around the groin using extra slabs. Final use of synthetic cast strengthens the spica and avoids the need for a connecting bar. **(Fig. 21.7)**
- Once the spica cast is applied, AP and lateral X-rays are done to confirm length and angular and rotational alignment. **(Fig. 21.8 and Table 21.1)**

For the single leg 'walking' spica, the long leg cast is applied with approximately 45° knee flexion, hip in 45° flexion and 15° external rotation and valgus. Hip should be reinforced anteriorly with multiple layers of extra fiberglass and the pelvic band should be fairly wide so that the hip is well controlled. The foot is left free, the cast stopping at supramalleolar area.

Table 21.1: Acceptability criteria for femoral shaft fractures

Age	*Varus/ valgus (angulation)*	*Anterior/ posterior (angulation)*	*shortening (mm)*
Birth-2 years	30°	30°	15
2-5 years	15°	20°	20
6-10 years	10°	15°	15
11years-maturity	5°	10°	10

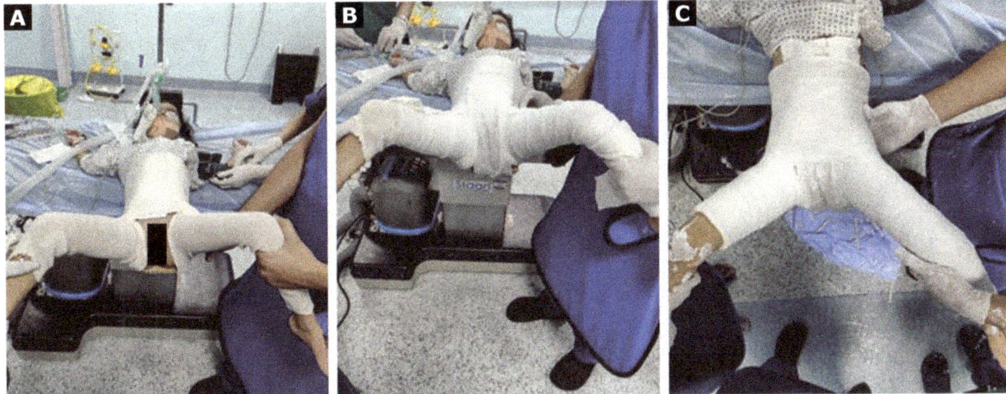

***Fig. 21.7**: Technique of spica cast application (A) Position on spica table: Hip in 60°-90° flexion, 30° abduction and 15° external rotation , application of stockinette (B) Application of softroll (C) Application of plaster with reinforcing slabs.*

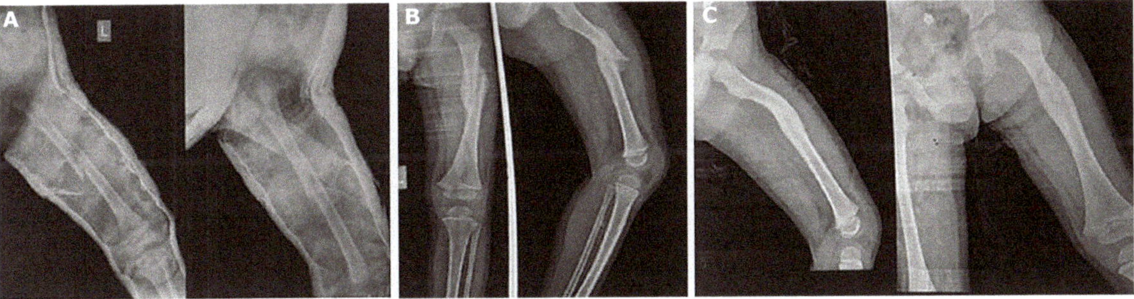

***Fig. 21.8**: (A) Well aligned fracture after reduction in spica cast (B) Fracture uniting with mild anterior angulation and varus at 6 weeks (C) Good union with remodelling at 3 months.*

- During follow up X-ray, if significant varus (>10°) or anterior angulation (>30°) or shortening (>2 cm) is present, fracture can be remanipulated and a new cast is applied or traction is advised, especially if shortening is >2 cm.
- Femoral shaft fracture healing depends on the age and fracture pattern, hence duration of spica cast may vary from 4 to 8 weeks.
- After cast removal, children are encouraged to stand and walk once comfortable, this may take a few days due to hip and knee stiffness. But formal physiotherapy is usually not needed.
- Follow up visits are needed in the first year after fracture to evaluate gait, leg length and joint range of motion(ROM).
- Risk of compartment syndrome is high with 90/90 spica cast. To minimise the complication, avoid traction on a short leg cast, leave the foot out and use less hip and knee flexion.
- Very rarely, in overweight larger children, flexible intramedullary nailing, traction or submuscular plating may be required.

School Going Children (6-11 years)

Flexible intramedullary (IM) nailing is the treatment of choice for mid shaft femur fracture in children between 6-11 years of age.

Advantages

- Safe
- Inexpensive
- Effective
- Ease of primary technique and later implant removal

Disadvantages

- Less rigid fixation
- For heavy children (>50 kg), more proximal and distal fractures and comminuted fractures - need for additional/hybrid fixation

Technique

Pre-operative planning

Ideal patient for flexible IM nailing is a child of age 6-11 years with

- Length stable femur fracture,
- In mid 80% of diaphysis,
- Body weight < 50 kg.,
- Transverse/short oblique fracture

Unstable fracture pattern treated with flexible IM nail may need supplemental immobilisation or use of additional external fixator to minimise the risk of shortening and angular malunion. **(Fig. 21.9)**

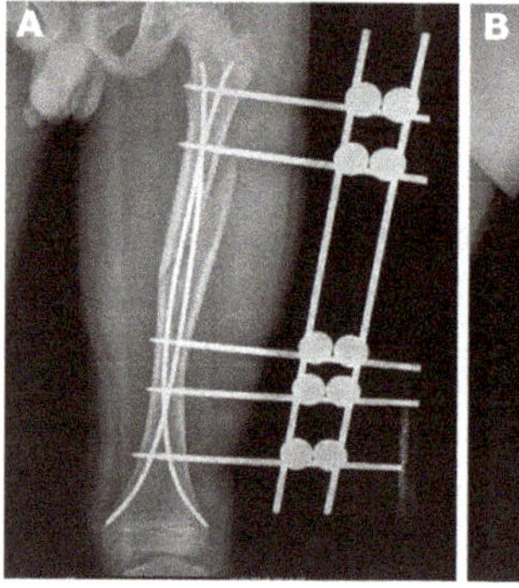

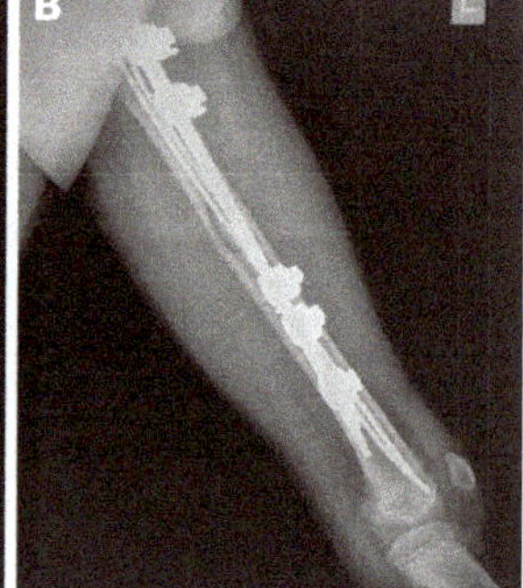

***Fig. 21.9**: Long oblique midshaft femur fracture treated with flexible IM nail and external fixator.*

Nail Size

Measure the minimum diameter of the diaphysis and multiply by 0.4. Hence two nails of such identical size are used to occupy 80% of canal diameter (most fractures require two 4 mm nails).

Titanium nails (though less stiff than steel) are preferred.

Nail Bending

The distance from the top of the inserted rod to the fracture site is measured and a gentle 30° bend (almost 3 times the diameter of the femur) is placed in the nail. Both the rods of identical size are bent at the same level, such that there is maximum spread of the nails in opposite directions at the fracture site, providing a 'pre stressed' fixation and spring effect that increases resistance to varus - valgus stress, as well as torsion. **(Fig. 21.10)**

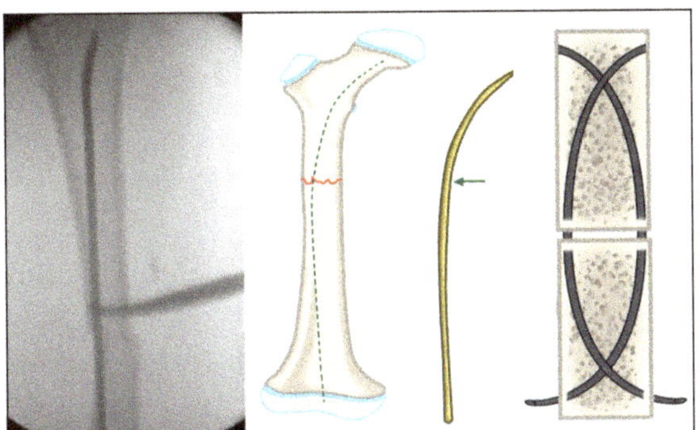

Fig. 21.10: *Pre-operative bending of the nail corresponding to the site of fracture in order to provide maximum spread of the two nails in opposite directions.*

Retrograde Insertion

Retrograde technique is preferred. The trolley is prepared with the instrument set necessary for the nailing technique **(Fig. 21.11)**

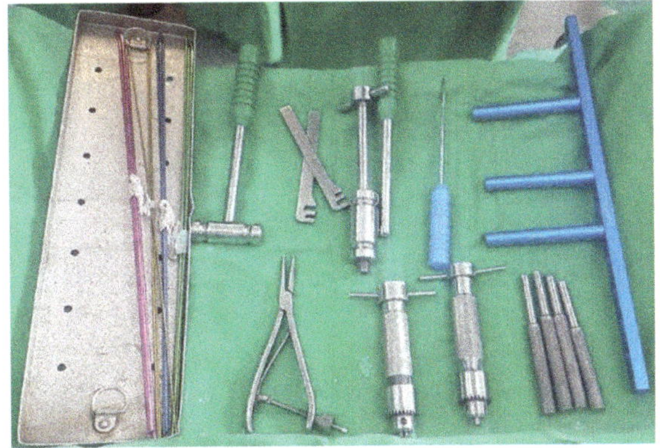

Fig. 21.11: *Instrumentation set for the flexible IM nailing technique.*

Position:

The authors' preferred position is using a fracture table **(Fig. 21.12)**, however radiolucent table is also used by some clinicians.

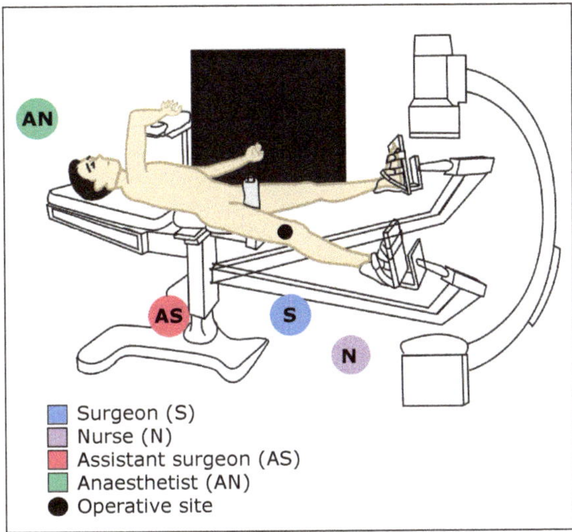

Fig. 21.12: *Position of the child on the fracture table for flexible intramedullary nailing.*

Steps:

The leg is prepared and draped with the thigh exposed from hip to knee. The image intensifier is used to localise the placement of skin incisions on the medial and lateral sides, about 2.5-3 cm proximal to the distal femoral physis.

The incision is about 2-3 cm long and proximal end should correspond to the nail entry site. A 4.5 mm drill bit/awl is used to make a hole in the cortex and open 2.5 cm distal femur metaphysis, by steeply making angle in the frontal plane to allow the passage of the nail through the dense paediatric metaphyseal bone. Initially the drill bit is placed in a perpendicular direction and once the cortex is entered, drill direction is changed to 45° oblique and medullary canal is entered. **(Fig. 21.13)**

Nail Advancement

Both medial and lateral nails' entry point should be at the same level and should be advanced simultaneously till the level

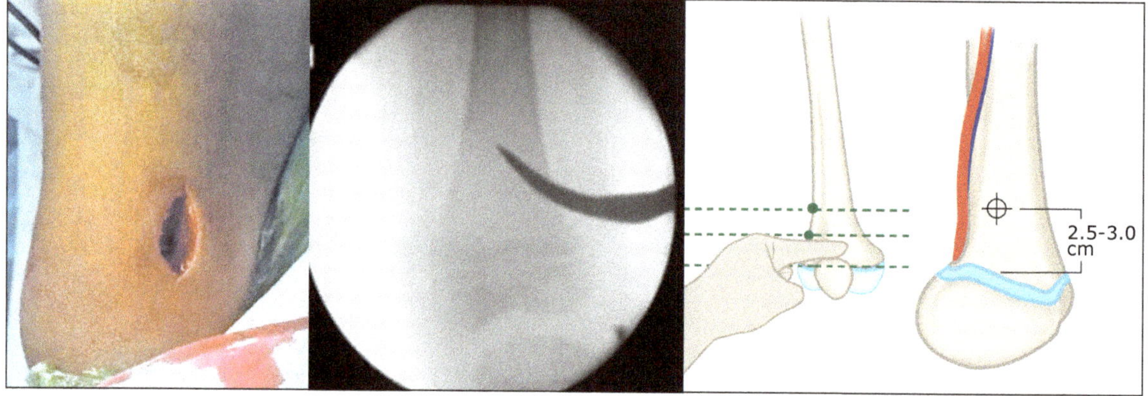

Fig. 21.13: *Safe entry point for the femur TENS- 2.5 to 3 cm. proximal to distal femoral physis.*

of the fracture. At this point, the fracture is reduced, if required with a radiolucent fracture reduction tool. Reduction is confirmed under image intensifier and the more difficult nail is passed first across the fracture site. The two nails are then driven into the proximal femur, one towards the greater trochanter and the other towards the femoral neck. Take care not to wind one nail around the other, while passing the second nail and rotating it. On the lateral view, one nail should have its tip pointing anteriorly, to avoid procurvatum. The nails are pulled back approximately 2 cm., the distal end of each nail is cut and then driven back with gentle hammering till the neck and greater trochanter. **(Figs. 21.14 and 21.15)**

The ends of the nails should lie adjacent to the distal femoral metaphysis, short enough to allow easy removal after fracture union and not irritate the perichondrium around the physis. Do not bend the exposed nail tip away from the metaphysis, as this may irritate the surrounding soft tissues and cause bursitis and knee stiffness **(Fig. 21.16)**

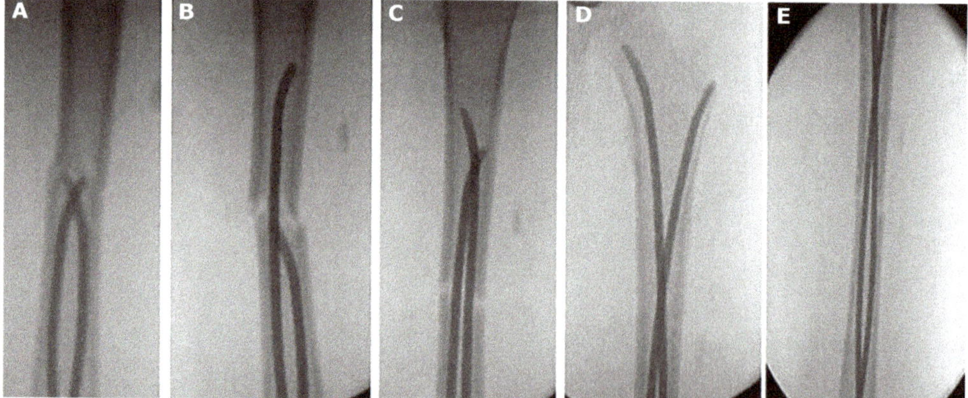

Fig. 21.14: *Steps of reduction and fixation of femur shaft fracture with TENS:*
(A) Passage of two nails till the fracture site; (B) Passage of more difficult nail across the fracture site after confirmation of reduction; (C) Passage of the other nail across the fracture; (D) Advancement of medial nail towards the femoral neck and lateral nail towards the greater trochanter; (E) Maximum spread of the nails at the fracture site.

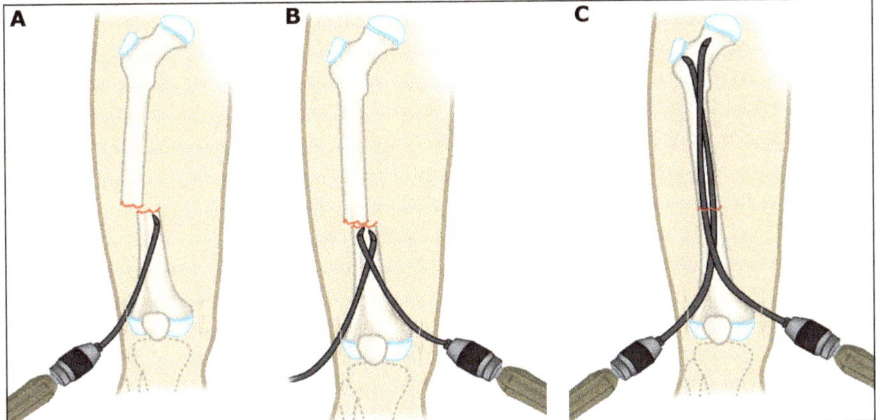

***Fig. 21.15**: Technique of femur TENS fixation: (A) Passage of the first nail till fracture site; (B) Passage of the second nail till fracture site; (C) Advancement of the nails after the reduction of fracture.*

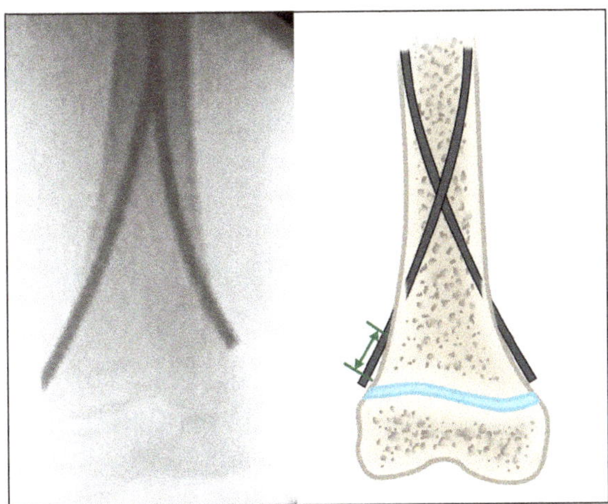

***Fig. 21.16**: Ends of the nails are cut such that they lie adjacent to the femoral metaphysis.*

In length unstable fractures, an end cap can be used to increase stability and lessen the risk of shortening and nail back out.

Stability comes from a proper technique:

- Torsional stability from divergence of nails in the metaphysis
- Resistance to sagittal and coronal bending from spreading of prebent rods through the diaphysis and also size and material properties of the rods.

Post-operative protocol

- A knee immobiliser is useful in the early post-operative period to reduce knee pain and quadriceps spasm.
- If used for unstable fracture, additional walking (one leg) spica is useful for 4-6 weeks till callus is visible on X-ray.
- For length stable fractures, touch down weight bearing can be started once the child is comfortable, with gradual resumption to full weight bearing by 6 weeks.
- Gentle knee ROM and quadriceps exercises are recommended.
- Functional knee brace may be helpful in cases of questionable stability.

Nail removal

6-12 months after the fracture has healed completely. **(Fig. 21.17)**.

Complications

Rare and mainly due to faulty technique or improper reduction.

- Malunion: To avoid it, pay attention to rotational stability after fixation and if needed, augment with a brace or external fixator.

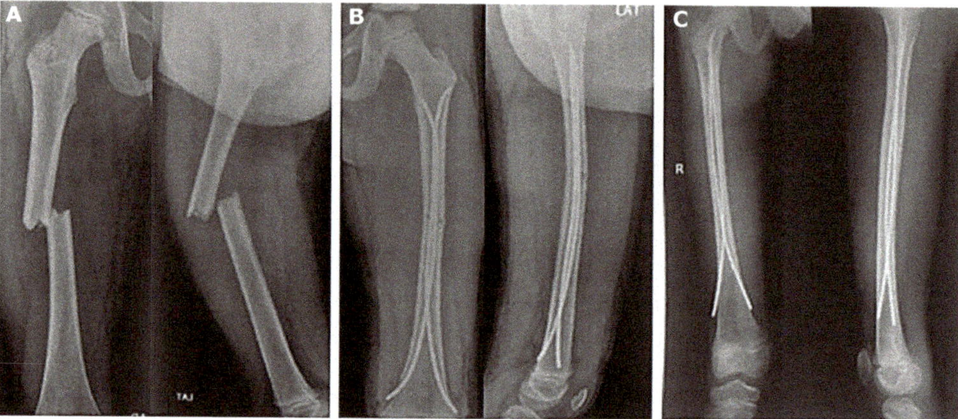

***Fig. 21.17**: (A) AP and lateral X-rays of mid shaft femur fracture in a 8-year-old child; (B) AP and lateral X-rays showing fixation with TENS; (C) At one year, showing good union and proximal migration of nails-time to remove the nails.*

- Overgrowth/shortening
- Bursitis due to prominent nail tip

External fixator

External fixation is used in femoral shaft fractures with

- Severe comminution
- Open wound
- Very proximal/distal location

Though being an effective and convenient method to align and stabilise the fractured femur, complications like pin tract infection, pin site scarring, delayed union and refracture are high.

Frame application technique

- Before the procedure, it is important to study the fracture pattern and any comminution. The size of the pins and the tubular rod should be determined as per the age and size of bone.
- The fracture table is preferred over a radiolucent table in order to obtain anatomical reduction, before prepping and draping.
- In all open fractures, a thorough debridement and irrigation should be done before frame application.
- The fracture is first reduced, both in length and angular and rotational alignment, before starting fixation.
- One pin is placed through the predrilled hole proximally in the shaft and another pin is placed distally, perpendicular to the long axis of the shaft. Minimum two pins should be placed proximally and distally, along with an intermediate or auxiliary pin if possible.
- Once all the pins are inserted, all fixation nuts are secured and sterile dressings are applied to the pins.
- Post-operative adequate pin care is important to avoid infection.
- Fixator is left in place until early callus stabilises the fracture (around 6-8 weeks) or till complete fracture healing.

11 years To Skeletal maturity

Trochanteric entry, locked intramedullary nail is currently the primary mode of treatment for femur fractures in preadolescent and adolescent age groups. ***(Fig. 21.18)***

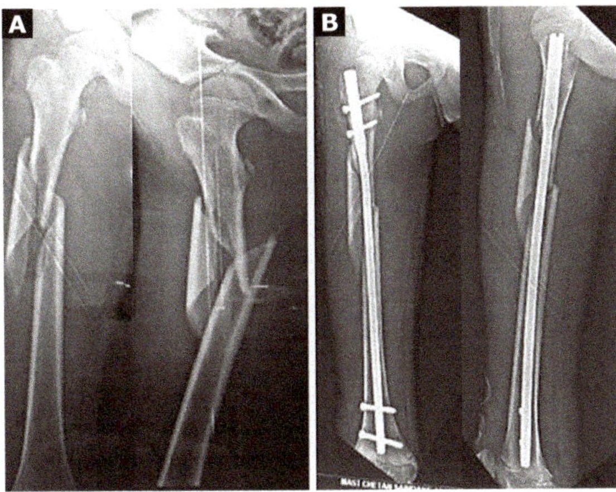

Fig. 21.18: (A) AP and lateral X-rays of femur showing comminuted femur shaft fracture in a 13- year-old male; (B) Treatment with closed reduction and fixation with trochanteric entry locked IM nail.

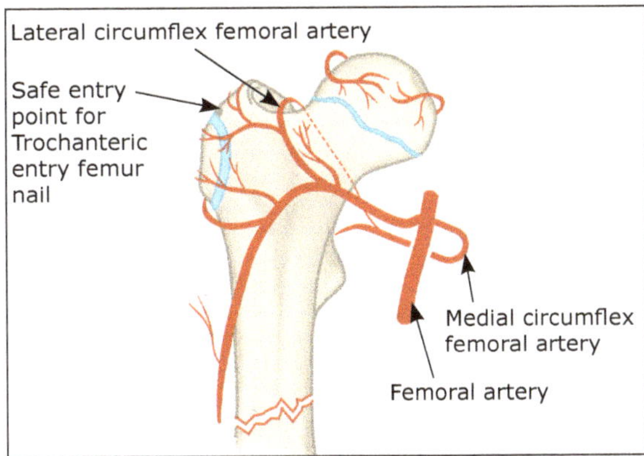

Fig. 21.19: Blood supply of proximal femur and correct entry point for femur nail in adolescents.

Technique

Position:

Supine or lateral decubitus position on a fracture table.

Incision:

About 3 cm longitudinal incision is placed over the greater trochanter.

Steps:

- The dissection should be limited to the lateral aspect of the greater trochanter, without extending to the capsule or mid portion of the femoral neck. This will avoid any injury to the lateral ascending cervical artery medial to the piriformis fossa. **(Fig. 21.19)**
- The nail is inserted through the lateral aspect of the greater trochanter. Smallest size (generally < 9mm) nail is chosen to avoid damage to the proximal femoral insertion area.
- Only one distal locking screw is necessary, but two can be used. Dynamisation is usually not necessary.
- Proximal 1 cm end of the nail should be left outside for possible later removal (9-18 months after fracture). Routine removal is not recommended in teenage patients.
- Nail with an expandable proximal cross section should be avoided. Nail should be angled proximally and specifically designed for transtrochanteric insertion.

Complications include avascular necrosis and proximal femur growth arrest with limb length discrepancy.

Submuscular bridge plating

Submuscular bridge plating allows for stable internal fixation, maintains vascularity of small fragments of bone and facilitates early healing. It is useful in subtrochanteric and supracondylar fracture as well as spiral oblique and comminuted fractures. **(Fig. 21.20)**

Technique

Position:

- The child is placed on a fracture table.
- Provisional reduction is obtained with gentle traction.
- 4.5 mm narrow long (10-16 holes) LC DCP/Locking plate for osteoporotic

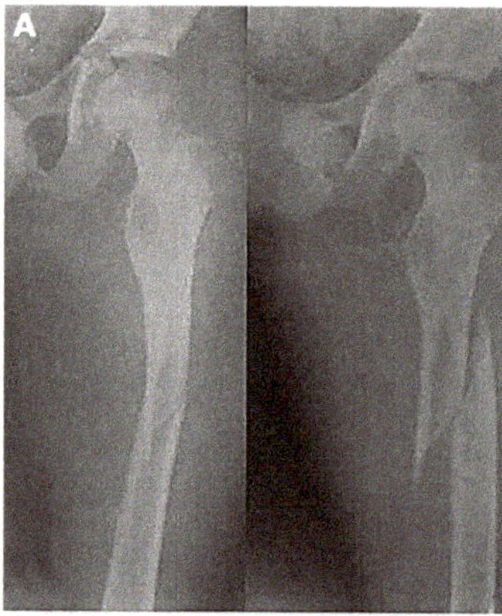

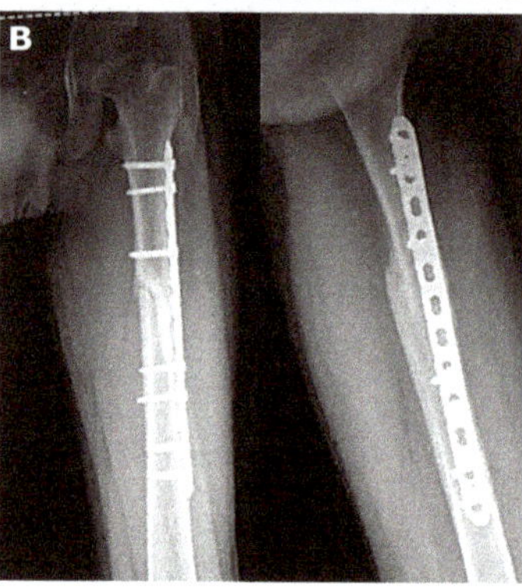

Fig. 21.20: *(A) AP and lateral X-rays of hip with femur showing long oblique subtrochanteric femur fracture in a 14-year-old child; (B) Treatment with open reduction and internal fixation using submuscular plating.*

children is used, based on the fluoroscopic evaluation with the plate placed over the anterior thigh. Minimum six screw holes should be present proximal and distal to the fracture. Distal contouring of the plate over the supracondylar region and proximal contouring over greater trochanter may be required using table-top plate bender.

Incision:

2 to 3 cm incision is made over the distal femur, just above the physis.

Steps:

- The periosteum is exposed below the vastus lateralis and plate is passed proximally in the submuscular plane.
- After AP and lateral fluoroscopic confirmation of the plate position and the fracture alignment, a K-wire is placed in the most proximal and most distal holes of the plate to maintain length.
- The principle of external fixation is used in choosing the screw sites. Greater spread of screws increases the stability of fixation. After proximal most and distal most screws are passed, central screws are placed using a free hand technique through stab incisions. Six cortices purchase on either side of fracture is essential.

Post-operative protocol

- Protected weight bearing with crutches is recommended.
- There is no need for a cast or knee immobiliser.
- Plate removal can be done in 1 year.

Complications: Rarely, refracture occurs through the screw hole/end of the plate.

Complications

1. Limb length discrepancy:

   Average overgrowth of around 0.9 cm occurs after femur shaft fractures, especially in children, 2-10 years of age after proximal third, oblique or comminuted fracture. The fractured femur may be initially short from overriding of the fragments at union and to 'make up' the difference, growth stimulation occurs, maximum during the first 2 years after fracture and to a much lesser degree for the next year or so. In fact due to such overgrowth, shortening of 2-3 cm during the initial cast is acceptable.

2. Angular deformity

   If the guidelines for acceptable alignment are not followed, angular deformity is likely after femur shaft fractures in children. Some amount of remodelling occurs based on age, site and plane of angular deformity, almost upto 5 years following fracture. 74% of the remodelling that occurs is physeal and much less is appositional. Varus-valgus remodelling is less compared to anterior-posterior remodelling. If significant angular deformity is present after fracture union, corrective osteotomy should be delayed for at least a year, to allow for maximum remodelling, unless severe deformity is present with functional impairment.

   Occasional genu recurvatum deformity of proximal tibia is reported after femur shaft fracture if proximal tibial physis is damaged during pin insertion for skeletal traction. Hence it is better to put a distal femur pin.

3. Rotational deformity:

   In infants and young children, some rotational deformity (~30°) can be accepted, because either true rotational remodelling occurs or functional adaptation allows resumption of normal gait. However the goal should be to restore rotational alignment within 10° in older adolescents, as no significant rotational remodelling occurs.

4. Delayed Union:

   Delayed union of femur shaft fractures is uncommon in children, unless there is open fracture or external fixator application or improper treatment. Time taken for femur fracture to unite is different as per age.

   Infants: 2-3 weeks

   < 5 years: 4-6 weeks

   5-10 years: 8-10 weeks

   Adolescents: 10-15 weeks

   For delayed union in younger children, prolonged cast immobilisation is recommended till bridging callus appears, whereas delayed union in older children and adolescents requires bone grafting and internal fixation with compression plate or locked IM nail.

5. Non union:

   Non union is rare in femur shaft fracture unless there is infection or severe soft tissue loss or segmental bone loss. Treatment consists of compression plating or locked IM nail, with bone grafting.

6. Neurovascular injury:

   Peroneal, femoral or sciatic nerve injuries are uncommon in femur shaft fractures in children. If present on initial evaluation in a closed fracture, observe as it may recover. But if nerve deficit occurs during reduction or treatment, exploration of the nerve is required. Also persistent nerve loss without recovery over 4-6 months is an indication for exploration.

   Vascular injury occurs in ~1.3% fractures and standard protocol of fracture stability followed by vascular repair is to be followed.

7. Compartment syndrome:

   It is occasionally reported after skin traction or spica cast or IM nailing. The treatment is fasciotomy.

Special fractures

Subtrochanteric fracture

Subtrochanteric fractures are challenging to treat as they heal slowly, have a tendency for varus angulation, are more prone for overgrowth and have limited internal fixation options due to short proximal fragment. Different treatment options are-

1. Traction for 2-3 weeks, followed by casting in valgus mould

Regular follow up and wedging as necessary

2. External fixator if there is place for at least 2 proximal pins followed by walking cast for 6 weeks
3. TENS with proximal and distal entry
4. Submuscular plating
5. Paediatric DHS **(Fig. 21.21)**

Supracondylar fracture

Supracondylar fractures are challenging to treat as gastrocnemius muscle insertion just above the femoral condyles constantly pulls the distal fragment into extension, hence it is difficult to maintain alignment in cast. Different treatment options are external fixator followed by walking cast, proximal entry intramedullary nail or submuscular plating. ***(Fig. 21.22)***

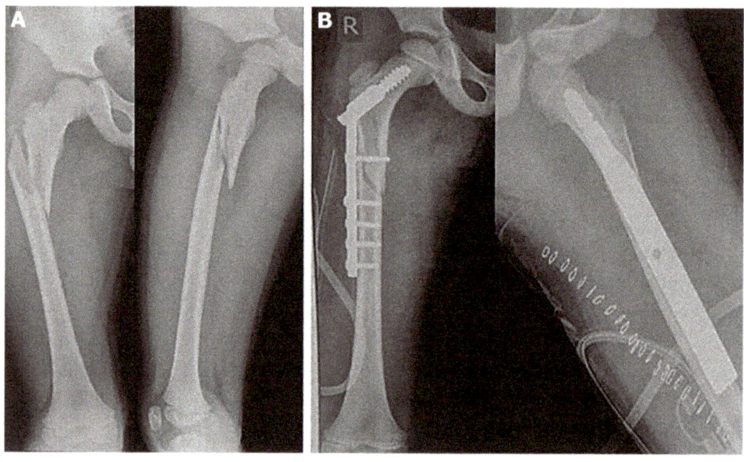

Fig. 21.21: *(A) Pre-operative and (B) post-operative X-rays showing subtrochanteric femur fracture treated with open reduction and internal fixation with paediatric DHS.*

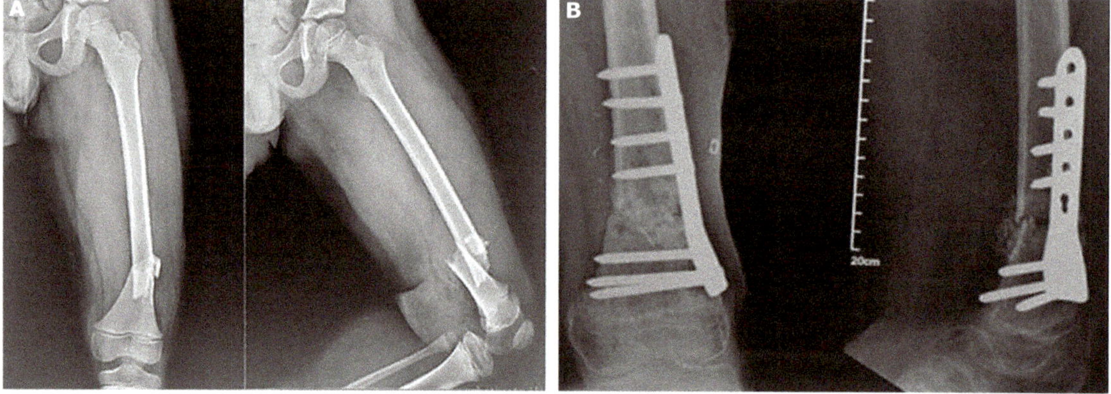

Fig. 21.22: *(A) AP and lateral X-rays of hip with femur showing supracondylar femur fracture; (B) Treatment with open reduction and internal fixation using distal femur submuscular plate.*

Flowchart 21.1

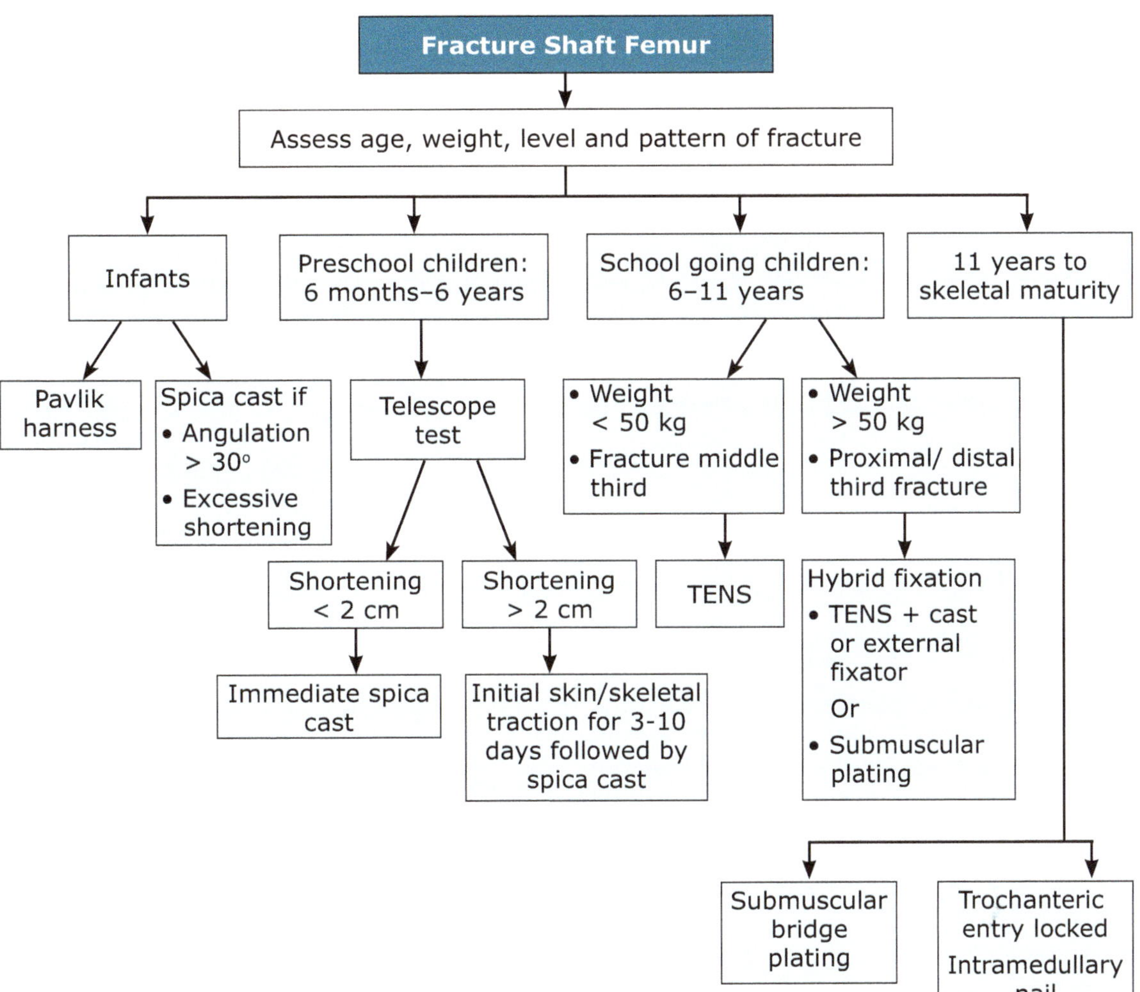

22 Fractures of the Distal Femoral Physis

Introduction

Fractures of the distal femoral physis are rare, constituting < 2% of all physeal injuries. But the rate of complications is high ~40-60% , the most common being growth arrest as distal femoral physis contributes to 70% growth of the femur and 37% growth of the lower limb.

Physeal Anatomy

- Distal femoral epiphysis is the first to ossify in the body.
- At birth, distal femur physis is flat and least stable. It becomes undulating and more convoluted with maturation. Distal femur physeal separation rarely occurs following birth trauma, especially in breech, difficult vaginal delivery or precipitate labour and delivery. But there is less damage to germinal cells and their blood supply. **(Fig. 22.1)**
- By 2-3 years, an intercondylar groove or central prominence is developed and sulci are formed that traverse medially and laterally proximal to each condyle, thus dividing the physis into four quadrants.
- Stability of physis is increased by such complex physeal geometry and large area. Also, circumferential perichondrial ring and knee ligaments provide additional resistance to injury. Hence, in 2-11 years old children, physeal injury occurs only after high energy trauma (45-50% due to motor vehicle accidents, 25% due to sports injury and 20% due to fall from height) and these injuries are associated with poor prognosis.
- During adolescence (>11-12 years), the perichondrial ring becomes thinner, thereby relatively weakening the physis. Hence injury occurs after low energy trauma like sports, varus-valgus stress from direct blow or buckling while landing from height. Also, due to irregular configuration of

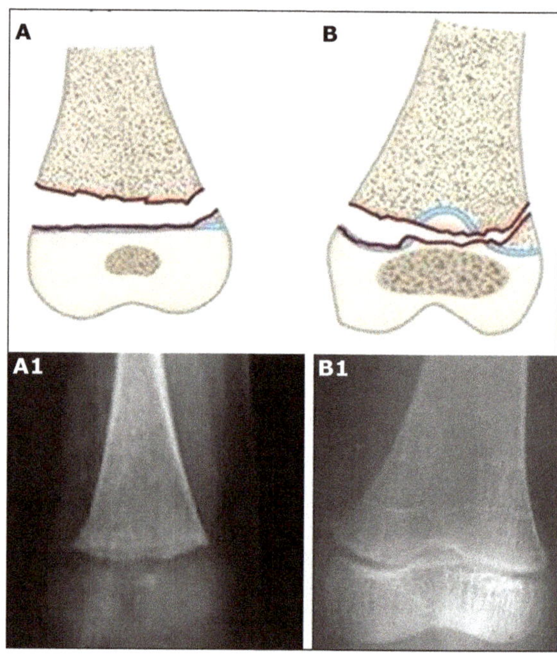

***Fig. 22.1**: Distal femur physeal shape and effect of physeal fracture on growth:*
A and A1 : Flat shape of the physis at birth, hence distal femur physeal separation may not disturb growth;
B and B1: Central ridge and Undulating physis with maturity, hence fracture likely to traverse through multiple zones of physis with likely growth arrest

the physis, there is high incidence of growth disturbance, mainly due to two reasons:

1. Fracture line, instead of clearly traversing the hypertrophic zone and area of provisional calcification, extends through multiple regions of physis and damages germinal cells regardless of fracture type. **(Fig. 22.1)**
2. During reduction of displaced fracture, the epiphyseal ridges may grind against metaphyseal projections and further damage cartilage producing resting cells.

Distal femoral physis is completely extra-synovial. The joint capsule and all of the major knee ligaments are attached to the epiphysis distal to the physis, but medial and lateral heads of gastrocnemius muscle originate from distal femur proximal to the joint capsule and physis and the pull of theses muscles may be a deforming force for the fractures of distal femur, mainly the metaphysis.

- Vascular anatomy of distal femur is important **(Fig. 22.2)**

Femoral artery travels through the adductor canal medially, just above the distal femoral metaphysis and then courses posteriorly behind the popliteal space.

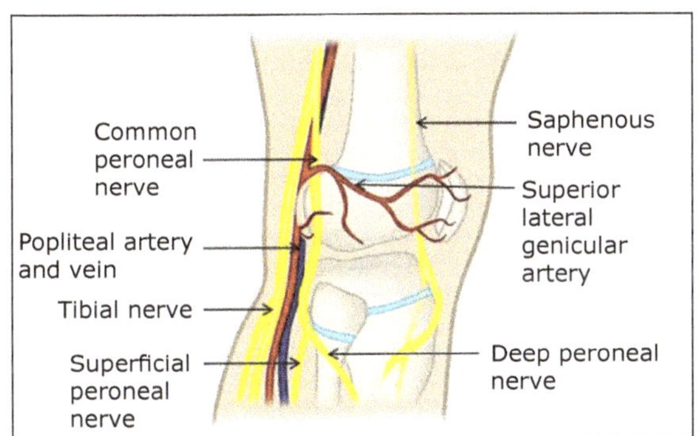

***Fig. 22.2**: Neurovascular anatomy of distal femur*

Popliteal artery trifurcates into the anterior interosseous, posterior interosseous and peroneal arteries and is vulnerable to injury from hyperextension force.

There is poor collateral circulation around the knee, hence popliteal artery injury frequently results in loss of viability of the leg.

- Common peroneal nerve lies superficial at the knee level and is vulnerable in direct trauma and varus stress injury with severe anteromedial displacement.

Clinical Features

- In high energy trauma, the initial survey should include ABC (Airway, Breathing, Circulation) of trauma. One must look for associated pelvis, spine and visceral injuries.
- In displaced fracture, the diagnosis is obvious from swelling, deformity, ecchymosis and may be tenting, puckering of skin.
- In undisplaced fracture, the diagnosis may be difficult. There is mild pain and swelling and painful limp. But there is point tenderness at the level of distal femur physis.
- Careful assessment of neurovascular status is important, especially in anteromedially displaced fracture.
- Associated ligamentous injuries occur frequently, with the most commonly involved ligament being the anterior cruciate ligament, followed by the lateral collateral ligament and then the medial collateral ligament. But often they are diagnosed late, after the fracture has healed and the child returns to activities.
- Pathological distal femur physeal injuries are common in neuromuscular disorders like cerebral palsy, spina bifida, arthrogryposis (during

manipulation of knee contractures) and in nutritional deficiency.

Imaging

- AP and lateral X-rays of the knee and entire femur, including the hip joint are essential.
- Additional oblique X-rays may be required to detect occult fracture of the epiphysis or metaphysis.
- CT scan is especially useful in S-H type III and IV injuries.
- MRI/Ultrasound may be required to diagnose S-H type I injuries in a newborn with limited ossification.

Classification (Fig. 22.3)

S-H I fracture:

~15% of distal femur physeal fractures

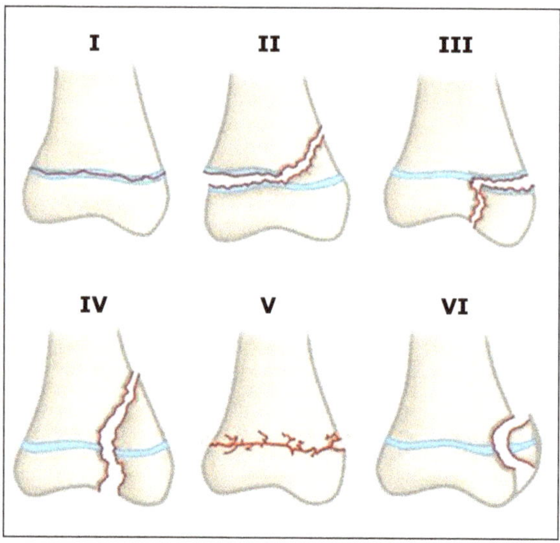

***Fig. 22.3**: Salter Harris classification of Distal femur physeal injuries.*

- These fractures can occur either following hyperextension injuries in which the distal fragment is displaced anteriorly or flexion injuries where the distal fragment is displaced posteriorly. **(Fig. 22.4)**

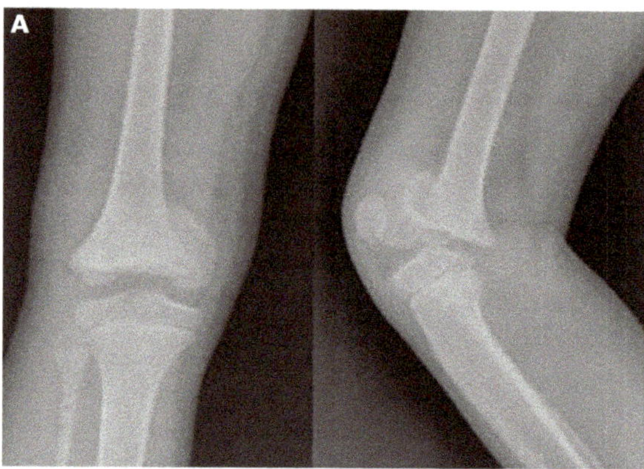

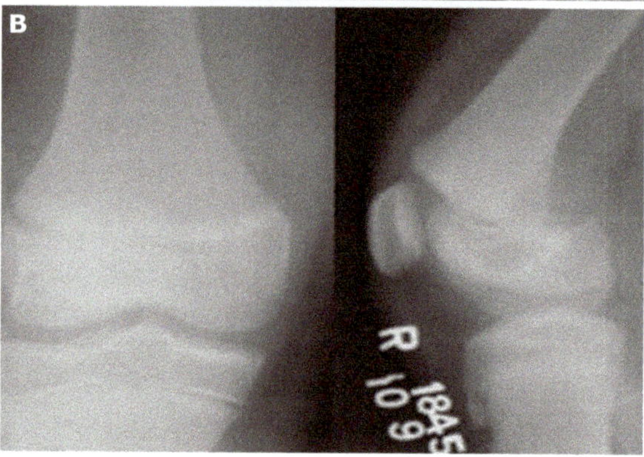

***Fig. 22.4**: AP and lateral X-rays of the knee showing S-H type I fracture of distal femoral physis (A) Hyperextension injury with anteriorly displaced physis (B) Flexion injury with posteriorly displaced physis.*

- Due to undulation of the distal femur physis, most of the distal femur physeal fractures don't propagate clearly across the zones of hypertrophy and provisional calcification, but also extend into germinal zone, hence growth arrest is likely even in S-H I and II injuries.
- The diagnosis is sometimes difficult and made in retrospect in undisplaced fractures. Displacement occurs usually in the sagittal plane in children < 2 years.

S-H II fracture:

Most common, includes > 57% of distal femur physeal fractures.

The metaphyseal spike in S-H II injuries (Thurston Holland fragment) occurs on the side of compression force and direction of displacement. **(Fig. 22.5)**

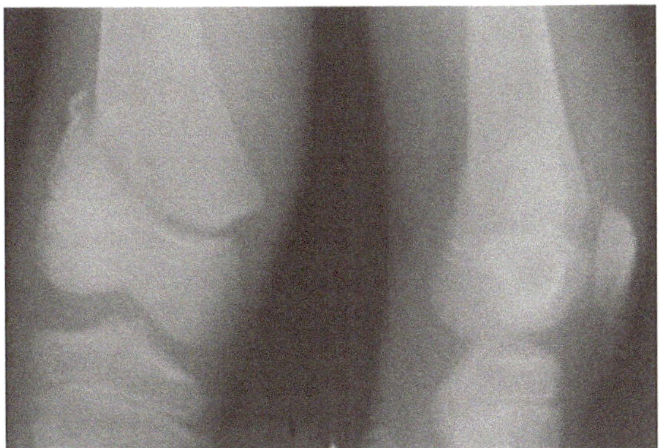

Fig. 22.5*: AP and lateral X-rays of the knee showing valgus injury leading to S-H type II fracture of distal femoral physis. Note the lateral metaphyseal fragment on the side of compression.*

S-H III fractures

~10 % of distal femur physeal fractures

- This injury occurs in older children, near skeletal maturity, when the central portion of the distal femoral physis begins to close before medial and lateral parts of the physis. **(Fig. 22.6)**

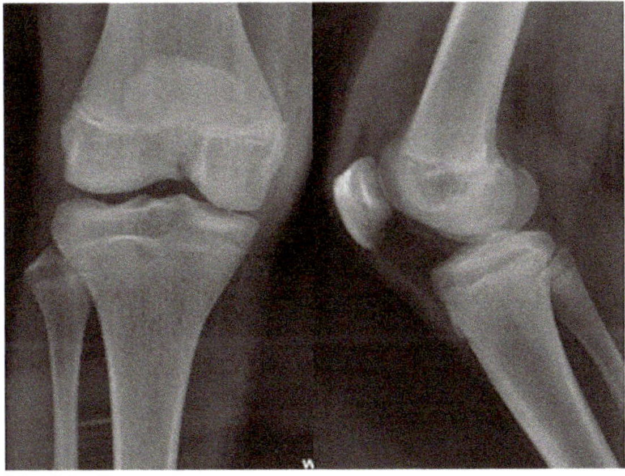

Fig. 22.6*: AP and lateral X-rays of the knee showing S-H type III fracture of medial distal femoral physis.*

- Occasionally, coronal fracture occurs in medial condyle, like Hoffa fracture of adults. This type and non displaced S-H III and IV are sometimes difficult to diagnose on X-ray and require MRI/CT.

S-H IV fracture

~12% of distal femur physeal fractures

Metaphyseal fragment may be small in some cases, making it difficult to differentiate from type III.

S-H V fracture

~ 3% of distal femur physeal fractures

This injury occurs due to axial loading, for example fall from height. It is difficult to diagnose acutely. MRI is helpful as it can show bone contusion on either side of the growth plate after the trauma.

S-H VI fracture

It is the avulsion fracture of periphery of physis, comprising a portion of the perichondrial ring of physis and small adjacent pieces of metaphysis and epiphysis. **(Fig. 22.7)**

Treatment

- The goal of treatment in distal femur physeal fracture is to stabilise the

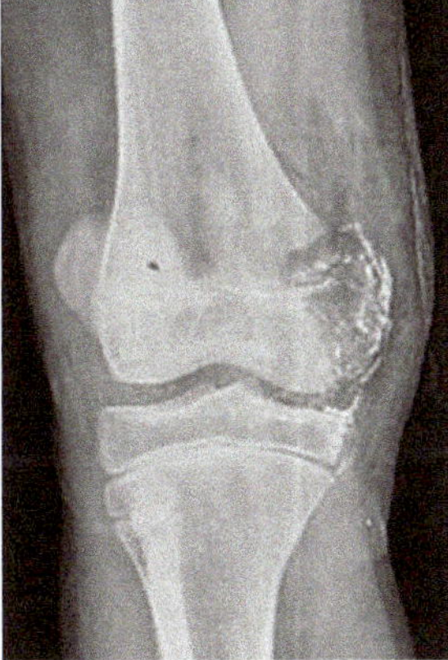

Fig. 22.7*: AP X-ray of the knee showing S-H type VI fracture of distal femur physis with avulsion of medial metaphysis and epiphysis .*

fracture in the position of anatomical reduction, without any iatrogenic damage to the physis and with preservation of knee range of motion (ROM).

- Non displaced or minimally displaced S-H type I/II and completely non displaced S-H type III/IV can be treated by closed reduction and casting/ fixation.
- In a younger child, acceptable alignment is < 20° sagittal angulation and < 5° varus/valgus angulation and no rotation deformity. However, in an older child (> 10 years), an anatomical reduction with stable fixation is a must.

Technique of closed reduction

- Reduction should be carried out under general anaesthesia with muscle relaxation.
- The reduction manoeuvre should be gentle and should consist of predominantly traction, followed by manipulation.
- It is important to check the neurovascular status routinely, both before and after reduction.
- In S-H type I fracture with antero-posterior type of physeal displacement, closed reduction can be done in supine position by gentle longitudinal traction followed by flexion of the knee **(Fig. 22.8)** or a better way is to do the reduction in prone position (manoeuvre like in extension type supracondylar humerus fracture) **(Fig. 22.9)**
- In S-H type I fracture with medial-lateral type of physeal displacement or S-H type II fracture, longitudinal traction is applied first and then the epiphysis (in type I) or the concave side of Thurston Holland fragment (in type II) with intact periosteum is gently manipulated to realign with the long axis of the shaft of femur. Counter pressure on the proximal segment in an opposite direction helps. **(Fig. 22.10)**
- Reduction can be checked under image intensifier. If stable, a long leg cast is applied with knee flexed 30°–60°.
- If unstable, it is better to fix the fracture with K-wires/screws, as the risk of redisplacement in cast is ~30%.

Technique of percutaneous pins/screw fixation

- After the reduction is confirmed, two crossed K-wires are passed in retrograde manner from the epiphysis (just off the articular margin) and directed anteriorly to avoid injury to posterior neurovascular structure.
- As per recent literature, it is preferred to pass the wires from proximal to distal.

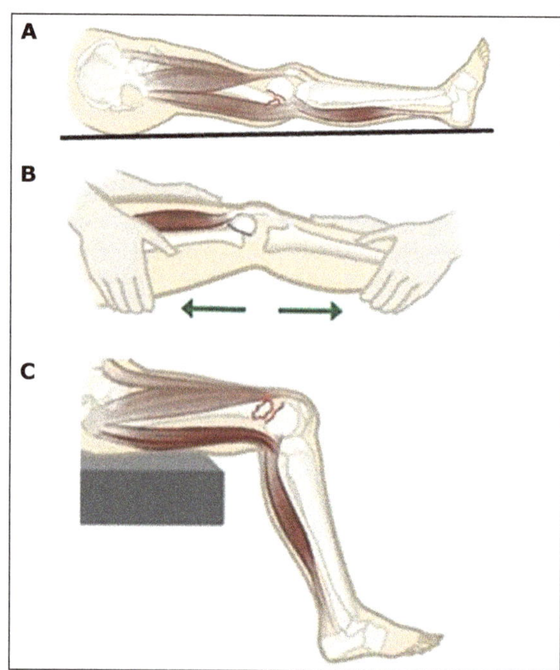

Fig. 22.8: *Technique of closed reduction of S-H type I distal femur physeal fracture in supine position: (A) Anteriorly displaced distal femur physis (B) Application of gentle longitudinal traction (C) Reduction by flexion of the knee*

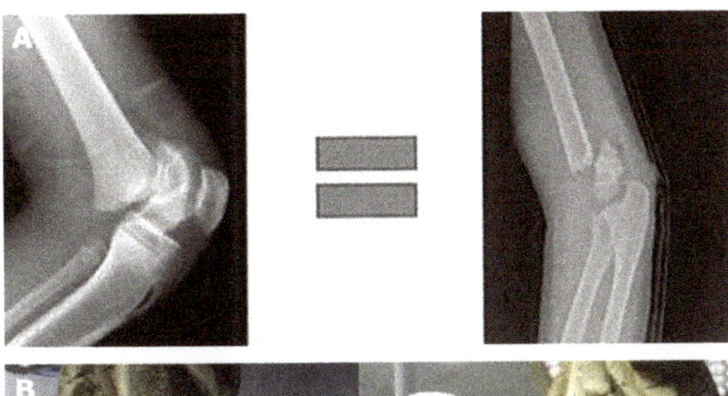

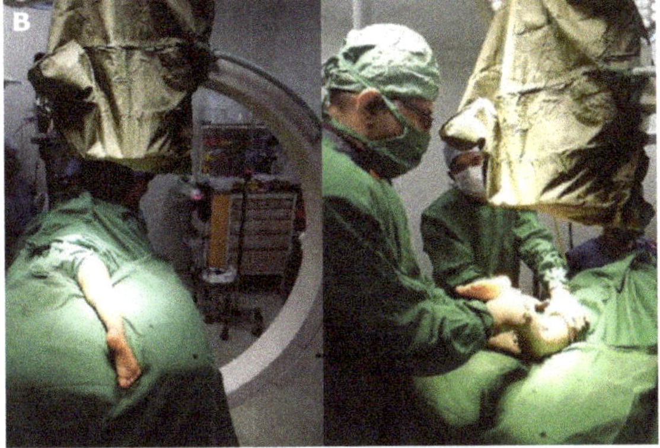

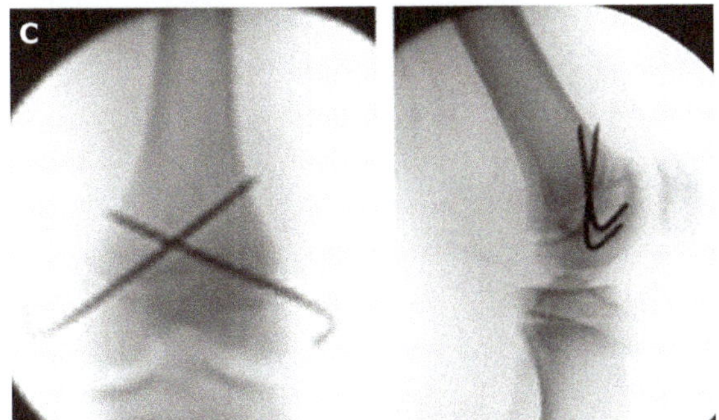

***Fig. 22.9**: Technique of closed reduction and percutaneous K-wire fixation in S-H type I distal femur physeal fracture in prone position (A) Consider hyperextension type S-H I injury equivalent to extension type supracondylar humerus fracture (B) Reduction manoeuvre in prone position by traction followed by flexion of the knee (C) Percutaneous crossed K-wire fixation after fluoroscopic confirmation of reduction*

- The first wire is usually from the concave side of the fracture pattern.
- Once both wires are inserted, the stability of fracture is assessed by gently stressing in varus-valgus and flexion-extension. K-wires are kept subcutaneously.

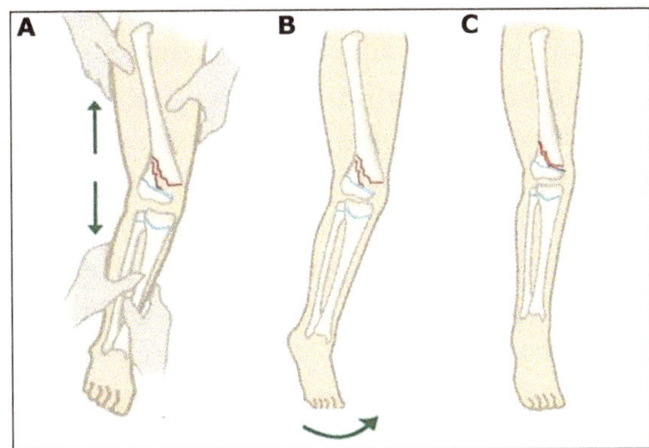

***Fig. 22.10**: Technique of closed reduction for valgus S-H type II distal femur physeal fracture*
(A) Gentle longitudinal traction
(B) Reversal of mechanism of injury-in this case, varus of distal fragment, while giving counter pressure on the proximal fragment on the opposite direction
(C) Reduction achieved

- After K-wire fixation, a non-weight bearing long leg cast is applied .
- K-wires are removed at 4 weeks. Partial weight bearing can be started, gradually progressing to full weight bearing by 6 weeks.
- In case of S-H type II fracture with a large metaphyseal fragment, fixation can be done with one or two 6.5 mm or larger screws from metaphysis to proximal fragment, passed parallel to physis using a small incision in the metaphysis over the Thurston Holland fragment **(Fig. 22.11)**. Sometimes one screw and one K-wire from the side opposite the entry of screw can be used.
- Postoperative protocol is similar as for pins.
- For S-H type III and IV, the use of reduction bone forceps or clamp is advisable to close down a gap or diastasis of the condyles. For S-H type III, two screws, one anterior and one posterior can be used. **(Fig. 22.12)**
- For S-H IV, one metaphyseal and one epiphyseal screw can be used.

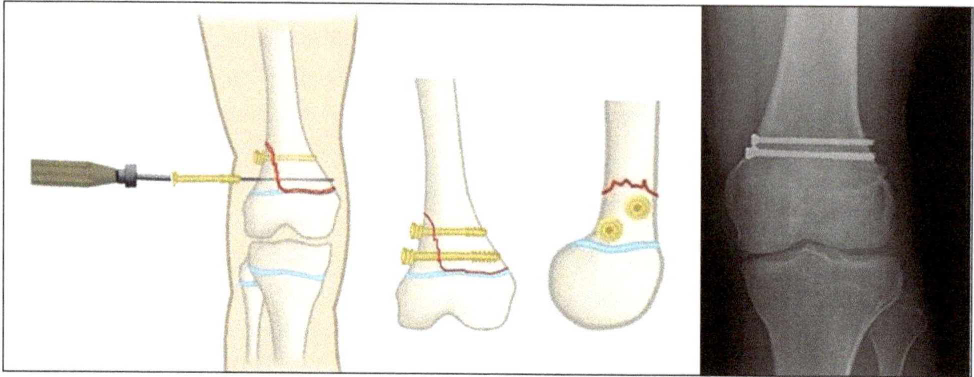

Fig. 22.11: *Fixation of S-H type II distal femur physeal fracture with metaphyseal cancellous screws passed parallel to the physis.*

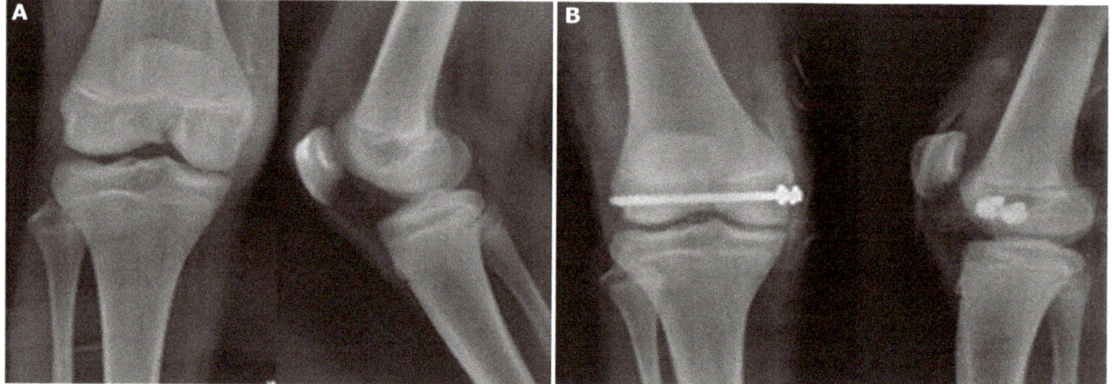

Fig. 22.12: *(A) AP and lateral X-rays of the knee showing S-H type III distal physeal fracture (B) Closed reduction and fixation using two screws-one anterior and one posterior.*

- Care is to be taken, not to place the screws too distal in epiphysis as they may impinge on the intercondylar notch.
- Various pin and screw configuration as per S-H types are shown in **Fig. 22.13.**

Technique of Open reduction and internal fixation:

In case the fracture is irreducible by closed means or there is articular or metaphyseal comminution, open reduction and internal fixation is indicated.

Position

Supine on a radiolucent table. Tourniquet is used. **(Fig. 22.14)**

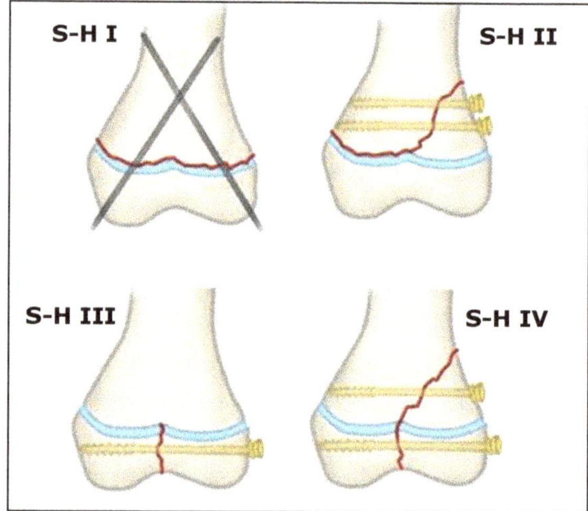

Fig. 22.13: *Different pin and screw configuration as per Salter Harris classification of distal femur physeal fractures.*

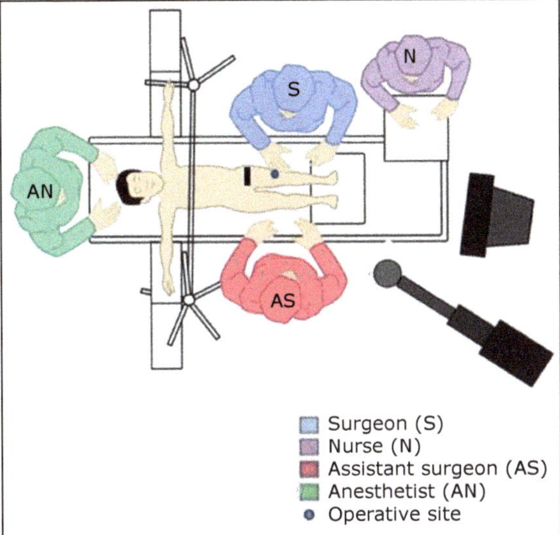

***Fig. 22.14**: Supine position on a radiolucent table for open reduction of distal femur physeal fracture.*

Incision

- Irreducible S-H type I and II fractures may have an interposed periosteum on the convex side of the fracture or the side of open physis, the incision is made over that area either medial or lateral.In case of S-H type III and IV fractures, a longitudinal incision is made anteriorly on the knee at the site of the intra-articular fracture. **(Fig. 22.15)**

Steps

- The periosteum should be carefully removed without causing any further damage to the physis by retractors or surgical instruments.

  Additional evacuation of the haematoma also may be needed in order to achieve anatomical reduction.

- The alignment of the physis and the joint are used to assess the reduction Once reduction is confirmed under image intensifier, it is fixed with K-wires or screws.

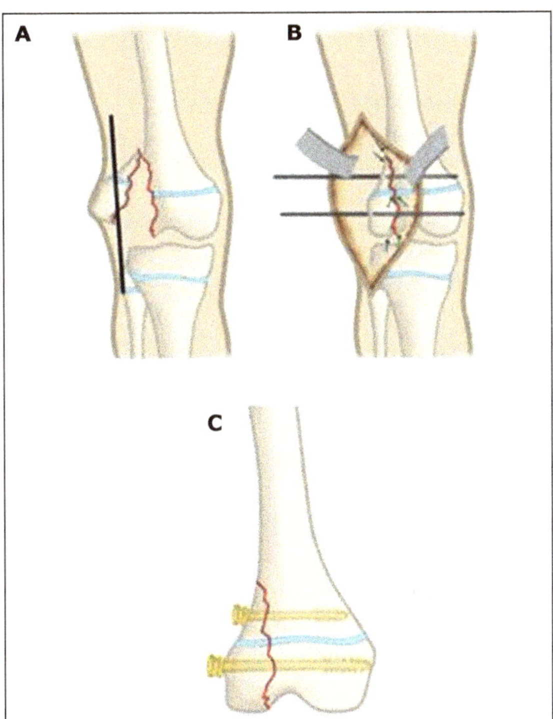

***Fig. 22.15**: Technique of open reduction and internal fixation for S-H type IV distal femur physeal fracture (A) Longitudinal skin incision anteriorly over the intra-articular fragment (B) After confirmation of physeal and articular alignment, guidewires placed parallel to the joint (C) Cannulated cancellous screw fixation in the metaphysis and epiphysis*

- For cannulated screw fixation, the guidewires are inserted parallel to the physis, above and below the physis. Then the cannulated screws with or without washers are inserted over the guide wires.

After open reduction, the chances of knee stiffness are high, hence early knee mobilisation, after 4 weeks is recommended.

Sometimes, S-H type III and IV fractures are fixed arthroscopically.

Complications

Immediate post-operative complications:

1. Loss of reduction

- Interposed periosteum sometimes causes physeal widening, prevents anatomical reduction, contributes to fracture instability and subsequent loss of reduction in the cast.
- Very common (30-70%) if immobilised in long leg cast, but reduced to 10 % if immobilised in hip spica. So, hip spica application is recommended for younger children treated with closed reduction.
- Also, additional internal fixation with pins/screws can provide stability to fracture.

2. Neurovascular injury

Vascular injury

Occasionally seen following hyperextension injury due to metaphyseal spike of proximal fragment.

- Prompt reduction in OR is advised in such cases.
- If post–reduction vascularity is good, admission for 24 hours for observation and serial check of vascularity is advised.
- If distal perfusion does not return within 15-20 minutes, after quick fracture fixation, exploration of the vessel by a vascular surgeon is recommended.
- If ischaemia time is > 6-8 hours, four compartment fasciotomy is done to minimise effects of reperfusion.

Peripheral nerve injury

- Mostly neuropraxia occurring due to traction or anteromedial displacement of physis. This usually recovers spontaneously within 6-12 weeks of injury.
- If persistent deficit > 3 months, nerve conduction study is advised and exploration may be needed.

Late complications

3. Ligament injury

- Symptomatic knee joint instability occurs in 8-40 %
- ACL injury is common after S –H III medial femoral condyle fracture. MRI is advised for diagnosis after fracture healing. Ligament reconstruction is best done after knee ROM has been restored.
- Meniscal repair is usually done soon after fracture healing to facilitate rehabilitation.

4. Knee stiffness

- This may occur in 30-35% patients due to muscle or capsule contracture or intra-articular adhesions.
- Treatment consists of physiotherapy. If unsuccessful, manipulation under general anaesthesia (MUGA) or open release may be required.

5. Growth Disturbance (Angulation/ Shortening/Both)

- Mostly occurs in 2-12 years age group, after displaced distal femur physeal fracture, especially if treated with transphyseal fixation and repeated reduction attempts. Sometimes, it occurs even in S-H I and II injury, due to typical physeal anatomy as described earlier.
- Growth arrest is typically evident 6 months post injury. Radiologically, Park-Harris growth arrest lines converge towards the site of growth arrest as mentioned in chapter 2.
- Full length bilateral lower limb scanogram is helpful in diagnosis of growth arrest.

- MRI/CT may be helpful to detect physeal bar, even at 2 months post-injury.
- Treatment of Growth Arrest:
  Principles of management of growth arrest are described in Chapter 2.

Flowchart 22.1

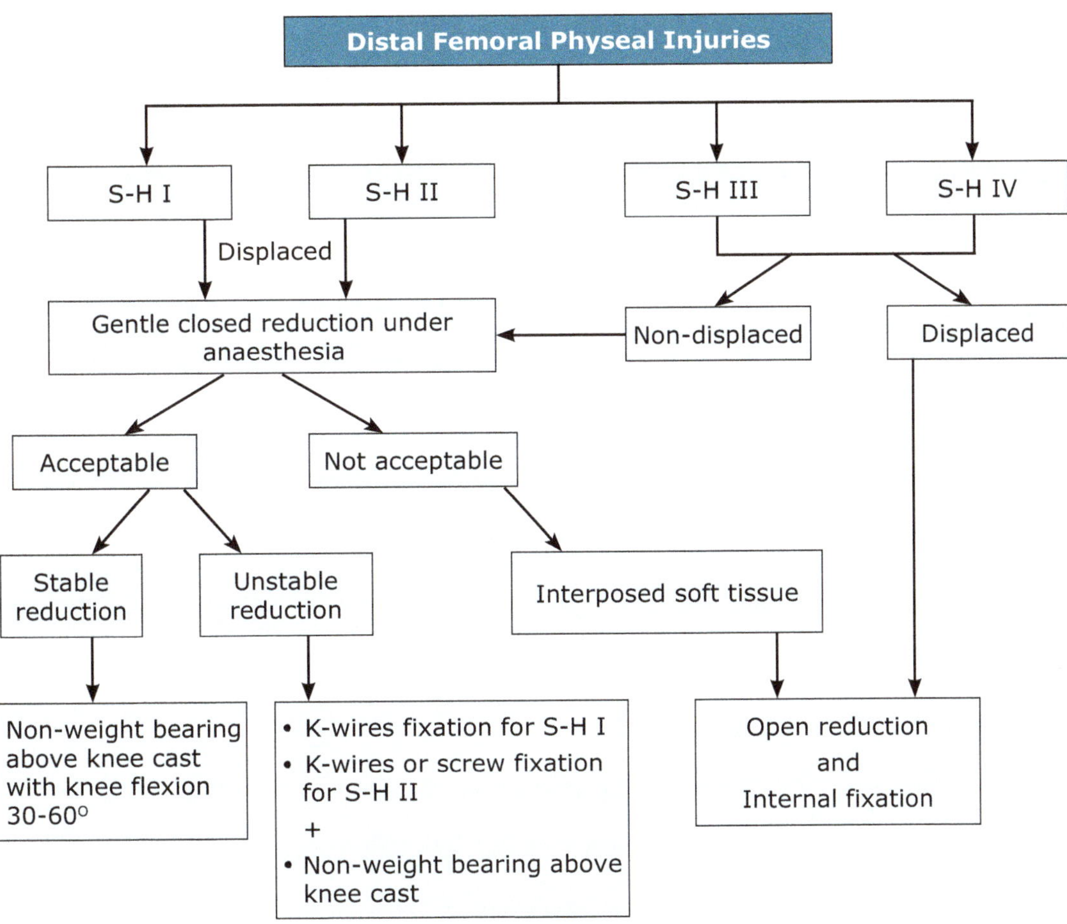

23 Intra-articular Injuries of the Knee

FRACTURE OF THE TIBIAL SPINE (INTERCONDYLAR EMINENCE)

Introduction

The tibial spine (Intercondylar eminence) is the region of the articular portions of the adjacent plateaus of the proximal tibia. It consists of medial tibial spine where Anterior Cruciate Ligament (ACL) is attached and lateral tibial spine **(Fig. 23.1)**. Fracture of the tibial spine is an uncommon injury, occurring due to chondro-epiphyseal avulsion of ACL insertion on the anteromedial tibial eminence, mainly due to forced valgus and external rotation of tibia.

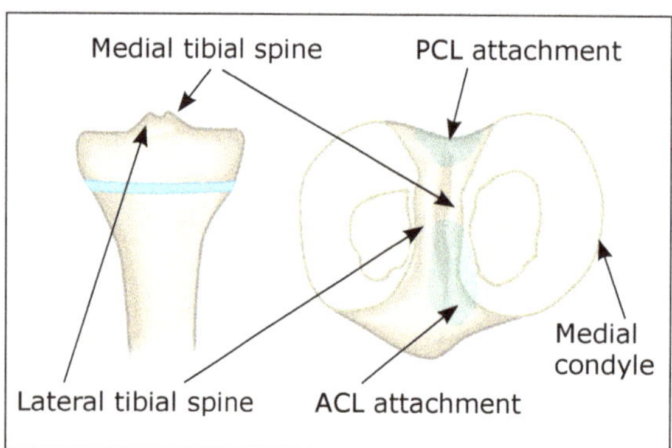

***Fig. 23.1**: Anatomy of Tibial plateau.*

Clinical Features

The child presents with a painful and swollen knee due to haemarthrosis resulting from the intra-articular fracture. There is limitation of knee movement and inability to bear weight.

Patients with non union complain of instability. They have a positive anterior drawer test and a positive Lachman test.

Patients with malunion of displaced tibial spine fracture have lack of full extension due to mechanical bony block.

Imaging

Standard anteroposterior (AP) and lateral X-ray views are diagnostic. **(Fig. 23.2)**

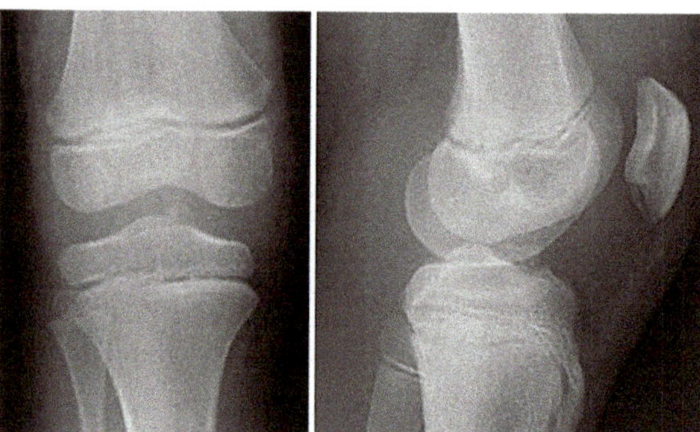

***Fig. 23.2**: AP and lateral X-rays of the knee showing ACL tibial bony avulsion fracture.*

Classification **(Fig. 23.3)**

Modified Meyer and McKeever classification:

Type I: Undisplaced fracture

Type II: Displacement of anterior part of the fragment that is lifted upward and hinged on its intact posterior border

Type III: Complete separation of the avulsed fragment from the proximal tibia epiphysis

Type IV: Comminution of tibial eminence fragment

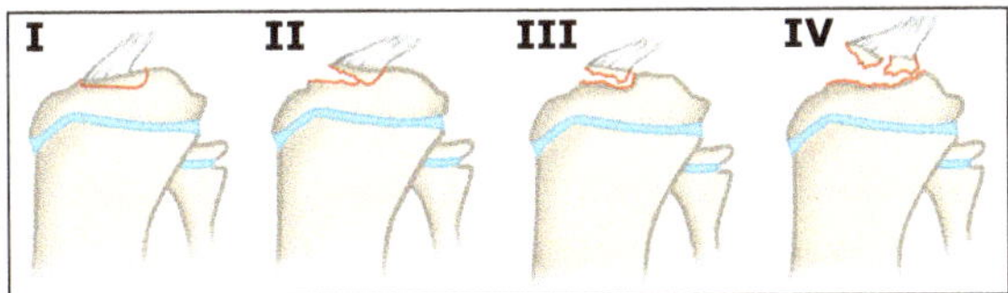

***Fig. 23.3**: Modified Meyers and McKeever classification of Tibial spine fractures.*

Treatment

Type I:

- Treatment is conservative in the form of long leg cast immobilisation in full extension in younger children and locked knee brace in adolescents and older children for a period of 4 to 6 weeks.

Type II:

- Closed reduction is attempted in full extension and a long leg cast is applied for 4 to 6 weeks. If there is marked pain and swelling, haemarthrosis is aspirated. Weekly check X-rays are done to rule out any displacement.
- Closed reduction may not be successful if there is interposition of the intermeniscal ligament. If there is failure or loss of closed reduction, arthroscopic or open reduction and fixation should be done.

Type III:

Arthroscopic reduction or open reduction through a medial parapatellar incision and fixation is essential. The fixation can be done with suture or screw **(Figs. 23.4 and 23.5)**. Mild residual knee laxity is frequently seen even after anatomical reduction and healing of tibial eminence fracture due to plastic deformation of ACL during the injury. This can be avoided by countersinking the tibial spine fragment within the epiphysis during reduction and fixation. After surgery, hinged knee brace and toe touch weight bearing is recommended for 6 weeks. Knee range of motion can be gradually started, with the aim to achieve full range of motion by 6 weeks.

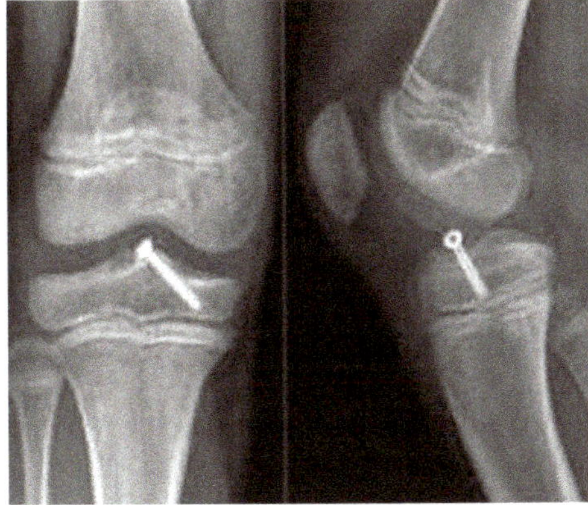

***Fig. 23.4**: AP and lateral X-rays of the knee showing ACL bony avulsion fracture treated with arthroscopic screw fixation.*

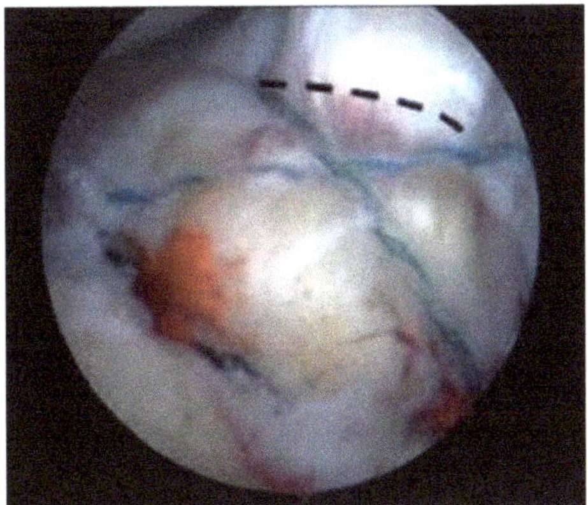

***Fig. 23.5**: Arthroscopic fixation of ACL bony avulsion using sutures.*

Complications

1. Malunion

   It can cause knee impingement during terminal extension leading to a flexion deformity. If the child is symptomatic, following treatment can be offered:

   - Osteotomy of the malunited fragment and refixation in anatomical but more recessed position.
   - Excision of the malunited fragment and reconstruction of ACL.

2. Non union

   Non union of the tibial spine fracture can cause knee instability. Arthroscopic or open reduction and internal fixation is recommended. For the non union in type IV fracture, excision of the fragment and ACL reconstruction is recommended in adolescents.

3. Arthrofibrosis and stiffness

   Prolonged immobilisation can result in arthrofibrosis and stiff knee. To prevent this, early mobilisation is recommended after conservative treatment or surgery. Arthroscopic lysis of adhesions and gentle manipulation under anaesthesia is done for stiffness not responding to physiotherapy for 6 weeks.

4. Hardware related complications

   Implant removal is recommended for screws that cross the proximal tibial physis as they may lead to growth disturbance and recurvatum deformity or shortening.

OSTEOCHONDRAL FRACTURES

Introduction

Osteochondral fractures are commonly seen in adolescents, associated with acute lateral patellar dislocation occurring due to a direct blow or flexion-rotation injury to the knee.Dislocation of the patella may tear the medial retinaculum and Medial Patello Femoral Ligament (MPFL), but the rest of the quadriceps muscle–patellar ligament complex continues to apply significant compression forces as the patella dislocates laterally. These forces are believed to cause osteochondral fractures at two common locations-infero-medial patellar facet or lateral aspect of lateral femoral condyle **(Fig. 23.6)**

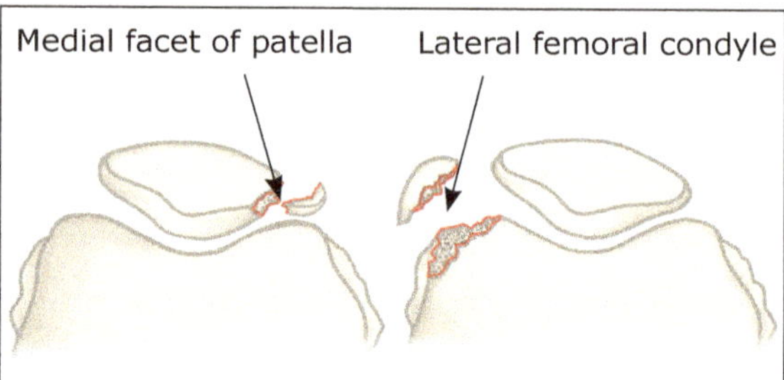

Fig. 23.6: *Osteochondral fractures associated with patella dislocation.*

Clinical Features

Child presents with pain, swelling due to haemarthrosis and difficulty in weight bearing. Child may present late with intermittent locking or catching of the knee due to loose osteochondral fracture fragment.

Imaging

In addition to AP and lateral views, skyline view is recommended **(Fig. 23.7)**. In 30-40% of the cases, the fracture is still difficult to visualise on X-ray.Hence it is recommended to do MRI in all cases of acute traumatic patellar dislocation even if the X-ray does not show any osteochondral fracture.

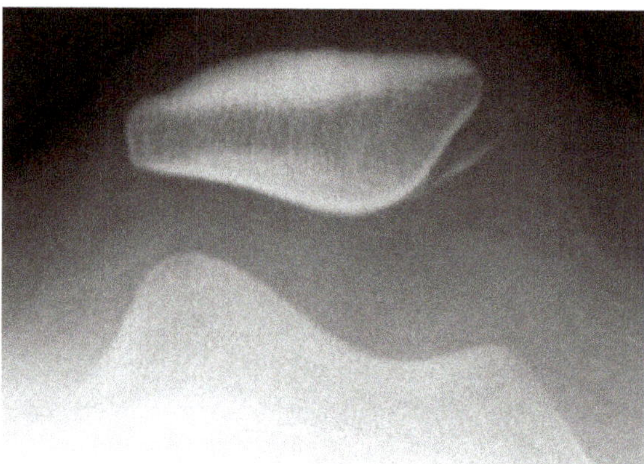

Fig. 23.7: *Skyline view of the knee showing osteochondral fracture associated with patella dislocation.*

Classification

Classification of the osteochondral fractures is based on the site, type and mechanism of injury **(Table 23.1)**.

Table 23.1: Classification of osteochondral fractures

	Site	*Mechanism of injury*
1.	Medial femoral condyle	Direct blow (fall) Compression and rotation (tibiofemoral)
2.	Lateral femoral condyle	Direct blow (kick) Compression and rotation (tibiofemoral) Acute patellar dislocation
3.	Patella (medial margin)	Acute patellar dislocation

Treatment

Treatment depends on the size and site of osteochondral fracture.

1. *Osteochondral fracture fragment < 5 mm:* For symptomatic patients, arthroscopic removal of the loose bodies is recommended.The site of origin of the loose body is managed by creating multiple holes of size 2 mm upto the subchondral bone (microfracture) in order to encourage fibrocartilage formation.

   MPFL repair is done in case of traumatic patellofemoral dislocation to reduce the risk of recurrent instability of patella. Repair is done using suture anchors either on the femoral or patellar side.

2. *Osteochondral fracture fragment >5 mm:* Fragment fixation is recommended.

   Osteochondral fracture fragment and fracture bed are debrided of fibrous tissue, anatomic reduction is done and fixation is done using headless screws, countersunk cannulated screws or suture bridge.

Complications

1. Recurrent patellar instability:

   This is the most common complication encountered.

2. Stiffness:

   Commonly seen after fracture fixation. Physiotherapy should be started immediately after surgery. For established cases of knee stiffness which have not responded to 3 months of physiotherapy, arthroscopic adhesiolysis and manipulation under anaesthesia is warranted.

3. Non union:

   The ununited fragment should be excised or re-fixed, followed by chondral resurfacing using marrow stimulation process (microfracture), osteochondral grafting (mosaicplasty) or autologous chondrocyte implant.

PATELLAR DISLOCATION

Introduction

Acute traumatic patella dislocation is commonly seen in adolescents due to flexion- rotation injury or rarely direct injury to the knee, mostly during athletic activities. Chronic atraumatic recurrent patellofemoral instability is mostly seen in adolescent females with underlying ligament laxity or other risk factors, like abnormal coronal and rotational alignment. Patellar dislocation may be associated with osteochondral fracture, bone bruise or MPFL tear.

Clinical Features

Child gives history of 'pop' associated with dislocation and sometimes a second 'pop' associated with spontaneous reduction after a twisting injury. There is diffuse parapatellar tenderness and pain on attempted lateral movement of patella with a positive apprehension test. If there is associated osteochondral fracture, large haemarthrosis and swelling is present. It is important to check for additional ligament injuries.

Imaging

In addition to AP and lateral views, a skyline view is important.

MRI is advocated in all cases of patellar dislocation as it can detect the associated ligamentous and chondral injuries. CT scan is helpful in assessment of potential risk factors for recurrence like trochlea and patellar dysplasia, torsional alignment and patella height.

Treatment

- *Acute patellar dislocation without osteochondral fracture:* They reduce spontaneously or can be reduced closed under sedation as follows.

  The hip is flexed to relax quadriceps and then the knee is gradually extended while gently pushing the patella medially back into position. The knee is immobilised in extension for 2 weeks followed by patello-femoral brace and physiotherapy for vastus medialis obliquus (VMO) strengthening and range of motion exercises. Return to sports is allowed after 12 weeks.

- *Acute patellar dislocation with associated osteochondral fracture:* The size of the osteochondral fracture should be assessed. If it is < 5 mm, it is excised, but if the size is > 5 mm, the fragment needs fixation. During surgery, MPFL repair or medial retinacular reefing can be done in order to prevent recurrent instability.

  Surgery is also indicated if there is complete avulsion of VMO and/or MPFL from medial patella.

Operative Procedure

Position:

Supine

Incision:

Anterior to the medial epicondyle in the distal portion of the VMO

- MPFL is identified deep to the fascial layer of the VMO.
- Direct repair of the MPFL, that is avulsed from the femur, can be performed via suture anchors.
- Sometimes an MPFL tightening procedure, referred to as reefing, imbrication or medial retinacular plasty procedure is required.
- In addition, lateral release is performed if there is residual patellar tilt.

In case of chronic dislocation, extensive realignment procedure is needed **(Fig. 23.8)**.

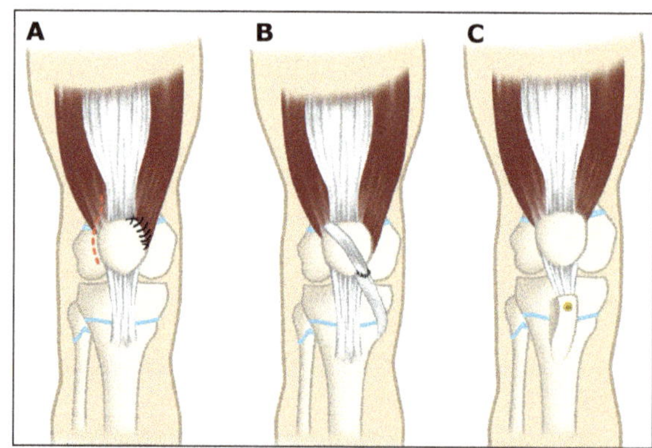

***Fig. 23.8**: Surgical techniques for chronic patella dislocation: Galeazzi procedure, consisting of -*
(A) Lateral release , medial plication and VMO advancement
(B) Semitendinosus tenodesis
(C) Elmslie Trillat procedure consisting of medial transfer of tibial tubercle

- In skeletally immature children, Galeazzi procedure is the preferred method. It comprises of

- Lateral retinacular release
- Medial retinacular and VMO advancement
- Semitendinosus transfer into the patella, to act as a check rein

- In skeletally mature patients, with abnormally high Q angle, Elmslie Trillat procedure with medial transfer of the tibial tubercle is the preferred method.

Complications

- Patella redislocation
- Patella instability
- Arthrofibrosis

PATELLA FRACTURE

Introduction

Patella fractures are rare, accounting for < 5% of all knee injuries in children. The diagnosis is sometimes difficult to make and often missed, eventually requiring late reconstruction that results in knee extensor lag and unsatisfactory outcome.

Classification

There are two basic patterns-

Primary osseous fracture:

Mainly transverse M/3 fracture, but some are vertical and stellate type fracture

Sleeve or avulsion fracture:

Most common, in the inferior part of the patella **(Fig. 23.9)**

Rarely in the proximal pole and medially, as in patella dislocation

Mechanism of Injury

- Direct trauma like MVA or fall onto the knee leads to transverse mid patella fracture.
- Indirect trauma like forceful contraction of quadriceps occurring at the start of a jump during sports like basketball or track field events leads to sleeve or avulsion fracture.

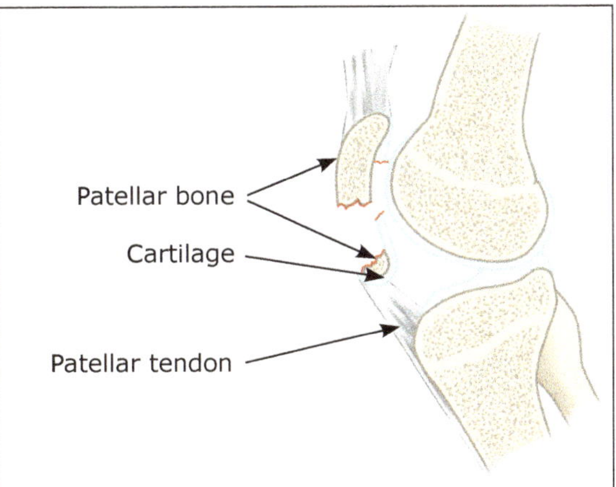

Fig. 23.9: *Patellar sleeve fracture.*

Clinical Features and Imaging

- In complete fracture or avulsion fracture, the clinical diagnosis is obvious from symptoms like pain and swelling of knee with inability to bear weight. There is tenderness, marked swelling, lack of full active knee extension and high riding patella with occasional palpable defect.
- In incomplete injury (undisplaced transverse patella fracture or minimally displaced inferior sleeve fracture), the clinical presentation is mild and hence often missed. Lateral X-ray of the knee in 30° flexion may reveal small bony fragments coming from the inferior pole of the patella, associated with patella alta. Even though the bone fragments appear small, there may be associated large cartilaginous fragment attached to the patellar tendon. If in doubt, a comparative X-ray of the opposite knee is helpful. The sleeve fracture must be differentiated from inferior accessory ossification centre. AP X-ray is important for diagnosis of vertical fracture and for differentiation from a bipartite patella.

Treatment

- Conservative treatment

  For undisplaced fracture with active knee extension possible (suggestive of intact retinaculum), conservative treatment is recommended in the form of long leg cast with almost full extension for 6-8 weeks, followed by progressive weight bearing.

- Operative treatment

  For displaced fracture with > 4 mm articular displacement or with articular step off >2-3 mm and for open fracture, surgical treatment is recommended.

For Sleeve fracture

- *Young child (<10 years):* Anatomical reduction and non absorbable suture repair, placed through cartilaginous sleeve and the patellar tendon, followed by long leg cast for 6-8 weeks.
- *Child > 10 years*: Anatomical reduction and fixation with 2 K-wires and tension band wiring (TBW), followed by long leg cast. Active SLR and weight bearing can be allowed after 2 weeks.
- *Late presentation (minimally displaced fracture):* If there is no extensor lag at the time of presentation, long leg cast in extension is recommended. If there is extensor lag, surgical intervention is required, as discussed above.

For transverse displaced fracture

Surgical treatment is recommended in the form of open reduction and internal fixation with 2 K-wires and tension band wiring.

Surgical steps

- Through a vertical incision over the patella, the fracture is reduced anatomically, held with a towel clip and 2 parallel K-wires are passed from inferior to superior.
- A loop of wire is then placed in a figure of eight fashion.
- The loop/knot is placed both medially and laterally to allow for compression across the fracture site. **(Fig. 23.10)**
- Some surgeons prefer to use sutures instead of TBW.

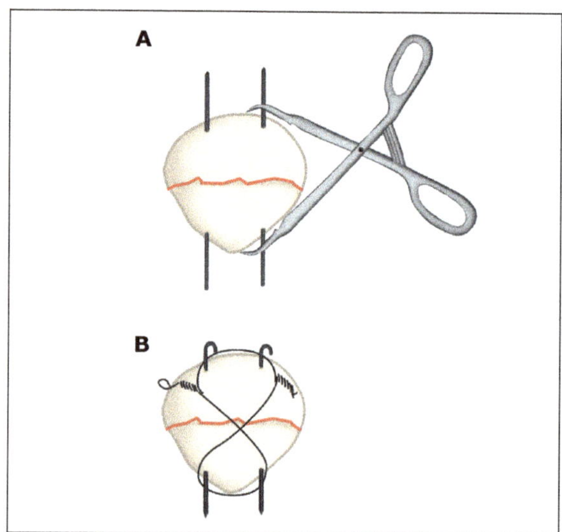

Fig. 23.10: *TBW fixation of transverse patella fracture:*
(A) Reduction held with a towel clip and two parallel K-wires
(B) A loop of wire placed in a figure of eight fashion, tightened both medially and laterally to allow for compression across the fracture site

For Comminuted fractures

- These fractures are difficult to treat and are associated with poor results.
- Treatment decision should be based on the fracture pattern.
- Anatomical reduction of the larger fragments should be performed and either excision of small non articular fragments or internal fixation of the remaining fragment to the larger fragment is done if possible.
- Avoid patellectomy as far as possible.

Complications

- Non union due to inadequate fixation
- Extensor lag
- Loss of flexion
- Rarely, AVN patella

MENISCAL INJURIES

Introduction

Meniscal injuries are rare in children younger than 10 years, unless associated with discoid meniscus. Medial meniscus is more commonly involved as compared to lateral meniscus and 50-90% are longitudinal tears. Most common mechanism is rotational injury during sports. These injuries may be associated with tears of the ACL.

Classification

Meniscal injuries are classified in different ways.

- *Based on the meniscus involved:*

  Medial or lateral

- *Based on the location of tear:*

  Posterior horn

  Body

  Anterior horn

- *Based on the pattern of tear* **(Figs. 23.11 and 23.12)**

  Vertical/Longitudinal

  Bucket-handle

  Horizontal cleavage

  Transverse/Radial

  Complex

- *Based on chronicity of tear*

  Acute (< 6 weeks)

  Chronic (> 6 weeks)

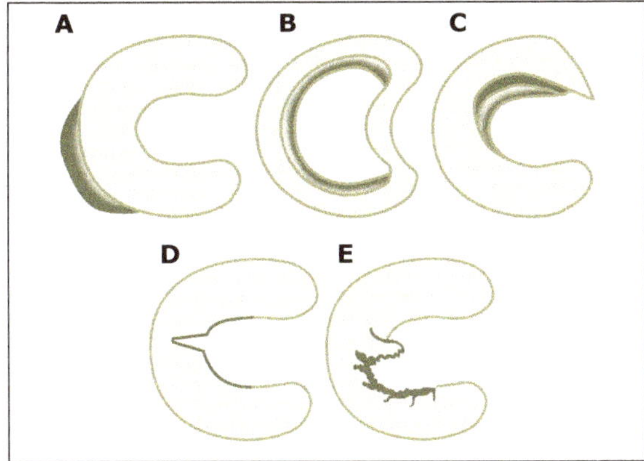

Fig. 23.11: *Types of meniscal injuries in adolescents*
(A) Peripheral
(B) Bucket handle
(C) Horizontal
(D) Transverse
(D) Complex

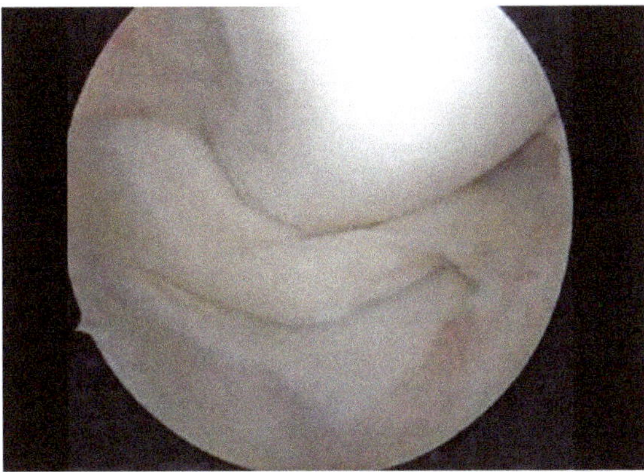

Fig. 23.12: *Arthroscopic picture of a bucket-handle tear of the medial meniscus.*

Clinical Features

Child presents with pain, swelling and mechanical symptoms like snapping, popping or catching. In case of a bucket handle tear, there may be locking of the knee with inability to extend the knee. McMurray's test is helpful in subacute or chronic cases. Clinical diagnosis is not always easy and accurate in acute cases. MRI is essential to make the correct diagnosis.

Imaging

MRI is the gold standard with 80-90% accuracy rate. Medial meniscus tear is identified when linear signal changes extend to the articular surface. The site and tear pattern and associated injuries can be diagnosed based on MRI.

Treatment

- Conservative treatment is indicated for asymptomatic meniscal tears. These tears are usually small (<1cm), stable and located in the peripheral vascular zone. Protected weight bearing in knee brace for 4-6 weeks and avoidance of pivoting and sports for 12 weeks is recommended.

  Radial tears do not heal with conservative treatment and may require surgery.

- Operative treatment is indicated for symptomatic meniscal tears. Meniscal repair is indicated for unstable meniscal tears located in the peripheral 2/3rd vascular zone. Various techniques (inside-out, outside – in or all inside) can be utilised for meniscal repair. **(Figs. 23.13 and 23.14)**

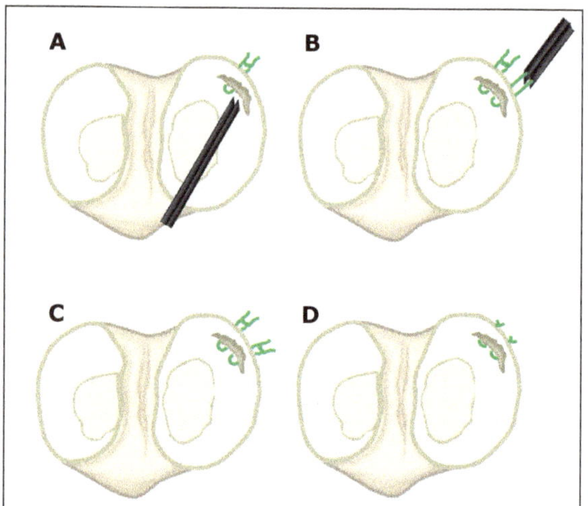

***Fig. 23.13**: Technique of meniscal repair A.Inside-out B. Outside-in C. Sutures placed in a horizontal manner D. Sutures tied on the outside*

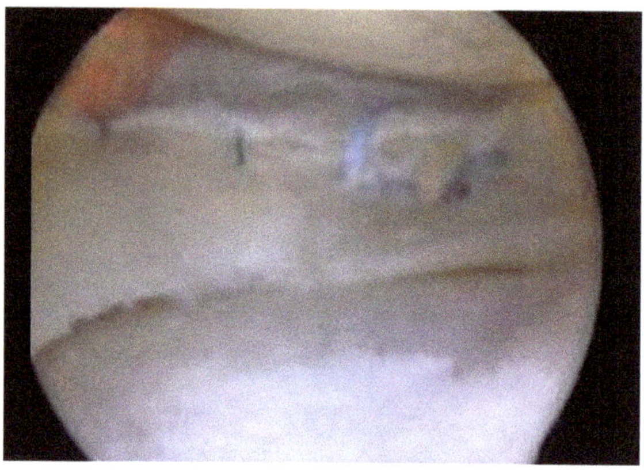

***Fig. 23.14**: Arthroscopic picture of repair of the medial meniscus.*

- Tears in the avascular zone (inner 1/3rd) require partial meniscectomy.
- In children and adolescents, emphasis should be on meniscal repair over meniscectomy.
- Bucket handle meniscal tear with a locked knee requires urgent treatment to allow for reduction and meniscal repair and avoid further injury to meniscus.
- Cases treated by meniscal repair require non weight bearing for 6 weeks.

Complications

- Haemarthrosis, persistent effusion, stiffness
- Failure to heal/retear of meniscus repair.

LIGAMENT INJURY

Introduction

Ligament structures work synchronously to provide stability to the knee joint. **(Fig. 23.15)**

- Anterior Cruciate Ligament (ACL) is the primary restraint to anterior translation whereas deep Medial Collateral Ligament (MCL) is a secondary restraint.

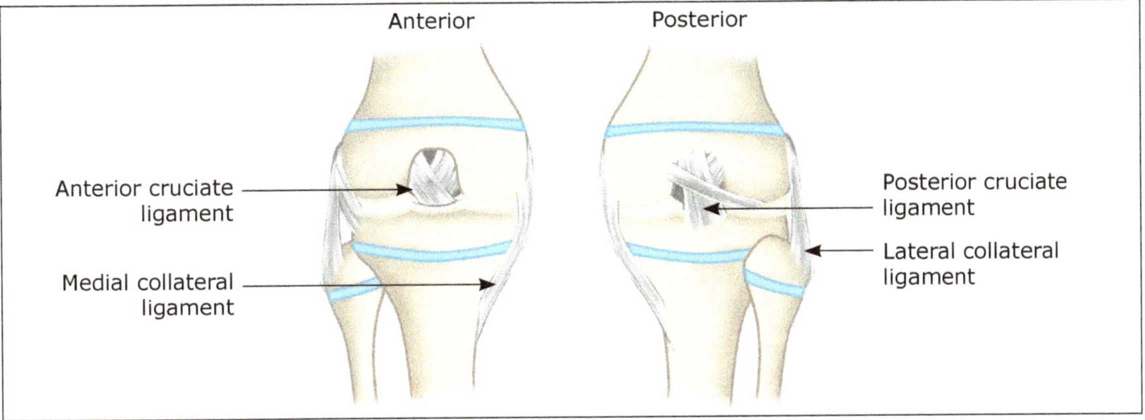

***Fig. 23.15**: Normal Ligaments around the knee.*

- Posterior Cruciate Ligament (PCL) is the primary restraint to posterior translation and Lateral Collateral Ligament (LCL), posterolateral complex and superficial MCL are secondary restraints. Ligament injuries are uncommon in children and may occur as a part of polytrauma. But in adolescents, these injuries can occur during contact sports or sports that require 'pivoting' manoeuvres while running. Isolated ACL and PCL injuries are more common.
- Hyperextension with internal rotation of tibia on femur leads to isolated ACL injury.
- Direct blow to the front of the tibia in a flexed knee position leads to isolated PCL injury. ACL injury may be associated with MCL tear and meniscal injury.
- LCL injury occurs with a varus displacement of the knee.
- MCL injury occurs due to valgus moment from a direct blow to the lateral aspect of the knee.

Clinical Features

- Patients with ACL tear describe a characteristic sudden movement in the knee with a 'give way' or 'shifting' sensation. 40-60% often describe injury with inability to continue sports, accompanied by a large effusion. Both lower limbs should be examined for comparison. ACL tear can be confirmed by anterior drawer test or Lachman/ Pivot shift test. **(Fig. 23.16)**

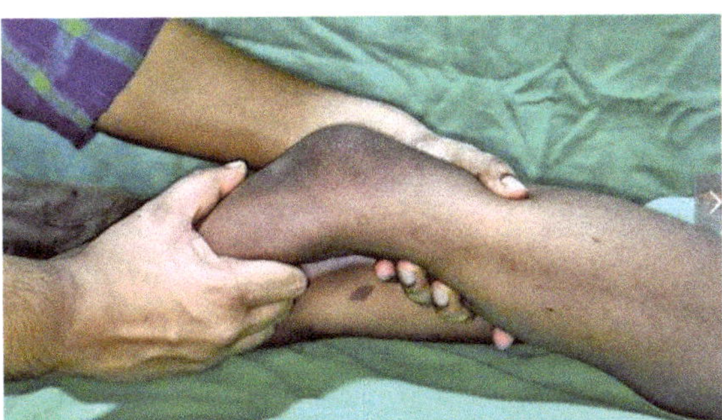

***Fig. 23.16**: Lachman test for anterior cruciate ligament: With the knee in 20-30° flexion and leg in slight external rotation, the examiner holds the child's distal thigh with one hand and stabilises the proximal tibia with the other keeping the thumb on the tibial tubercle.. An anteriorly directed force is then applied to the proximal tibia. The amount of anterior displacement of the tibia is determined to grade the anterior instability. Grade 1: 1 to 5 mm, Grade 2: 6 to 10 mm, Grade 3: 11 to 15 mm, Grade 4: 16 to 20 mm*

- PCL injury is diagnosed by posterior drawer test, posterior sag sign and quadriceps active test. **(Fig. 23.17)**

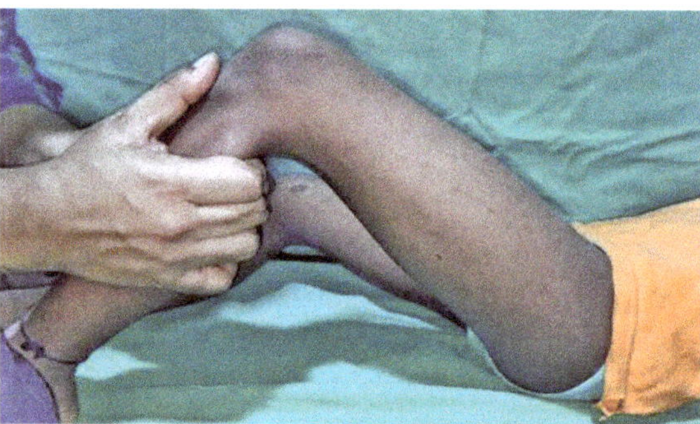

Fig. 23.17: *Posterior drawer test for posterior cruciate ligament: The child's knee is flexed to 90° and the examiner can sit lightly on the distal aspect of foot. The examiner grasps the proximal aspect of tibia with both the hands while placing the thumbs on the tibial tubercle. A posteriorly directed force is then applied to the proximal tibia and the amount of posterior displacement is graded as in the Lachman test.*

- MCL/LCL injuries can be diagnosed by checking for tenderness at origin/ insertion of collateral ligaments and varus/valgus stress tests in 20° flexion and full extension. **(Figs. 23.18 and 23.19)**

Classification

I. *Based on severity of injury:*

1. First degree:

- Tear of few fibres of ligament

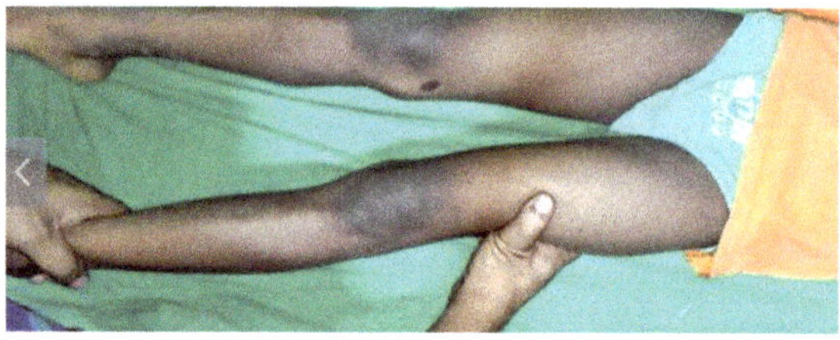

Fig. 23.18: *Valgus stress test for medial collateral ligament : With the knee in full extension, a valgus stress is applied to the knee. Opening on the medial aspect of the knee in this position indicates a substantial tear of the MCL along with the medial capsule and one or both cruciate ligaments. Repeating the same test with the knee in 10-15° flexion to relax the posterior capsule allows specific testing of the MCL.*

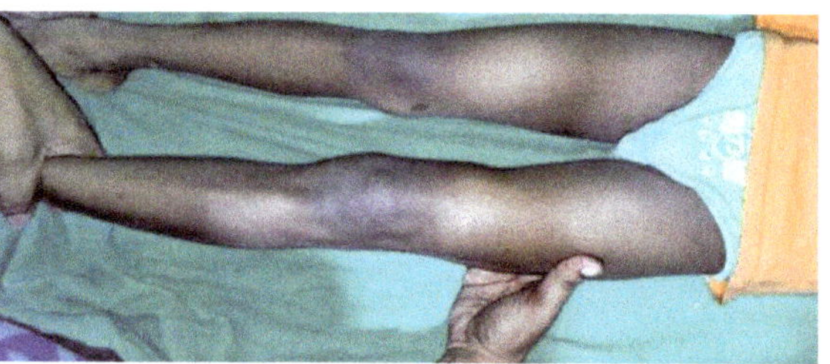

Fig. 23.19: *Varus stress test for lateral collateral ligament: With the knee in full extension,a varus stress is applied to the knee. Opening on the lateral side in this position indicates tear of the LCL.*

- Only localised tenderness
- No instability
- < 5 mm separation of joint on stress testing

2. Second degree:

- Disruption of more fibres of ligament
- Asymmetry with stress testing
- Minor instability
- 5-10 mm separation of joint on stress testing

3. Third degree:

- Complete disruption of ligament
- Gross instability
- > 10 mm separation of joint on stress testing

II. *Anatomical* **(Fig. 23.20)**

1. Femoral attachment avulsion
2. Midsubstance/interstitial tear
3. Tibial attachment avulsion

III. *Based on plane of instability:*

1. One plane instability (simple/straight)
2. Rotary instability (Anteromedial/ Anterolateral/Posteromedial/Postero-lateral)
3. Combined instability (AL-PL, AL-AM, AM-PM)

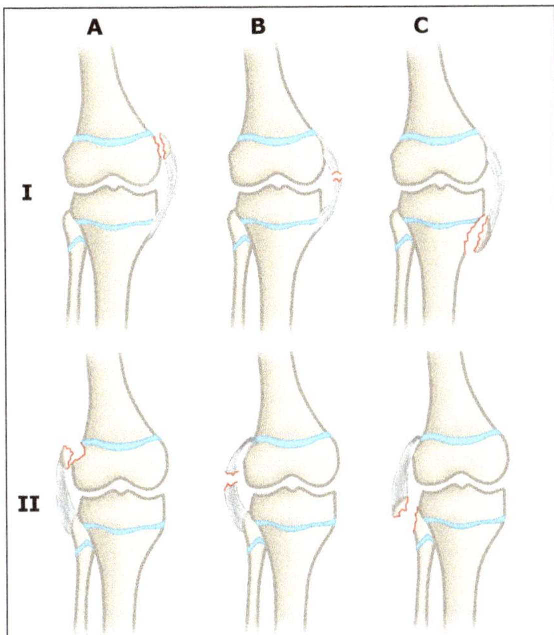

***Fig. 23.20**: Classification of:*
I. Medial collateral ligament and
II. Lateral collateral ligament injuries based on the level of tear
A. Femoral attachment
B. Mid substance
C. Tibial/Fibular attachment

Imaging

- AP and lateral X-ray: Look for epiphyseal/physeal fracture, tibial spine fracture, avulsion fracture around MCL/LCL insertion.
- Stress X-rays help in evaluation of degree of ligament strain, but may be difficult in an acute setting.
- MRI is the most important imaging modality for diagnosis of ligament injuries.

Treatment

MCL and LCL

- Isolated grade I or II injuries are treated conservatively with hinged knee brace and crutch walking for 4 weeks. Once a painless full range of motion is achieved, the child can be allowed to run and gradually resume athletic activities.
- Isolated grade III disruption requires 6 weeks immobilisation in hinged knee brace followed by rehabilitation of quadriceps muscles and knee range of motion exercises.

  If MCL injury is associated with ACL injury, ACL reconstruction should be delayed at least 4-6 weeks to allow time for early MCL healing and achieve full range of motion.

ACL

- Partial ACL tear (< 50 % fibres, with negative pivot shift test and no instability) can be treated conservatively.
- In children, acute ACL reconstruction should not be performed within the first 3 weeks of injury, to minimise the risk of arthrofibrosis. During these 3 weeks,rehabilitation is performed to reduce swelling and regain range of motion.
- If additional bucket-handle medial meniscus tear is present, meniscal repair should be done, followed by ACL reconstruction.
- Treatment of complete ACL tears is done according to the chronological, physiological (Tanner staging system) and skeletal age.
- In prepubescent patients (M < 12 years, F < 11 years, Tanner 1 or 2), physeal sparing combined intra and extra-articular reconstruction is recommended.
- In adolescents with growth remaining (M: 13-16 years, F: 12-14 years, Tanner 2 or 3), transphyseal reconstruction with hamstrings and metaphyseal fixation is advised.
- In older adolescents with closing physes (M > 16 years, F > 14 years, Tanner

5), adult type ACL reconstruction with interference screw fixation, using patellar tendon or hamstrings is advised.

PCL

- PCL injuries are quite rare. PCL tibial bony avulsion is more common in adolescent age group.
- For skeletally immature children, arthroscopic suture repair of bony avulsions is done through small bony tunnels, with the limbs of suture tied over a cortical bone bridge.
- For skeletally mature adolescents, PCL reconstruction with adult-based technique is used.

Complications

- Persistent instability
- Arthrofibrosis
- Graft failure
- Infection
- Donor site morbidity

Flowchart 23.1

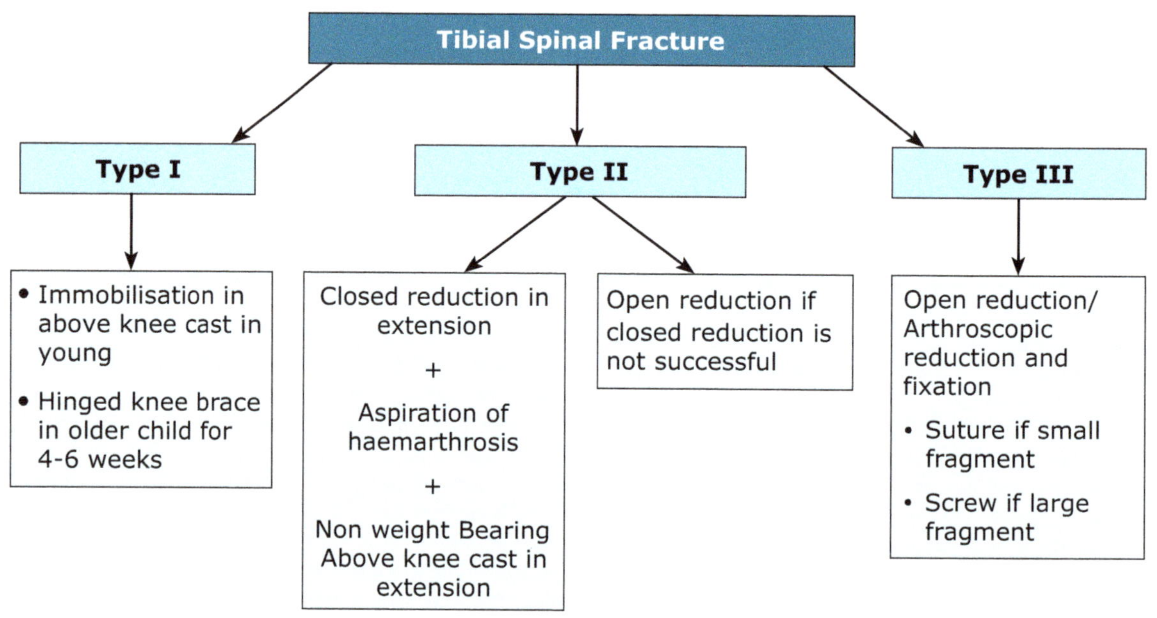

Flowchart 23.2

Osteochondral Knee Fracture
Assess the size and site of fragment
≤5 mm osteochondral fracture
and
Chondral shear fracture
or
Fracture involving NWB area
or
Chronic loose bodies
>5 mm osteochondral fracture
and
Chondral fracture in WB area
Fixation of fracture
• Removal of loose bodies
• In symptomatic patients, perforation of underlying subchondral bone
+ MPFL repair/proximal medial retinacular reefing if traumatic patellar dislocation

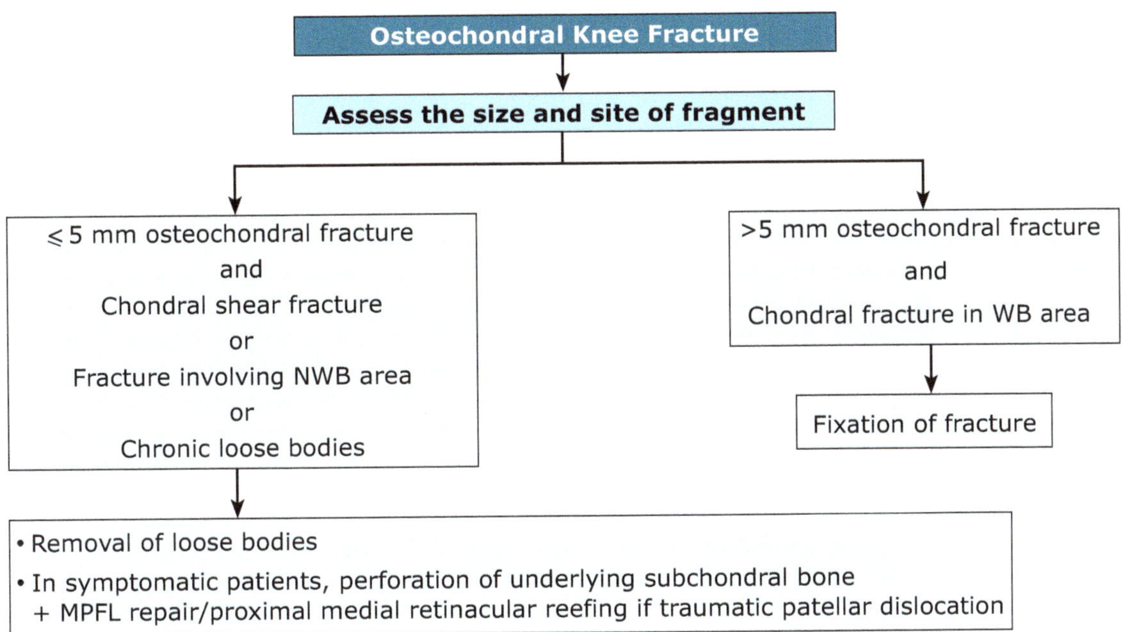

Flowchart 23.3

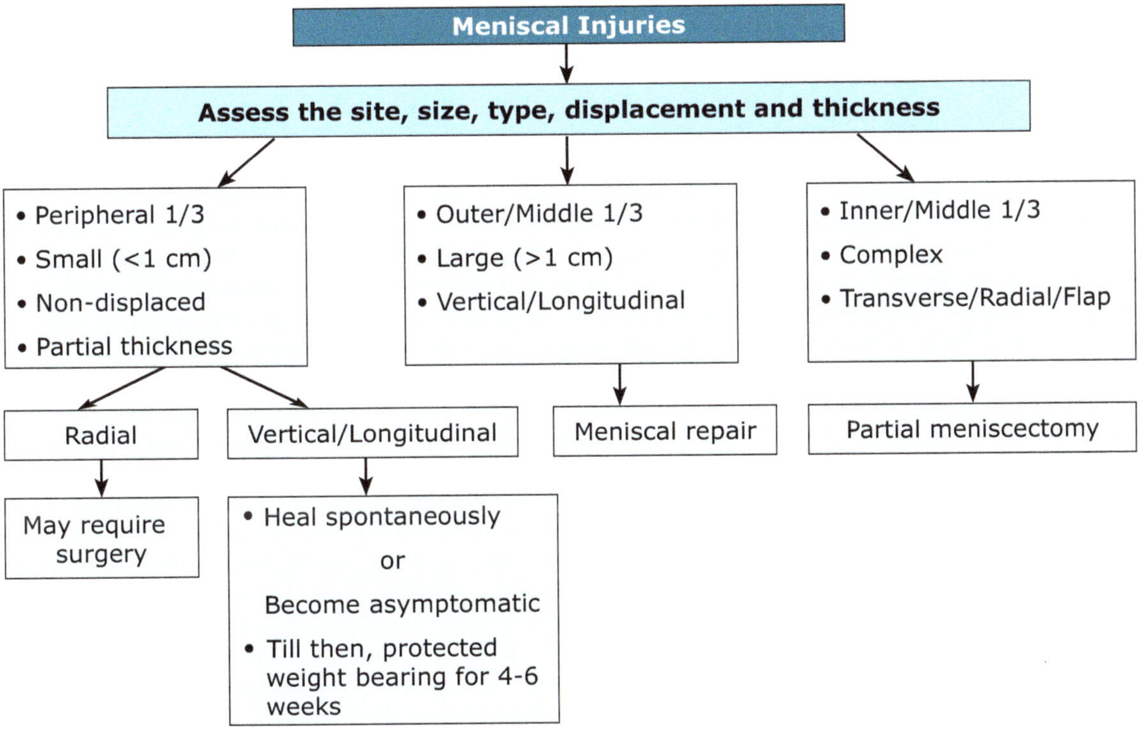

Meniscal Injuries
Assess the site, size, type, displacement and thickness
• Peripheral 1/3
• Small (<1 cm)
• Non-displaced
• Partial thickness
• Outer/Middle 1/3
• Large (>1 cm)
• Vertical/Longitudinal
• Inner/Middle 1/3
• Complex
• Transverse/Radial/Flap
Radial
Vertical/Longitudinal
Meniscal repair
Partial meniscectomy
May require surgery
• Heal spontaneously
or
Become asymptomatic
• Till then, protected weight bearing for 4-6 weeks

Flowchart 23.4

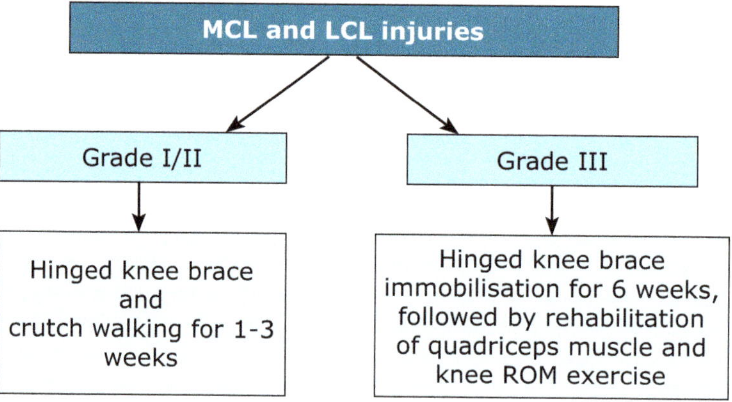

Flowchart 23.5

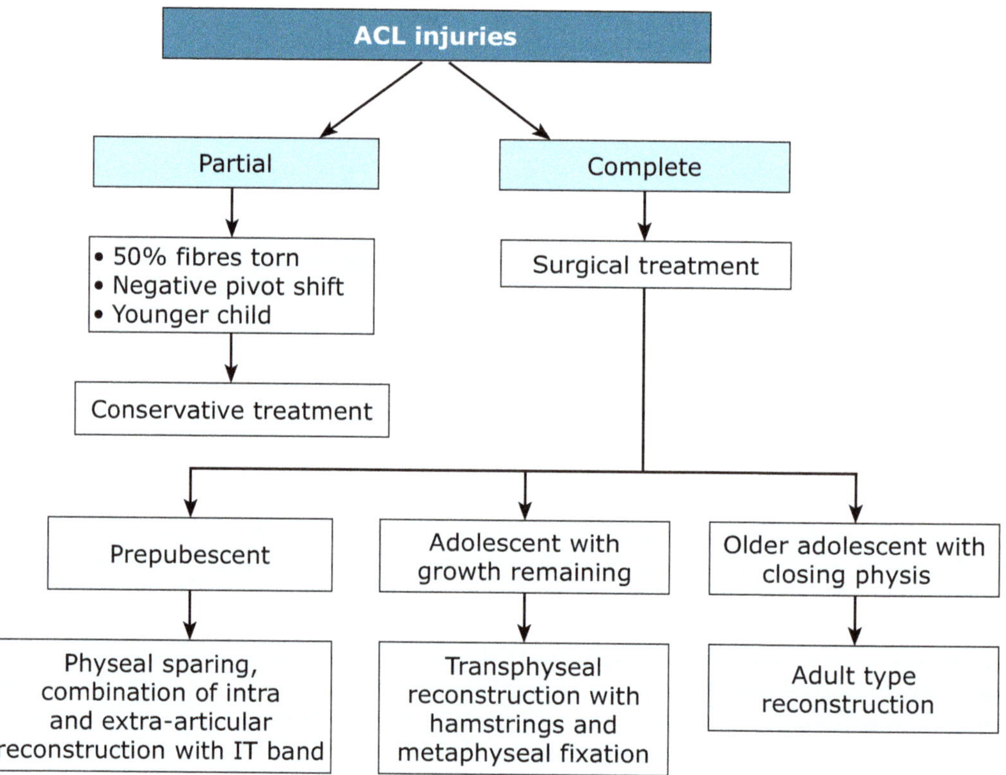

24 Proximal Tibial Physeal Fractures

Introduction

Proximal tibial physis has intrinsic stability because of collateral ligaments and lateral fibular buttress, hence significant force is required for it to fracture. Due to this, proximal tibial physeal injury is rare, seen in < 1% of all physeal injuries. But the most critical feature is its proximity to the popliteal artery and possibility of development of compartment syndrome. The most common mechanism of injury is hyperextension, resulting in the metaphyseal portion of tibia displacing posteriorly towards the popliteal artery **(Fig. 24.1)**. Also, there may be injury to anterior tibial recurrent artery with bleeding into anterior compartment with development of compartment syndrome. Associated ligamentous injuries and internal derangement of the knee may be seen in 30-40% of Salter-Harris (S-H) type III and IV proximal tibial physeal fractures.

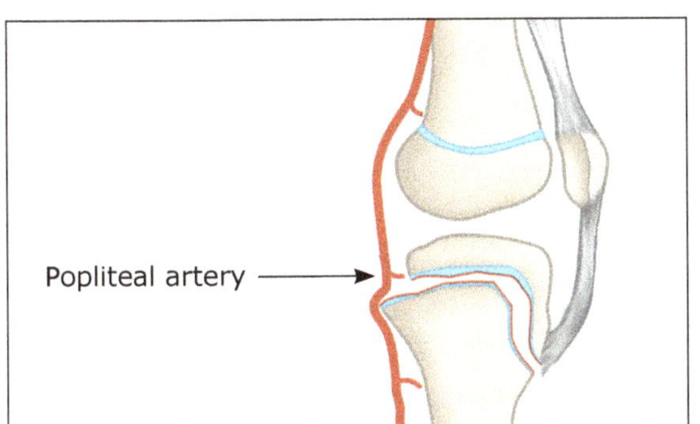

***Fig. 24.1**: Hyperextension type of proximal tibial physeal injury with the metaphyseal fragment displacing posteriorly towards the popliteal artery*

Clinical Features

The child presents with pain and swelling in the knee joint. There is knee effusion, haemarthrosis, hamstring spasm and restriction of knee range of motion. Tenderness distal to the joint line refers to physeal injury whereas tenderness anterior to the joint line refers to tibial tubercle injury. With posteriorly displaced proximal metaphysis, concavity may be palpated anteriorly. As vascular injury is relatively common, careful palpation of dorsalis pedis and posterior tibial artery and careful evaluation for compartment syndrome is necessary.

Imaging

- X-rays: AP, lateral and oblique views of the knee with tibia are necessary.
- CT scan may be needed in S-H type III and IV injuries to assess the joint incongruity, fracture line orientation and fracture displacement.
- MRI is helpful for diagnosis of additional ligament injury.

Classification

Fractures of the proximal tibial physis can be classified in two ways.

1. *Based on mechanism of injury*

Indirect (Avulsion) injury: **(Fig. 24.2)**

- Valgus/Varus (common in younger children: 3-9 years)
- Extension/Flexion

  Extension injury is the most common mechanism, with an indirect blow to a hyperextended knee when the lower leg is in a fixed position

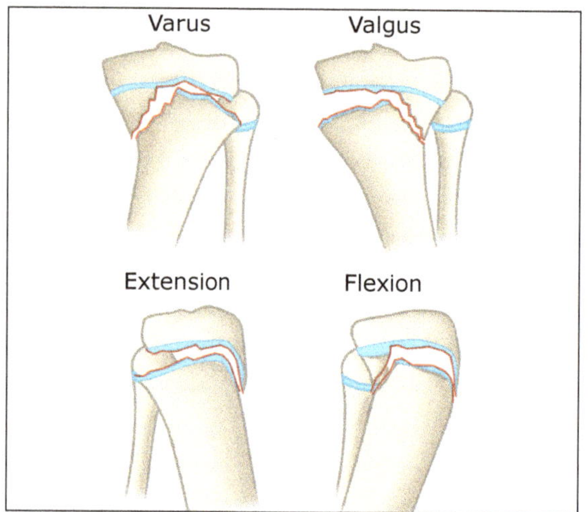

***Fig. 24.2**: Types of proximal tibia physeal fractures as per mechanism of injury.*

Flexion injury is a rare mechanism due to jumping activity that can produce avulsion, shear and compression stresses and produce this fracture.

Direct Injury: Run over in MVA or sports injury like football.

2. *Salter Harris classification*

S-H I: ~ 15 %

Majority (~ 50 %) S- H I fractures are non displaced due to overhanging tubercle preventing anterior displacement and fibula preventing lateral displacement of metaphysis.

S-H II: ~35-40%

About 2/3rd S-H II fractures are displaced with medial opening and lateral Thurston Holland fragment, with valgus deformity and associated proximal fibula fracture.

S-H III: ~ 20-25%

Majority are displaced fractures and require surgical intervention.

Two types of fractures occur. The first one, more common, involves either the medial or the lateral plateau, best seen on AP X-ray. The second one, involving both the tibial tubercle and the anterior aspect of the proximal tibial epiphysis, is best seen on the lateral X-ray.

S-H IV: ~ 15-20%
Requires surgical intervention

S-H V: Rare, often recognised only after physeal arrest has occurred.

Treatment

The goal of treatment is to obtain and maintain an anatomical reduction without causing any further damage to the physis. Careful evaluation of the distal vascular status is a must before undertaking any treatment.

Stable S-H type I and II fractures with <2-3 mm. displacement can be treated by closed reduction and casting.

- Prior to closed reduction, tense knee effusion may be aspirated using sterile technique under LA/conscious sedation/GA.
- It is important to give gentle traction during reduction to minimise the risk of damage to the physis.
- Reduction is performed by an anteriorly directed translation of the metaphyseal fragment for the extension type and varus force for the valgus type of fracture.
- Knee is then flexed to obtain and maintain the reduction.
- Cast is applied with the knee in less than 60^{0} flexion for 4-6 weeks.
- Child should always be admitted for observation and gentle elevation should be given to monitor for high incidence of vascular injury and compartment syndrome.
- Cast should be univalved/bivalved to permit swelling.
- Post reduction X-ray and follow up X-ray at 1 week are mandatory.

- Cast removal is done 4-6 weeks after injury if the fracture demonstrates clinicoradiological union.
- ROM and quadriceps strengthening are initiated at 6 weeks following injury.
- Return to normal activities can take at least 4 weeks.
- Status of the physis to look for growth arrest should be checked every 4-6 months post injury with periodic X-rays.

Unstable S-H type I and II injuries with more than 2-3 mm displacement require closed reduction and cross pinning with smooth K-wires, if metaphyseal fragment is small and percutaneous compression screw if metaphyseal fragment is large.

Pin size depends on the size of tibia, usually ranging from 2-2.5 mm. Pins should start from the metaphysis and aim from slightly anterior to posterior. Pins should be bicortical and should not cross at fracture line.

If there is widening / interposition of soft tissue (pes anserinus/ periosteum), open reduction may be necessary.

S-H type III and IV injuries

- Open reduction and fixation is required via arthrotomy or arthroscopy to assess articular reduction and intra articular pathology.
- Midline incision is taken and the fracture bed is cleared of any debris such as fracture haematoma or entrapped periosteal flap.
- Fracture reduction is done utilising the same manoeuvre as in closed reduction, that is using axial traction and leverage in an appropriate direction to reduce the displacement.
- Smooth pins or screws are used depending on fracture pattern and size.
- Sometimes tension band wire is used, especially when fracture fragments are comminuted or too small for secure fixation to tibial metaphysis.
- During open reduction, anterior compartment fascia is released to reduce the risk of compartment syndrome and a drain is placed in the anterior compartment.
- When circulation is questionable, CT angiogram may be helpful.
- Fracture fixation should be done prior to vascular repair.

  Extended medial approach will allow open reduction of fracture and vessel management by vascular surgeon. Alternatively, posterior approach can be used for easier access to popliteal space and it can be combined with percutaneous fixation of fracture.

Complications

- Compartment syndrome and vascular injury (3-7%)
- Growth disturbance (10-20%) in the form of limb length discrepancy or recurvatum
- Knee instability (due to associated ligament injuries as in S-H III and IV)
- Loss of reduction
- Arthrofibrosis and loss of ROM
- Prominent and painful implant and bursitis (50% require implant removal later and parents to be counselled about it)

TIBIAL TUBERCLE FRACTURE

The tibial tubercle is the most anterior aspect of the proximal tibial epiphysis and contributes to the growth of the proximal tibia. It serves as an insertion site of the patellar tendon. Upto 9-10 years, it is cartilaginous. Then 2 to 3 centres of ossification appear at 8-12 years in girls and 10-14 years in boys. They unite with the proximal tibial epiphysis at approximately 15 years. Its fracture mainly occurs in the adolescent age group between 13 to 16 years, when the proximal tibial physis is in the process of closure. Fusion of the proximal tibia physis follows a definite pattern of posterior to anterior and medial to lateral with simultaneous proximal to distal closure of the tubercle apophysis. **(Fig. 24.3)**

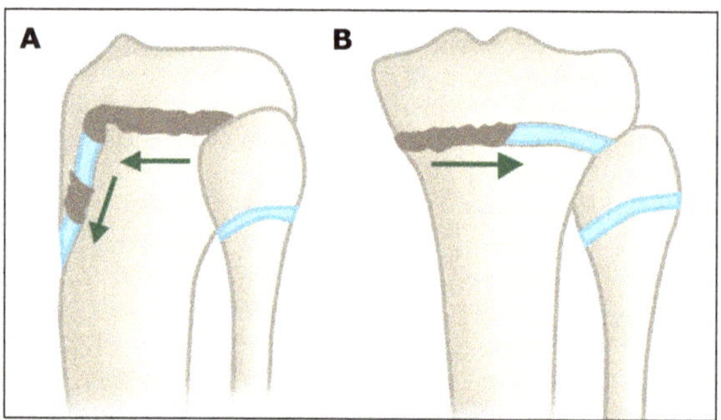

Fig. 24.3: *Closure of Proximal tibial physis: A. Posterior to anterior and for tubercle apophysis-Proximal to distal, B. Medial to lateral.*

Tibial tubercle fracture occurs during jumping activities as a result of active extension of the knee with sudden, strong contraction of the quadriceps **(*Fig. 24.4*)**

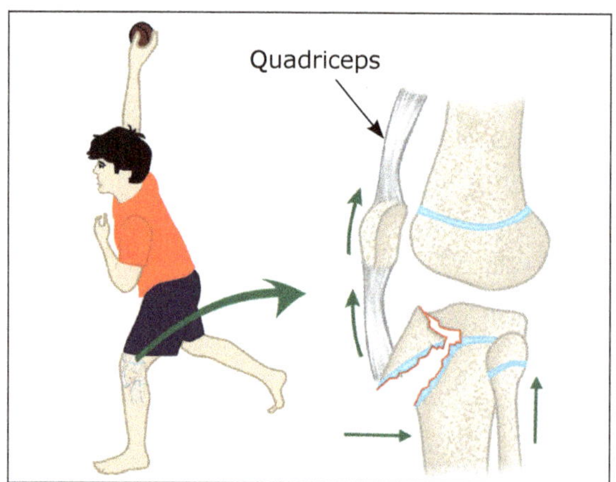

Fig. 24.4: *Tibial tubercle fracture due to sudden quadriceps contraction during jumping activity.*

or with acute passive flexion against a contracted quadriceps, as occurs in football players. This fracture may be associated with cruciate and collateral ligamentous injuries or rupture of patellar ligament and quadriceps tendon.

Classification

Ogden modification of Watson–Jones classification (Fig. 24.5)

Type I: Fracture distal to the normal junction of the ossification centres of the proximal end of the tibia and tuberosity

I A: Minimal displacement

I B: Hinged anteriorly and proximally

Type II: Fracture at the junction of the ossification of the proximal end of the tibia and the tuberosity

II A: Simple

II B: Comminuted

Type III: Fracture extends to the joint and is associated with displacement of the anterior fragment and discontinuation of the joint surface

III A: Single fragment

III B: Comminuted fragment

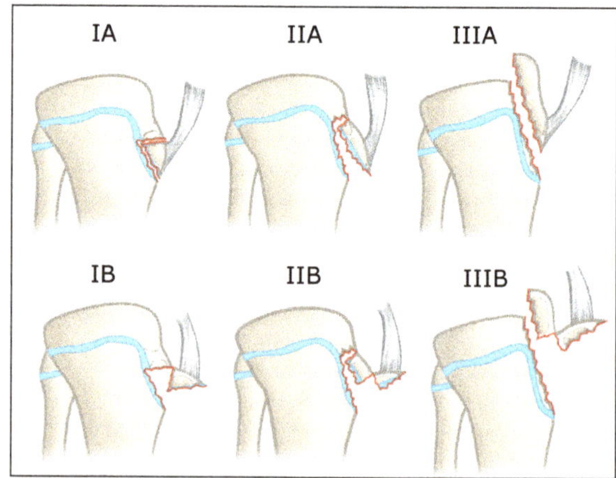

Fig. 24.5: *Ogden modification of Watson–Jones classification of Tibial tubercle fracture.*

Clinical Features

- Pain, swelling and tenderness over the tibial tubercle, with knee usually held in 20-40° flexion.
- With small tibial tubercle avulsion, the child may be able to extend the knee actively through intact retinacular tissue, but with a large fragment, active extension is impaired.
- In type II and III, a defect can be palpated at the level of the tibial tubercle.
- In displaced fracture, the patella rides abnormally high on femur with inability to extend the leg.
- In displaced high energy fractures, the child may have severe pain and swelling suggestive of compartment syndrome.

Imaging

- AP and lateral X-rays of the knee with proximal tibia along with comparative opposite side X-rays are necessary.
- Level of the patella is an important indicator of the degree of displacement of tibial tubercle.

  If Insall ratio (Patella height/distance between lower pole of patella to tibial tubercle) is < 0.8, it may suggest some disruption of patellar ligament or tibial tubercle.

Treatment

- Ogden type I fracture with minimal displacement can be treated with closed reduction and casting for 6-8 weeks. The initial cast should be in full extension and later flexed to 30°.
- Ogden type II and III fractures require surgical treatment for decompression of the fracture haematoma, anatomical reduction and stable internal fixation.

  Assessment and management of intra-articular pathology is important in type III.

Technique

Position

Supine on a radiolucent table. Tourniquet used. ***(Fig. 24.6)***

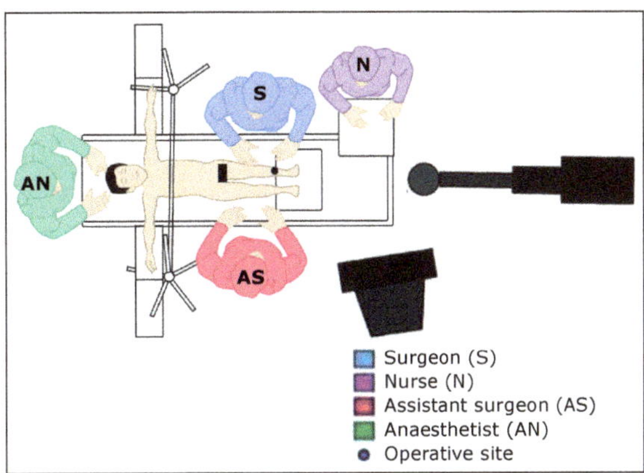

***Fig. 24.6**: Supine position on a radiolucent table with tourniquet applied, for open reduction of left tibial tubercle fracture.*

Incision

Long incision medial or lateral to patellar tendon **(Fig. 24.7)**

Steps

- The fracture haematoma is thoroughly evacuated.
- The fracture bed is cleared of any interposed soft tissue.
- The fracture is anatomically reduced with the knee extended.
- The fracture is fixed with two 4 mm/6.5 mm cancellous screws placed parallel to the joint surface with washers, to prevent screw head penetration of the anterior cortex.
- The patellar tendon is sutured to its lateral attachment.
- In a comminuted fracture, multiple screws/TBW may be necessary.

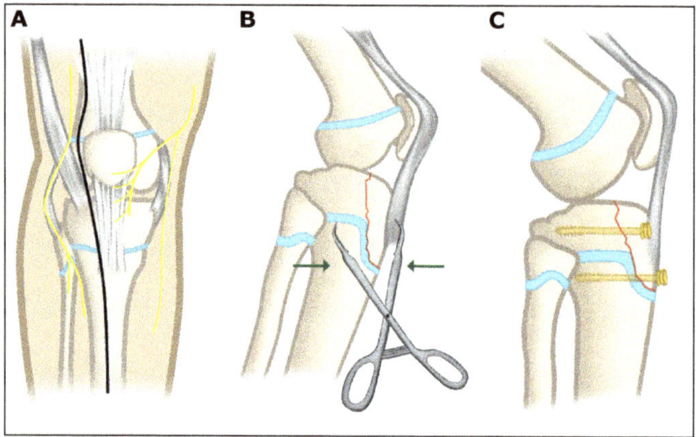

***Fig. 24.7**: Surgical treatment of Tibial tubercle fracture: A. Lateral parapatellar incision, B. Type III A fracture reduction held with a towel clip, C. Cancellous screws passed parallel to the joint*

- The screws may be passed across the physis if required for stability. (as these fractures occur nearing maturity)

Post operatively a long leg/cylinder cast is given for 6-8 weeks.

Sports activities are avoided for additional 6-8 weeks.

Flowchart 24.1

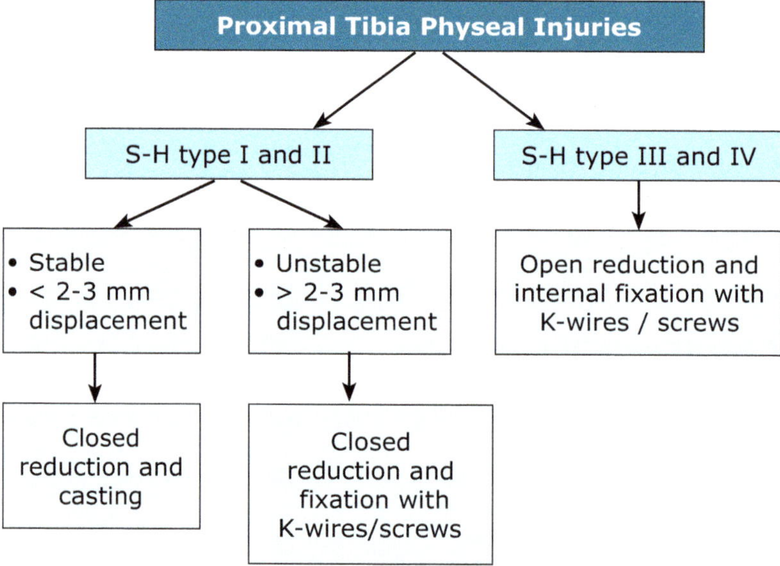

Flowchart 24.2

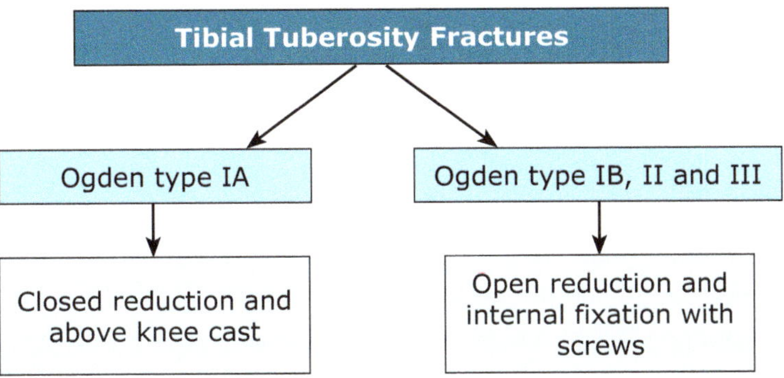

25 Fractures of the Shaft of Tibia and Fibula

Introduction

Tibia shaft fractures are the third most common long bone fractures in children and second most common long bone fracture in children with non-accidental trauma. Around 9% are open fractures. Occasionally the fracture may be pathological through an underlying bone lesion (e.g. Non ossifying fibroma, Aneurysmal bone cyst, Osteomyelitis etc.). Careful assessment of distal neurovascular status becomes important, not only due to proximity of neurovascular structure but also due to likelihood of raised compartment pressure in tibia-fibula fractures.

Relevant Anatomy

Popliteal artery divides into anterior and posterior tibial arteries in close proximity to tibia at the distal border of popliteus. Common peroneal nerve traverses around the fibular neck before dividing into superficial and deep peroneal nerves and can be injured during the actual trauma as well as during the surgical exposure of the fibula. **(Fig. 25.1)**

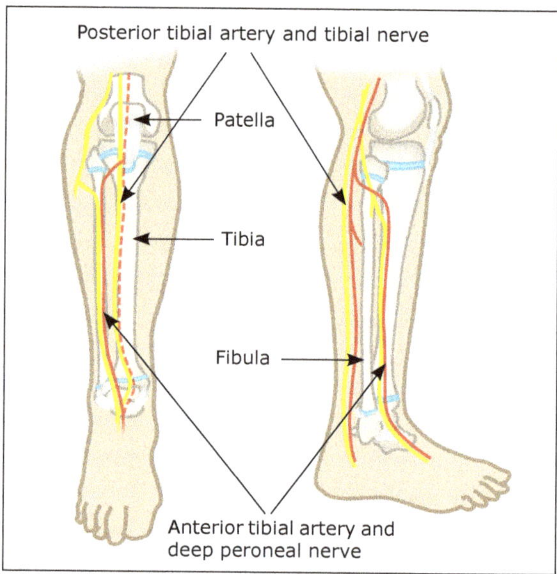

***Fig. 25.1**: Neurovascular anatomy of tibia-fibula.*

Classification

Clinical presentation and management is based on the classification of fractures.

1. Fractures of Proximal tibia Metaphysis (Least common)
2. Diaphyseal fractures of Tibia and Fibula (20-40%)
3. Fractures of Distal Tibia Metaphysis (50-70%)

Special consideration is required for

A. Open Tibia Fracture

B. Toddler's Fracture

C. Stress Fracture

FRACTURES OF PROXIMAL TIBIA METAPHYSIS

This type of fracture is mostly seen in young children, with peak at 3-6 years. Usually these fractures occur due to low energy force, applied to the lateral aspect of the extended knee (valgus moment), resulting in incomplete greenstick fractures. Fibula generally escapes injury, though plastic deformation may occur.

Clinical Features

Careful assessment of neurovascular

status is important, in addition to typical presentation like any other fracture.

Imaging

AP and lateral X-rays are sufficient for diagnosis of proximal tibial metaphyseal fractures.

Treatment

Even though proximal tibial metaphyseal fractures appear simple to treat, one must be aware and explain the relatives about a possible sequela known as "***Cozen phenomenon***" described by Cozen in 1953. It is the development of progressive valgus deformity in children following proximal tibia metaphyseal fracture. Proposed aetiologies for this valgus deformity are-

- Overgrowth of medial proximal tibia physis/Physeal arrest of lateral tibial physis
- Inadequate reduction
- Interposed soft tissues (Medial collateral ligament/Pes anserinus)
- Loss of tethering effect of pes anserinus
- Tethering effect of fibula
- Premature weight bearing
- Hypertrophic callus formation

Natural history of Cozen phenomenon

- Valgus deformity usually appears 4-6 months post injury and may progress for upto 18-24 months.
- Thereafter gradual restoration of normal alignment occurs over time.
- However in some children, there is persistent tibia valga 18 months post injury, with MAD(Mechanical Axis Deviation) >10°. Bracing does not have any role in this deformity correction. It requires proximal medial tibial hemiepiphysiodesis or corrective osteotomy, depending on the number of years of growth remaining. **(Fig. 25.2)**

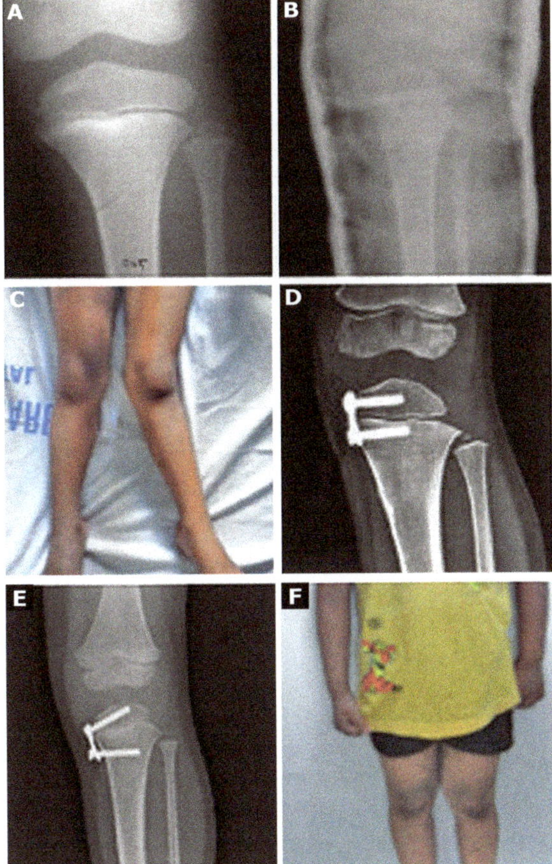

Fig. 25.2: *Cozen phenomenon (A) Undisplaced proximal tibia fracture in a 4-year-old male child (B) Treatment in above-knee cast (C) Development of progressive valgus deformity (Cozen phenomenon) (D) Treatment with growth modulation surgery using proximal medial tibial 8 plate (E) Gradual correction of deformity as evident by divergence of the screws (F) Good clinical result with correction of deformity.*

Undisplaced Proximal tibia metaphyseal fracture

Conservative treatment in long leg cast with knee in 5-10° flexion and with varus mould.

Displaced Proximal tibia metaphyseal fracture

- Closed reduction under anaesthesia
- If not successful, it may require

open reduction and removal of any interposed soft tissue and repair of the pes anserinus plate if disrupted.

- After closed/open reduction, immobilisation in long leg straight knee cast with varus mould is required. Rarely, smooth pins or external fixator may be required.
- Regular follow up is essential. In case of loss of reduction, cast wedging or repeat reduction may be necessary.

DIAPHYSEAL FRACTURES OF TIBIA AND FIBULA

- 70% paediatric tibia fractures are isolated injuries. Most of these fractures in children less than 11 years of age are oblique or spiral and are caused by torsional force, when the body rotates with the foot in a fixed position on the ground. ***(Fig. 25.3)*** Sometimes transverse or comminuted fractures are seen caused by direct trauma.

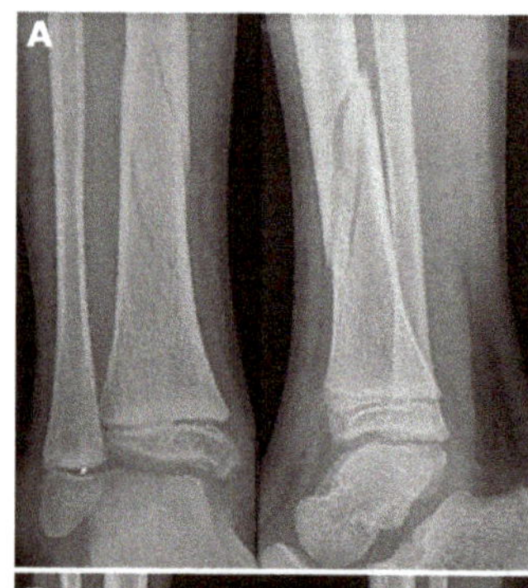

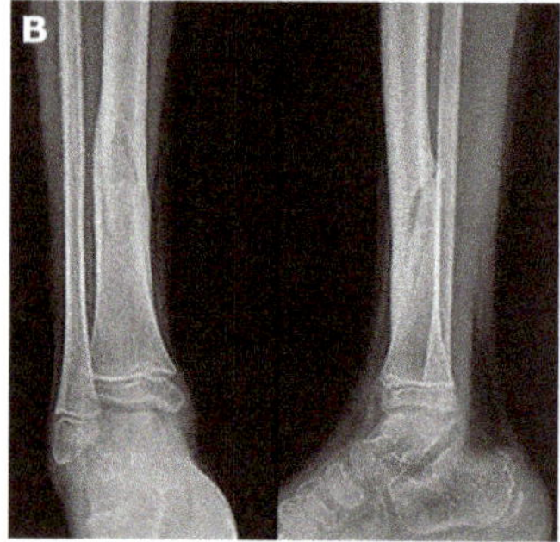

Fig. 25.3: *(A) AP and lateral X-rays of isolated spiral fracture of the tibial shaft, (B) Good union after conservative treatment in above knee cast. Shortening is prevented due to intact fibula.*

Shortening is prevented in these fractures due to intact fibula, but varus angulation occurs in around 60% children in the first 2 weeks post injury.

- 30% paediatric tibial shaft fractures are associated with fibula fracture that may be complete/incomplete or plastic deformation.

These fractures are prone for shortening and valgus malalignment.

- Rarely, fractures involve only fibula. These are mostly undisplaced fractures and treated by immobilisation in cast/ splint or sometimes symptomatically.

Clinical Features

Clinical presentation varies with severity and mechanism of injury. In addition to pain, swelling and deformity, children have refusal to walk. Careful neurological assessment, especially of common peroneal nerve is required in case of fibula neck fracture. Dorsalis pedis and posterior tibial pulsations need to be checked and if found absent, Doppler study needs to be done for assessment of perfusion. Diaphyseal fractures of tibia and fibula are prone for compartment syndrome and one must be vigilant about its symptoms and signs.

Treatment

Conservative

Majority of diaphyseal tibia-fibula fractures can be treated by casting.

Non- displaced: In situ above-knee cast

Displaced: It requires reduction under anaesthesia followed by above-knee cast. Manipulation technique is based on review of the deforming forces associated with specific fracture pattern ***(Fig. 25.4)***.

First a short leg cast is applied, extending proximally till inferior aspect of patella

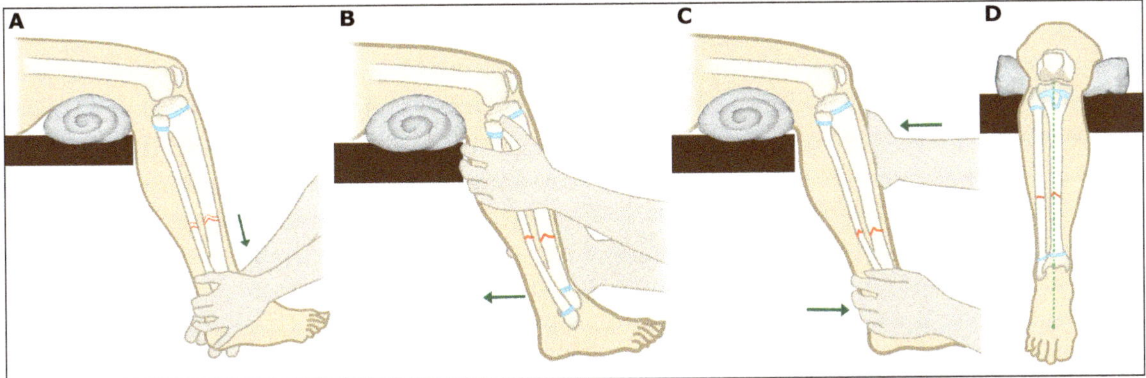

***Fig. 25.4**: Closed reduction technique for tibia shaft fracture: (A) Longitudinal traction, (B) Correction of mediolateral alignment, (C) Correction of anteroposterior alignment, (D) Correction of rotational alignment.*

anteriorly and 2 cm. distal to the popliteal flexor crease posteriorly. The plaster should be moulded well with either varus or valgus mould, depending on fracture pattern and alignment. **(Fig. 25.5A)** Ankle should initially be in some plantar flexion (20° for M/3 and L/3, 10° for U/3) to prevent generation of apex posterior angulation at fracture site.After application of such short leg cast, reduction should be confirmed under fluoroscopy.

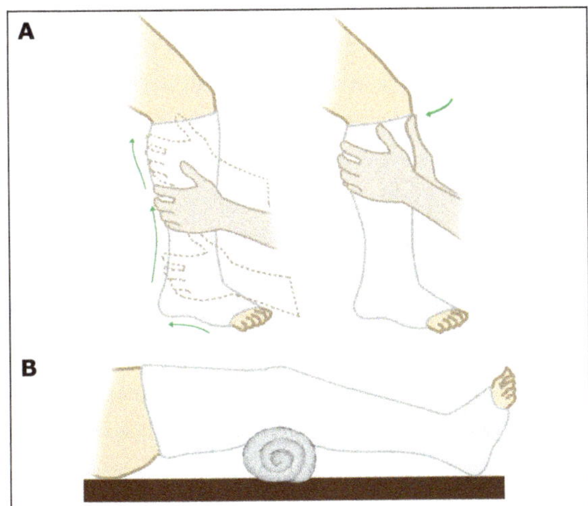

***Fig. 25.5**: Plaster application technique for tibia shaft fracture: (A) Application of below-knee cast with proper moulding. (B) Conversion to above knee cast after fluoroscopic confirmation of reduction.*

Acceptable alignment as per age is given in **Table 25.1**:

Table 25.1: Acceptability criteria for diaphyseal fractures of tibia

Age	< 8 years	≥ 8 years
Valgus	5°	5°
Varus	10°	5°
Anterior angulation	10°	5°
Posterior angulation	5°	0°
Rotation	5°	5°
Shortening	10 mm	5 mm

Moderate translation is acceptable in young children and upto 50% in adolescents.

If reduction is acceptable, the cast is converted to above-knee cast with knee in some flexion, in order to control rotation at fracture site and to ensure non-weight bearing status during initial healing phase. **(Fig. 25.5B)**

Weekly check X-rays are recommended for 3 weeks followed by one at the time of plaster removal at around six weeks.

If there is loss of reduction on follow up, cast wedging or repeat manipulation is recommended. For cast wedging, open wedge technique is preferred. Post wedging, there may be residual leg swelling and some pain. Parents are to be warned regarding this and the child should be observed for a short time for evidence of compartment syndrome.

After 4-6 weeks, cast can be changed to short leg weight bearing cast or patellar tendon bearing cast in older children **(Fig. 25.6).**

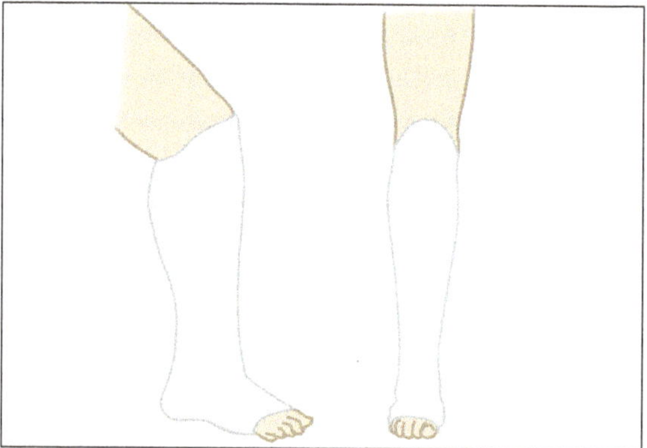

Fig. 25.6: *Patellar Tendon Bearing cast.*

Length of immobilisation varies with the child's age and type of fracture, with a younger child with an undisplaced or a minimally displaced fracture requiring only about 4 weeks of immobilisation while an older child with a displaced fracture may require 6-8 weeks of immobilisation. **(Fig. 25.7)**

Surgical

Surgical treatment is recommended for

- Unstable fractures where it is difficult to obtain or maintain alignment
- Open fractures
- Fractures with associated compartment syndrome
- Floating knee, multiple long bone fractures, multiple system injuries
- Fractures in children with spasticity (cerebral palsy, head injury)

Elastic stable intramedullary nailing (ESIN) is the preferred choice of implant, but in comminuted or highly unstable or open fractures, external fixation is used rarely, with a minimum of two pins each in proximal and distal segments of the bones. Alternatively, plate osteosynthesis is used, but it has a higher rate of wound complications.

Technique of Intramedullary nailing for Tibia shaft fracture

Position: **(Fig. 25.8)**

- Child is placed supine on a radiolucent table with a bump under the ipsilateral pelvis, to counter external rotation of the femur, so that the patella is pointed

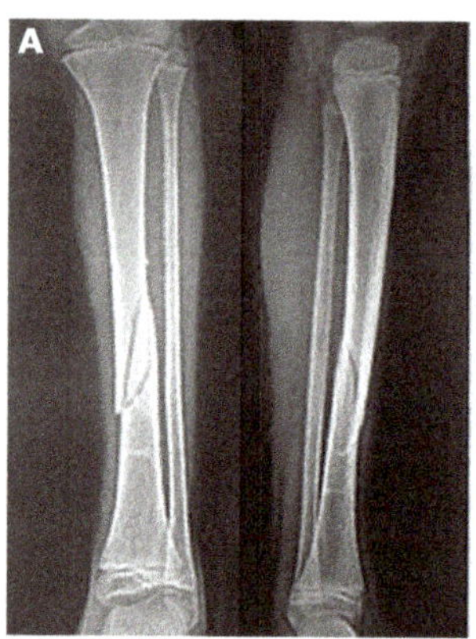

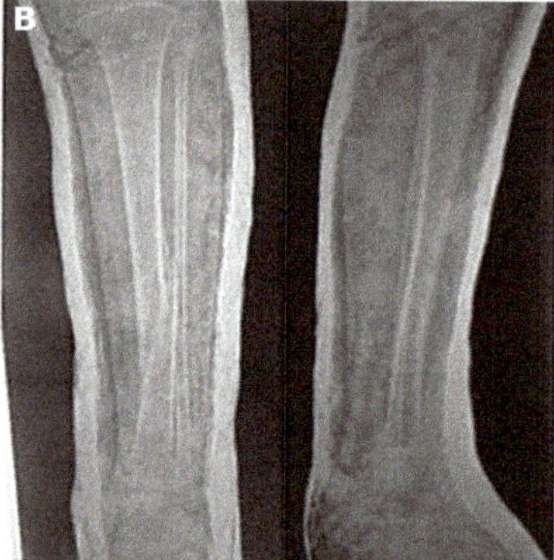

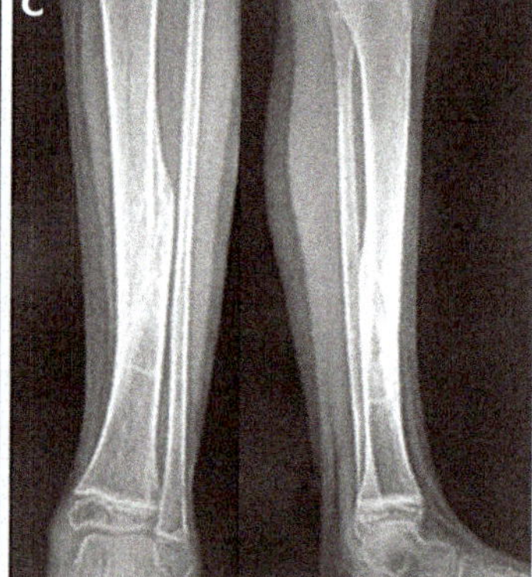

Fig. 25.7: *(A) AP and lateral X-rays of a 10-year-old child showing isolated oblique fracture of tibial diaphysis (B) Treatment with closed reduction and above-knee cast for 6 weeks (C) Union with mild varus due to the presence of intact fibula.*

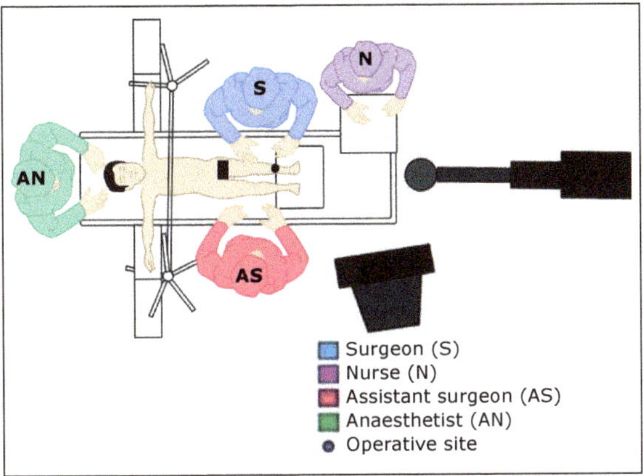

Fig. 25.8: *Supine position of the child on a radiolucent table for intramedullary nailing.*

straight vertically. The C-arm can be brought in from the opposite side of the table so that it is out of the surgeon's way.

- Tourniquet is used

Incision

Medial and lateral proximal tibial incisions are taken such that the entry point of the nail is at the distal end of the incision.

Steps

- Entry is made just proximal to the level of the tibial tubercle, at least 1 cm. distal to the proximal tibia physis **(Fig. 25.9)** and 2 cm. posterior to tibial tubercle physis, medially and laterally using drill/awl.
- The drill should be 1 to 1.5 mm. larger than the diameter of the nail.

Selection of Nail

- Stainless steel/Titanium
- Size: Two nails of equal diameter are selected such that together they occupy 80% of canal diameter.

  Nails are contoured such that there is a C shape with its apex at the fracture site and around three times the canal diameter. This will cause cortical contact at the apex, yielding 3 point fixation (proximal,cortical at fracture site and distal) **(Fig. 25.10)**

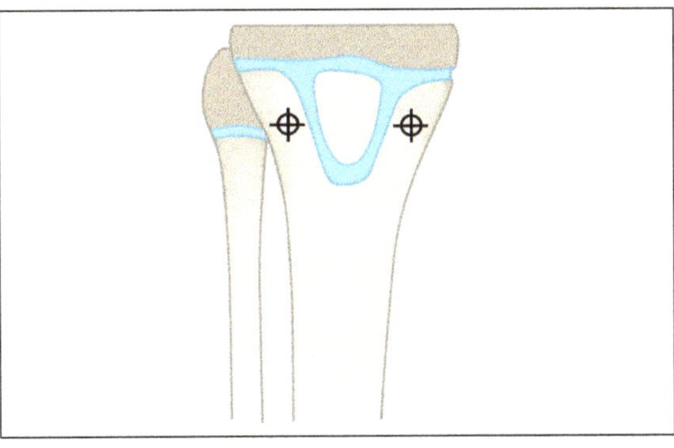

Fig. 25.9: *Entry points for the medial and lateral tibia nails at least 1 cm. distal to proximal tibial physis.*

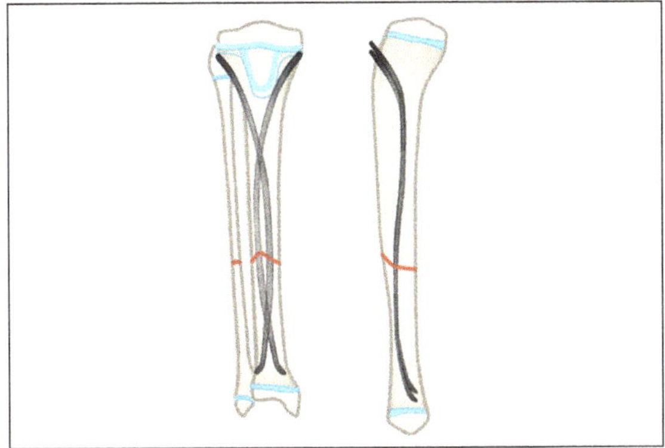

Fig. 25.10: *Fixation of tibia shaft fracture with two C-shaped elastic nails with the apex at the fracture site, yielding 3 point fixation.*

- Precontoured nails are passed till the fracture site medially and laterally using to-and-fro rocking movements and/or gentle hammering if required.
- Fracture is reduced using traction and manipulation, reduction is confirmed fluoroscopically.
- To pass the nails across the fracture, it is helpful to consider the initial deformity of the fracture.For example, if the fracture is in valgus, pass the medial nail first to apply varus force. Nails are then advanced beyond the fracture into distal metaphyses. Proximally, nails are cut close to the bone, keeping around

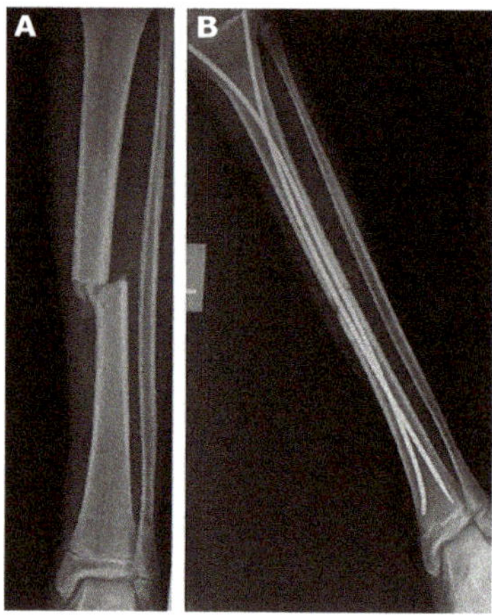

Fig. 25.11*: (A) AP X-ray showing midshaft tibia fracture in a 10-year-old child. (B) Closed reduction and fixation using elastic stable intramedullary nails.*

2 cm. out to allow easy removal later **(Fig. 25.11)**.

Post–operative Protocol

Post-operative cast application is used depending on the stability of the fracture post fixation and kept for around 3-4 weeks. Gradual weight bearing is allowed after the removal of cast.

Nails are removed 6-9 months after injury, as the nails will become completely intramedullary with significant, continued growth, thus making later removal very difficult.

FRACTURES OF DISTAL TIBIA METAPHYSIS

These fractures usually occur secondary to axial load on a dorsiflexed foot, resulting in greenstick type fracture with impaction of anterior cortex and displacement of posterior cortex under tension with a tear of overlying periosteum. This results in recurvatum and valgus deformity.

Treatment

Undisplaced fractures are immobilised in the above-knee or below-knee cast.

Displaced fractures are reduced under anaesthesia/sedation and immobilised in above-knee cast, with foot in moderate plantar flexion initially to prevent recurvatum deformity. Foot can be brought to neutral after 3-4 weeks and then short leg walking cast can be applied.

If reduction is unstable, percutaneous pinning or antegrade flexible nail can be used **(Fig. 25.12)**. Sometimes open reduction of tibia and associated fibula fracture may be required to prevent malalignment.

SPECIAL FRACTURES

Open Tibia Fractures

Though the general principles of treatment

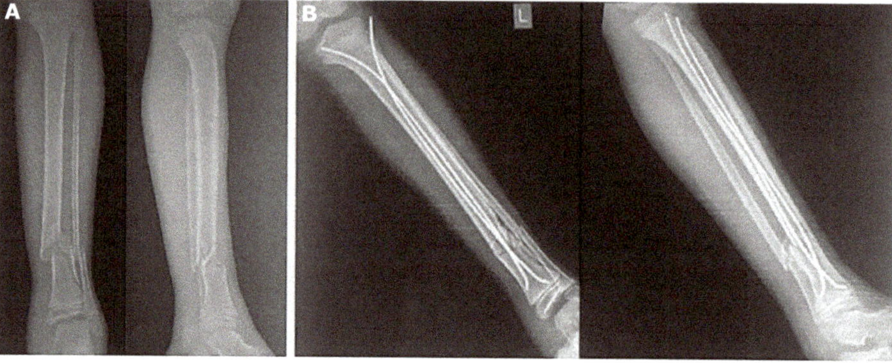

Fig. 25.12*: (A) AP and lateral X-rays of the distal tibia fibula metaphyseal fracture (B) Treatment with antegrade elastic nails.*

of open tibia fractures in children are similar to adults, there are following differences:

- In children especially <11 years, comparable soft tissue and bony injuries heal more reliably.
- Devitalised bone that is not contaminated and that can be covered with soft tissues can incorporate into fracture callus, hence can be left within the wound in some cases.
- In younger children, retained periosteum can regenerate bone even after segmental bone loss.
- In uncontaminated grade I open wounds, primary closure may be done after thorough irrigation and debridement, without any increased risk of infection.

The safe zones at different levels of the leg for the insertion of pins of external fixator are shown in **Fig. 25.13.**

- External fixator can work as definitive treatment and can be maintained if necessary until fracture consolidation. **(Fig. 25.14)**
- Use of negative pressure dressings can be effectively used in the management of open tibia fractures.

Vascular injuries are seen in around 5% of open tibia fractures. Management principles are similar to adults (Rate of amputation is around 79%). Isolated anterior tibial and peroneal artery injuries have good prognosis, whereas posterior tibial and popliteal artery injuries have poor prognosis and more commonly require vascular repair

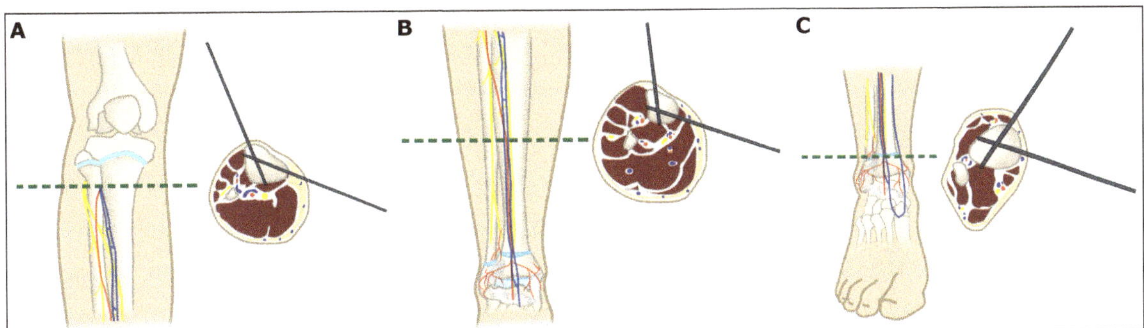

Fig. 25.13: *Safe zones for insertion of pins of external fixator: (A) Proximal third, (B) Mid shaft, (C) Distal third.*

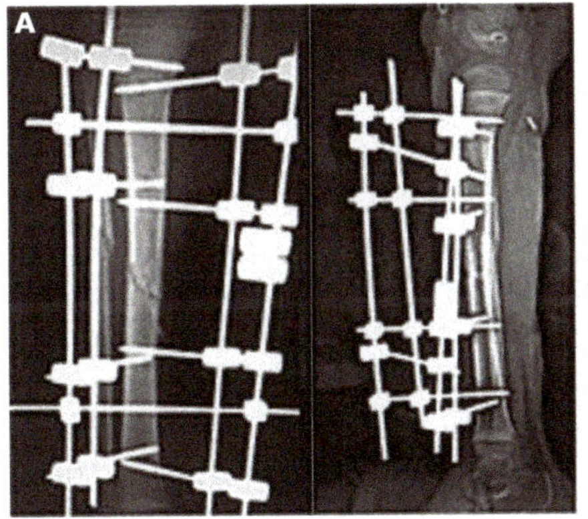

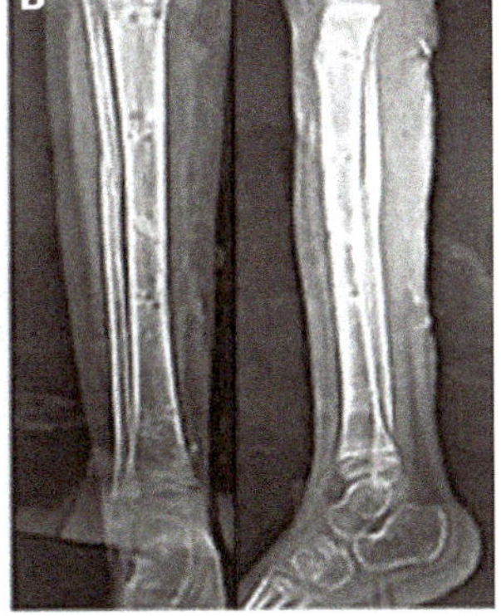

Fig. 25.14: *(A) Compound M/3 tibia-fibula fractures treated with external fixator, (B) External fixator removed after fracture union.*

or reconstruction. It is important to stabilise the fracture with external/ internal fixation before vascular reconstruction.

Toddler's Fractures

- In children < 6 years, a minor twisting injury with external rotation of foot in a flexed knee leads to spiral fracture of tibia, mostly distal metaphysis, without a concomitant fibula fracture. This is known as Toddler's fracture.
- Clinical presentation is usually subtle with minimal swelling, tenderness and limp/refusal to bear weight.
- In addition to AP and lateral X-rays, internal oblique X-ray may be required to diagnose undisplaced fracture.
- Treatment consists of immobilisation in below/above-knee cast (as per age) for 3-4 weeks. In case of stable fracture, weight bearing is permitted once the child is comfortable.

Stress Fracture

Stress fractures occur mainly in proximal third tibia or occasionally distal third fibula, following repetitive stress. Clinically, it presents as insidious onset of dull aching pain, worsening with sports activities and associated with minimal swelling. X-rays may be normal initially, but may show periosteal new bone formation, endosteal thickening and radiolucent cortical fracture line after 2 weeks. CT scan/MRI may be helpful for differentiating from infection/sarcoma/ soft tissue injury.

Stress fracture is treated by activity modification and walking boot for 4-6 weeks with gradual resumption of activities.

Complications

1. Compartment syndrome

   This can occur after any type of tibia fracture like minor, closed fracture to severe, comminuted and open fracture. Children treated with flexible intramedullary nails, especially in heavy weight children (>50 kg.) and more complex or comminuted fracture patterns may also develop compartment syndrome.

   The typical clinical presentation, as described in chapter no. 5 should be looked for and treated as per the provided guidelines. Otherwise late complications occur in the form of clawed toes, dorsal bunion, limited subtalar movements secondary to necrosis and fibrous contracture of deep posterior compartment muscles.

2. Vascular injuries: Uncommon

   Displaced proximal tibial metaphyseal fractures are most frequently associated with anterior tibial artery injury where it passes between fibula and tibia into the anterior compartment. Also, in posteriorly displaced distal tibia fracture, anterior tibial artery can be injured by the anterior spike of proximal fragment. Hence careful clinical evaluation and appropriate treatment is mandatory.

3. Angular deformity

   The goal of treatment in tibia shaft fractures should be to obtain as close to anatomic alignment as possible, since remodelling of an angular deformity is often incomplete (especially for valgus >5-7° and recurvatum >10° and also in cases of multiplanar deformities). Also, spontaneous remodelling occurs only in the first 18 months after fracture.

   As per literature, angular correction occurs upto 50% in 9-12 years old girls and 11-12 years old boys whereas angular correction occurs only upto 25% in children >13 years.

4. Malrotation

- There is no spontaneous rotational

correction after malunion, hence it should be avoided.

- CT scan is required to measure the amount of rotational deformity.
- >10° malrotation is functionally significant and may require supramalleolar derotational osteotomy.
- Additional fibula osteotomy is required for > 20° rotational correction.

5. Limb length discrepancy

Just like in femur shaft fracture, hyperaemia associated with tibia fracture (especially in younger children with comminuted fracture) can stimulate physes and cause lengthening of average 4-5 mm.

6. Delayed union and Non union

- More common after high energy tibia fracture.
- Inadequate immobilisation or use of an external fixator in open fracture may lead to delayed /non union.
- In case of suspected delayed /non union, 1 cm. fibulectomy may increase compression at the non union site with weight bearing and often induce healing.
- If an external fixator is being used, dynamise the fixator at the earliest to maximise bone healing.
- Posterolateral bone grafting is another useful technique for achieving union.
- In older children/adolescents nearing skeletal maturity, reamed intra-medullary nail, fibula osteotomy and correction of angulation at the non union site is recommended.

7. Anterior tibial physeal closure

This can occur due to damage to physis while passing K-wire or external fixator or due to concomitant physeal injury.

It leads to genu recurvatum deformity and may require corrective osteotomy.

Flowchart 25.1

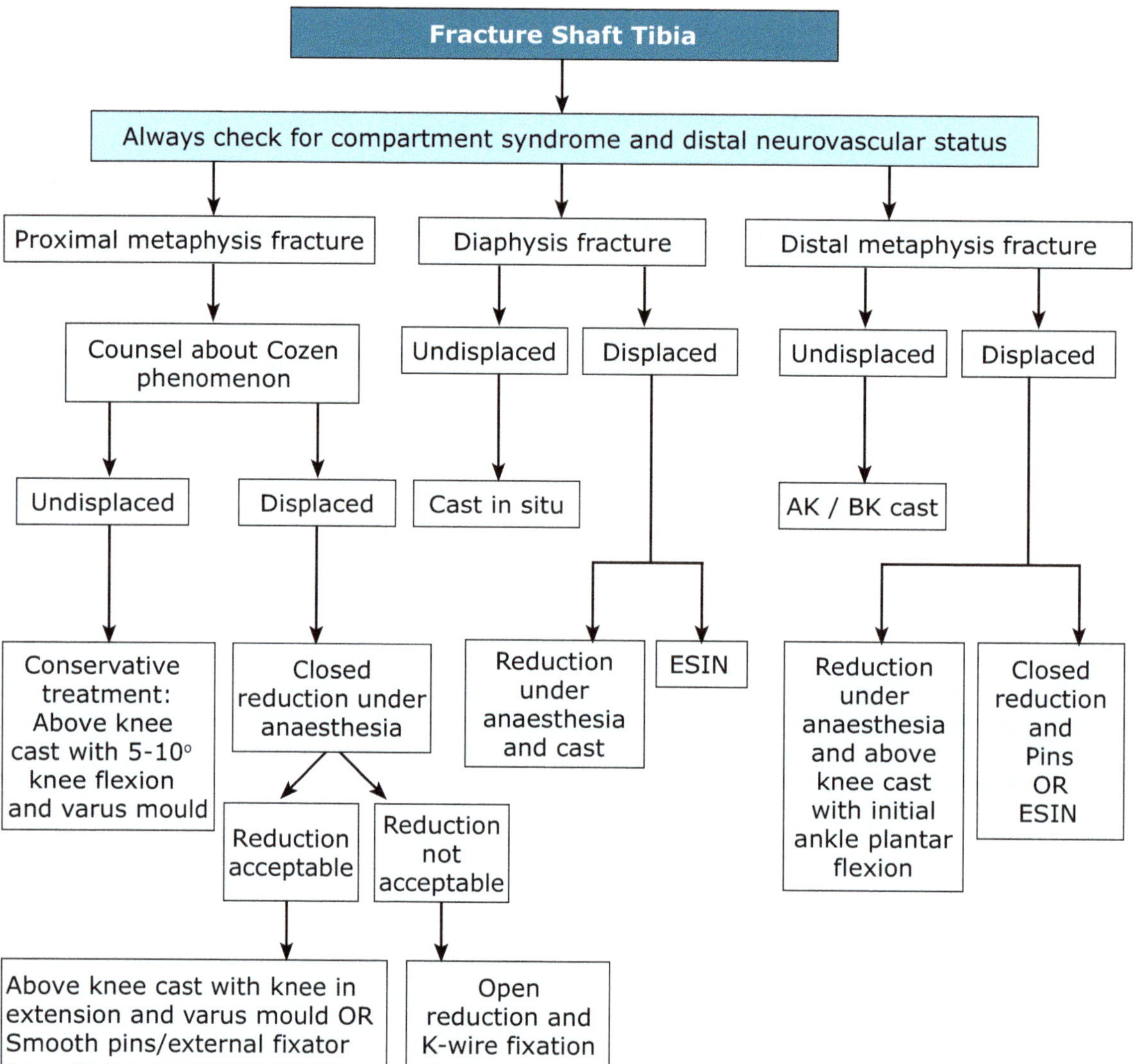

26 Fractures Around the Ankle

Introduction

Ankle injuries are the third most common physeal injuries, comprising 25-38% of all physeal fractures. Ankle injuries are common between 10–15 years of age, usually require operative intervention and are prone for premature growth arrest.

Relevant Pathoanatomy

Ankle is a hinge joint, where distal tibia and fibula are stabilised into ankle mortise by four ligamentous structures, of which three are in the syndesmosis and one is the interosseous ligament.

- *Syndesmotic ligaments:*

1. Anterior inferior tibiofibular ligament (important in pathomechanics of 'transitional' ankle fracture)
2. Posterior inferior tibiofibular ligament
3. Inferior transverse ligament

   Syndesmotic injuries are uncommon in children.

- The Interosseous ligament is important in pathomechanics of incisural fracture.

  Additionally, there are medial deltoid and lateral collateral ligaments that originate distal to tibial and fibular physes. **(Figs. 26.1 and 26.2)** These ligaments are stronger than the physes and hence physeal fractures are more common than ligament injuries in children.

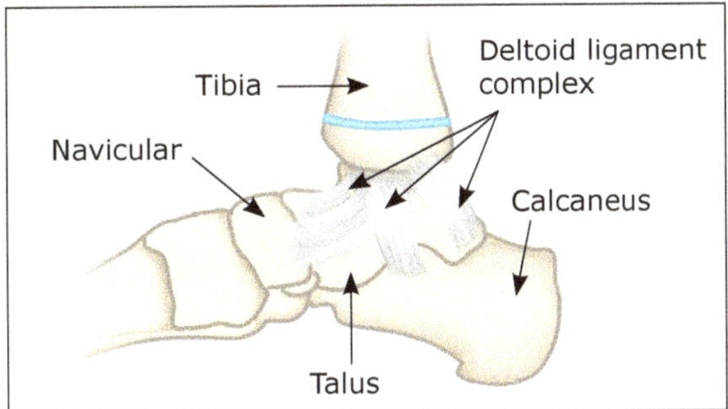

***Fig. 26.1**: Medial collateral ligaments around the ankle.*

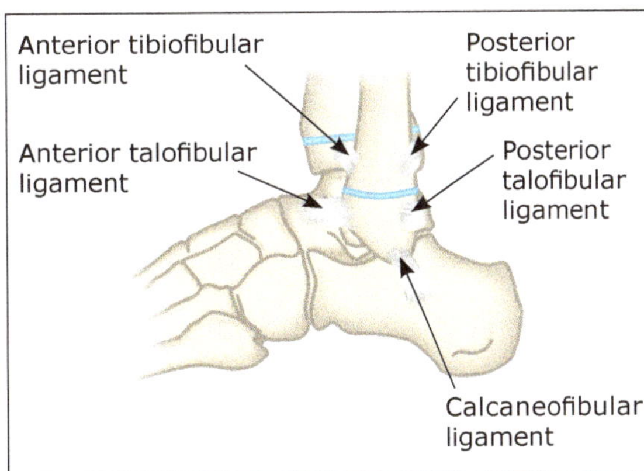

***Fig. 26.2**: Lateral collateral ligaments around the ankle.*

Classification and Mechanism of Injury

The most widely used classification based on mechanism of injury is by *Dias and Tachdjian*. There are four main types. In each type, the first word describes the position of the foot at the time of injury and the second word describes the force that produced the injury. **(Fig. 26.3)**

1) Supination–Inversion (SI)

- This injury occurs when an inversion force is applied to the supinated foot **(Fig. 26.4)**
- Grade I : Inversion/adduction force

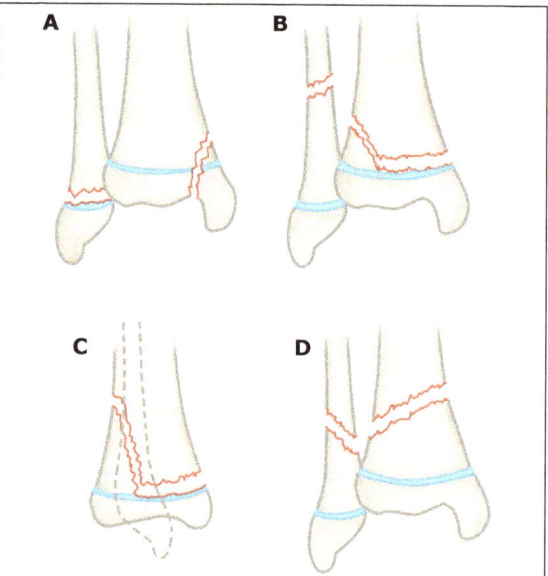

Fig. 26.3: *Dias –Tachdjian classification of ankle fractures:*
(A) Supination Inversion
(B) Pronation Eversion External rotation
(C) Supination Plantar flexion
(D) Pronation External rotation

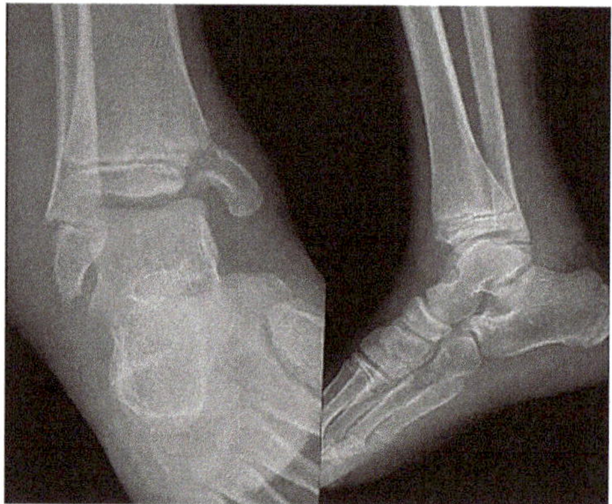

Fig. 26.4: *Supination–Inversion(SI) injury with S-H type I fracture of distal fibula and S-H type IV fracture of distal tibia.*

leads to avulsion of the distal fibular epiphysis (S-H type I or II)

Rarely, there is transepiphyseal fracture or failure of lateral ligament.

- Grade II : Further inversion leads to tibial fracture, mostly S-H type III or IV

Rarely, there is S-H type I or II fracture or fracture is trans epiphyseal through medial malleolus.

2) Pronation–Eversion–External Rotation (PEER)

- This injury occurs when an eversion and external rotation force is applied to the fully pronated foot. **(Fig. 26.5)**

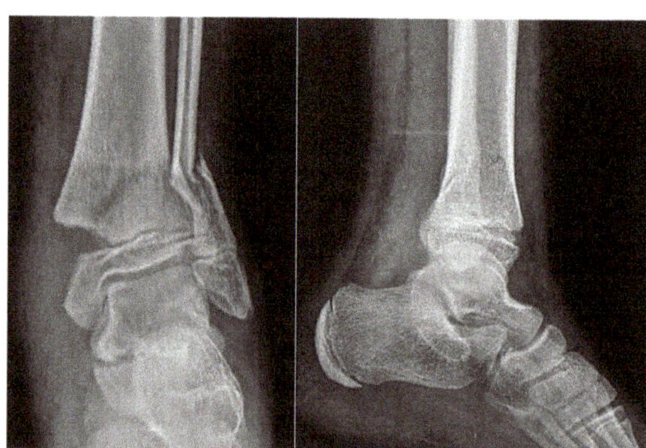

Fig. 26.5: *Pronation- Eversion- External rotation (PEER) injury with S-H type II fracture of distal tibia and short oblique fracture of fibula.*

- This mechanism leads to S-H type I or II fracture of distal tibia, with lateral/posterolateral displacement of metaphyseal fragment.
- Rarely, there is trans-epiphyseal fracture through medial malleolus (S-H type II).
- There is simultaneous transverse or short oblique fibula fracture, located 4-7 cm. proximal to the tip of the lateral malleolus.
- PEER injuries can rarely be associated with diastasis of the ankle joint.

3) Supination – Plantar flexion (SPF)

- This injury occurs when the foot is fixed in full supination while a plantar flexion force is exerted on the ankle. **(Fig. 26.6)**

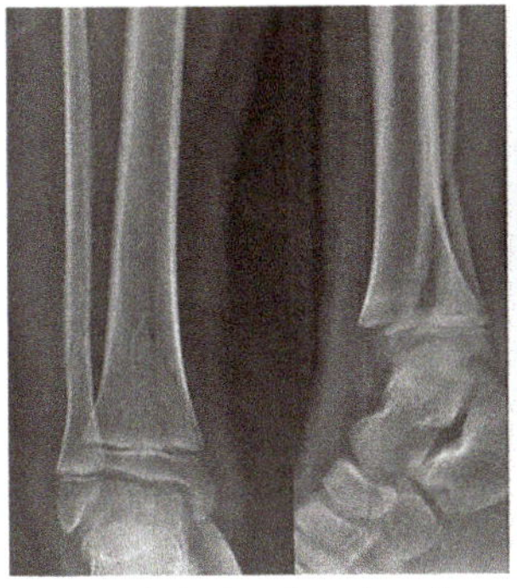
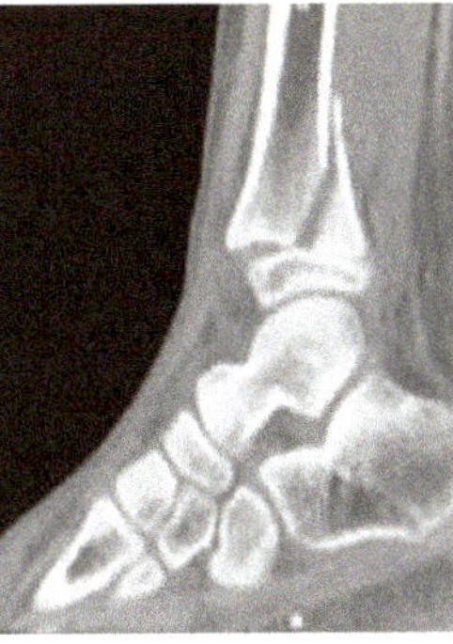

Fig. 26.6*: Supination- plantar flexion(SPF) injury with posteriorly displaced S-H type II fracture of distal tibia and an associated fibula fracture.*

- Plantar flexion leads to S-H type I or II fracture of distal tibia, with posterior displacement. It may be difficult to see this fracture on AP X-ray.
- Rarely there is an associated fracture of fibula.

4) Supination –External rotation (SER)

- This injury occurs when the foot is fixed in full supination while an external rotation force is exerted on the ankle. **(Fig. 26.7)**
- Grade I: External rotation force leads to S-H type II fracture of distal tibia, with posterior displacement, with fracture line extending proximally and medially (Unlike in Supination –Plantar flexion type, metaphyseal fragment is visible on AP X-ray).
- Grade II: Further external rotation leads to spiral fracture of fibula, fracture line extending from anteroinferior to posterosuperior.

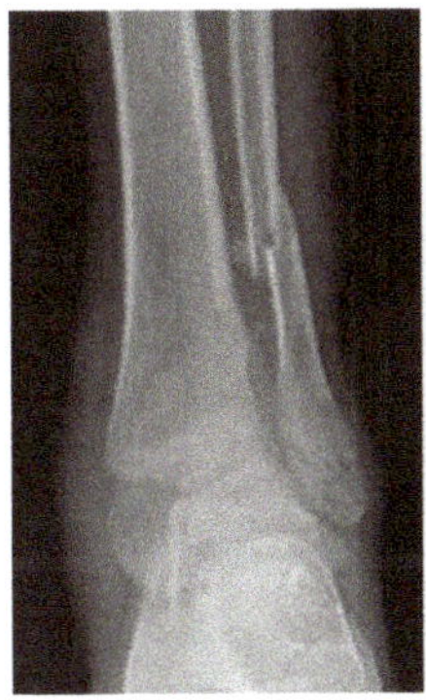
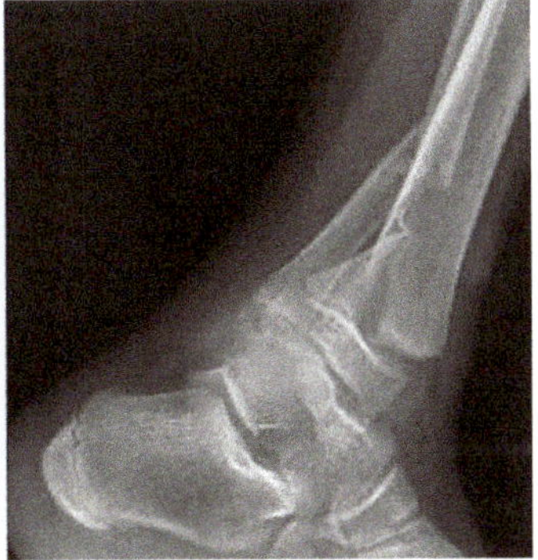

Fig. 26.7*: Supination-external rotation (SER) injury with posteriorly displaced S-H type II fracture of distal tibia and fracture of fibula, with fracture line extending from anteroinferior to posterosuperior.*

Axial compression (Rare, < 1% of ankle injuries)

This is S-H type V injury of distal tibia physis, usually diagnosed late when there is growth arrest, as initial X-ray may not show any abnormality.

Transitional Fractures

As the name suggests, these fractures occur during the transition from a skeletally immature to skeletally mature ankle during 18 months period of asymmetric closure of distal tibial physis (central-medial-lateral-complete). **(Fig. 26.8)**

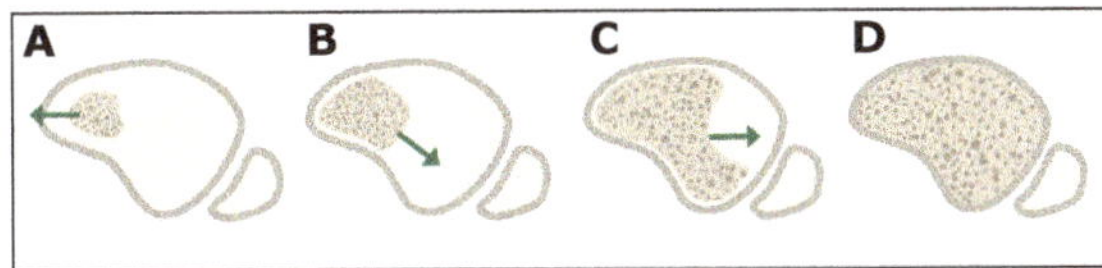

Fig. 26.8*: Pattern of closure of the distal tibial physis: (A) Central, (B) Medial, (C) Lateral, (D) Complete.*

Juvenile Tillaux fractures (Named after French surgeon Tillaux)

External rotation of foot causes S-H type III fracture involving anterolateral distal tibia, due to avulsion of anteroinferior tibiofibular ligament. Here, portion of the physis not involved in the fracture is closed. **(Fig. 26.9)**

Triplane fracture

Triplane fractures are a unique group of fractures appearing as S-H type III fracture on AP and S-H type II fracture on lateral X-ray but in reality are S-H type

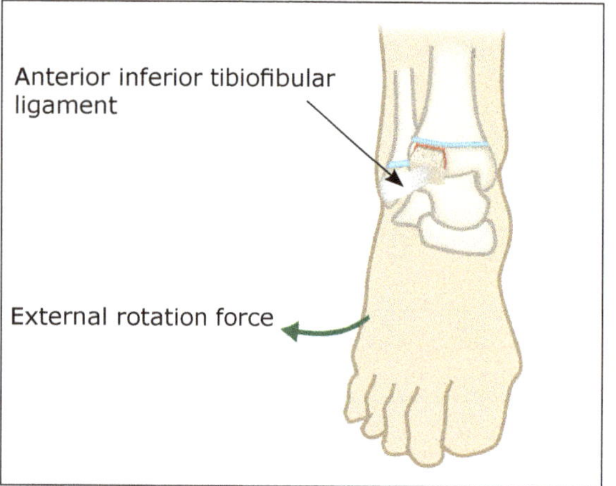

***Fig. 26.9**: Mechanism of injury of Tillaux fracture-External rotation of foot with avulsion of anteroinferior tibiofibular ligament leading to S-H type III fracture of anterolateral distal tibia.*

IV fractures as a whole. **(Figs. 26.10 and 26.11)**

Adolescent pilon fracture

This is a very rare injury in children which involves a tibial plafond fracture with articular and physeal involvement, variable tibial and fibular involvement, variable comminution and usually with greater than 5 mm displacement.

Incisura fracture

This is an avulsion fracture of the distal tibia by the interosseous ligament (variant of adult tibio-fibular diastasis injury). Though it looks like Tillaux fracture on standard X-ray, the size of the fragment

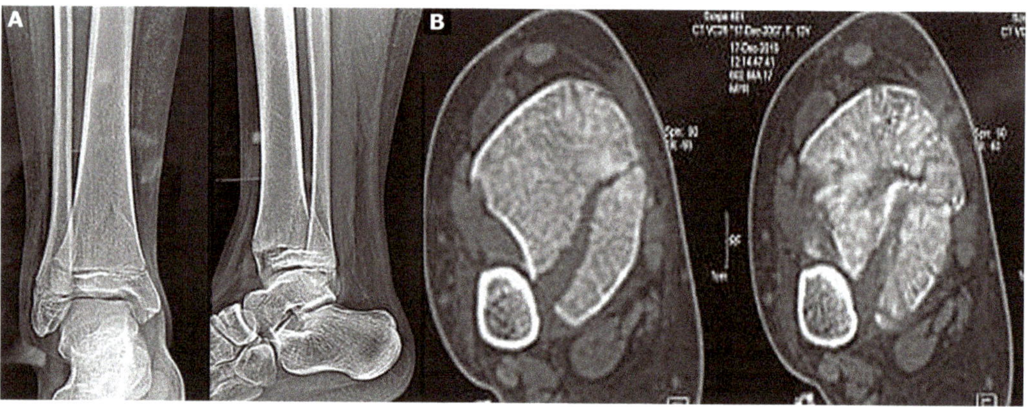

***Fig. 26.10**: (A) Displaced triplane fracture in a 14-year-old male, appearing as S-H type III in AP and S-H type II in lateral view. (B) CT scan is helpful in demarcating the fracture pattern.*

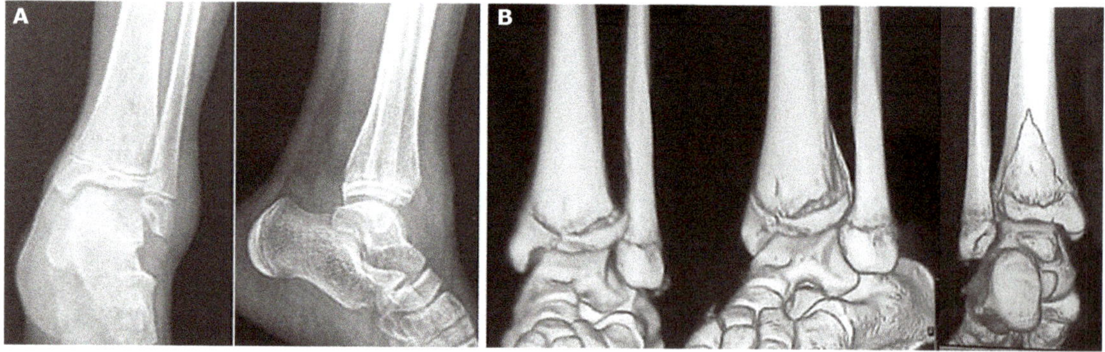

***Fig. 26.11**: (A) AP and lateral X-rays of the ankle showing minimally displaced Triplane fracture in a 13-year-old girl. (B) 3-D CT scan confirms the fracture pattern.*

is smaller and fracture does not include attachment of anterior-inferior tibiofibular ligament.

Syndesmotic injury of distal tibia and fibula

It is a rare injury, usually associated with proximal and distal fibular fracture, Tillaux fracture and S-H type I fracture of tibia.

Clinical Features

- Displaced fractures can be easily diagnosed with severe pain, swelling and typical deformity.
- The type of deformity and position of the foot in relation to the leg can give an idea about the mechanism of injury and guide regarding reduction manoeuvre.
- Compartment syndrome is likely in very severe injuries and proper examination of neurovascular status is important.
- Local skin condition needs to be checked for decision regarding timing of surgery.

Imaging

- In children with obvious deformity/ suspected displaced fracture, AP, lateral and Mortise view have to be taken.
- In children with subtle clinical presentation/suspected non displaced fractures, X-rays need to be taken if there is pain near a malleolus with inability to bear weight or tenderness to palpation at the malleoli.

To avoid overtreatment/undertreatment, it is also important to know certain normal radiological variants in some children:

- There are accessory ossification centres (~20% on the medial side and ~1% on the lateral side) **(Fig. 26.12)**

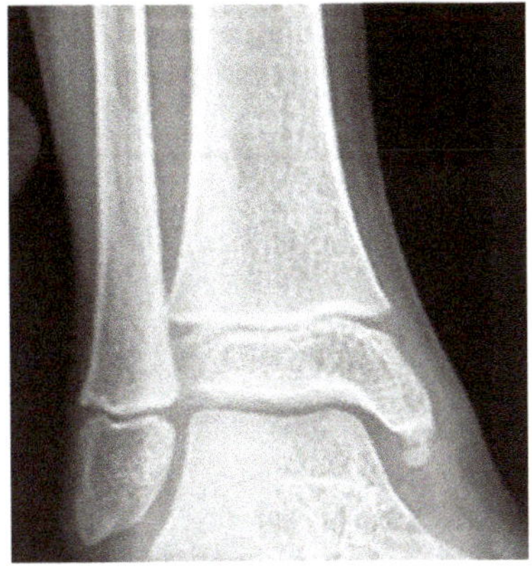

***Fig. 26.12**: AP X-ray of the ankle showing accessory ossification centre of the medial malleolus. Note the smooth margin of the fragment to differentiate it from a fracture.*

- There are clefts on the lateral and medial sides of distal tibial epiphysis. These may be confused with fractures.
- Bump on the distal fibula may simulate a torus fracture.
- Apparent offset of distal fibular epiphysis may simulate a fracture.

For occult fractures, USG can be helpful. For complex fracture of distal tibia and ankle and rare osteochondral injuries, MRI is helpful.

CT scan and 3-D reconstruction are essential for intra-articular fractures, especially juvenile Tillaux and Triplane fractures. **(Fig. 26.13)**

Treatment

The goal of treatment is to restore anatomy and function of the ankle. The treatment is based on the age of the child, location of fracture and degree of displacement.

Distal Tibia Fractures

S-H Type I Fracture

- S-H I fracture of distal tibia is rare (~15%) and can occur by any of the four

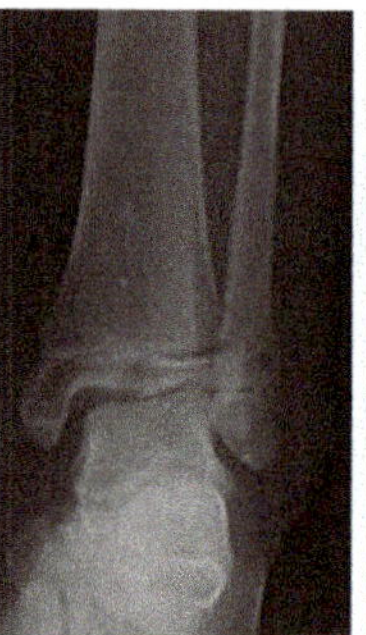
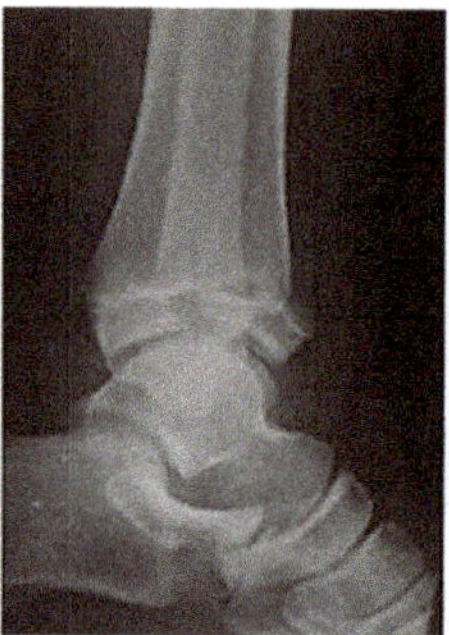
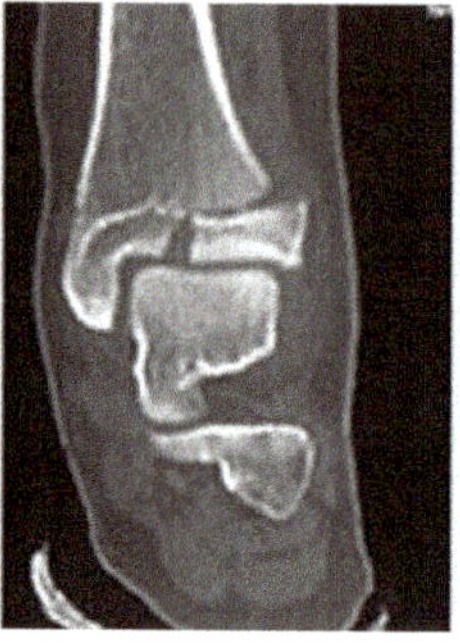
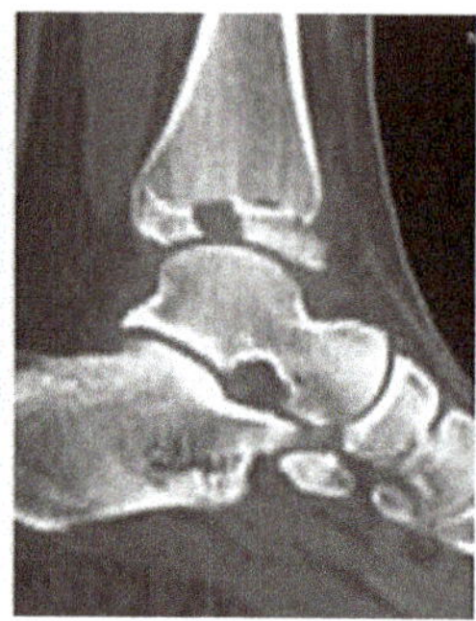
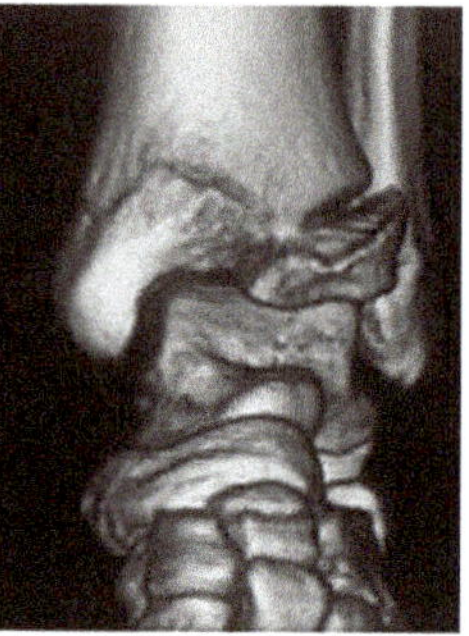

***Fig. 26.13**: AP and lateral X-rays, CT scan and 3 D reconstruction images showing Tillaux fracture.*

mechanisms- SI, SER, PEER and SPF. Associated fibula fracture is seen in ~ 25% of cases.

- The mechanism of injury can be known by direction of displacement of distal tibial epiphysis (for example, posterior in SPF, posteromedial in SER and posterolateral in PEER) and types of associated fibula fracture (lower spiral in SER, high/oblique/transverse in PEER and usually no fracture in SPF).
- Treatment consists of gentle closed reduction with reversal of original mechanism of injury and above-knee non-weight-bearing cast for 3-4 weeks, followed by below-knee walking cast for additional 2 weeks. In unstable fracture, K-wire fixation is essential, followed by below-knee cast and pins are removed by 2-3 weeks.

S-H Type II Fracture

- S-H II fracture of distal tibia is the most common (~ 40%).

  Associated fibula fracture is seen in ~ 20% of cases.
- S-H type II fracture of distal tibia also can occur by any of the four mechanisms- SI, SER (most common, >50%), PEER and SPF.
- The mechanism of injury can be known by the direction of displacement of metaphyseal Thurston- Holland fragment.

  Lateral fragment: PEER

  Posteromedial fragment: SER

  Posterior fragment: SPF
- Non-displaced fractures can be treated in the initial above-knee cast for 3-4 weeks, followed by below-knee cast for another 3-4 weeks.

Technique of Closed Reduction for displaced S-H type I and II distal tibia fracture

A gentle closed reduction should be performed under sedation or general anaesthesia (GA) to allow muscle relaxation so that further injury to the physis is limited.

Position

- Flex the knee 90° and plantar flex the foot to relax the triceps surae.
- An assistant applies countertraction to the thigh while the surgeon holds the foot at the heel and stabilises the distal tibia with the opposite hand.

Steps

- First apply axial traction on the distal segment in line with the deformity.
- Then, reduce the fracture by manipulating the distal fragment in a direction opposite the initial deforming force, for example in SI injury, the foot is pronated and everted. **(Fig. 26.14)**

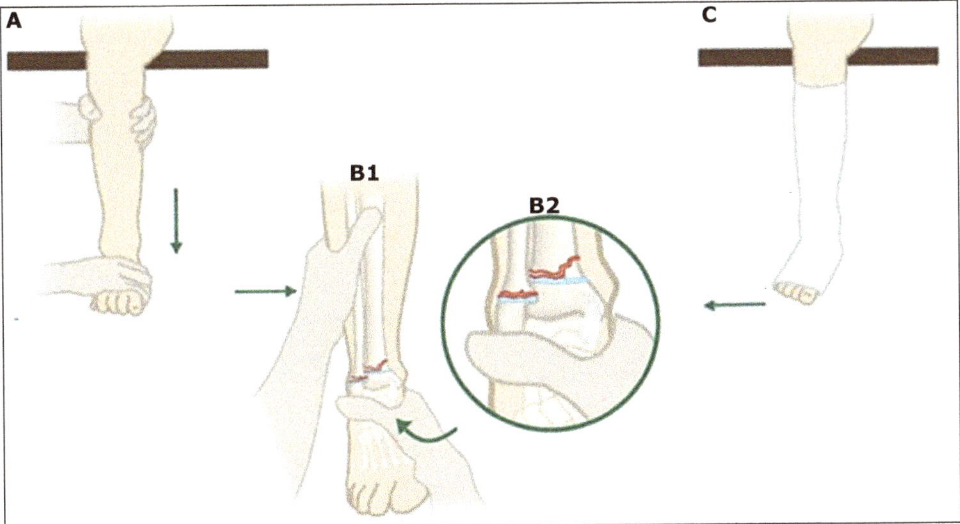

Fig. 26.14: *Technique of closed reduction of displaced S-H I and II distal tibia fractures:*
(A) Gentle traction
(B) Reversal of the mechanism of injury (pronation and eversion for supination-inversion injury)
(C) Initial application of below-knee cast

- Confirm reduction under fluoroscopy.
- There is controversy regarding acceptable limits and need for reduction.

  For displaced fractures in children with at least 3 years growth remaining, following residual deformities are acceptable.

  10-15° plantar tilt for posteriorly displaced fracture

  5-10° valgus for laterally displaced fracture

  0° varus for medially displaced fracture

  For <2 years of growth remaining, acceptable angulation is <5° for all.
- First, a below-knee cast is applied and then extended above the knee. **(Fig. 26.15)**
- After closed reduction, if the fracture is unstable, smooth pins or percutaneous screw fixation in the Thurston Holland metaphyseal fragment can be used to stabilise the fracture. **(Fig. 26.16)**

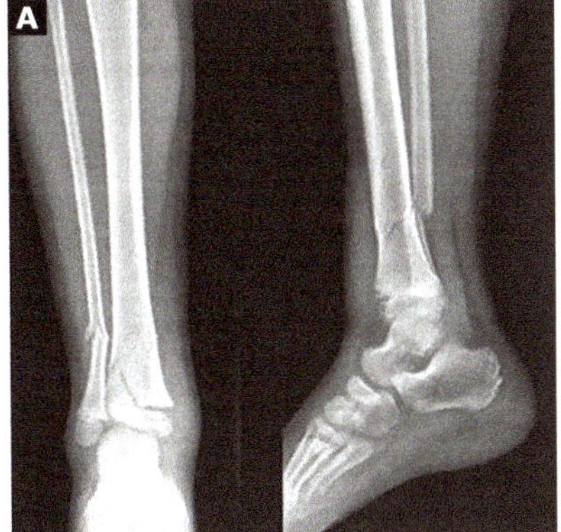

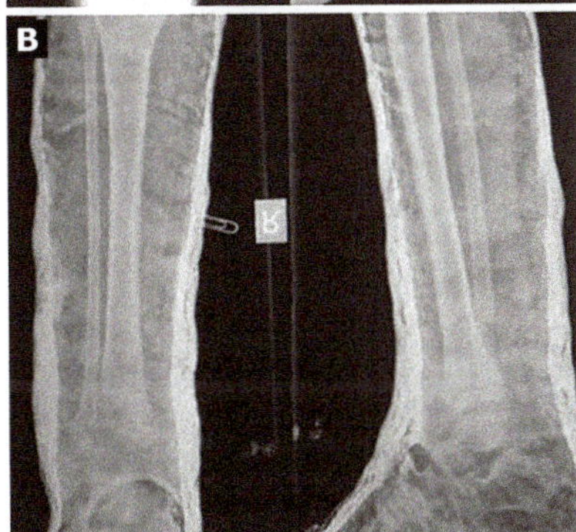

Fig. 26.15: *(A) Minimally displaced PEER injury with S-H type II distal tibia fracture and transverse distal fibula fracture (B) Treatment with closed reduction and above-knee cast.*

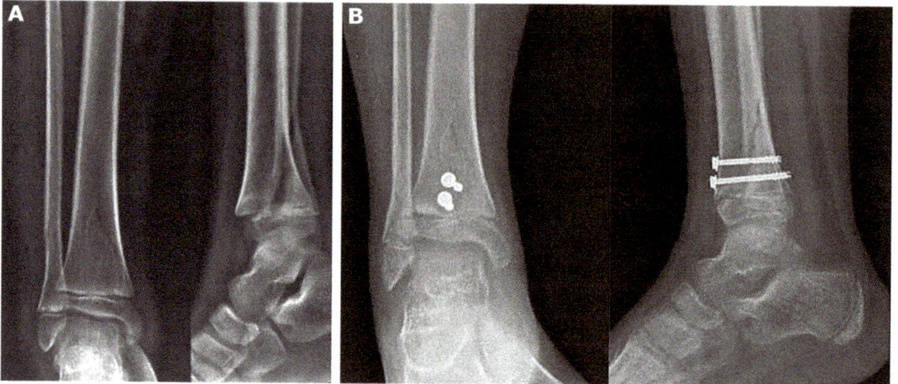

Fig. 26.16: *(A) AP and lateral X-rays of the ankle showing SPF injury with posteriorly displaced S-H type II fracture of distal tibia (B) Closed reduction and percutaneous fixation with two 4 mm cancellous screws.*

- After closed reduction, if there is physeal widening, it may be due to interposed periosteal flap or neurovascular structures. Open reduction is required to remove the interposed soft tissue **(Fig. 26.17)**. The risk of premature physeal closure is ~60% with >3 mm and ~17% with < 3 mm physeal widening.
- If the fracture presents after 7-10 days, it is better to leave it alone and do a corrective osteotomy later as the risk of iatrogenic physeal damage and arrest are high.
- Multiple variables like energy of initial injury, amount of displacements, number of reduction attempts and age of the patient determine the possibility of early physeal closure.

S-H Type III and IV Fracture

- S-H type III and IV fracture constitutes 20% of all distal tibia fractures in children. Associated fibula fracture occurs in ~ 25% of cases.
- S-H type III and IV fracture of distal tibia occurs in supination-inversion injury. The epiphyseal fracture component is always medial (unlike Tillaux fracture)

For non displaced fracture, CT scan is a must to confirm the fracture configuration. It can be treated in a non-weight-bearing above-knee cast for

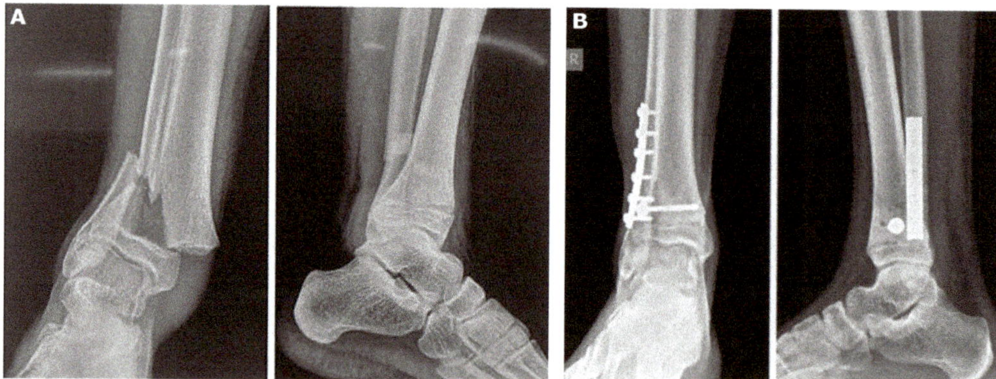

Fig. 26.17: *(A) AP and lateral X-rays of the ankle showing PEER injury (B) Open reduction and internal fixation with metaphyseal 4 mm cancellous screw for distal tibia and 3.5 mm reconstruction plate for distal fibula.*

4-6 weeks, followed by a short leg cast for another 4 weeks. The initial plaster cast should be placed with the foot in around 10° eversion with a good mould on the medial aspect of the ankle. Serial check X-ray/CT scan may be required in the first 2 weeks.

- For >2 mm displaced fracture, anatomical reduction is a must, otherwise articular incongruity may lead to post traumatic arthritis, child may become symptomatic 5-8 years after skeletal maturity.

Technique of open reduction (Fig. 26.18)

Position

Supine. Tourniquet is used.

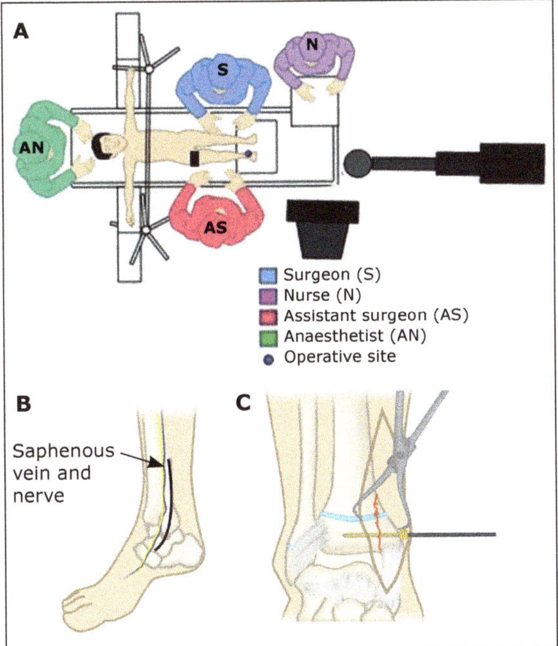

Fig. 26.18: Open reduction and internal fixation of type IV S-H distal tibia fracture:
(A) Supine position with tourniquet
(B) Medial approach to ankle
(C) Reduction held with a bone-reduction forceps and cannulated screw passed over guide wire in the epiphyseal fragment, parallel to the joint

Incision

- For S-H type III fracture, reduction may be attempted by mini open arthrotomy through a small 3-4 cm. incision in the interval between extensor digitorum longus (EDL) and extensor hallucis longus (EHL).
- For S-H type IV fracture, open reduction and internal fixation through medial approach is recommended.A curvilinear skin incision is taken over medial aspect of ankle such that it allows direct viewing of the intra-articular as well as metaphyseal fragment.

Steps

- The saphenous vein and nerve are identified and retracted posteriorly .
- The intra-articular and metaphyseal fragments are clearly identified.
- The reduction is performed with a bone-reduction forceps and confirmed under fluoroscopy.
- The fracture is fixed with smooth pins/3.5 or 4 mm cancellous screws/ bioabsorbable pins or screws. The screws should be parallel to physis, within epiphysis/metaphysis **(Fig. 26.19)**
- Post-operatively, a long-leg cast immobilisation is required for 3-4 weeks,followed by a short-leg cast for additional 3 weeks with progressive weight bearing.
- After S-H III and IV fractures, monitoring of the distal tibial physis with serial X-rays and/or scanogram is recommended every 6 months. If growth arrest is suspected, screw removal followed by CT or MRI is necessary to know the status of the physis.

S-H Type V Fracture

- Extremely rare

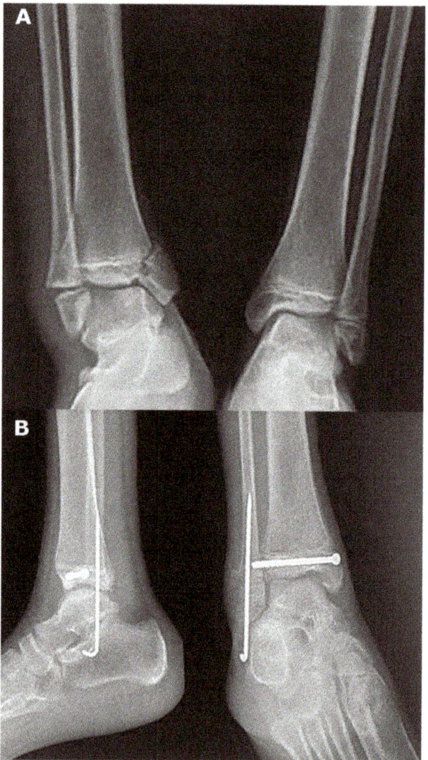

Fig. 26.19: *Open reduction and internal fixation of SI injury with epiphyseal 4 mm cancellous screw for S-H type IV fracture of distal tibia and K-wire fixation for S-H type I fracture of distal fibula.*

- Due to damage to the germinal layer of physis, growth arrest is likely after this fracture.

Diagnosis in the acute stage is difficult and no specific treatment is recommended.

Juvenile Tillaux Fracture

Mortise view or CT scan is required for diagnosis of this fracture.

- Non displaced/< 2 mm displaced fractures can be treated in above-knee cast with knee in 30° flexion and foot in neutral/internal rotation.
- > 2 mm displaced fractures require closed reduction by internal rotation of foot and manual pressure over anterolateral tibia. Once reduction is achieved, percutaneous K-wire or screw can be used for providing stability **(Fig. 26.20)**.

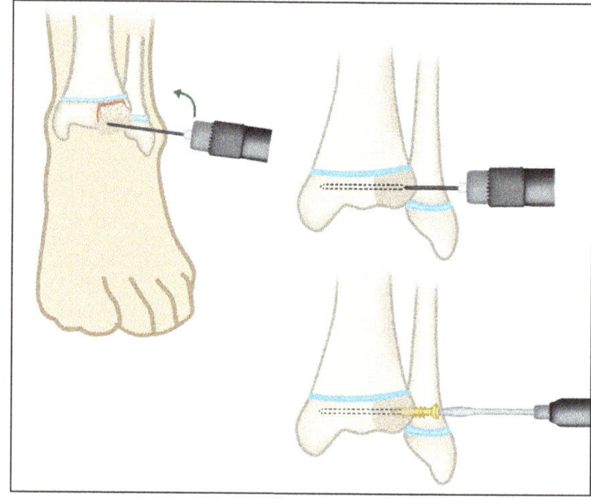

Fig. 26.20: *Technique of closed reduction by internal rotation of foot and percutaneous K-wire or screw fixation for Tillaux fracture.*

- If the fracture cannot be reduced closed, open reduction/percutaneous reduction with K-wires as joystick or arthroscopic assistance can be used. It is better to use a 4 mm. partially threaded screw for compression across the fracture site if the fragment is large **(Fig. 26.21)**.
- Open reduction is performed through an anterior approach between EDL and EHL tendon interval to allow direct observation of the fracture fragment.

Fracture of the incisura

- Long period (~12 weeks) of immobilisation is required, but still radiological non union may persist even if the child is asymptomatic.
- In c/o syndesmotic injury, reduction and internal fixation is required.

S-H Type I and II Distal Fibula Fracture

- S-H type I distal fibula fracture is the

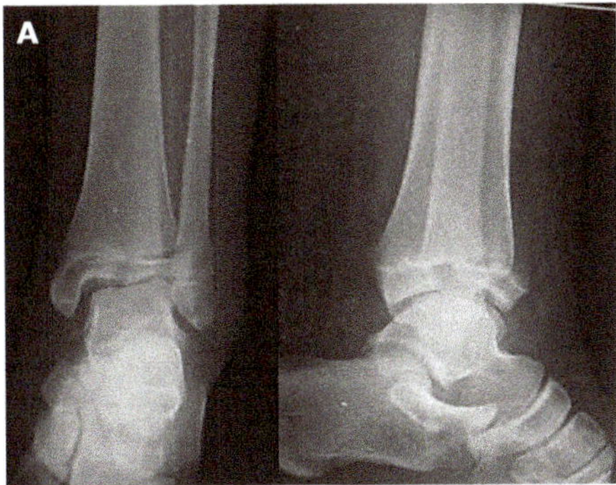

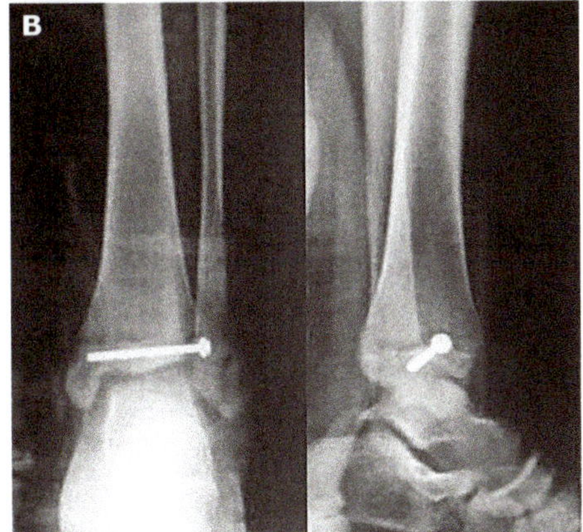

Fig. 26.21: *(A) AP and lateral X-rays of the ankle showing Tillaux fracture (B) Treatment with open reduction and internal fixation using 4 mm cancellous screw*

most common fracture of the ankle in children occurring due to SI injury and often misdiagnosed as ankle sprain.

- High index of suspicion and careful examination for tenderness/swelling over fibular physis is necessary for diagnosis.
- Isolated non displaced S- H type I distal fibula fracture is treated in a short leg walking cast for 4 weeks.
- Displaced fracture requires closed reduction and short-leg non-weight-bearing cast for 4 to 6 weeks.
- S-H type II fracture is treated with a short-leg non-weight-bearing cast for 4 to 6 weeks.
- Displaced distal fibula fracture associated with distal tibia fracture usually reduces once tibia fracture is reduced. If the reduction is stable, it does not require any internal fixation.

Complications

1. Premature closure of the physis:

- Though rare, it is the most common complication following displaced S-H type III and IV injury of distal tibia physis in spite of anatomical reduction, mainly due to significant injury to the growth plate at the time of trauma.
- The adduction force imparted to these fractures leads to injury to the medial aspect of the distal tibial physis, producing an asymmetrical growth arrest and varus deformity.
- It is important to follow these children closely during the first 2 years after injury and ideally upto skeletal maturity for diagnosis of growth arrest.
- Diagnosis and Management: Similar principles as mentioned in Chapter 2.

2. Delayed union and Non union: very rare

- May occur in the adolescent with a distal tibia fracture
- Treatment involves open reduction, debridement of fibrous tissue and bone grafting with internal fixation.

3. Malunion with valgus deformity:

- Due to inadequate reduction of PEER fracture
- Any valgus >15-20° will not remodel.
- Treatment consists of medial epiphysiodesis or corrective osteotomy.

TRIPLANE FRACTURE

Introduction

- Triplane fractures are transitional fractures occurring mainly in adolescents (10-16 years), consisting of three major fragments

1. Tibia metaphysis
2. Anterolateral quadrant of distal tibia epiphysis
3. Medial and posterior portion of the epiphysis, in addition to posterior metaphyseal spike.

- Mechanism of injury is an external rotation force applied to a supinated foot.
- Based on the extent of physeal closure at the time of injury, 2-part, 3-part and 4-part fractures are described based on CT **(Fig. 26.22)**.

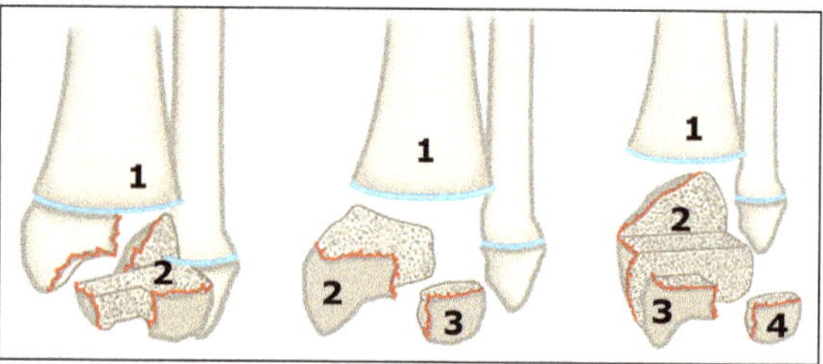

***Fig. 26.22**: Different types of Triplane fractures: 2-part, 3-part, 4-part.*

- Triplane fractures are usually associated with fibula fracture (48%). Associated proximal fibula fracture and syndesmotic injury are known as Maisonneuve equivalent. Proper identification and treatment of this type is important to prevent chronic instability.
- For planning of fixation, CT scan is mandatory and it helps the surgeon to determine the exact modality of fixation and the direction and configuration of screws.

Treatment

The goal of treatment is to achieve an anatomical reduction of the distal tibial articular surface and to avoid early degenerative arthritis.

- Non displaced, < 2 mm displaced and extra-articular fractures can be treated with closed reduction with axial traction on the ankle and internal rotation of the foot with the patient under anaesthesia. Fracture is immobilised in non-weight-bearing above-knee cast with knee in 30-40^{0} of flexion and foot in internal rotation for lateral fracture and eversion for medial fracture for 3 to 4 weeks, followed by a short leg cast for additional 2 to 3 weeks. Serial follow up X-ray and CT scan is required for confirmation of reduction. **(Fig. 26.23)**
- >2 mm displaced fractures are reduced under general anaesthesia and fixed percutaneously with screws.
- If closed reduction is not successful, open reduction is done through an anterolateral approach for lateral triplane or anteromedial approach for medial triplane fractures. Percutaneous clamp, arthroscopic assistance or additional incisions may be necessary for adequate exposure and reduction.
- Two 4 mm cancellous screws are inserted from medial to lateral or anterior to posterior or both, based on the fracture pattern. **(Fig. 26.24)**
- Arthroscopic assistance or percutaneous clamps may be of additional help.
- 3 or more part fracture may require additional exposure for reduction and internal fixation.

A stab incision is used in the posterior aspect of the ankle, just lateral to the tendo achilles (TA) or a formal posterolateral incision lateral to TA, developing the interval between the flexor hallucis longus (FHL) and the peroneus brevis. **(Fig. 26.25)**

Reduction and internal fixation is done in a stepwise manner. S-H type II fracture is first reduced by provisional fixation to distal tibia through metaphyseal fragment and S-H type III fragment can later be reduced and provisionally fixed to the already

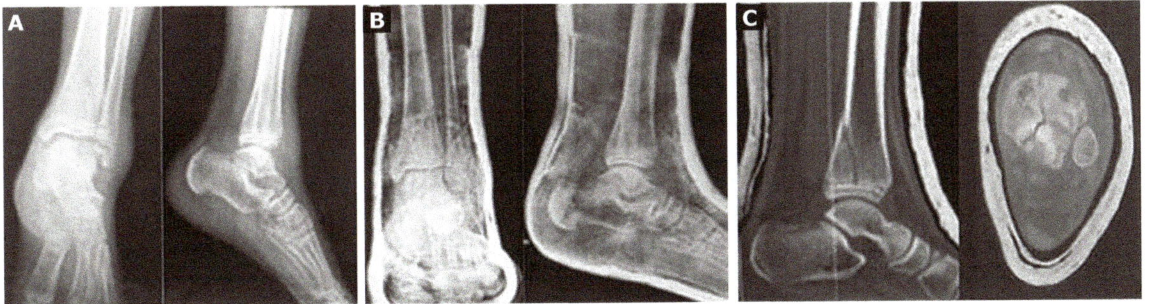

Fig. 26.23: (A) AP and lateral X-rays of the ankle showing non displaced triplane fracture (B) Conservative treatment in above-knee cast. (C) CT scan is done to confirm the reduction.

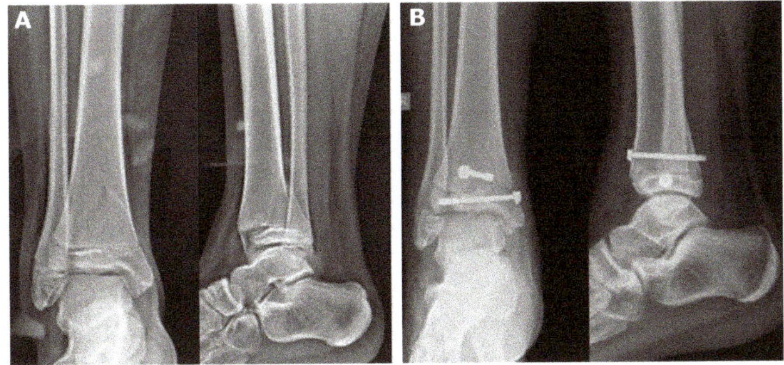

Fig. 26.24: (A) AP and lateral X-rays of the ankle showing displaced 2-part triplane fracture (B) Treatment with open reduction and internal fixation using two 4 mm. cancellous screws from medial to lateral and anterior to posterior

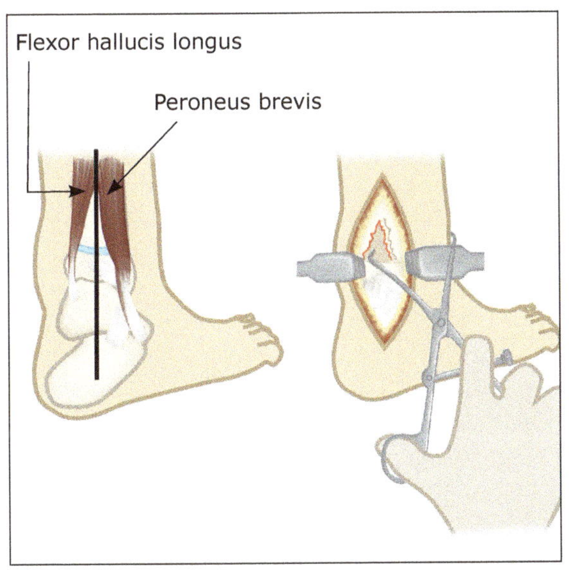

Fig. 26.25: Open reduction of metaphyseal fragment through posterior approach in a 3 or 4 part Triplane fracture.

stabilised type II fragment. (Order of fixation can be reversed also)

The leg is immobilised in a non-weight-bearing above-knee cast for 4 weeks, followed by a below-knee cast for additional 2 to 3 weeks.

- Associated Greenstick or displaced fracture of the fibula may make reduction difficult because the strong ligamentous attachments to the fibula maintains the angular deformity and the resultant shortening of the attached tibial fragment. Therefore it is necessary to reduce the fibula fracture before attempting any reduction of the tibia.

The results of treatment of triplane fractures are generally good in the short term, but the long term outcome is not fully defined.

Flowchart 26.1

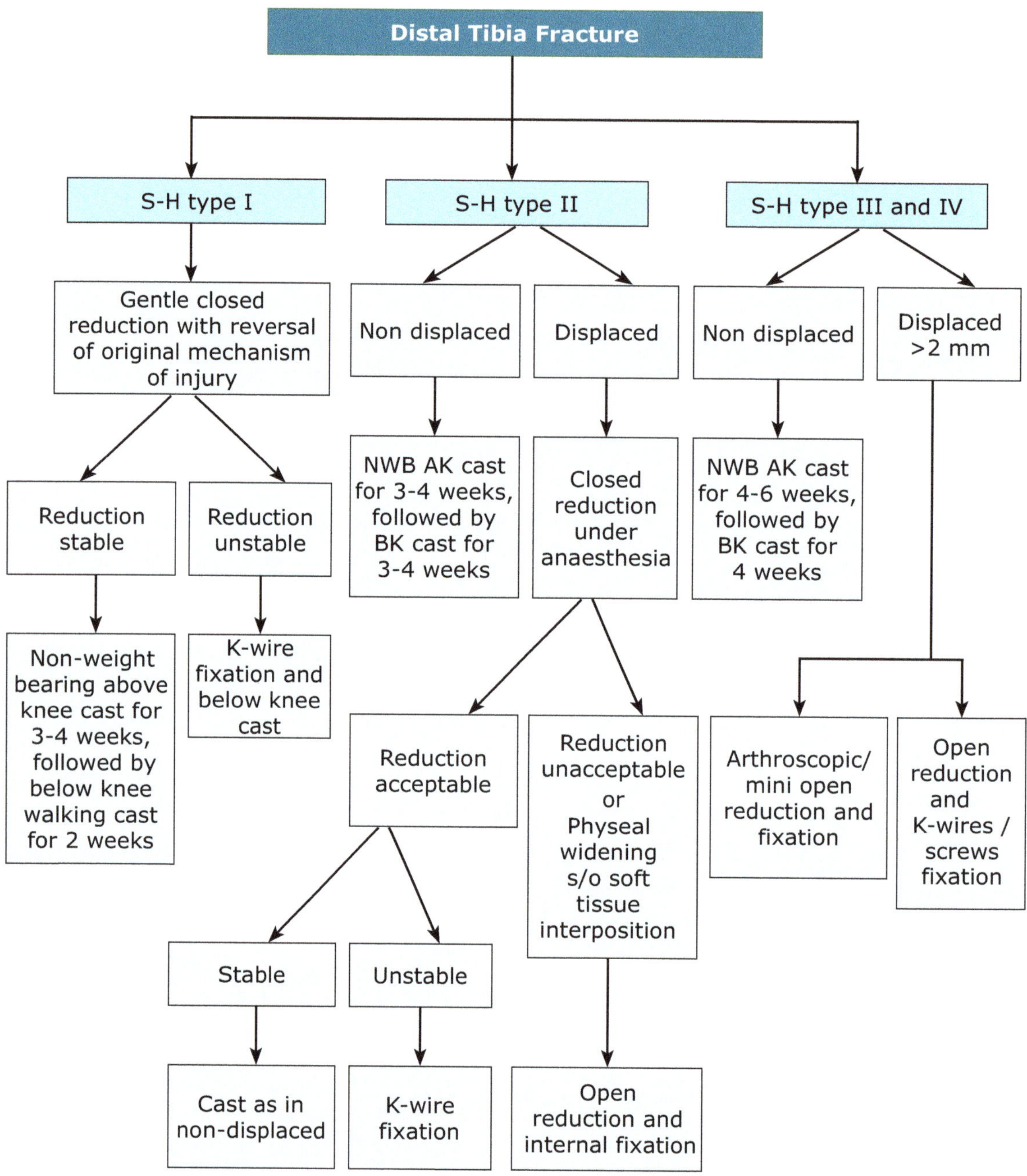

Flowchart 26.2

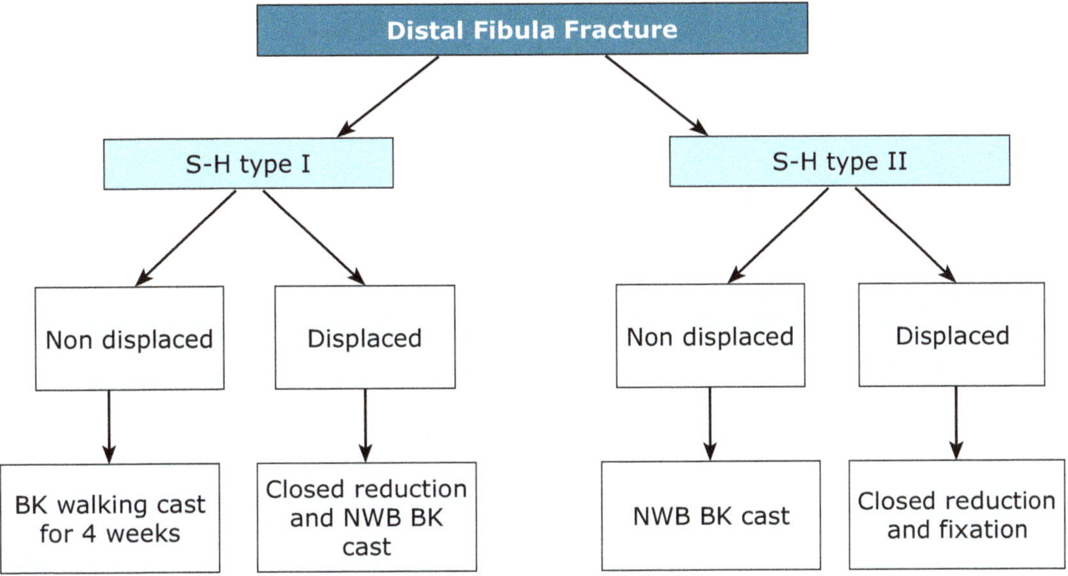

Flowchart 26.3

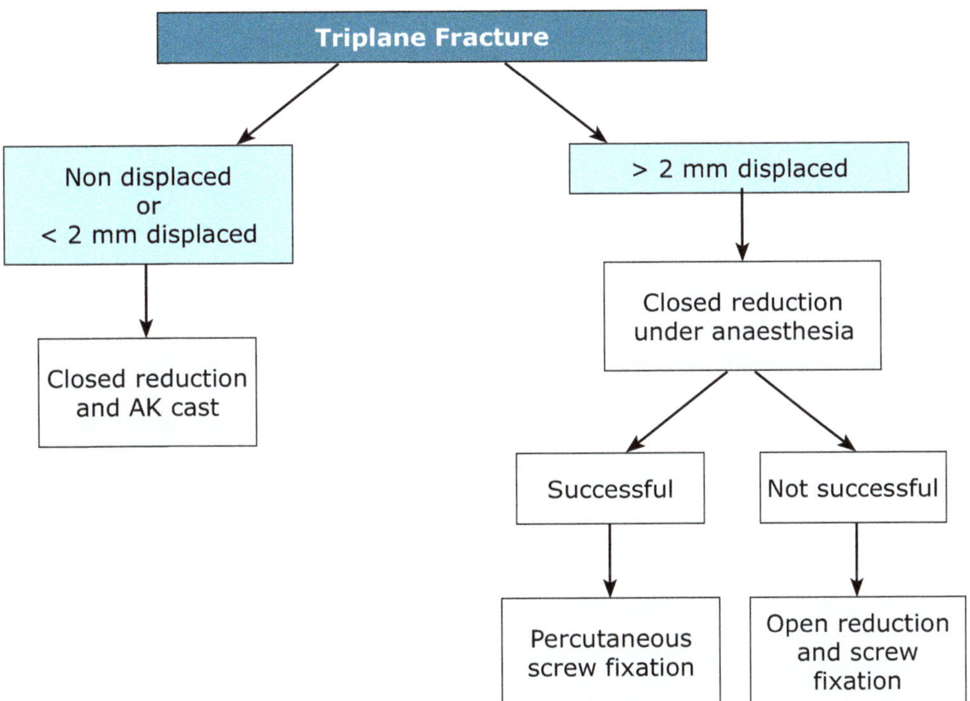

27 Fractures and Dislocations of the Foot

Trauma to the paediatric foot used to be traditionally treated non–operatively, considering that foot bones are mainly cartilaginous and would remodel as the child matures. In recent times, the trends have changed. More involvement of children in sports and activities of greater physical intensity has led to more complex fractures and dislocations and need for surgical interventions for early rehabilitation. Child's foot is largely cartilaginous and there are certain unique features of paediatric foot fractures.

- As the energy of injury is dissipated by elasticity of the cartilage, fractures in children are less severe as compared to adults.
- At birth, only calcaneus and talus are ossified. Cuboid ossification centre appears shortly thereafter and navicular ossifies at around 3 years. Hence interpretation of imaging becomes more difficult.
- There are many accessory bones and secondary centres of ossification that makes X-ray interpretation difficult.
- Due to remodelling potential of cartilage, some displacement and angulation of fractures is acceptable in children.

CALCANEUS FRACTURES

Introduction

Calcaneal fractures are rare injuries in children. But they are often missed, particularly in young children < 4 years with undisplaced extra-articular fractures. So in cases of persistent limp beyond a week, re-investigation and repeat X-ray is advisable. Also, a secondary ossification centre (crescentic epiphysis) that is seen posteriorly at 6-8 years should not be mistaken for a fracture.

Clinical Features

- Careful palpation for tenderness can guide about the site of fracture.
- Extreme swelling and bruising around the heel and dorsum of the foot is usually evident.
- It is essential to look for clinical features of compartment syndrome.
- Also, assessment of associated injuries in spine, pelvis, upper and lower limb is important.

Table 27.1: Anatomical structures visualised in various calcaneal views

Postero-anterior view	Calcaneo-cuboid and Talo-navicular joint
Lateral view	Congruity of posterior articular facet Calculation of Bohler angle
Axial view	Tuberosity, Body, Sustentaculum tali, Posterior facet of calcaneus
Oblique view	Anterior process, Subtalar joint
Broden view	Articular surface of the posterior facet

Imaging

Postero-anterior, lateral, oblique and axial views of the calcaneus are essential for diagnosis and management of calcaneal fractures. The anatomical structures seen in various views are as follows: **(Figs. 27.1, 27.2 and Table 27.1)**

Calculation of the following angles on the lateral view is important to judge the articular congruity. **(Fig. 27.3)**

Bohler angle: between a line drawn from the highest point of the anterior process to the highest point of the posterior facet and a line drawn tangent to the highest point of the calcaneal tuberosity.

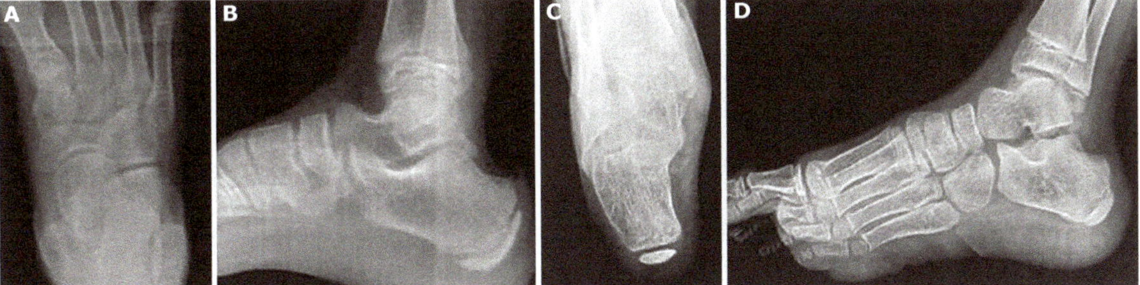

Fig. 27.1: *(A) Posteroanterior, (B) Lateral, (C) Axial and (D) Oblique views of the calcaneus*

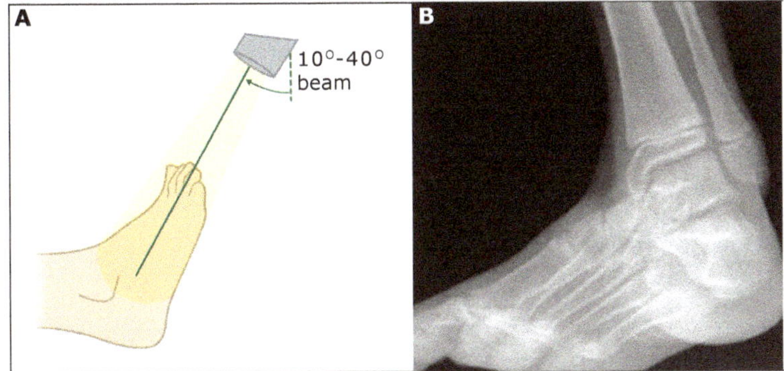

Fig. 27.2: *Broden's view: 40° internal rotation view with the beam angled 10-40° towards the head. It demonstrates the articular surface of the posterior facet clearly.*

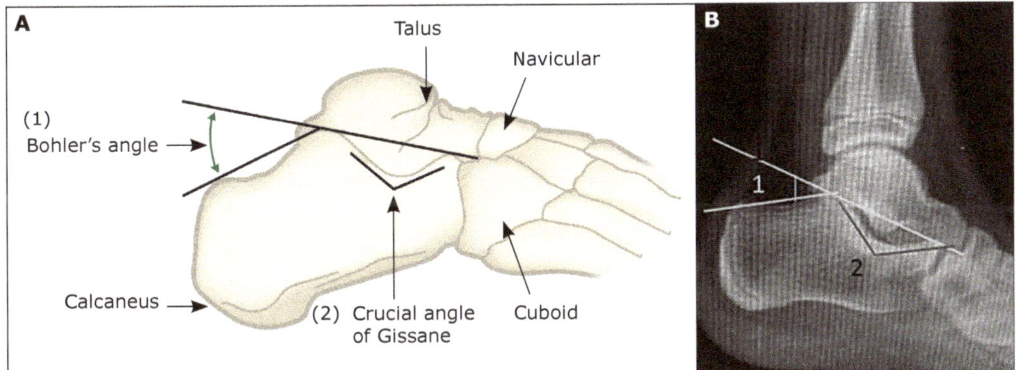

Fig. 27.3: *(A) Schematic diagram and (B) Lateral X-ray showing Measurement of (1) Bohler's angle and (2) Crucial angle of Gissane.*

Normal in Adults: 20-40°

Children: slightly less

Crucial angle of Gissane: angle formed by two strong cortical struts seen on the lateral X-ray, one along the lateral margin of the posterior facet and the other running up to the anterior process of the calcaneus.

Normal: 95-105°

In doubtful cases, CT scan or MRI in very young children is helpful.

Classification

Schmidt and Weiner classification is used for calcaneal fractures in children. **(Fig. 27.4)**

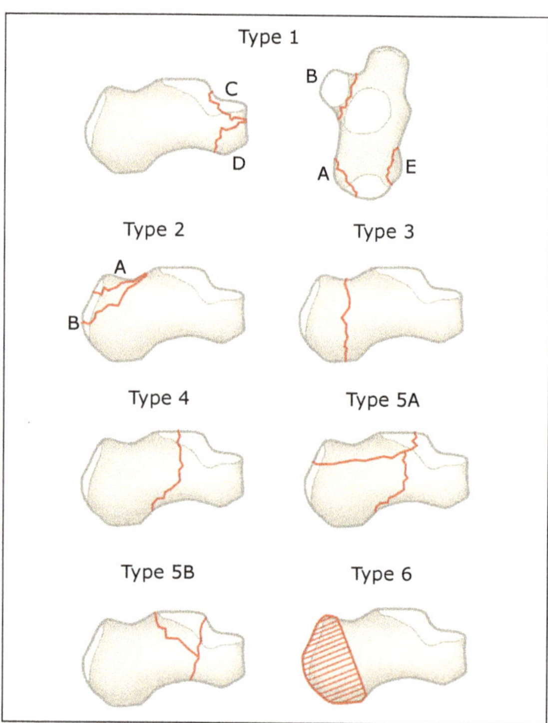

Fig. 27.4: *Schmidt and Weiner classification of calcaneal fractures:*
Type 1,2,3: Extra-articular fractures
Type 4, 5: Intra-articular fractures
Type 6: Fracture with significant bone loss

Extra-articular

Type 1:

A. Fracture of tuberosity or apophysis

B. Fracture of sustentaculum tali

C. Fracture of anterior process

D. Fracture of distal inferolateral aspect

E. Small avulsion fracture of body

Type 2:

A. Beak fracture

B. Avulsion fracture of insertion of Achilles tendon

Type 3:

Linear fracture not involving subtalar joint

Intra-articular

Type 4:

Linear fracture involving subtalar joint

Type 5:

Compression fracture of subtalar joint

A. Tongue type

B. Joint depression type

Type 6:

Significant bone loss of posterior aspect with loss of Achilles tendon insertion

Treatment

- Almost all closed fractures, including intra-articular displaced fractures, in children < 10 years and extra-articular fractures in children >10 years can be treated non operatively, due to marked remodelling potential. Below-knee cast immobilisation for 6 weeks is recommended and once the child is comfortable at 2-3 weeks, weight bearing can be started.
- Intra-articular, displaced fractures in adolescents require operative treatment, but undisplaced fractures

can be treated in below knee non-weight bearing cast for 6-8 weeks till fracture heals.

- In *tongue type* fracture, if the posterior gap is > 1 cm and tendo achilles has been significantly shortened by proximally displaced fracture, percutaneous reduction by technique described by Essex-Lopresti can be useful. **(Fig. 27.5)** A pin is inserted into the tongue fragment to be used as a joystick to manipulate the fragment into a better position. For this, downward force is applied on the pin and forefoot is plantar flexed. Once reduction is confirmed under fluoroscopy, the pin is driven across the fracture to maintain reduction.

- For severely displaced, *Joint depression type* intra-articular fracture in adolescents, open reduction and internal fixation with plate and screw is recommended once the swelling has subsided and fracture blisters have resolved.

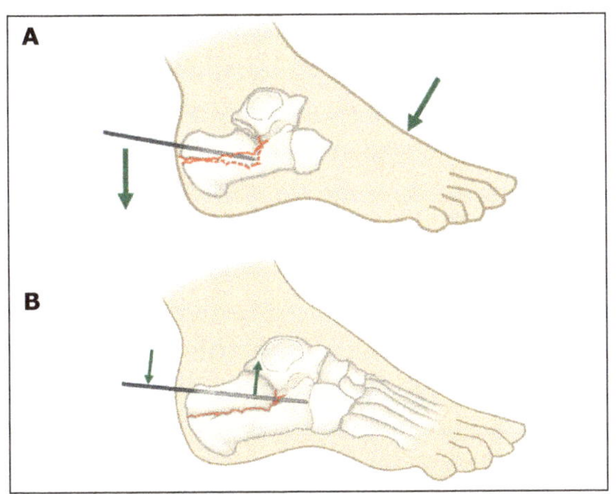

Fig. 27.5: *Essex Lopresti manoeuvre to reduce Tongue type intra-articular calcaneal fracture*
(A) Pin inserted into the tongue fragment, to be used as a joystick.
The fragment is manipulated with downward force applied on the pin while the forefoot is plantar flexed
(B) After fluoroscopic confirmation of reduction, the pin is advanced across the fracture.

Technique of Open Reduction and Internal Fixation

Position **(Fig. 27.6)**

- Lateral position with the knee and the hip flexed 45°

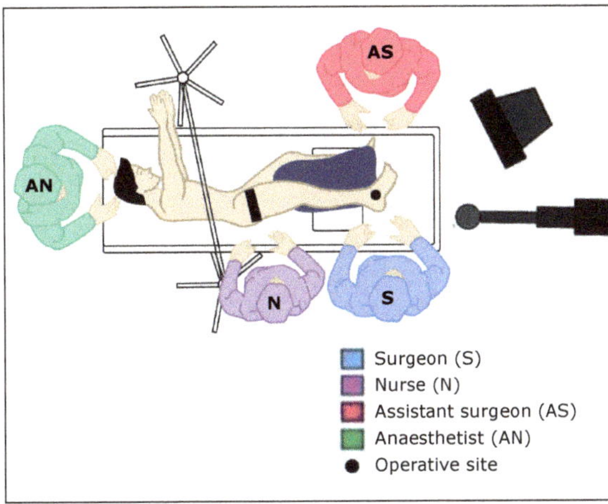

Fig. 27.6: *Lateral position with the hip and the knee in flexion for open reduction and internal fixation for calcaneal fracture.*

Incision **(Fig. 27.7)**

- Under tourniquet, L shaped incision is taken anterior to the lateral border of tendo achilles, curved at apex, extending from 3 cm. cephalad to tip of fibula and distally extending to 5th metatarsal base.

Steps

- Short saphenous vein and sural nerve should be identified and protected proximally by blunt dissection with scissors.

- Care should be taken to create thick skin flaps by sharp dissection and subperiosteal elevation with no. 15 blade directly to the lateral wall of the calcaneus. Peroneal tendons and attachment of calcaneofibular ligament are to be reflected dorsally, for exposure of anterior process and calcaneo-cuboid joint.

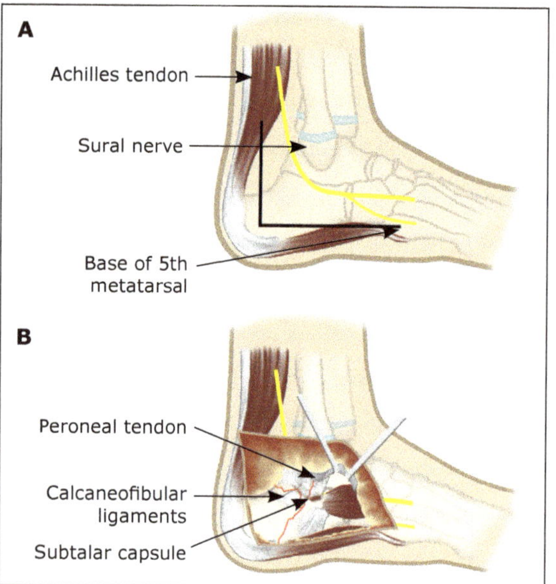

***Fig. 27.7**: Open reduction of joint depression type intra-articular calcaneal fractures*
(A) L shaped incision
(B) Exposure of the fracture after dorsal reflection of peroneal tendons and calcaneofibular ligaments.

- Dorsally elevated flap can be maintained by K-wires into the neck and body of the talus and fibula and it exposes the posterior facet of the calcaneus and sinus tarsi.
- Tourniquet can be deflated once exposure is complete.
- Fracture can be reduced by applying traction on the Schanz pin placed in the inferior aspect of posterior tubercle. Reflect the lateral wall laterally, if needed. Reduce anterior to posterior, medial to lateral and dorsal to plantar, that is, anterior process first, then posterior facet and finally restore alignment of os calcis by confirming reduction and alignment of the crucial angle.
- Provisional fixation with multiple K-wires can be checked with image intensifier. Once reduction is confirmed, 2.7 mm. reconstruction plate can be fixed on the lateral wall of the calcaneus **(Fig. 27.8)**. Posterior facet reduction can be maintained with interfragmentary screws.
- If there is a bony defect/void, bone grafting can be used as per guidelines as in adults.
- 2-layered closure over drain and post-operative elevation to reduce swelling and wound complications is advisable.
- Below knee slab and restricted mobility is continued till suture removal.

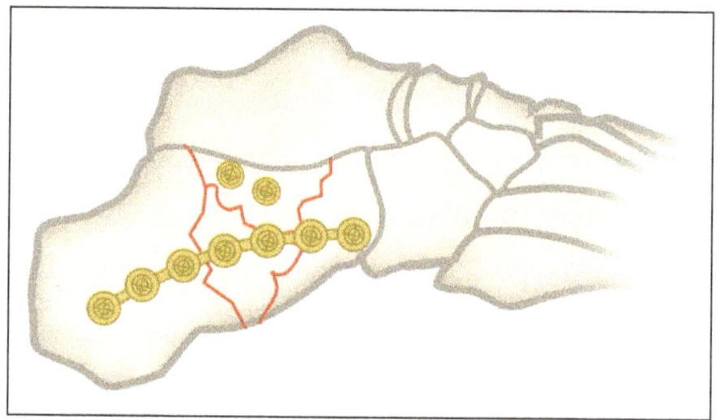

***Fig. 27.8**: Fixation of intra-articular calcaneal fracture using 2.7 mm reconstruction plate.*

Complications

1. Wound complications:

   Rare as compared to adults, due to fewer risk factors like smoking, obesity and diabetes mellitus.

   If superficial, the wound can be managed with antibiotics and immobilisation.

   If deep, wound debridement and vacuum assisted closure (VAC) may be helpful. It is advisable to take help from a plastic surgeon.

2. Complex regional pain syndrome:

   This complication is more commonly seen in children, especially in girls, just before puberty. It manifests as pain out of proportion, pain even on touch, grey discolouration, cold clammy skin, reduced hair growth and disuse calf atrophy. Treatment requires a multidisciplinary team approach including anti-inflammatory, gabapentin, amitriptyline, sometimes sympathetic blocks and also functional rehabilitation and physiotherapy. Response to treatment is good, but recurrence rate is high.

3. Peroneal tendonitis/dislocation:

   Laterally displaced wall in conservatively treated fractures or prominent hardware in surgically treated fractures can present with peroneal tendonitis or subluxation. Early implant removal may be needed in symptomatic children.

FRACTURES OF TALUS

Introduction

Fractures of the talus are very rare in children and adolescents and mostly occur through the neck and sometimes the body. Branches of three major vessels- anterior tibial, posterior tibial and peroneal artery perforate the short talar neck circumferentially and are prone for injury during fracture. Avascular necrosis (AVN) is more prevalent in innocuous fractures when compared to adults with similar injury. Children less than 6 years of age generally have a better prognosis.

Classification

Fractures of the Talar Neck

A fall from height, leading to forcible dorsiflexion of the foot results in shear force with neck of the talus impinging against anterior lip of distal tibia and resultant vertical/slightly oblique fracture at the junction of the talar neck and body. Fracture can also occur in crushing injuries/vehicular accidents. The force required to fracture a child's talus is almost twice that required to fracture other ankle/foot fractures. Hence, there is a high incidence of associated injuries like calcaneus, malleoli, tibia and lumbar spine and hence during clinical examination, these sites should be specifically examined.

Clinical Features

- History of the exact mechanism of injury should be asked for.
- The ankle and foot appear extremely swollen and careful palpation around the talus may be needed.
- The foot should be closely evaluated for compartment syndrome.
- In addition to AP, lateral and oblique X-rays, Canale and Kelly pronated oblique view(foot placed into equinus, pronated ~15° and the X-ray beam angled 75° to the horizontal) is helpful in diagnosis of fracture. Due to largely cartilaginous talus, MRI may be needed for diagnosis of fracture in children <10 years of age. Also, CT scan is useful in assessment of fracture anatomy and pre-operative planning.

Modified Hawkins Classification **(Fig. 27.9)**

Type I: Stable undisplaced talar neck fracture

Type II: Displaced talar neck fracture with subtalar subluxation or dislocation

Type III: Displaced talar neck fracture with subluxation or dislocation of both the ankle and subtalar joint

Type IV: Very rare, basically a type III with talonavicular joint displacement.

Treatment

Treatment of talar neck fracture in children is based on the severity of fracture and age of the child. In children <8 years, a less than perfect reduction can be accepted due to remodelling potential.

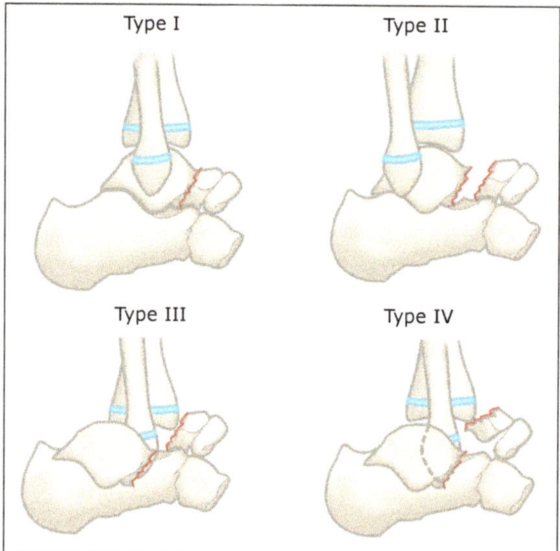

***Fig. 27.9**: Modified Hawkins Classification of talar neck fractures.*

But in adolescents, the fracture is treated on similar principles as in adults.

Hawkins Type I fracture

This fracture can be treated in non-weight bearing below-knee cast for 6-8 weeks. Once radiological union is confirmed, full weight bearing can be started.

The rate of AVN is only 0-10% as theoretically there is damage to only one vessel entering the neck.

Hawkins type II fracture

- This fracture requires immediate closed reduction of the dorsomedially displaced distal fragment. The reduction is done under general anaesthesia, by gentle plantar flexion and pronation of foot.
- If stable reduction is achieved, a well moulded below-knee cast is applied, with initial 4 weeks in plantar flexion and next 4 weeks in neutral position. Post reduction serial X-rays or CT scan may be required to monitor the loss of reduction, if any.
- If the reduction is achieved but the fracture is unstable, fixation with two percutaneous K-wires from dorsomedial incision, medial to extensor hallucis longus (EHL) are recommended.
- If the reduction is not acceptable (>few mm. of offset and >10° angulation), open reduction may be required.
- Risk of AVN in type II fractures is 20-50 %, as the blood supply from two or three sources (neck vessel and the one entering the tarsal canal) are lost.

Hawkins type III/IV fracture

Type III/IV fractures are a result of serious injury and all three sources of blood supply are affected. Hence, urgent surgery is required for open reduction and internal fixation. Risk of AVN is very high, 80-100%.

Surgical approaches

The choice of surgical approach depends on the condition of the soft tissues and familiarity of the approach.

1. *Posterolateral:*

- In supine position, incision is made lateral to tendo achilles(TA). Care should be taken to avoid damage to sural nerve. The posterior joint capsule is opened and the posterior process of talus is identified.
- Posterior screws are more stable biomechanically and hence one or two 4.5/6.5 mm. titanium partially threaded cancellous screws are passed to provide compression across fracture.

2. *Anteromedial* **(Figs. 27.10 and 27.11)**

- This approach is useful for direct visualisation of talar neck and direct reduction of fracture.
- It is potentially less harmful to the blood supply of talus, when compared to anterolateral approach as it avoids

damage to the deltoid branch of posterior tibial and medial branch of anterior tibial artery.

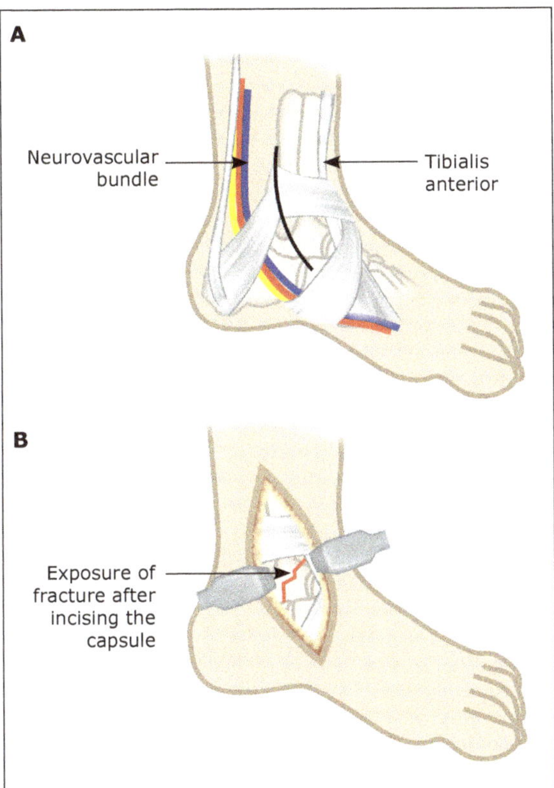

Fig. 27.10: *Anteromedial approach for open reduction of talar neck fracture:*
(A) Incision anterior to medial malleolus
(B) Capsule incised in the interval between tibialis anterior and tibialis posterior to expose the fracture

Position:

Supine

Incision:

Incision is made from just anterior to medial malleolus, directed distally down the midfoot.

Steps:

- Deeper dissection is done medial to tibialis anterior and extensor hallucis longus (EHL)
- The capsule is exposed and opened in the interval between tibialis anterior and tibialis posterior.
- The fracture is exposed, reduced and fixed with screws.

3. *Anterolateral:*

- The advantage of anterolateral approach is that it allows excellent exposure of lateral talar neck that is usually not comminuted (unlike medial), thereby allowing anatomical reduction and also good access to subtalar joint.
- The disadvantage is that it may disrupt the blood supply more than any other approach.
- The incision is from the tip of the lateral malleolus to the base of the 4th metatarsal. Care should be taken to avoid damage to the sural nerve and artery of sinus tarsi.

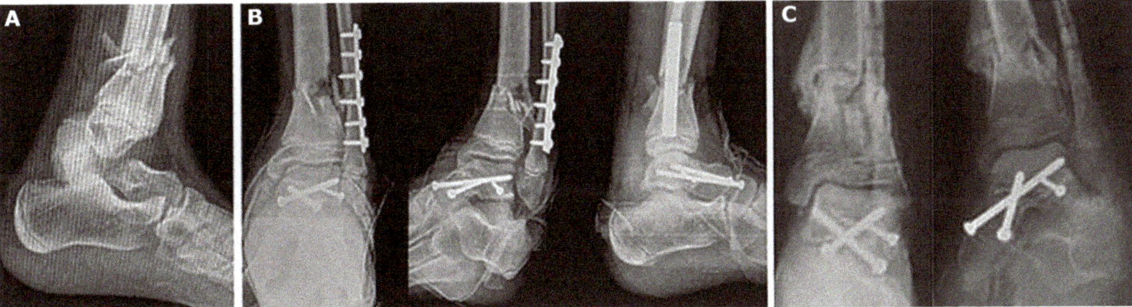

Fig. 27.11: *(A) Lateral X-ray of the ankle showing talar neck and distal tibia-fibula fracture (B) AP, Lateral and Mortise view showing fixation of talar neck fracture with cancellous screws and fixation of fibula fracture with reconstruction plate (C) AP and Mortise view at 3 months showing healing of fractures.*

Post-operative protocol

- Child should be non-weight bearing in below-knee cast for 6-8 weeks.
- Serial X-rays are done to evaluate fracture healing and presence or absence of *'Hawkins sign'*.

  Hawkins described a subchondral lucent line, that indicates normal blood flow to the talar body. The absence of this lucency may indicate the development of osteonecrosis.
- Progressive weight bearing can be started if the fracture is healing and Hawkins sign is present, suggesting adequate blood supply and less chance of AVN.
- Non-weight bearing to be continued until subchondral lucency is present.
- If it is still not present beyond 3 months, MRI is recommended for accurate assessment of vascularity.
- AVN of the talus sometimes takes 18-24 months to revascularise. So the decision on the amount of weight bearing in the presence of altered blood supply (to prevent premature collapse of the body) is controversial.

Fracture of the Talar Body and Dome

- These are rare fractures in children.
- Sneppen classification system of talar body fractures **(Fig. 27.12)**

Table 27.2: Sneppen classification

Group	Fracture type
I	Transchondral/Osteochondral
II	Coronal, sagittal or horizontal shear
III	Posterior tubercle
IV	Lateral process
V	Crush fracture

- Undisplaced fractures are treated in non-weight-bearing below-knee cast for 6-8 weeks.

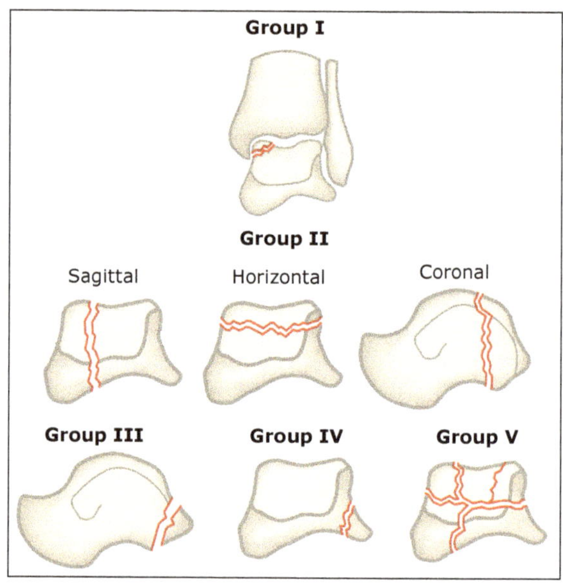

***Fig. 27.12**: Sneppen Classification of talar body fractures.*

- Displaced fractures require open reduction and internal fixation. Displaced lateral process fractures are best visualised on Mortise view or CT scan. Anatomical reduction is required in case of intra-articular fracture with >2-3 mm. joint incongruity. A single compression screw through lateral approach and immobilisation in below-knee cast for 6 weeks is recommended.

Osteochondral Fractures

The initial X-rays following an ankle injury in a child should be closely assessed for an osteochondral injury. If pain and swelling persist beyond 2 months after an 'ankle sprain', then further investigations are needed to look for an osteochondral lesion. Further X-rays, MRI or MR arthrogram may be needed.

- If the loose fragment becomes trapped within the joint, mechanical symptoms of locking and catching, swelling and effusion may be evident.

Classification of Osteochondral Fractures of Talar Dome

Bendt and Harty classification: **(Fig. 27.13)**

Stage I: Subchondral trabecular compression fracture (not seen on X-ray)

Stage II: Incomplete separation of an osteochondral fracture

Stage III: The osteochondral fragment is unattached but undisplaced

Stage IV: A displaced osteochondral fragment

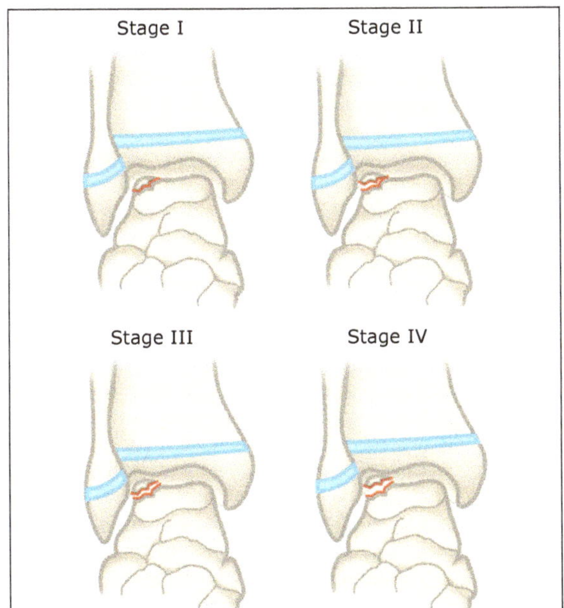

***Fig. 27.13**: Berndt and Harty classification of talar osteochondral lesions.*

Stage I, II and III lesions can be treated symptomatically with 6 weeks below-knee cast immobilisation and later elastic ankle support and activity modification till 6 months. Repeat MRI can be done and if the stage has worsened, arthroscopic debridement and microfracture or stabilisation can be done.

Stage IV displaced fragments require arthroscopic removal and microfracture or repair/internal fixation with bioabsorbable screws, bone grafting.

MIDTARSAL INJURIES

Introduction

Midtarsal area includes the navicular, cuboid and 3 cuneiform bones, that are linked together by strong ligaments especially on the plantar surface, lateral side of the midfoot being more stable than medial side. Due to this inherent stability, larger force is required to fracture these bones. Hence isolated fractures of midtarsal bones are rare and usually associated with Chopart joint dislocation (Calcaneo-Cuboid/Talo-Navicular) or the more severe Lisfranc injury.

Navicular Fracture

It is a rare injury and the treatment is conservative with below-knee cast, but it is important to differentiate this fracture from other conditions that mimic fractures.

- Kohler disease (AVN of the navicular): common in 2-5 years.
- Stress fracture (Sagittal fracture in the middle third): Diagnosis mostly on bone scans, CT and MRI
- Accessory navicular (Edges are rounded and smooth)

Cuboid Fracture

It is a rare injury. The diagnosis is by 'nutcracker manoeuvre': After stabilising the heel with one hand, the forefoot is abducted with the other hand-Pain in the lateral aspect of the foot usually suggests fracture of the cuboid.

CT scan may be required if the fracture is not evident on X-ray.

2 types of fractures are seen (Weber and Locher)

Type 1: Distal impaction shear type

Type 2: Burst fracture

Treatment is by below-knee cast for 2-3 weeks.

TARSOMETATARSAL INJURIES/ LISFRANC FRACTURE-DISLOCATION

Introduction

Lisfranc injury is less common in children and difficult to diagnose, especially in case of a subtle disruption of the Lisfranc ligament and if left untreated can develop into chronic painful foot.

Surgical Anatomy

- Tarsometatarsal joint complex consists of tarso-metatarsal (TMT) joints, inter-tarsal joints and inter-metatarsal joints.
- It is divided into two columns:

  Medial column: Continuation of talus and navicular and includes cuneiforms and medial three metatarsals.

  Lateral column: Continuation of calcaneus and includes cuboid and 4th, 5th metatarsals.
- TMT joint complex represents the apex of the longitudinal and transverse arches of the foot, hence both structural integrity and mobility are equally important for normal foot function.
- Inter-metatarsal ligaments bind the lateral four metatarsal fragments, but are absent between 1st and 2nd metatarsal. Instead, 2nd metatarsal is connected to medial cuneiform by 'Lisfranc ligament' (medial interosseous ligament) .The plantar ligaments are extremely strong. **(Fig. 27.14)**

  Stability is also provided by the 2nd metatarsal that is 'keyed' into the step formed by the cuneiforms. Tibialis anterior and peroneus longus insertion on the base of 1st metatarsal also provide added stability to 1st metatarsal.

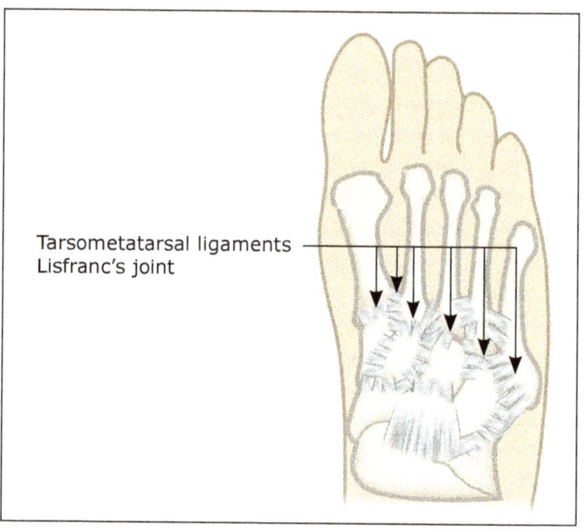

***Fig. 27.14**: Tarsometatarsal ligaments of the Lisfranc's joint.*

- Dorsalis pedis and deep peroneal nerve are likely to be damaged by Lisfranc injury. Hence careful assessment during examination and care during internal fixation is very important.

Mechanism of Injury

TMT injuries can be caused either by a direct blow to the foot, secondary to fall of a heavy load or indirectly, where there is forced plantar flexion of the forefoot in combination with a rotational force. The indirect injuries are commonly through the following mechanisms: **(Fig. 27.15)**

1. Traumatic impact in the tiptoe position (jumping) and landing on toes.
2. Heel-to-toe compression (load on heel with child in kneeling position)
3. Fixed forefoot (Falling backward with the forefoot pinned)

Clinical Features

- High index of suspicion is important after a typical mechanism of injury.
- Subtle injuries may be difficult to diagnose due to minor pain and swelling over 1st and 2nd metatarsals. Plantar

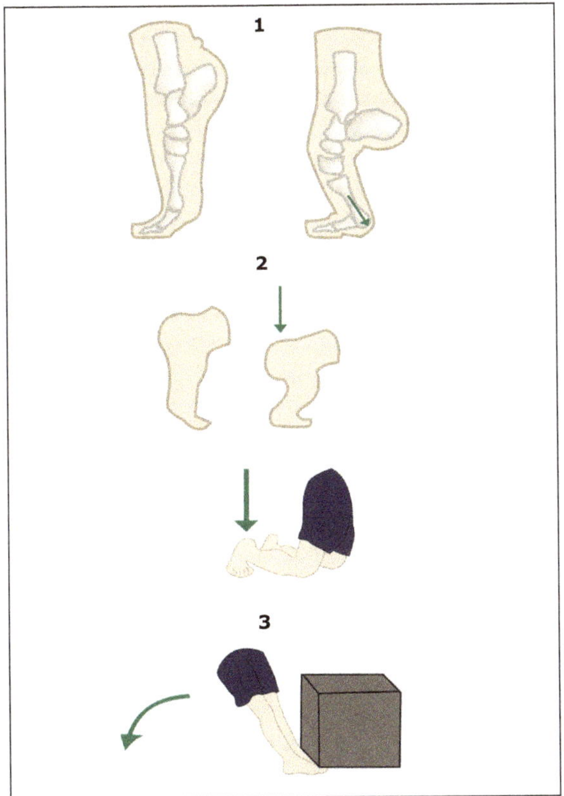

Fig. 27.15: *Various mechanisms of injuries producing Lisfranc fracture-dislocation*
1. *Indirect injury with the impact load applied to a tip-toed foot*
2. *Direct injury with the load applied to the posterior heel in a kneeling position*
3. *Injury due to the child falling backwards from a fixed forefoot.*

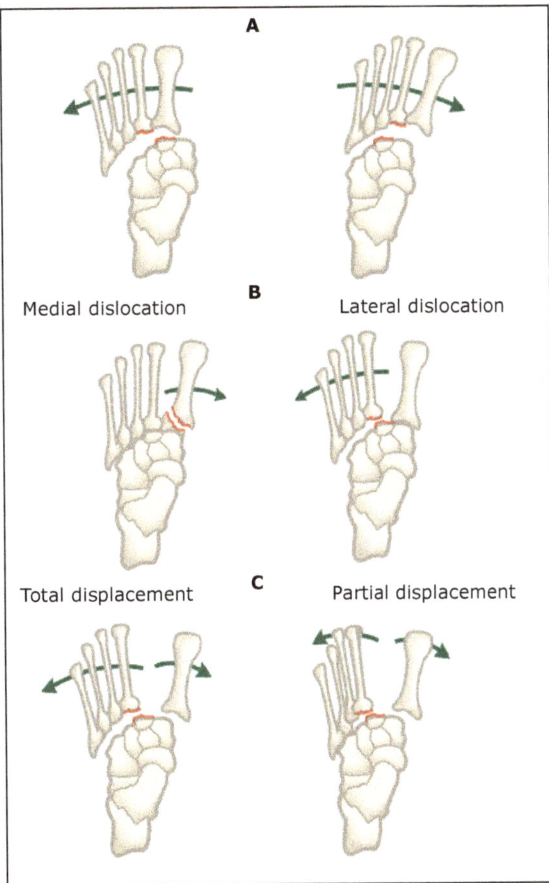

Fig. 27.16: *Hardcastle classification of Lisfranc injuries:*
Type A: Total incongruity
Type B: Partial incongruity
Type C: Divergent

ecchymosis sign along the midfoot (due to torn TMT ligament) may be helpful in diagnosis. Child can be asked to do a single limb heel lift. Pain in the midfoot area suggests TMT injury.

- In case of significant trauma, there is greater ligamentous injury and more swelling. It is important to check for compartment syndrome in such cases.

Classification

Hardcastle et. al. **(Fig. 27.16)**

Type A: *Total incongruity*

Total incongruity of the entire metatarsal joint in a single plane- coronal, sagittal, or combined.

Type B: *Partial incongruity* (more common)

Medial displacement of 1st metatarsal due to Lisfranc ligament disruption or base of metatarsal fracture or lateral displacement of the four lateral metatarsals.

Type C: *Divergent pattern*

1st metatarsal displaces medially and any combination of the four lateral metatarsals may be displaced laterally, associated with partial or total incongruity.

Imaging

- AP, lateral and oblique views of the foot (weight bearing, preferred) are essential.
- Comparative weight bearing X-ray of the opposite foot is helpful.
- In order to diagnose subtle Lisfranc injuries, it is of utmost importance to understand the normal alignment on various views:

Normal alignment on AP view: **(Fig. 27.17)**

Lateral border of 1st metatarsal should be in line with the lateral border of medial cuneiform.

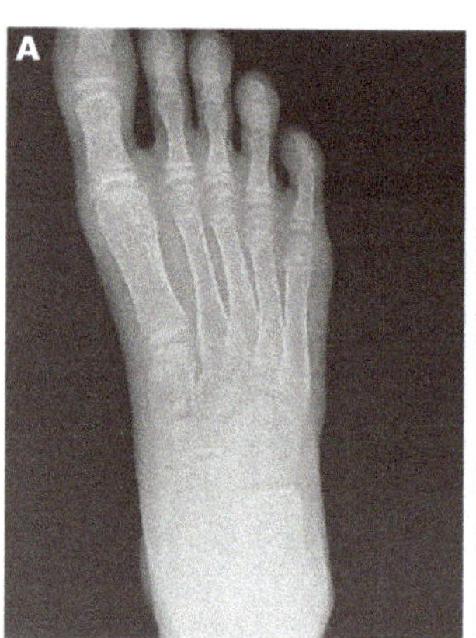

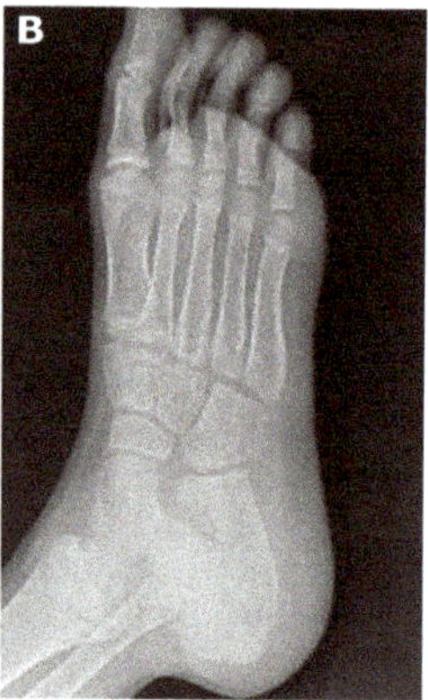

Fig. 27.17: *Normal foot X-rays - AP and oblique views.*

Medial border of 2nd metatarsal should be in line with the medial border of middle cuneiform

Normal alignment on oblique view:

Medial border of 4th metatarsal should be in line with the medial border of the cuboid.

Look for disruption in these lines or diastasis of > 2 mm between the base of 1st and 2nd metatarsals.

- Fracture of 2nd metatarsal base with/ without associated cuboid fracture should raise a suspicion of Lisfranc injury.
- If the diagnosis is not clear on X-ray, CT scan or MRI should be done.

Treatment

The goal of treatment is to achieve anatomical congruency of TMT joint complex that is stable on weight bearing.

- Undisplaced or minimally displaced (<1-2 mm.) fractures or clinically diagnosed 'sprain' of the foot can be treated in below-knee non-weight-bearing cast for 6 weeks. Weight bearing X-rays are taken on removal of the cast to assess stability and repeated 6 weeks later, once pain free weight bearing is achieved to confirm maintenance of reduction.
- If TMT joint displacement is >1-2 mm., closed reduction under anaesthesia is done, once acute swelling has subsided. By applying traction on toes using 'finger traps', displaced metatarsal is manipulated into place.
  - If stable anatomical reduction is confirmed radiologically, below-knee non-weight- bearing cast is advised with weekly check X-rays, for confirming maintenance of reduction.
  - If unstable, 1.5-2 mm K-wires/screw fixation is recommended, based on direction of displacement of metatarsals and the number of metatarsals involved. **(Fig. 27.19 A and B)**

The sequence of reduction and stabilisation of TMT fracture- dislocation should be as follows: **(Fig. 27.18)**

- First, stabilise the 1st ray by aligning 1st metatarsal, medial cuneiform and navicular.
- Next, stabilise Lisfranc ligament i.e. 2nd metatarsal to medial cuneiform (this is the most important wire) and also medial to middle cuneiforms.

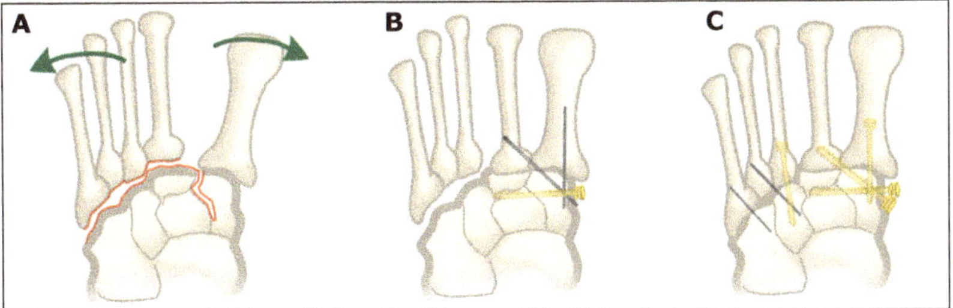

***Fig. 27.18**: Technique of fixation of Lisfranc injury:*
(A) Divergent type Lisfranc injury
(B) Stabilisation of 1st ray, Lisfranc ligament and medial-middle cuneiforms
(C) Stabilisation of 3rd to 5th metatarsals to their corresponding tarsals

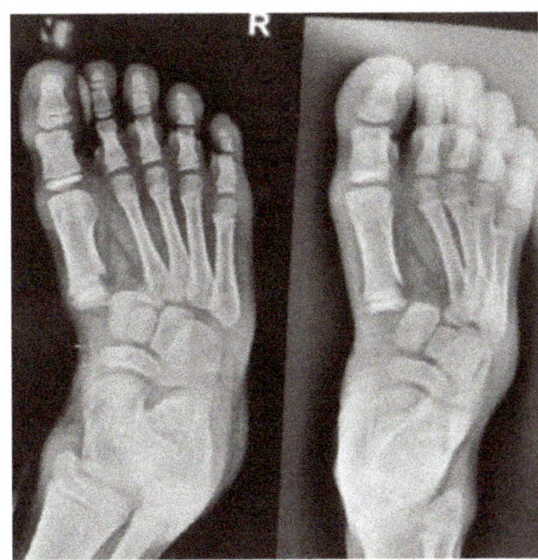

***Fig. 27.19A**: AP and Oblique X-rays of the foot showing Divergent pattern of Lisfranc injury in a 10-year-old child with medially displaced first metatarsal and laterally displaced fracture of the base of 2nd metatarsal.*

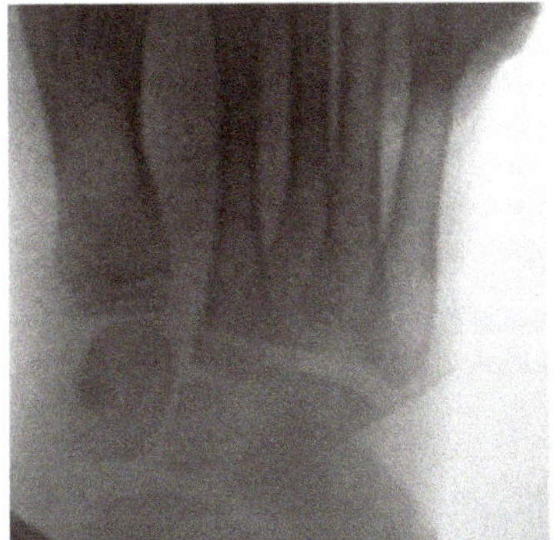

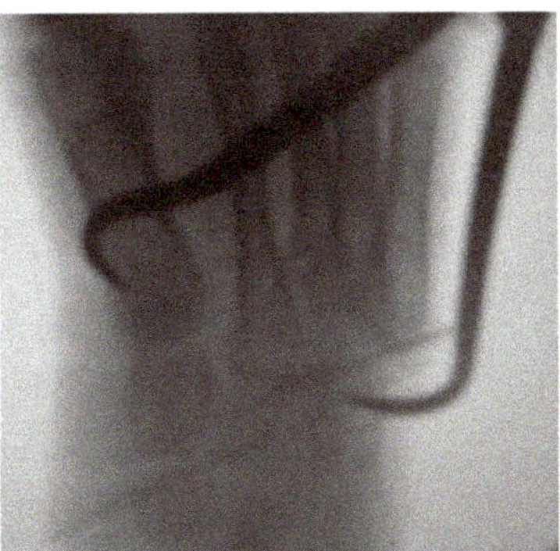

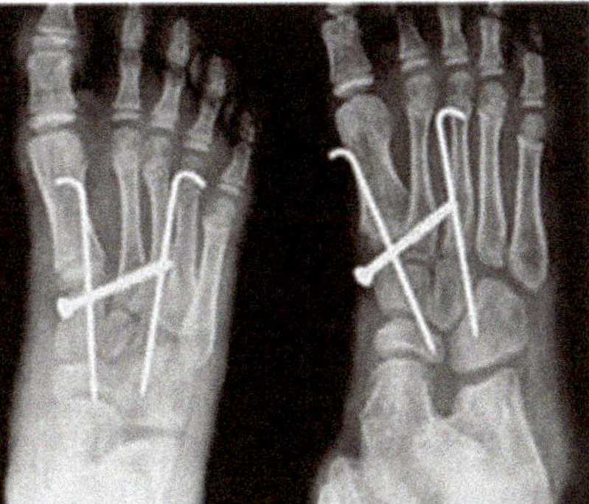

***Fig. 27.19B**: Closed reduction and percutaneous fixation of Divergent pattern of Lisfranc injury.*

- Lastly, stabilise 3rd to 5th metatarsals to their corresponding tarsals.
- Additional wire can be passed from 1st to 2nd metatarsal if required.

Percutaneous K-wires/screws can be removed 4-6 weeks after radiological confirmation of healing on weight bearing X-rays. Weight bearing can be started after this.

- Rarely, closed reduction may not be achieved due to interposed tibialis anterior tendon or interposed fracture fragment in 2nd metatarsal-middle cuneiform articulation. Open reduction is required in such cases using two longitudinal incisions- First over 1st-2nd intermetatarsal space and second in line with 4th metatarsal for lesser TMT joints. After open reduction, K-wire or 3.5 mm. screw fixation can be done and small osteochondral fragments can be excised whereas larger osteochondral fragments can be repaired. **(Fig. 27.20)**

Be careful to avoid injury to the proximal growth plate of 1st MT, if screw is used. Screws can be removed once pain free weight bearing is established, within 3 months, as beyond this time, there are chances of screw breakage and damage to the joint.

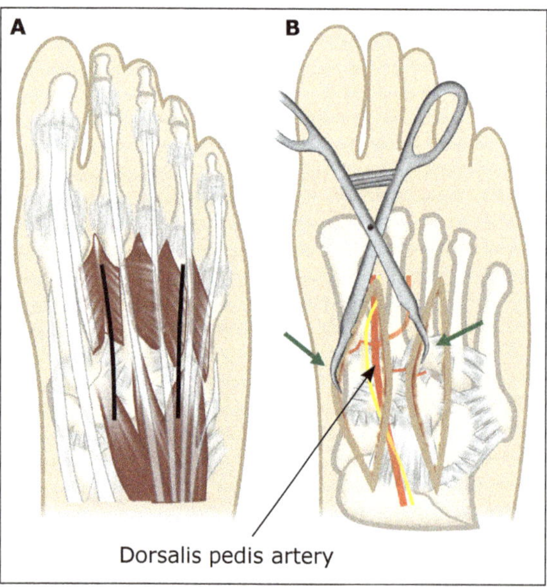

***Fig. 27.20**: Open reduction of Lisfranc injury*
(A) Two incisions- first along the 1st - 2nd intermetatarsal space and second along the 4th metatarsal
(B) Exposure of the 2nd metatarsal- medial cuneiform interval

Complications

Post-traumatic arthritis is a common complication in case of missed injury or delayed diagnosis > 6 weeks or due to loss of reduction or sometimes due to damage to articular cartilage from initial trauma. If conservative treatment fails, arthrodesis of TMT joints may be required in rare cases. But one must be careful to avoid arthrodesis of lesser TMT joints as their mobility is important for long term function of foot.

METATARSAL FRACTURES

Introduction

Metatarsal fractures are the most common paediatric foot fractures, comprising 60 % of all foot fractures in children. Fractures of the first metatarsal and fifth metatarsal base usually occur as isolated injuries but need special consideration. Second metatarsal neck is a common site for stress fracture.

Clinical Features

- Crush injury or direct injury due to fall of heavy load on the foot usually leads to mid diaphyseal fractures of the metatarsals and manifests as significant bruising and swelling. One must carefully assess for compartment syndrome.
- Indirect injury due to axial loading or torsional force leads to spiral fracture of proximal shaft or neck and manifests with minimal swelling.
- Always look for associated injuries in talus, cuboid etc.

Imaging

AP, lateral and oblique X-rays are routinely done.

If in doubt, CT scan may be required or repeat X-rays after 10-14 days may be performed.

Treatment

- Majority of metatarsal fractures can be treated conservatively in a below-knee cast. Child needs to be admitted in case of displaced fractures and monitored for pain, swelling and compartment syndrome.
- Closed reduction under anaesthesia and K-wire fixation is required for severely angulated fractures (dorsal angulation > 20°) or 'tenting' of the skin.
- First metatarsal is important in maintaining longitudinal arch of the foot and position of the first metatarsal head in relation to lesser metatarsal heads. Hence, it is important to treat first metatarsal fracture properly, especially in adolescents.
- Closed reduction is indicated for all fractures with > 10° dorsal angulation and any shortening. Translation is acceptable if there is no shortening. Intramedullary K-wire fixation **(Fig. 27.21)** or K-wires across fractured metatarsal to adjacent non fractured metatarsal both proximal and distal to fracture is recommended.

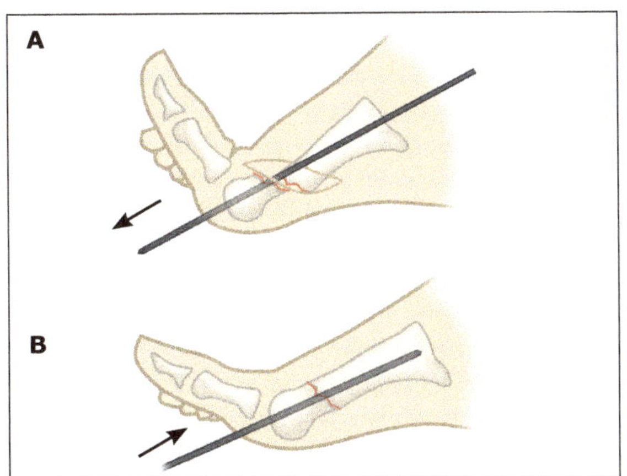

***Fig. 27.21**: Technique of open reduction of displaced 1st metatarsal fracture:*
(A) Retrograde insertion of the K-wire from the fracture site.
(B) Intramedullary advancement of the K-wire after reduction of fracture.

Fracture of the Base of 5th Metatarsal

This is the most common, accounting for 50% of all metatarsal fractures in children.

Surgical Anatomy

- Proximal apophyseal growth centre appears at 9 years and fuses at 12-15 years. This is often confused for a fracture. Hence, it is important to note that this growth centre is oriented longitudinally, almost parallel to the metatarsal shaft and has a smooth contour, as against a fracture.
- Nutrient artery enters the 5th metatarsal shaft at the junction of proximal and middle third and sends intra osseous branches proximally and distally. There is a small watershed area (zone 2) where there is overlap of metaphyseal vessels and proximal vessels from nutrient artery. There is a high rate of delayed union or non union of fracture in this area, especially in children close to maturity. **(Fig. 27.22)**
- There are many tendinous insertions on the base of 5th metatarsal. These may play a role in displacement of fracture.
- Peroneus brevis and abductor digiti minimi tendon insert on the dorsal

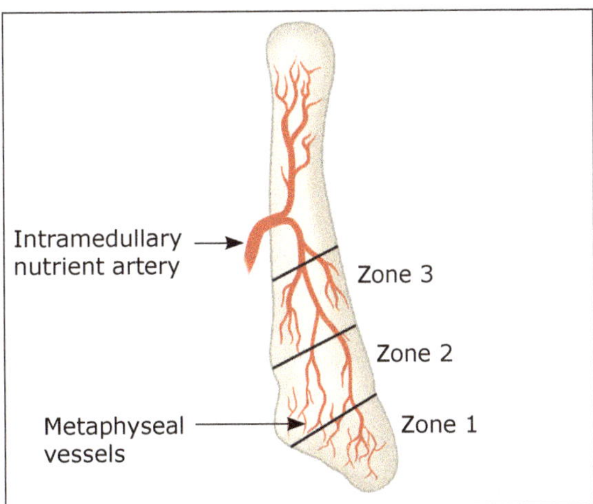

***Fig. 27.22**: Blood supply and zones of proximal 5th metatarsal*

aspect of 5th metatarsal at metaphyseal-diaphyseal junction. Plantar aponeurosis inserts on the plantar aspect of the tuberosity at the base.

Classification

Zone 1: Cancellous tuberosity that includes the insertion of the peroneus brevis tendon, abductor digiti minimi tendon and strong calcaneometatarsal ligament of plantar fascia.

Zone 2: Distal aspect of tuberosity (metaphyseal-diaphyseal junction), where the dorsal and plantar ligaments to the 4th metatarsal insert. Jones' fracture (oblique fracture in watershed area at metaphyseal diaphyseal junction) is included in this zone.

Zone 3: Distal to above ligamentous attachment to approximately mid – diaphyseal area.

Treatment

Zone 1 (Fig. 27.23)

Majority fractures in zone 1 being traction injuries can be treated conservatively with below-knee weight-bearing cast for 3-6 weeks. Most patients become asymptomatic by 3 weeks but radiological union takes longer.

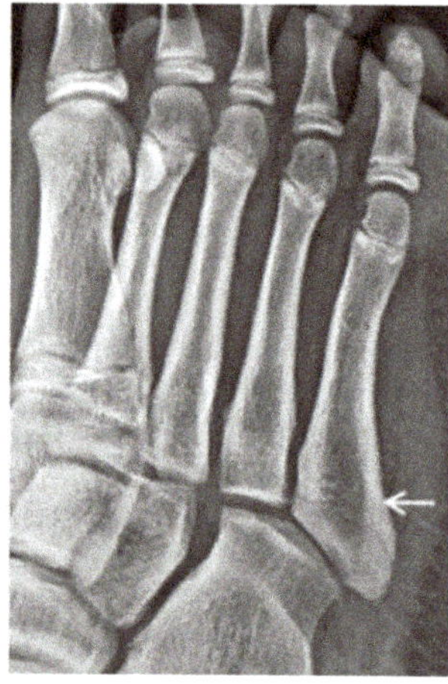

***Fig. 27.23**: Undisplaced fracture in zone 1 of the base of 5th metatarsal.*

Intra-articular, displaced > 3-4 mm. fractures in young active children require open reduction and fixation with 3.5 mm. partially or fully threaded screws inserted perpendicular to fracture line with bicortical hold. Direct lateral approach can be used. The fracture can be approached through the plane between peroneus brevis and peroneus tertius tendon insertion. Care is to be taken to protect the sural nerve.

Zone 2

This includes Jones' fracture typically seen in adolescents, caused by a combination of vertical loading and coronal shear forces. Acute fractures are treated by short leg non-weight-bearing cast for 6 weeks. Serial X-rays are important to monitor healing. Protected weight bearing can be started once callus is seen. In painful symptomatic chronic fracture, presenting 3 months post injury, a trial of below-knee non-weight-bearing cast can be given for 6 weeks. But if it fails to unite the fracture, internal fixation is recommended using 4 mm/6.5 mm cancellous screw from proximal to distal after thorough debridement of sclerotic medullary canal. **(Fig. 27.24)** Bone grafting also may be needed in selected cases.

Zone 3

This includes stress fractures seen in active athletes. Acute fracture requires a similar line of treatment as in zone 2, i.e. below-knee non-weight-bearing cast for 6 weeks, followed by protected weight bearing in hard soled shoes for 4 weeks. Chronic stress fractures may not respond to above treatment and may require surgical intervention, similar to zone 2.

PHALANGEAL FRACTURES

Phalangeal fractures are less common consisting ~18% of paediatric foot injuries.

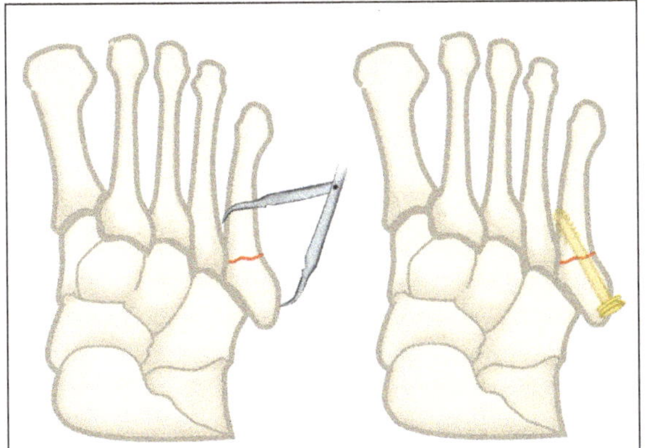

***Fig. 27.24**: Internal fixation of Jones' fracture with 4 mm cancellous screw.*

Injury to proximal phalanx is more common compared to distal phalanx and injuries of the great toe are more common than injuries of the lesser toes. The mechanism of injury can be direct trauma due to fall of a heavy object or indirect trauma due to twisting.

'Stubbing' injuries to the great toe are relatively common in children when they play outdoors barefoot without wearing protective footwear or even indoors due to the toe striking against a hard object. This can lead to fracture of the distal phalanx that often involves the physis. This physis is at the level of the root of the nail where the dermis of the skin is attached directly to the periosteum and there is no intervening subcutaneous tissue. Hence, any physeal injury of the distal phalanx of the great toe should be considered an open injury even if there is no evidence of bleeding from or around the nail. Due to barefoot playing, chances of contamination leading to osteomyelitis are high. Hence, early detection and prompt treatment is essential for this open distal phalanx physeal injury in the form of irrigation, debridement and antibiotics. Delay in the diagnosis or treatment can lead to complications like osteomyelitis, growth arrest and nail deformity.

Clinical Features

During clinical examination, one should check the site of tenderness, swelling, ecchymosis, obvious deformity and also rotational alignment. Always check for any breakdown of skin at the nail base, which indicates open physeal injury with associated nail bed injury. This requires a similar line of treatment as in fingers, with thorough debridement, nail bed repair, IV antibiotics and K-wire stabilisation of fracture.

Imaging

Standard AP and lateral X-rays are sufficient for diagnosis of phalangeal fractures. Sometimes it is difficult to assess the fracture on lateral X-ray due to overlap of toes. The remaining toes can be dorsiflexed with a towel for better visualisation.

Treatment

Majority of closed phalangeal fractures can be treated by ' buddy strapping ' with the adjacent toe, as the angulated coronal and sagittal plane fracture remodels well if the growth plate is still open, as in young children.

In adolescents however, K-wire fixation is preferred. In case of a great toe, intra-articular Salter-Harris type III and IV fractures are more common. These fractures may be treated with 'buddy strapping'. But if intra-articular displacement is more than 2-3 mm. and if > 25 % articular surface is involved, closed reduction is required for correction of axial and rotational alignment and then reduction can be maintained with strapping or K-wire fixation. **(Fig. 27.25)** Very rarely, open reduction may be required via dorsal/midlateral incision.

SESAMOID FRACTURE

There are many sesamoid bones in the

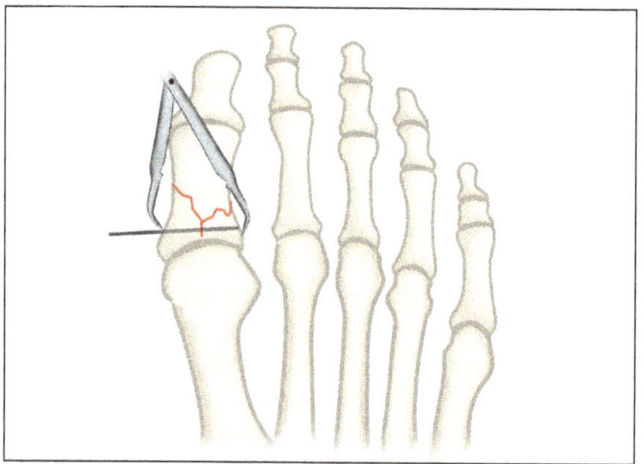

***Fig. 27.25**: K-wire fixation of intra-articular displaced fracture of the proximal phalanx of the great toe*

foot, but the two, medial and lateral sesamoid bones within the plantar plate of the 1st metatarsophalangeal joint and in the flexor hallucis brevis (FHB) tendons are most important, not only for shock absorption, but also to provide a fulcrum to improve the biomechanical function of the tendons of the first toe. These 2 sesamoid bones can get injured with forced dorsiflexion of the great toe. Such acute sesamoid bone fracture is rare in children but diagnosis can be difficult sometimes due to variable anatomy of these bones. Also, one has to differentiate fracture from partite sesamoid, that is seen approximately 10 times higher in medial sesamoid compared to lateral and seen bilaterally in 25-85 % children. Also, it is important to differentiate it from stress fracture/sesamoiditis as seen in runners and dancers due to repetitive dorsiflexion.

Imaging

AP and lateral weight bearing X-rays and tangential X-rays are required.

X-ray of the opposite side is helpful for comparison.

It can help in differentiating acute from chronic sesamoid injuries. Acute fracture has sharp corners and 'jagged' appearance, usually transverse and not widely displaced as fragments are contained within the plantar plate.

Treatment

Sesamoid fracture is treated by immobilisation in the below-knee plaster with the toe plate for 4-6 wks. Stress fracture may require a longer period of immobilisation. Surgery in the form of open reduction with bone grafting or excision of smaller fragment is rarely required in cases of symptomatic non union. One should be careful to avoid damage to the plantar plate.

Flowchart 27.1

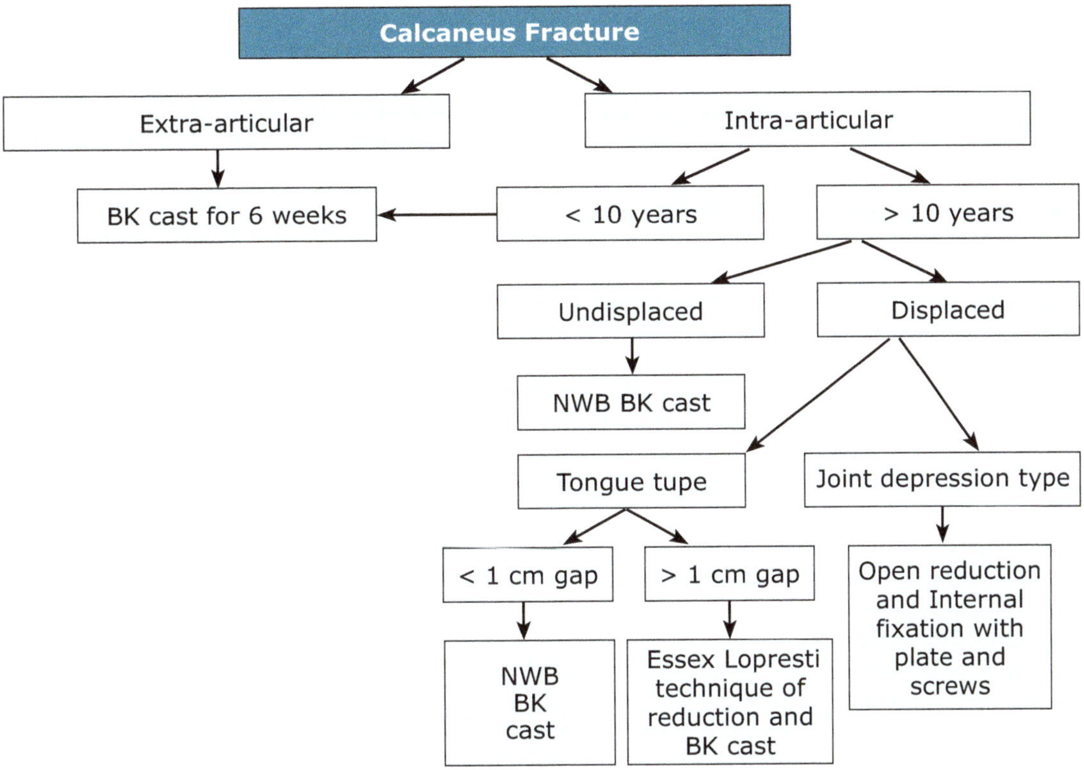

Calcaneus Fracture
Extra-articular
Intra-articular
BK cast for 6 weeks
< 10 years
> 10 years
Undisplaced
Displaced
NWB BK cast
Tongue tupe
Joint depression type
< 1 cm gap
> 1 cm gap
Open reduction and Internal fixation with plate and screws
NWB BK cast
Essex Lopresti technique of reduction and BK cast

Flowchart 27.2

Talar Neck Fracture
Type I
Type II
Type III
Type IV
NWB BK cast for 6-8 weeks
Immediate closed reduction under anaesthesia by plantar flexion and pronation of foot
Urgent open reduction and internal fixation
Stable reduction
Unstable reduction
NWB BK cast for 4 weeks in plantar flexion and for 4 weeks in neutral
Percutaneous K-wire/screw fixation and BK cast

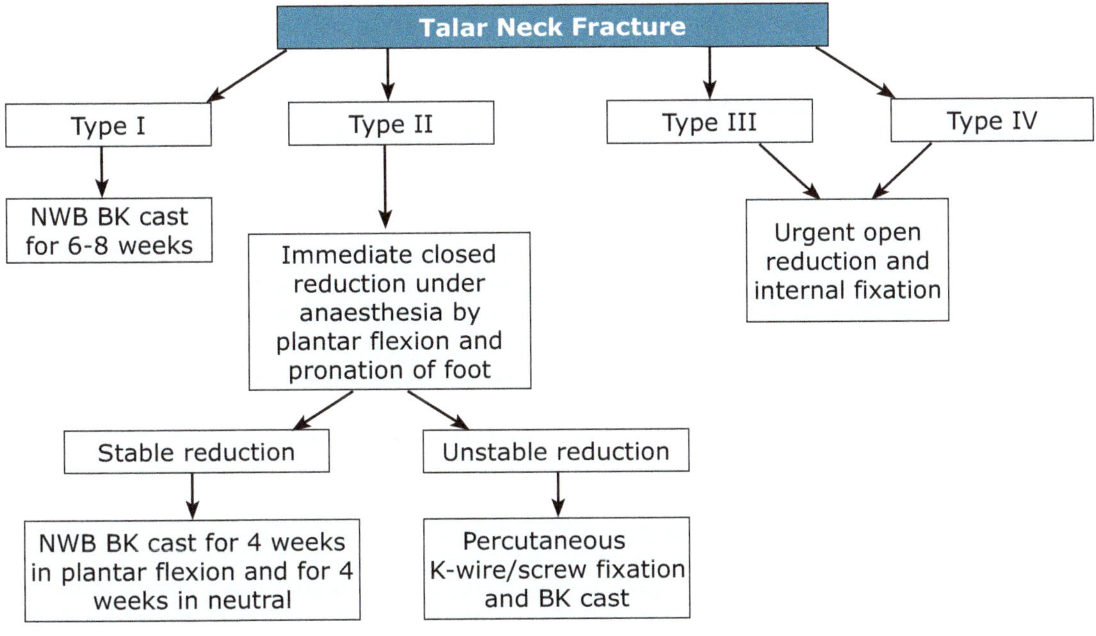

Flowchart 27.3

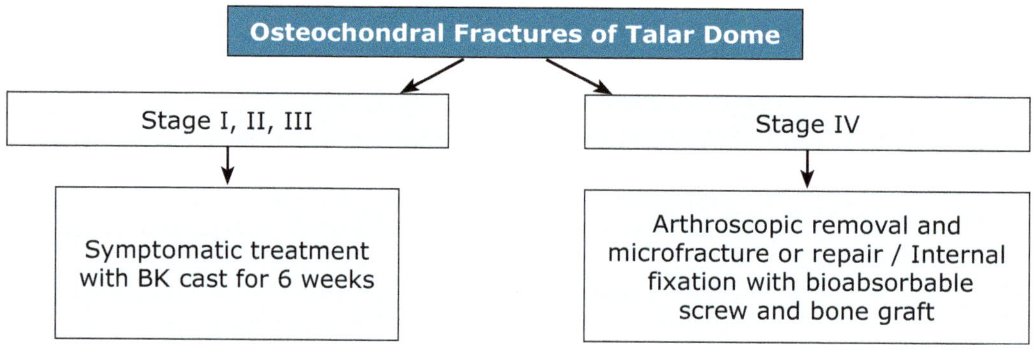

Flowchart 27.4

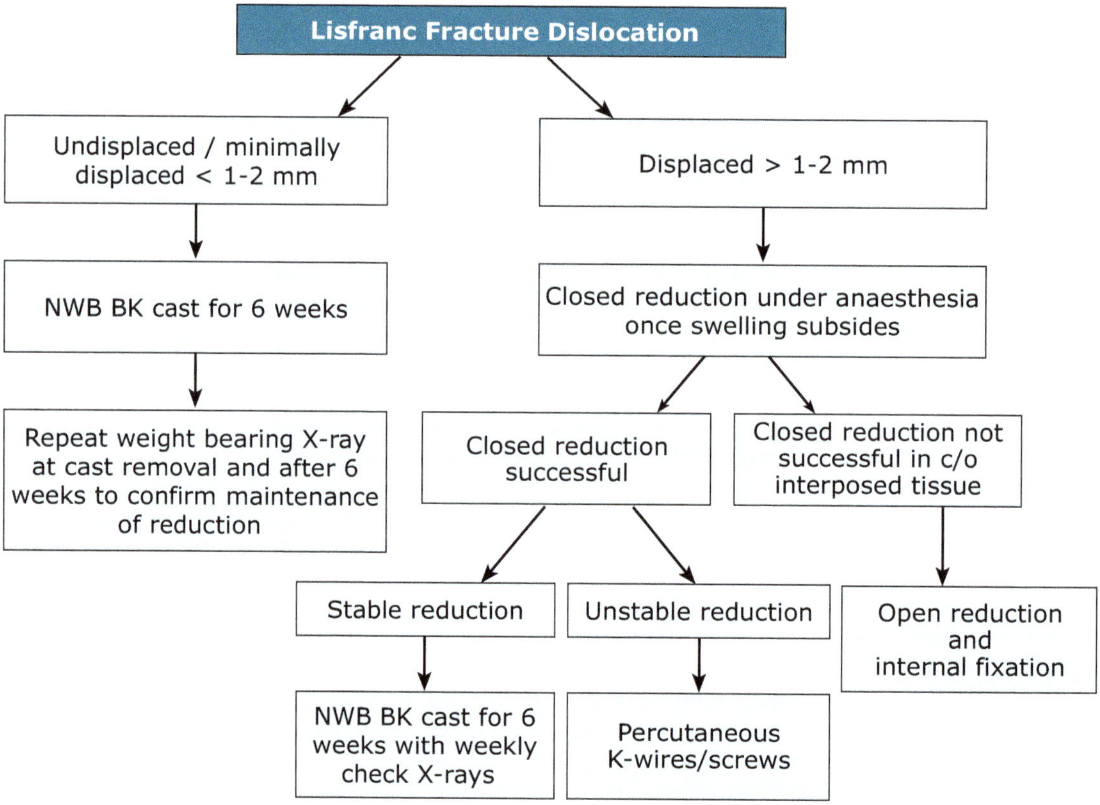

Lisfranc Fracture Dislocation

- Undisplaced / minimally displaced < 1-2 mm
  - NWB BK cast for 6 weeks
    - Repeat weight bearing X-ray at cast removal and after 6 weeks to confirm maintenance of reduction
- Displaced > 1-2 mm
  - Closed reduction under anaesthesia once swelling subsides
    - Closed reduction successful
      - Stable reduction
        - NWB BK cast for 6 weeks with weekly check X-rays
      - Unstable reduction
        - Percutaneous K-wires/screws
    - Closed reduction not successful in c/o interposed tissue
      - Open reduction and internal fixation

Flowchart 27.5

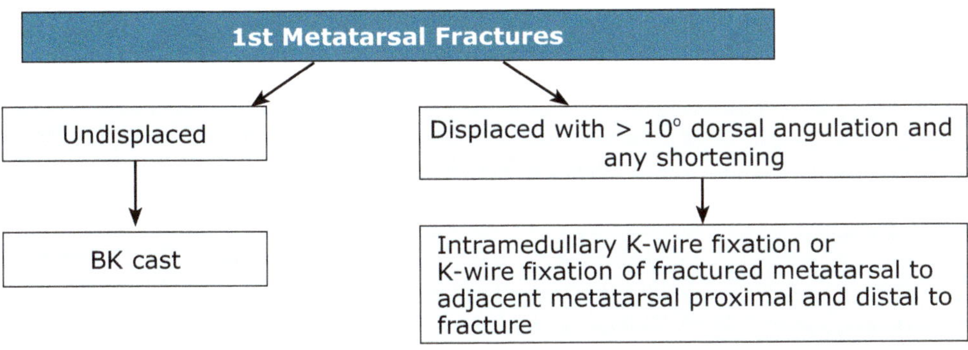

Flowchart 27.6

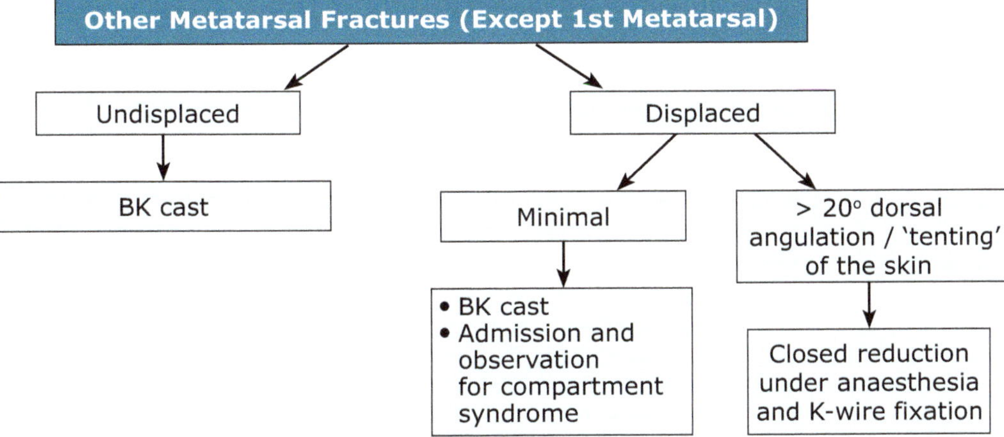

Flowchart 27.7

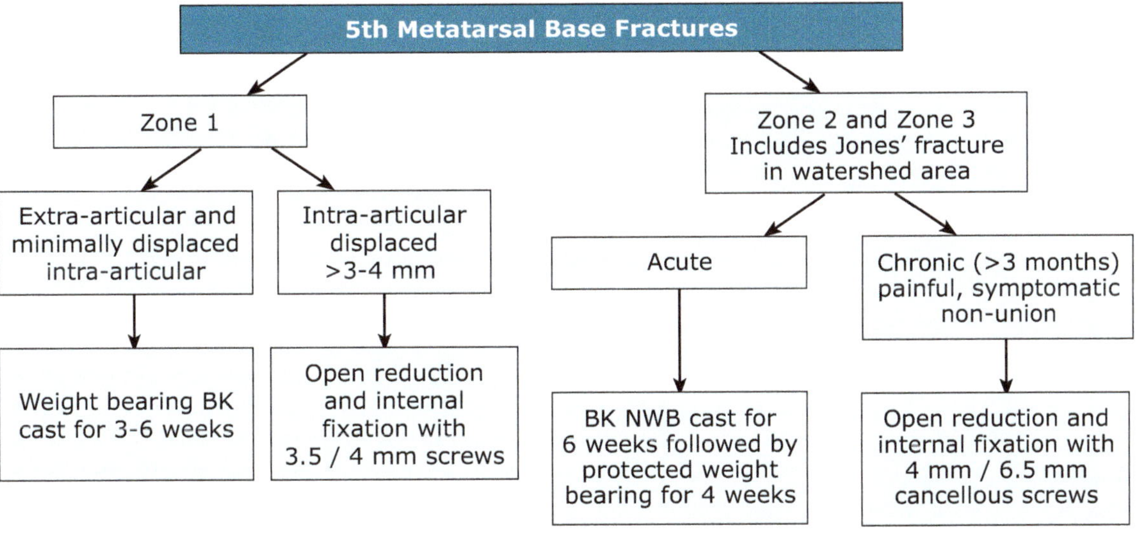

Flowchart 27.8

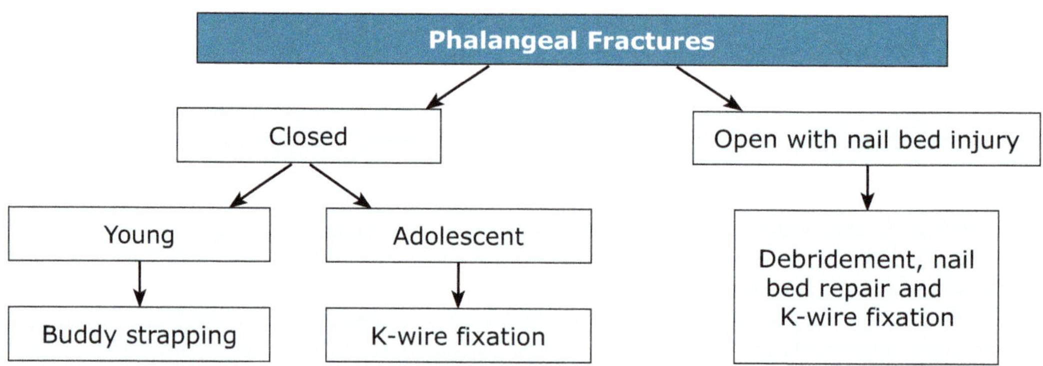

28 Fractures and Dislocations of the Cervical Spine

Introduction

- Cervical spine injuries are rare in children, accounting for <1% of all paediatric fractures and < 2% of all spine injuries. Children < 8 years are more prone for upper cervical spine injuries, due to large head translating forward on a hypermobile immature spine with ligament laxity and also due to horizontally oriented facet joints.
- Children are less prone for neurological deficit from cervical spine injury and if at all incomplete deficit occurs, they have better prognosis for recovery.
- The common mechanisms of injuries are high velocity motor vehicle accidents (MVA), fall from height, athletics, gymnastics, diving, birth trauma, child abuse etc. Associated facial and traumatic brain injuries are seen with cervical spine injuries.
- Spinal cord injury without radiographic abnormality (SCIWORA) is defined as clinical symptoms of traumatic myelopathy with no radiographic or computed tomographic (CT) features of spinal fracture or instability. SCIWORA commonly occurs in children < 8 years as the vertebral column can elongate upto 2 inches without disruption, whereas the spinal cord can rupture with even a quarter inch of elongation.

Clinical Features

- Children present with neck pain, headache, inability to move the neck, torticollis, subjective feeling of instability, neurological symptoms, respiratory distress etc.
- Physical examination should include a full assessment conducted from head to toe and evaluation of all organ systems. Examination of neck to elicit tenderness, muscle guarding or the presence of a gap in spinous process and complete neurological evaluation should be done.

Cervical spine clinical clearance decision rules for identifying trauma patients who require C-Spine imaging

National Emergency X-ray Utilization Study (NEXUS) 2000

- Midline cervical tenderness
- Focal neurological deficit
- Alertness
- Non–intoxicated state
- Absence of apparent injuries

NEXUS criteria has high sensitivity and negative predictive value in 9-17 years old.

Children below 3 years can clear C spine after trauma if

- No neurological deficit
- No cervical tenderness
- No distracting injuries
- No unexplained hypotension
- No MVA / fall from height >10 feet or Non-Accidental trauma

Children above 3 years can clear C spine after trauma if

- Alert
- No neurological deficit

- No midline tenderness
- No painful distracting injuries
- No unexplained hypotension
- Not intoxicated

Imaging

Plain X-ray:

- AP, lateral and open mouth view (>9 years)
- AP, lateral (<9 years)
- Supervised lateral flexion/extension view only in alert, cooperative child, never in an obtunded child

One should be aware of the normal radiological features in children that mimic fractures-

- Synchondrosis at the base of odontoid and

  Apparent anterior wedging of the vertebral body in a young child may mimic a *Fracture.*
- Apical ossification centre of odontoid and

  Secondary ossification centres at the tips of transverse and spinous processes may mimic an *Avulsion fracture.*
- Pseudo subluxation of C2-C3,

  Absent ossification centre of anterior arch of C1 in the first year of life and AAD upto 4.5 mm may mimic *Instability.*

Certain Specific Normal Radiological parameters on Lateral X-ray

Atlanto Occipital Junction: (Fig. 28.1)

- Distance between occipital condyles and facet joints of atlas should be < 5 mm. Any distance > 5 mm. suggests Atlanto- Occipital disruption.
- Distance between basion (anterior cortical margin of foramen magnum) and tip of dens should be < 12 mm

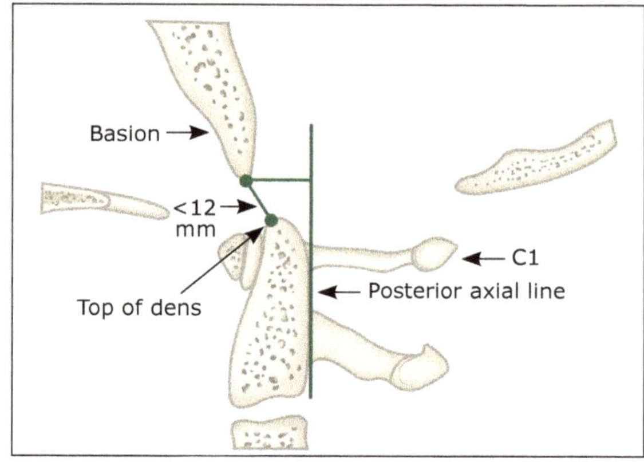

***Fig. 28.1**: Normal radiological parameters of Atlanto-occipital junction.*

Powers ratio

A line is drawn from the Basion (B) to the posterior arch of the atlas (C). A second line is drawn from the Opisthion (O) to the anterior arch of the atlas (A). Powers ratio is obtained by dividing the length of the line BC to the length of the line OA. **(Fig. 28.2)**

- Normal: Between 0.7 and 1

  Higher: Anterior subluxation

  Lower: Posterior subluxation
- **Wackenheim Line**

  This line is drawn along the posterior aspect of the clivus. If the line does not intersect the tip of the odontoid tangentially and if this line is displaced

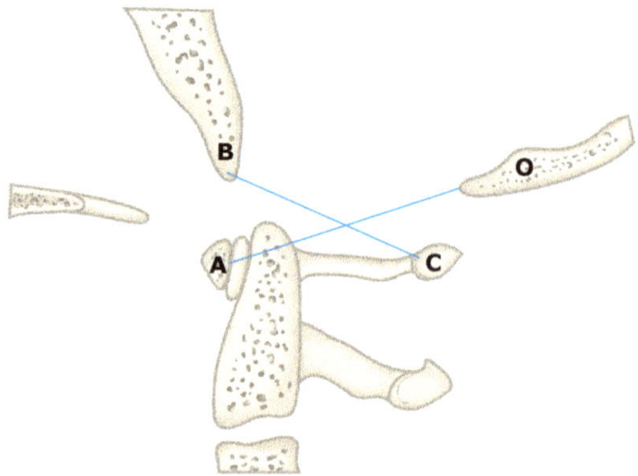

***Fig. 28.2**: Measurement of Powers ratio-BC/OA.*

anteriorly or posteriorly, disruption or increased laxity about the Atlanto Occipital joint should be suspected.

Atlanto-Axial Joint:

- ADI (Atlanto-Dens Interval): Normal upto 4.5 mm **(Fig. 28.3)**
- SAC (Space Available for Cord): Steel's rule of thirds **(Fig. 28.4)**

  ⅓rd occupied by the odontoid

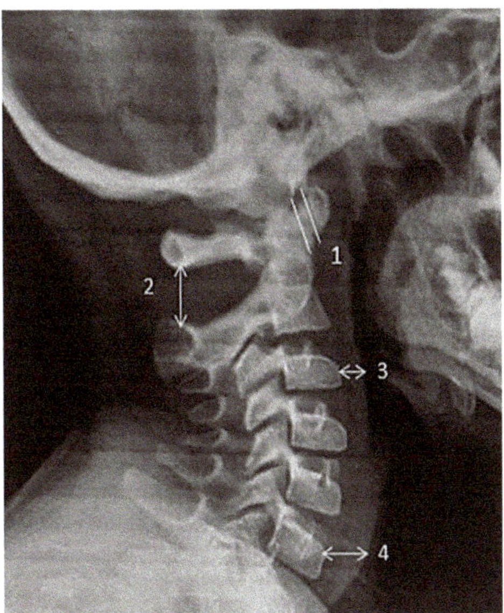

***Fig. 28.3**: Normal lateral X-ray of cervical spine in a 5-year-old child. Note: 1. ADI (Atlanto-Dens Interval) 2. Interspinous distance between C1 and C2 3.Prevertebral shadow at C3 and 4. at C6.*

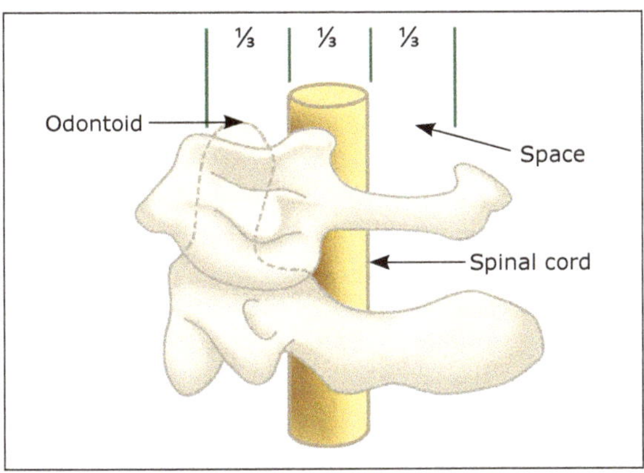

***Fig. 28.4**: Steel's rule of thirds.*

  ⅓rd occupied by the spinal cord

  ⅓rd is the free space available for the cord

- Interspinous distance between C1 and C2 should be <10 mm. If more, it is suggestive of ligament injury **(Fig. 28.3)**.

Upper cervical spine:

- C2 to C3 and C3 to C4: Displacement upto 3-4 mm in flexion and reducing on extension is normal.
- **Swischuk's line** (Spinolaminar line) is used to determine pseudosubluxation of C2 on C3. **(Fig. 28.5)** A line is drawn from the anterior cortex of the spinous process of C1 to the spinous process of C3. Anterior cortex of the spinous process of C2 should normally be within 3 mm of this line.

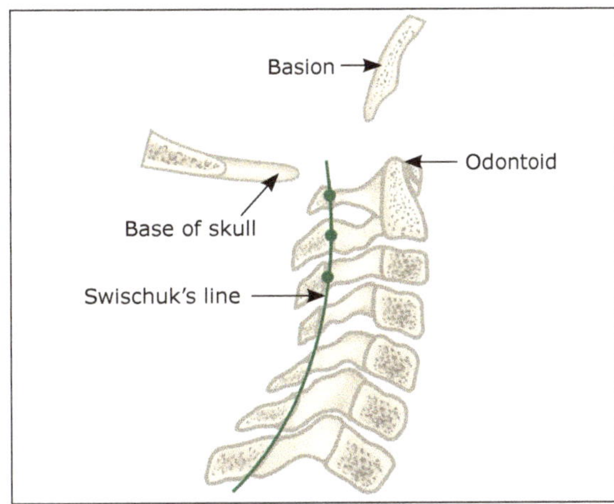

***Fig. 28.5**: Swischuk's line to determine pseudo-subluxation of C2 on C3.*

Lower cervical spine:

- The overall alignment can be evaluated by the smooth and continuous lines as seen on the lateral cervical spine X-ray. **(Fig. 28.6)**
- Interspinous distance should be no more than 1.5 times the distance at adjacent levels

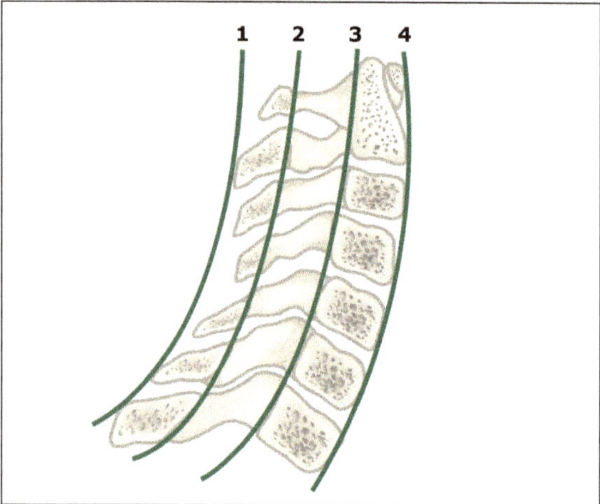

Fig. 28.6: *Assessment of overall alignment of lower cervical spine.*
1. Line adjoining the Spinous processes
2. Spinolaminar line
3. Posterior vertebral line
4. Anterior vertebral line

- Normal retropharyngeal (pre-vertebral) soft tissue space: **(Fig. 28.3)**

  < 6 mm at C3

  < 14 mm at C6

CT scan and MRI (including MR angiography) are helpful in case of doubtful diagnosis on X-ray. They can confirm ligament injuries, marrow oedema, intra spinal haemorrhage, SCIWORA, disc pathology etc.

Treatment

- Initial management of suspected cervical spine injury is very important to avoid further damage in unstable spine and spinal cord.
- Immobilisation should be done in the field in a modified backboard with a cut out to accommodate the large head of a child, while avoiding undue flexion.
- It is advisable to use a rigid cervical collar along with sandbags or taping on either side of head for better immobilisation or a custom made cervico-thoracic brace/ halo vest can be used if available.
- When ventilatory support is required, gentle in-line traction with orotracheal or nasotracheal intubation is safe and does not lead to further neurological injury.

Non-surgical Treatment

- Use of methylprednisolone is recommended as in adults.
- The recommended dose is 30 mg/kg loading dose over 3 hours, followed by 5.4 mg/kg over 24 hours, if the child presents within 3 hours of injury and over 48 hours if the child presents between 3-8 hours of injury.

Surgical Treatment

The surgical treatment varies as per the level of injury.

Occipital- C1 Injuries

Occipital Condyle Fracture

- This is a very rare injury requiring a high index of suspicion and is associated with high mortality rate.
- It is very difficult to diagnose on X-ray and requires CT scan with multiplanar reconstruction, especially if occipital condyle fracture is suspected in presence of lower cranial nerve deficits, associated head injury, basal skull fracture or significant neck pain.
- *Classification and Treatment*: **(Fig. 28.7)**

Type 1 and 2A are stable fractures and can be treated with a cervical orthosis.

Type 2B are unstable fractures due to associated disruption of tectorial membrane or alar ligament and require occipital cervical fusion with/without fixation. Post-operatively, the patient is

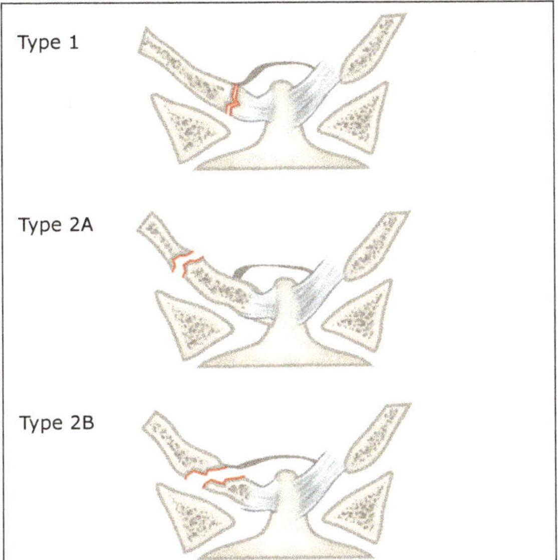

***Fig. 28.7**: Tuli classification of occipital condylar fractures based on displacement and stability of the occiput/C1 to C2 complex:*
Type 1: Undisplaced fracture
Type 2: A - Displaced but stable
B - Displaced and unstable

immobilised in a halo vest jacket or halo cast upto 3-4 months.

Atlanto-occipital instability

- Atlanto occipital dislocation can occur due to sudden acceleration or deceleration force where the head is thrown forward, causing sudden craniovertebral separation.
- Significant anterior soft tissue swelling on lateral X-ray should raise suspicion of atlanto occipital instability. This can be confirmed by some radiological parameters **(Figs. 28.1 and 28.2)**

  MRI is helpful to confirm the diagnosis.
- Atlanto occipital instability can be of three types: longitudinal distraction with axial occipital separation, rotational injury and anterior/posterior displacement
- Surgical stabilisation is the treatment of choice.

C1 – C2 injuries

Fracture of the Atlas

- *Jefferson fracture* (fracture of the ring of C1) is a rare injury and constitutes < 5% of all cervical spine fractures in children.
- Mechanism of injury is an axial load applied to the head, with the force transmitted through the occipital condyles to the lateral masses of C1 and causing disruption of C1 ring. **(Fig. 28.8)**
- In children, fractures can occur through normal synchondrosis or there can be plastic deformation of the ring with no obvious fracture. CT scan can be helpful to detect fracture and progressive healing.

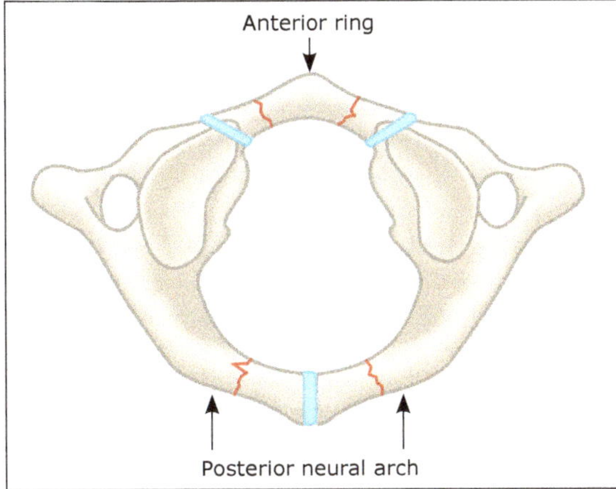

***Fig. 28.8**: Jefferson fracture.*

On AP X-ray, if the two lateral masses are widened >7 mm beyond the borders of the axis, an injury to TAL (transverse atlantal ligament) is suspected in the form of either rupture or avulsion that can be diagnosed on MRI. This can lead to atlanto-axial instability, which requires surgical management.

Majority of atlas fractures can be treated conservatively with immobilisation in an orthosis [rigid collar or SOMI (Sternal

Ocipital Mandibular Immobiliser) brace] or Minerva cast/halo brace for 8 weeks. After healing, stability is to be confirmed with flexion/extension lateral views.

Odontoid Fracture

- Odontoid fracture is a relatively common injury accounting for almost 10% of cervical spine fractures and dislocations in children.
- The most common fracture occurs through the synchondrosis of C2 distally at the base of the odontoid, appearing like S-H type I injury, commonly with anterior displacement.
- Odontoid fracture can occur after a severe injury like fall from a significant height or MVA, or sometimes after a relatively minor injury like a fall from bed in a younger child (<4 years).
- Clinical sign suggesting odontoid fracture is strong resistance to extend the neck and resistance to attempts of passive manipulation unless the head is supported by the examiner.
- If the X-ray is not clear, CT scan with 3-D reconstruction or MRI may be needed for diagnosis. **(Figs. 28.9 and 28.10)**
- Odontoid fracture is classified as in adults after fusion of C2 synchondrosis (3-6 years)

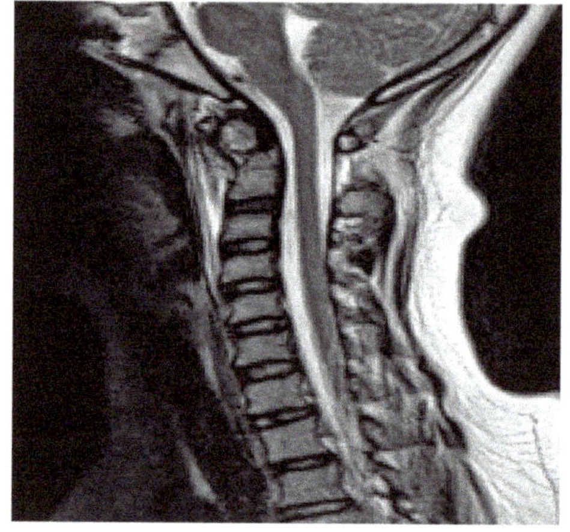

***Fig. 28.10**: MRI showing displaced odontoid fracture and no cord compression.*

Type I: Fracture at the tip of dens at the insertion of alar ligament

Type II: Fracture at the base of dens at its attachment to body

Type III: Subdentate fracture through the body of C2

- Majority odontoid fractures can be treated conservatively by closed reduction (slight hyperextension of neck) with the aim to achieve at least 50% apposition. After closed reduction, immobilisation in Minerva or halo cast or custom orthosis for 8-12 weeks is recommended.
- After healing, stability should be documented by flexion–extension X-rays.

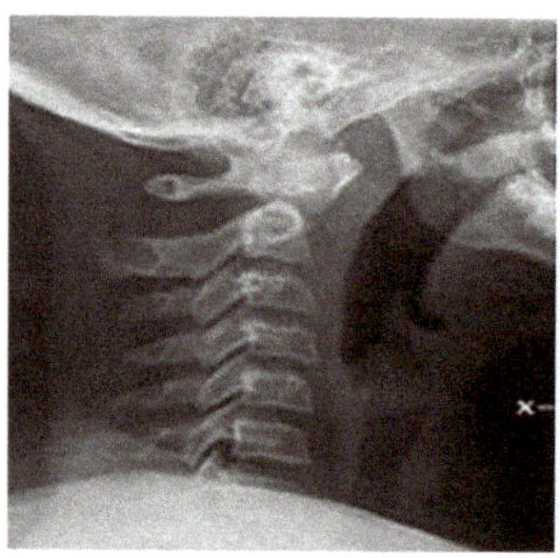

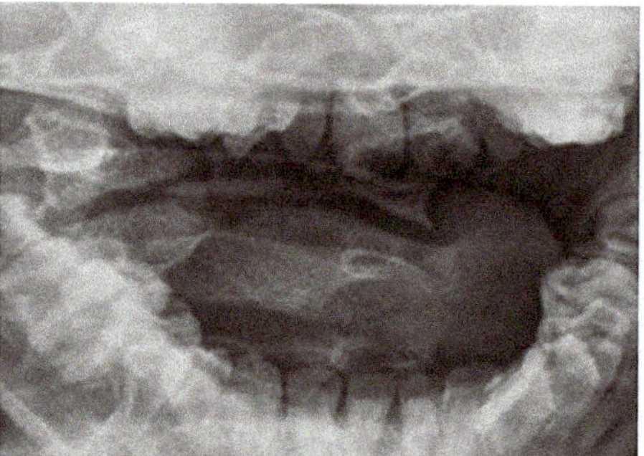

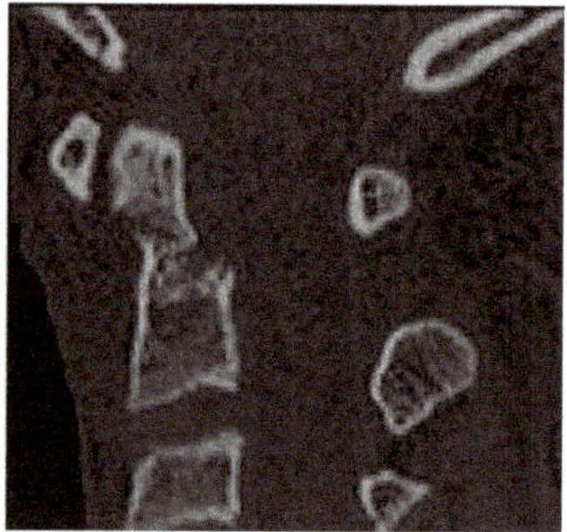

***Fig. 28.9**: Lateral and open mouth X-rays and CT scan showing Type II odontoid fracture.*

- Rarely, in a grossly unstable fracture, posterior C1-C2 fusion and fixation may be required.

Os odontoideum

- This is an anatomic variant when the dens and the body of C2 are separate.
- There may be associated atlanto-axial instability **(Fig. 28.11)**
- There are two types: orthotopic with a normal position and dystopic or displaced.
- It is seen as a well rounded ossicle above the hypoplastic dens.

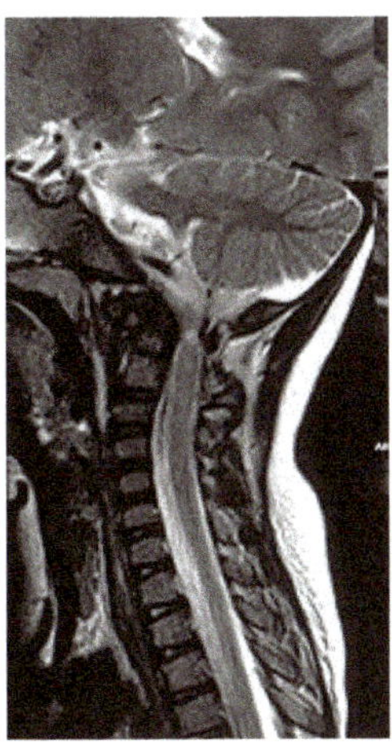

Fig. 28.11: *MRI showing os odontoideum with severe cervical stenosis.*

Traumatic Atlanto Axial Dislocation (AAD)

- AAD occurs as a result of injury to the transverse ligament and the alar ligament, especially in children with predisposing conditions like Down's syndrome, Larsen's syndrome, Juvenile Rheumatoid arthritis and other bony dysplasias. **(Fig. 28.12)**
- X-rays can be useful for diagnosis if the Atlanto-Dens interval is > 4.5 mm.
- Surgical stabilisation is required when anterior translation is > 8-10 mm. or when neurological deficit is present.

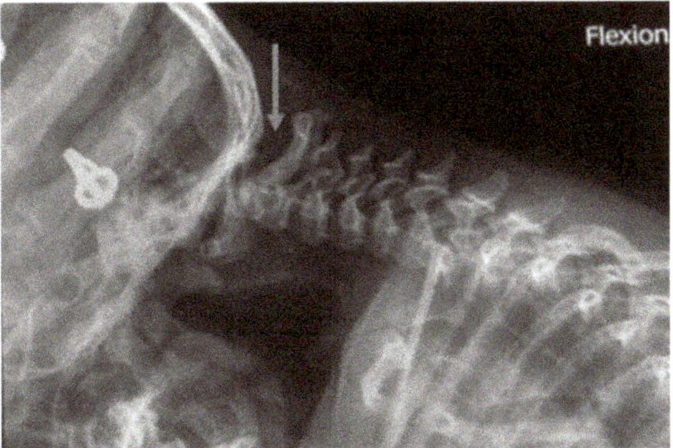

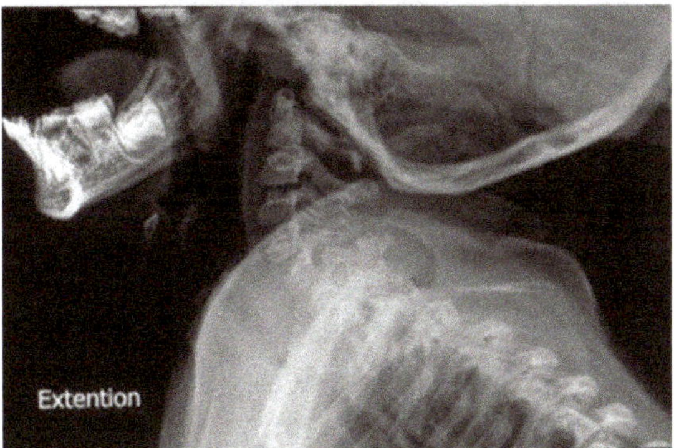

Fig. 28.12: *Flexion extension X-rays in a child with Down's syndrome with atlantoaxial instability.*

Atlanto axial arthrodesis: different options

1. Using sublaminar wires/cables: Brooks and Jenkins
2. Using wires passed under lamina of atlas and the spinous process of axis: Gallie **(Fig. 28.13)**

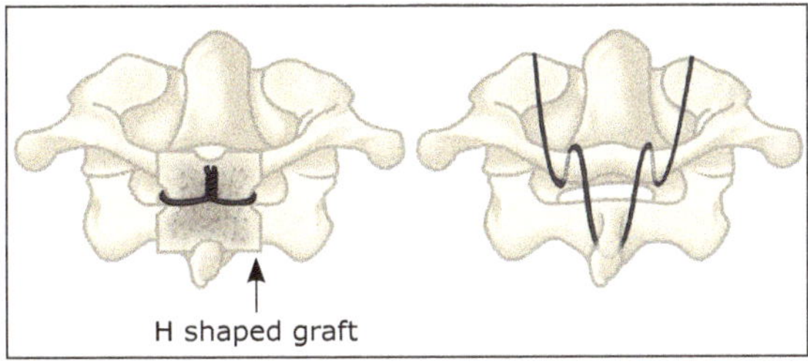

Fig. 28.13: *Gallie fusion technique of atlanto-axial arthrodesis.*

3. Posterior C1-C2 transarticular screw fixation **(Fig. 28.14)**

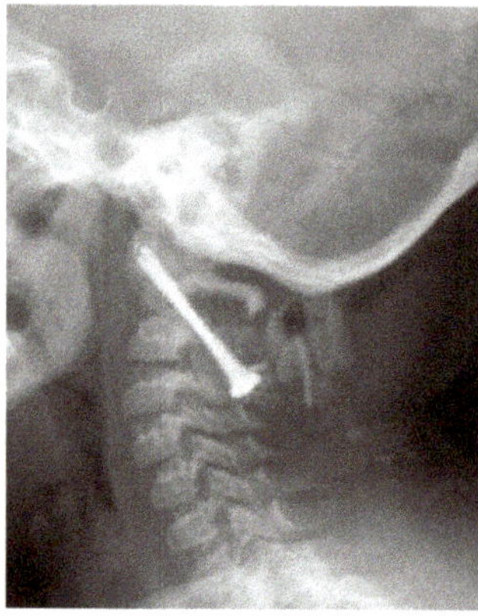

Fig. 28.14: *C1-C2 transarticular screw fixation for atlanto-axial instability.*

4. Posterior C1-C2 polyaxial screw and rod fixation **(Fig. 28.15)**

- In young children, posterior fusion using Gallie/Brooks technique is preferred, followed by immobilisation in halo vest or halo cast.
- In older children (>11 years), stable fixation with transarticular 3.5 mm C1-C2 screws is preferred.

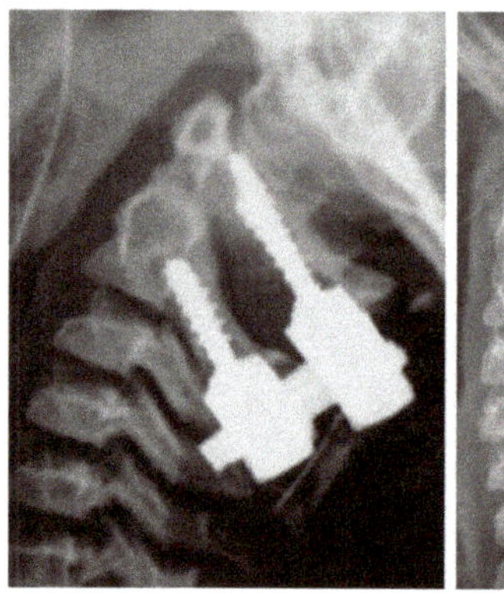

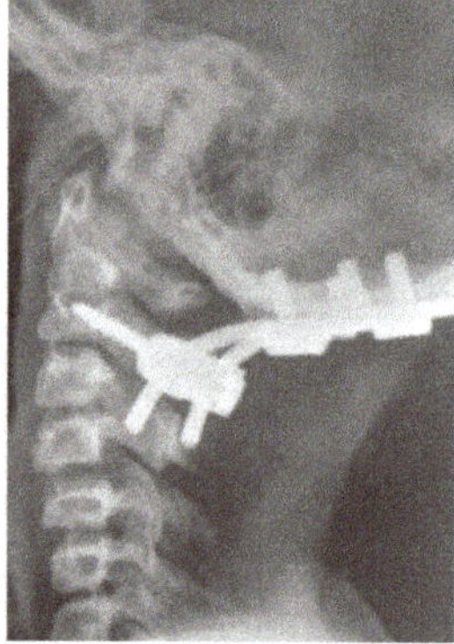

Fig. 28.15: *C1-C2 fixation and occipitocervical fixation using polyaxial screws and rods.*

C2-C3 injuries

Hangman's Fracture: (pedicle fracture of C2 with spondylolisthesis of C2 over C3)

- Hangman's fracture is common in children due to a large head with poor muscle control and hypermobility.
- Child abuse should be suspected in children less than 2 years.
- Mechanism of injury is forced hyperextension and axial loading.
- It is recommended to look for associated head/face injury.
- It is important to differentiate this fracture from congenital spondylolysis (persistent synchondrosis) which presents with symmetrical osseous gap with smooth well defined cortical margins, no prevertebral soft tissue swelling and no signs of instability.
- CT/MRI is important to differentiate and fully define the extent of fracture and the amount of displacement.

Treatment

Stable fracture (with < 3 mm. C2-3 subluxation) can be treated conservatively with immobilisation in Minerva jacket/ halo or cervical orthosis for 8-12 weeks.

Unstable fracture /nonunion are to be treated with anterior/posterior arthrodesis.

Subaxial (C3–C7) injuries

- These are rare injuries.
- Usually, the inferior end plate fractures, as the superior end plate is protected by the uncinate process.
- Fracture can be S-H type I where the end plate breaks completely through the cartilaginous portion or S-H type II where fracture exits through the bony edge.

Various types of subaxial injuries are as follows:

1. Posterior ligament disruption

- It occurs due to flexion- distraction injury
- The X-ray shows loss of lordosis and

increase in posterior interspinous distance. >7° kyphotic angulation between adjacent vertebral bodies is suggestive of unstable injury **(Fig. 28.16)**

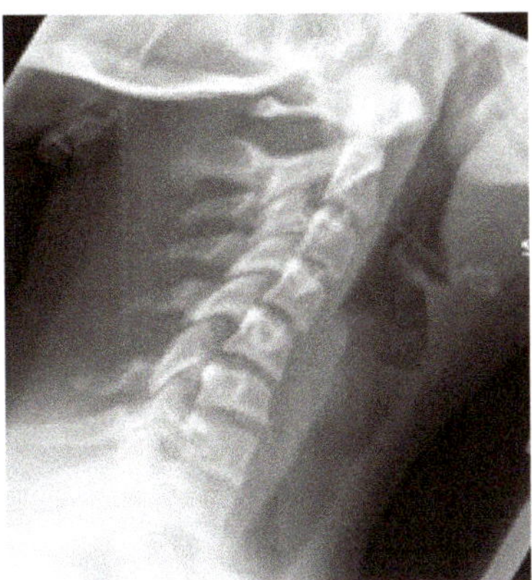

***Fig. 28.16**: C5-6 flexion distraction injury in an adolescent with cervical kyphosis and interspinous widening.*

- CT is corroborative **(Fig. 28.17)**
- MRI is helpful in diagnosis of ligament damage.

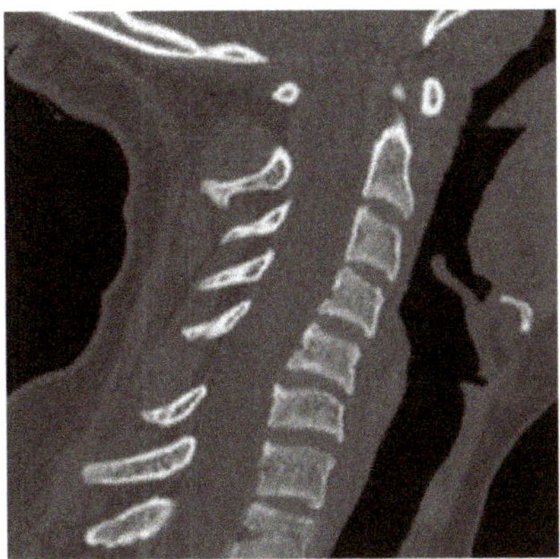

***Fig. 28.17**: CT scan showing C5-6 wedging and posterior ligament injury with interspinous widening .*

SLIC (Subaxial Cervical Spine Injury Classification) and severity score **(Table 28.1)**

Three major injury characteristics are used to describe subaxial cervical injuries – morphology, discoligamentous complex integrity and neurological status.

Table 28.1: Subaxial cervical spine injury classification (SLIC) and severity score

	Points
Morphology	
No abnormality	0
Compression	1
Burst	2
Distraction	3
Rotation or translation	4
Discoligamentous complex	
Intact	0
Indeterminate	1
Disrupted	2
Neurological status	
Intact	0
Root injury	1
Complete cord injury	2
Incomplete cord injury	3
Presence of continued cord compression in the setting of spinal cord injury	+1

Treatment:

Treatment recommendations are based on scoring:

≤3: conservative treatment in the form of immobilisation in extension orthosis with close follow up for any development of instability

4: indeterminate

≥5: surgical treatment in the form of posterior arthrodesis

2. Compression fracture

- It is the most common type of fracture occurring due to pure flexion moment with axial loading, without significant rotatory or axial loading.
- Neurological injury is rare.

- It is a stable fracture and heals within 3-6 weeks.
- Careful X-ray examination for reduction in vertebral body height is important.
- Majority are treated conservatively in the cervical collar for 3-6 weeks. Assessment of stability with flexion/extension films after 2-4 weeks is recommended.
- In children < 8 years, vertebral body height gets restored with growth, provided there is < 20° kyphosis.

3. Unilateral and bilateral facet dislocations

- It is the second most common subaxial injury, especially seen in adolescents, occurring due to a range of injury mechanisms like hyperflexion, hyperextension, and/or axial rotation from MVA/falls/diving accidents.
- Bilateral dislocations are usually associated with cord injury. Unilateral dislocations have minimum localised pain or no symptoms.
- X-ray shows 'perched facet' due to the overlapped cartilage. CT scan can confirm the fracture/dislocation. **(Fig. 28.18)**

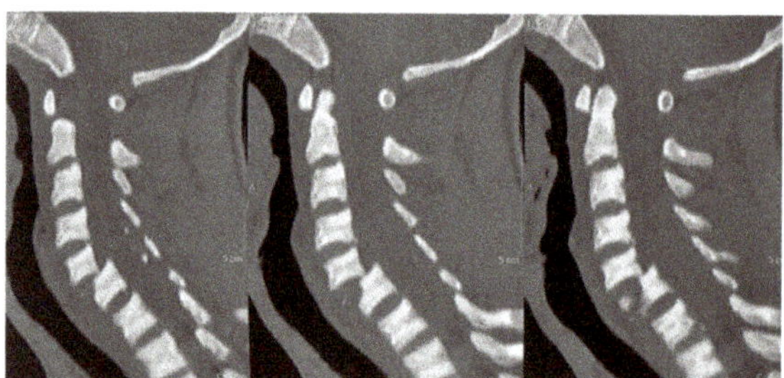

Fig. 28.18: *CT scan showing C5-6 fracture dislocation.*

- Treatment:

  Unilateral dislocation can be treated with skeletal traction and reduction.

  Bilateral dislocation is more unstable and associated with neurological deficit. It requires emergent reduction followed by immediate MRI to check for epidural haematoma or herniated disc. Anterior or posterior instrumentation and arthrodesis is required after reduction.

  There is a risk of neurological deterioration during reduction, so careful evaluation and neuro-monitoring is essential.

4. Burst fracture

- It is a rare injury, occurring due to axial loading of the slightly flexed head, usually after a high energy trauma.
- Characteristic fracture pattern includes anterior displacement of the antero inferior aspect of the body- the 'teardrop' fracture.
- It is mostly associated with neurological deficit.
- X-ray shows the loss of body height.

  CT scan is helpful to check retropulsed fragment or occult laminar fractures. **(Fig. 28.19)**

  MRI is helpful to assess disc injury, herniation and posterior ligament injury.

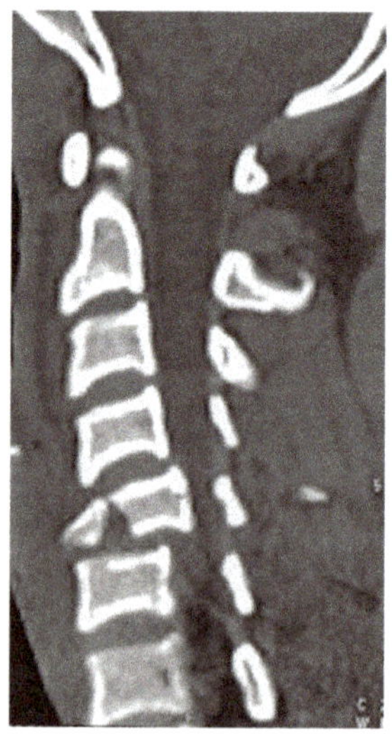

Fig. 28.19: *CT scan showing C5 fracture with retropulsed fragment.*

- Treatment:

  Traction followed by halo immobilisation is recommended if there is no neurological deficit/no significant canal compromise.

  If there is significant canal compromise, anterior decompression and arthrodesis is rarely recommended (as it damages anterior growth potential and kyphotic deformity may occur due to continued posterior growth). Anterior instrumentation and stabilisation is mainly used in older children and adolescents. **(Fig. 28.20)**

  When an anterior burst fracture is associated with significant posterior ligament instability, a posterior stabilisation procedure is necessary.

5. Spondylolysis and listhesis

- It occurs due to hyperextension or flexion-axial loading injury.
- AP, lateral and oblique views are required for diagnosis.
- CT/MRI is helpful to differentiate this injury from normal synchondrosis.
- Treatment:

  For stable injuries, cervical orthosis/halo brace is recommended.

  For unstable injuries or nonunion, surgical stabilisation in the form of posterior arthrodesis using K-wire and 16 gauge wire or lateral mass screw or translaminar screw is recommended.

  In older paediatric patients and adolescents, anterior arthrodesis is recommended based on similar principles as in adults.

Complications

General

- Pulmonary insufficiency
- Gastrointestinal haemorrhage
- Deep vein thrombosis
- Urinary tract infection
- Pressure sores

Local

- Late spinal deformity (very high chance) especially if child is < 10 years at the time of injury.

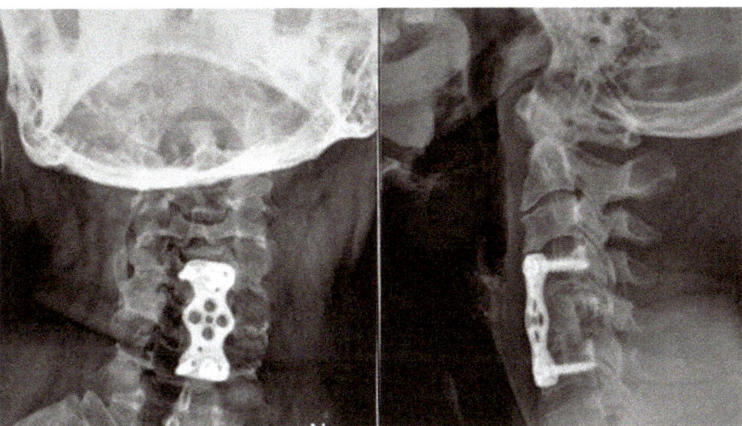

Fig. 28.20: *C5 corpectomy and C4 to C6 anterior cervical plate fixation and fusion with bone graft.*

Cervical Spine Injuries

Flowchart 28.1

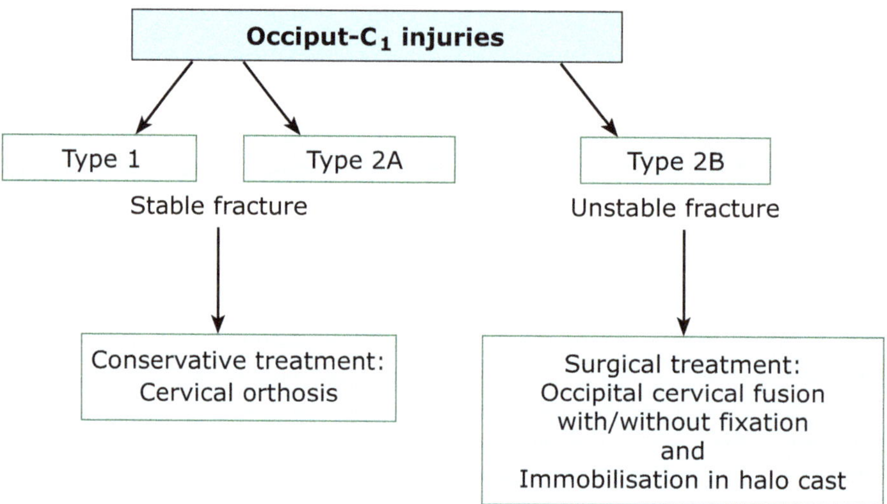

Flowchart 28.2

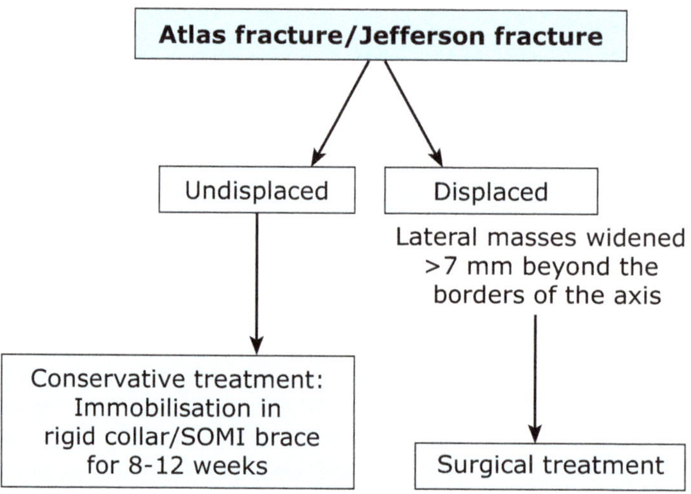

Flowchart 28.3

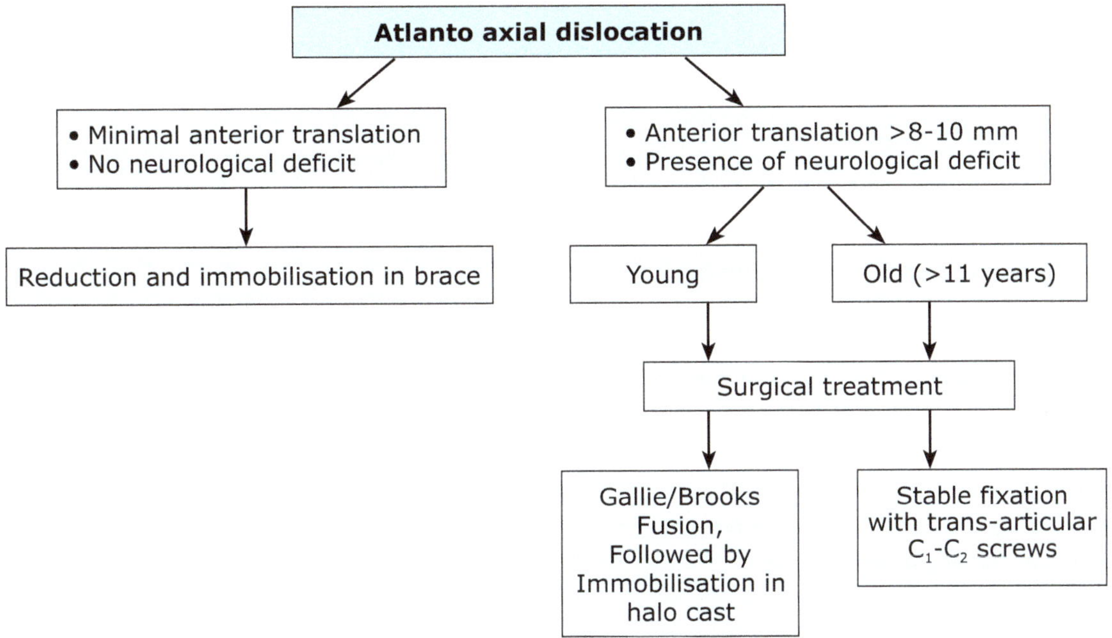

Flowchart 28.4

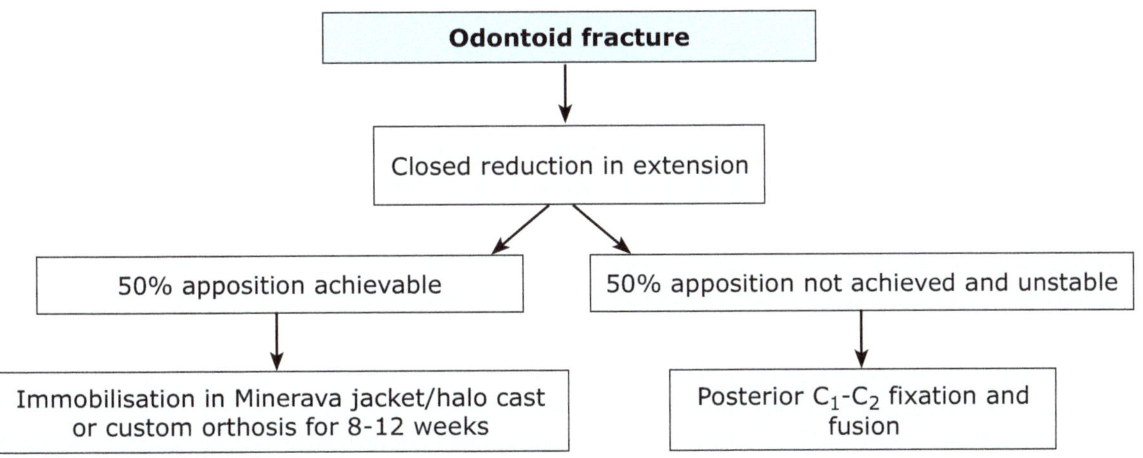

Flowchart 28.5

C_2-C_3 Injuries
Stable fracture (<3 mm C_{2-3} subluxation)
Unstable fracture (>3 mm subluxation)
Immobilisation in Minerava jacket/halo cast or custom orthosis for 8-12 weeks
Anterior or posterior arthrodesis

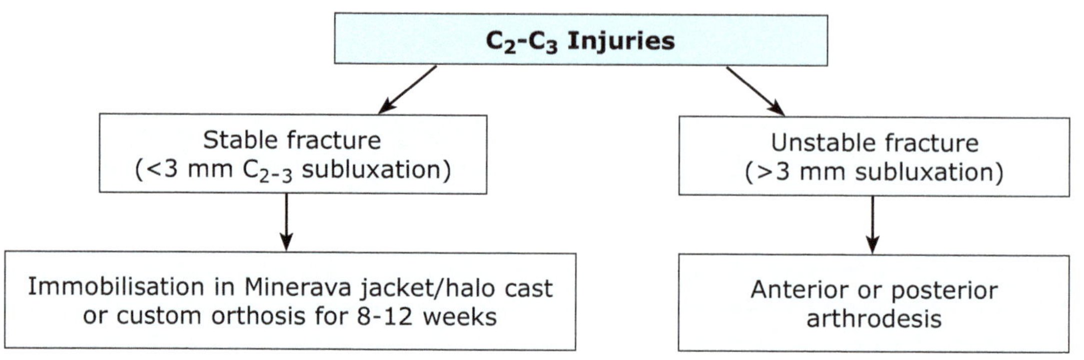

Flowchart 28.6

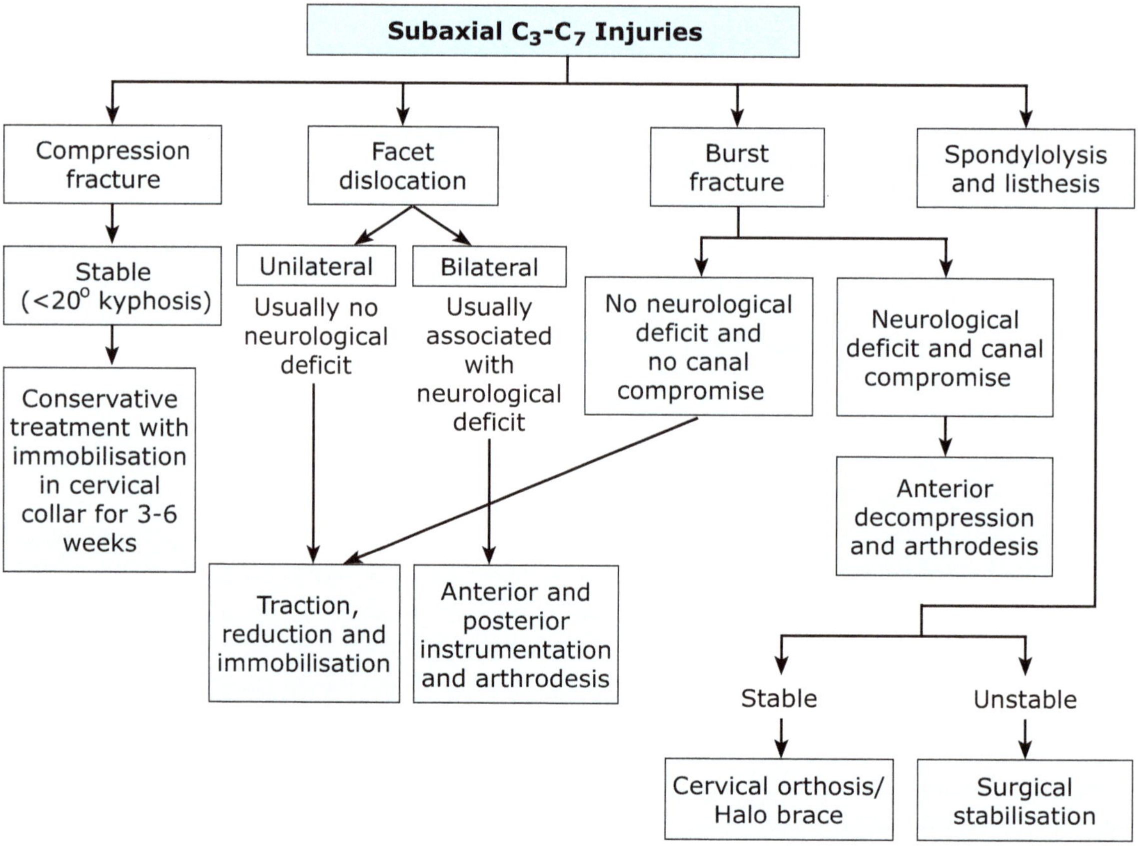

Subaxial C_3-C_7 Injuries
Compression fracture
Facet dislocation
Burst fracture
Spondylolysis and listhesis
Stable ($<20^o$ kyphosis)
Conservative treatment with immobilisation in cervical collar for 3-6 weeks
Unilateral
Usually no neurological deficit
Bilateral
Usually associated with neurological deficit
No neurological deficit and no canal compromise
Neurological deficit and canal compromise
Anterior decompression and arthrodesis
Traction, reduction and immobilisation
Anterior and posterior instrumentation and arthrodesis
Stable
Unstable
Cervical orthosis/ Halo brace
Surgical stabilisation

29 Fractures and Dislocations of the Thoracolumbar Spine

Introduction

- Thoracolumbar spine injuries are relatively uncommon injuries, less frequent than cervical spine injuries. The junction between the stiffer thoracic spine and more flexible lumbar spine is a common site of injury, being the transition zone between two regions with different inherent stability.
- Healing potential of the completely torn posterior ligament complex (PLC) is limited, as against bony fracture which is more likely to heal with resultant stability.
- The spinal cord terminates at L1 or L2 level. Hence injury below L1 level is less likely to be associated with permanent neurological deficit.

  Though less common compared to adults, the potential for recovery of spinal cord function is greater than in adults.

Relevant anatomy

Denis Three-column concept

Denis in 1983 described the three-columns, anterior, middle and posterior, comprising different anatomical components of the vertebral column. The knowledge of these three columns provides the basis for classification and rational approach to the management of thoracolumbar injuries. The exact details of the three columns are described in **Fig. 29.1.** Instability in flexion requires not only rupture of the posterior ligament, but also disruption of the middle column.

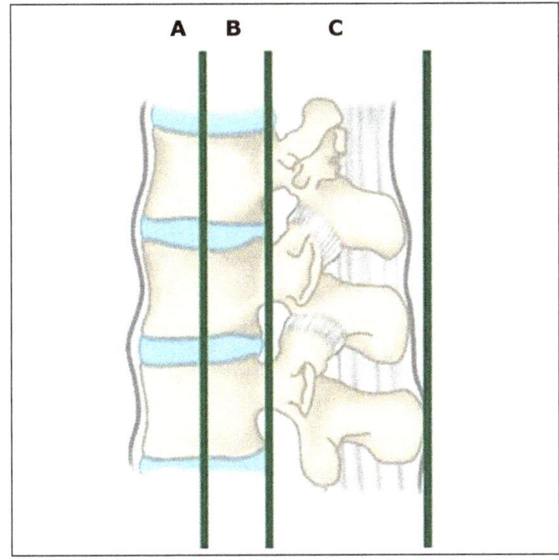

Fig. 29.1*: Denis three-columns:*

A. *Anterior column:*
   Anterior longitudinal ligament
   Anterior annulus fibrosus
   Anterior vertebral body

B. *Middle column:*
   Posterior longitudinal ligament
   Posterior annulus fibrosus
   Posterior vertebral body

C. *Posterior column:*
   Posterior arch
   Posterior ligamentous complex
   (Supraspinous and interspinous ligaments, facet joint capsules, Ligamentum flavum)

Mechanism of injury and Associated injuries

- Motor vehicular accidents, especially 'seat belt' injury is the most common mechanism of flexion distraction type of injury in all age groups. Almost 50% are associated with abdominal injuries and require careful evaluation.

- Fall from height, resulting in axial loading of the spine can lead to wedge compression or burst fracture.
- Pathological fracture after trivial trauma is also common, especially after chronic corticosteroid use for rheumatological/malignant conditions or primary lesions like Langerhans cell histiocytosis, tumours or infections.
- Rarely, unstable fracture dislocation injuries are found in non-accidental trauma.
- Associated head injury and limb injuries are common and require further evaluation.
- All patients with spinal column fracture or dislocation require a careful neurological examination to detect spinal cord injury(SCI). 85% children are neurologically intact and out of rest 15%, 5% have incomplete, whereas 10% have complete SCI. Occasionally, there is SCIWORA (Spinal Cord Injury Without Obvious Radiological Abnormality) due to flexibility of the paediatric spine.
- Neurological injuries are classified as primary or secondary.
- Primary are the result of direct injury to the neural elements and may be caused by contusion, stretch, compression or laceration.

  Contusion injuries are most common and have a poor prognosis for recovery.

  Compression produces injury through direct neuronal damage or secondary by altering vascular perfusion.
- Secondary injuries are the result of ischaemia and are most common in the watershed area of the thoracic spine (T7 to T10).

  Ischaemic injury may be exacerbated by systemic hypotension associated with shock from other traumatic injuries.

Clinical Features

- Thoracolumbar fractures usually result from serious injuries and careful evaluation of ABC (Airway, Breathing and Circulation) should be the first step of clinical assessment. After cardiovascular stabilisation, clinical assessment of pain, site of tenderness, swelling, deformity and ecchymosis should be done. Clinical evaluation of associated injuries (head injury, abdominal injuries) and a complete neurological evaluation is essential. The differentiation between complete and incomplete spinal cord injury and progressive or improving neurological injury are important in decision making regarding surgery.
- A complete injury is defined as the absence of motor and sensory function below the level of SCI.

  Spinal shock should have resolved before classifying the injury as complete or incomplete. Return of bulbocavernosus reflex which usually occurs within 24 hours indicates that S3-4 region of the conus medullaris of the spinal cord is physiologically and anatomically functional and there is resolution of spinal shock.
- Presence of some neurological function below the level of injury defines the injury as incomplete that has better prognosis for recovery.

  Sacral sparing evidenced by perianal sensation, voluntary rectal motor function and great toe flexion may be the only evidence of an incomplete lesion at the time of initial examination.

Imaging

- Plain radiographs AP and lateral views of the entire spine are important for classification and detecting presence of multiple fractures. Loss of vertebral height, widening of interpedicular distance or interspinous distance can give clue to the mechanism of injury and type of fracture. But plain radiographs alone can diagnose fractures in only 70% cases.

- CT scan is 100% sensitive for diagnosis of thoracolumbar fractures. **(Fig. 29.2)** MRI is helpful for evaluation of the disc, spinal cord and posterior ligament complex injuries and can also differentiate between spinal cord haemorrhage and oedema.

Classification

Denis' 5 part classification based on three-column biomechanical concept of spine divides thoracolumbar fracture spine into major and minor, with further subdivision of major injuries into four types. **(Fig. 29.3)**

Major Injuries

1. **Compression fracture:** Stable injury **(Fig. 29.4)**

- Due to axial load with flexion
- Mild wedging of anterior vertebral body
- Posterior vertebral height and posterior cortex intact

2. **Burst fracture:** Stable or unstable

- Due to severe axial compression
- Involvement of both anterior and middle column with loss of height throughout vertebral body
- AP X-ray will show loss of vertebral body height and widened interpedicular distance **(Fig. 29.5)**
- May be associated with retropulsion of posterior aspect of vertebra into spinal canal (best seen on CT scan) with cord

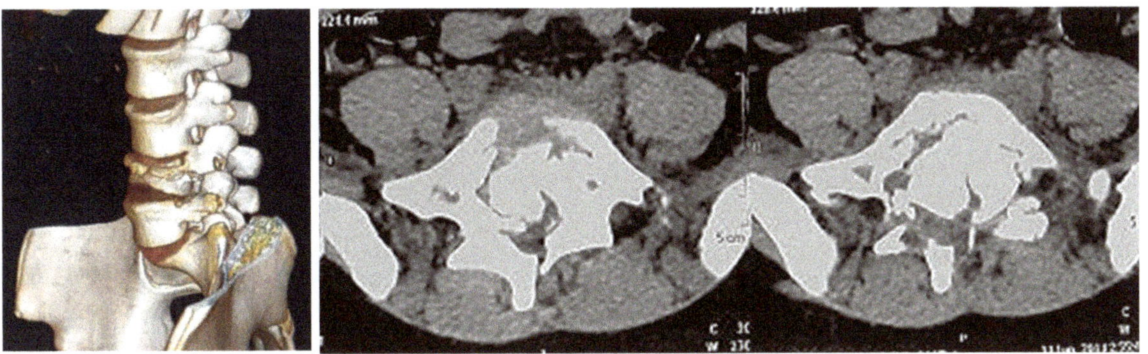

***Fig. 29.2**: 3-D CT scan and axial CT scan showing characteristic pattern of L4 fracture.*

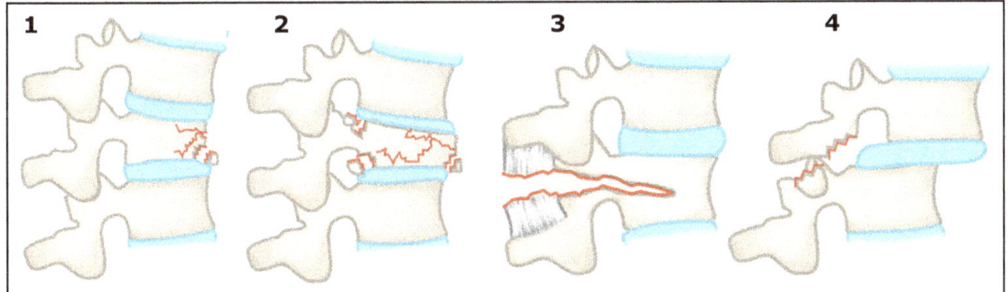

***Fig. 29.3**: Classification of thoracolumbar fractures:*
1. Compression fracture 2. Burst fracture 3. Flexion-Distraction fracture 4. Fracture-Dislocation

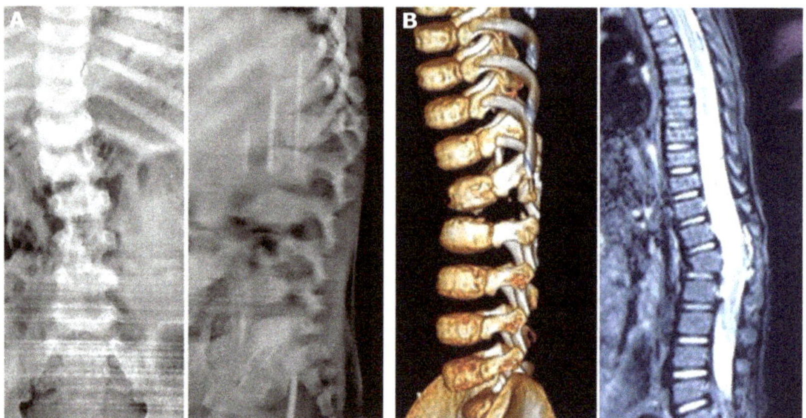

Fig. 29.4: *(A) AP and lateral X-rays (B) 3-D CT scan and MRI dorsolumbar spine showing L1 compression fracture in a 4- year-old child.*

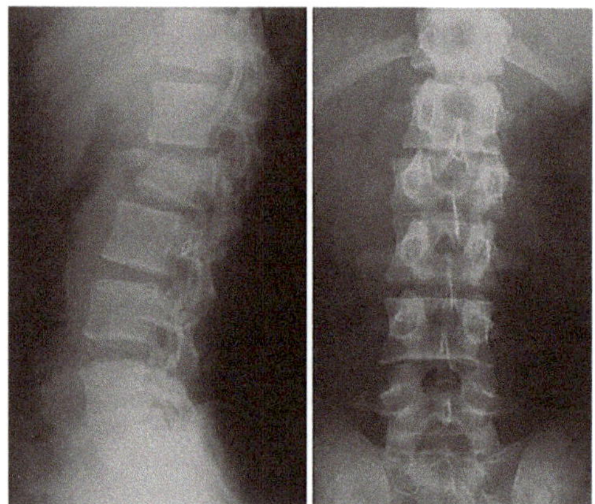

Fig. 29.5: *AP and lateral X-rays of lumbar spine showing L2 burst fracture in a 16-year-old male. Note the loss of height of the anterior and middle columns and widened interpedicular distance.*

compression (best seen on MRI) **(Fig. 29.6)**

- In addition, posterior vertebral fracture or ligament injury may occur

3. **Flexion–Distraction injuries:** Generally Unstable injury

- Common after classic 'seat belt' injury, especially when shoulder strap is lacking.
- Disruption of posterior elements- may occur entirely through bony(chance) or ligamentous elements (Smith).
- Both posterior and middle columns fail in tension and the anterior column

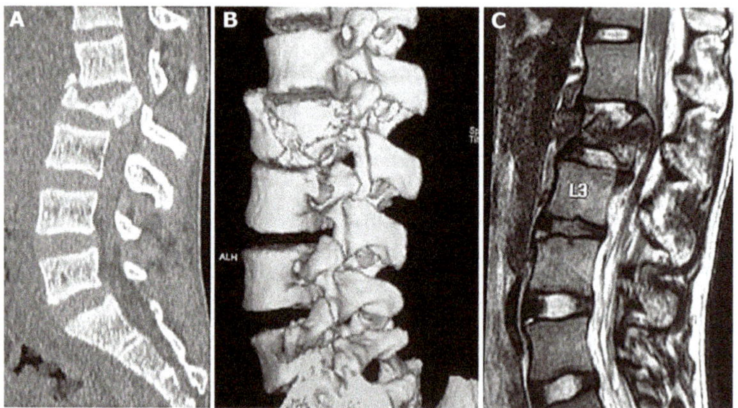

Fig. 29.6: *(A) Sagittal CT scan and (B) 3-D CT scan showing retropulsed fragment of L2 vertebral body and (C) MRI showing cord compression.*

may remain intact or may fail in compression.

- One classic finding is the 'empty facet' sign (when the inferior articular process of the superior vertebra is no longer in contact with the superior articular process of the inferior vertebra, the facet appears empty in the transverse CT image).
- MRI is helpful in diagnosis of PLC injuries.

4. **Fracture – Dislocation:** Unstable three column injury

- Complex injury with severe loading mechanism
- These injuries represent failure of all three columns in compression, tension, rotation or shear
- Translation of one vertebra over another
- Commonly associated with spinal cord injury

Minor Injuries

Fractures of the spinous and transverse processes, facets and pars interarticularis.

Special Injuries

1. Apophyseal injuries

   Flexion injuries in adolescents, where a portion of the posterior corner of the vertebral body (ring apophysis) fractures and displaces into the spinal canal. Clinical presentation is like in disc herniation.

2. SCIWORA

- Injury resulting from spinal cord stretch or vascular disruption/infarction
- MRI is helpful in diagnosis of cord oedema/haemorrhage
- Presence of late/subtle neurological deficit should be looked for.

Treatment

- The goal of treatment is to maximise neurological recovery and to provide stability to the spinal column to protect against future spinal cord injury.
- Patients with minor fractures can be treated symptomatically with a few days of bed rest and bracing for pain relief, followed by gradual return to normal activities.
- In general, $>25^{\circ}$ kyphosis (15° if there is >50% collapse of the anterior vertebral body) or 50% canal compromise is considered as an indication for surgical treatment.

1. Compression fractures

Conservative

- Isolated, stable compression fractures with intact posterior soft tissues and kyphosis $<40^{\circ}$ can be treated conservatively with immobilisation in a thoracolumbosacral orthosis (TLSO) for 4-6 weeks. For fractures proximal to D6, a Minerva brace is used.
- Moulding the brace into slight hyperextension at the fracture site may be beneficial.
- Serial X-rays in the first few weeks are essential to check the sagittal alignment.
- Asymmetric growth at the end plates allows some correction in the wedged alignment over time.

Operative

Compression fractures with $>30\text{-}40^{\circ}$ local kyphosis or fractures with neurological deficit require surgery in the form of posterior fixation and fusion and decompression if required.

2. Burst fractures

Burst fractures can be stable or unstable, based on the degree of comminution, loss of vertebral height, integrity of PLC and degree of kyphosis.

Conservative

A stable burst fracture with intact posterior soft tissues and normal neurological status can be treated in a TLSO or cast in hyperextension for 3 months, if local kyphosis is < 20°.

Operative

- In unstable burst fracture with posterior soft tissue disruption (with intact neurology), posterior instrumentation is preferred. **(Fig. 29.7)**
- Additional anterior decompression is required if canal compromise is > 50% and neurological deficit is present. **(Fig. 29.8)**

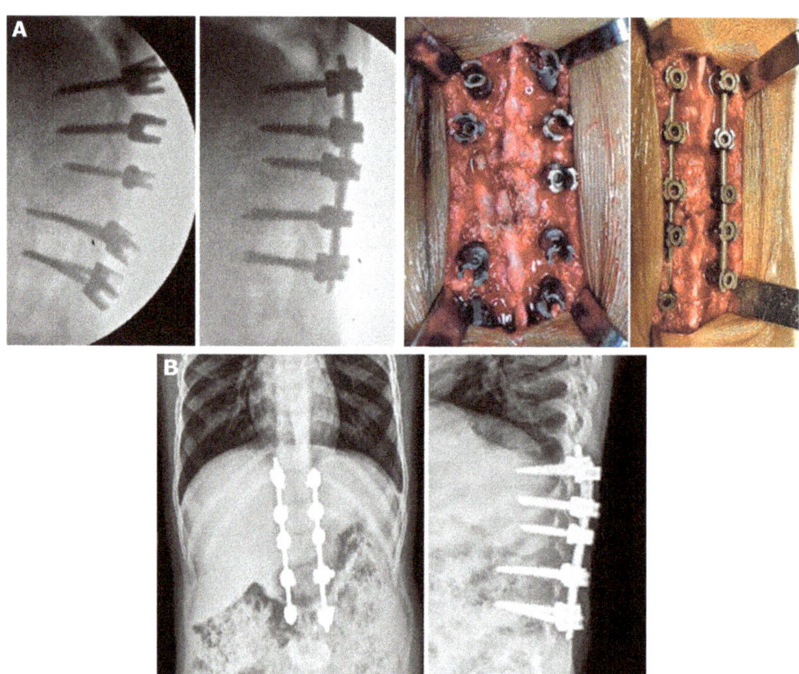

Fig. 29.7: *(A) Intra-operative fluoroscopic and clinical photos and (B) Post-operative X-rays of reduction of L2 burst fracture and posterior instrumentation with pedicular screws and rod fixation from D12 to L4 .*

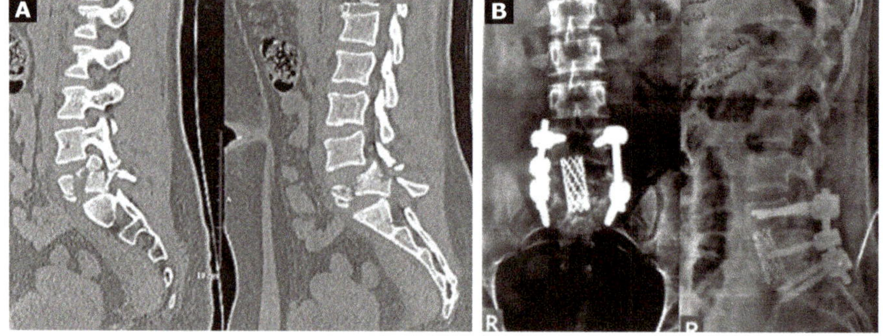

Fig. 29.8: *(A) CT scan showing L5 burst fracture with significant canal compromise leading to neurological deficit. (B) Posterior fixation from L4 to S1 and anterior decompression and fusion with cage and bone graft*

- There is controversy regarding anterior or posterior approach, but usually depends on the surgeon preference and features of the fracture.

3. Flexion – Distraction injuries

Treatment depends on the injury pattern and associated abdominal injuries.

Conservative

A young child (<10 years) with chance fracture, without significant intra-abdominal injury or ligament injury can be treated in hyperextension cast extending upto thigh or TLSO.

Operative

- In children with greater degree of ligament/facet disruption or greater degree of kyphosis, posterior fixation and fusion is recommended.
- Length of fusion is controversial and depends on the age of the child and magnitude and location of injury.
- Restitution of appropriate sagittal balance is the more important factor in the long term prognosis than the length of the fusion.

4. Fracture-Dislocation

These are highly unstable injuries and almost always require surgery in the form of posterior instrumented fusion at least two levels above and below the fracture.

Medical Treatment with Steroids

- The goal is to interrupt the cycle of oedema and ischaemic injury.

Recommendations in presence of neurological involvement (SCI):

- As per NASCIS II criteria (second national acute spinal cord injury study)

If the child is brought

- *Within 3 hours of injury:*

  Bolus of 30 mg/kg methylprednisolone, followed by hourly infusion of 5.4 mg/kg for 24 hours.

- *Between 3 and 8 hours:*

  Infusion of the same dose continues for 48 hours.

- *After 8 hours:*

  No steroid recommended.

Timing and necessity of spinal decompression for SCI remains debated. But early decompression of an incomplete SCI is always beneficial.

Complications

Complications are rare in injuries without neurological deficit:

- Growth arrest and deformity due to end plate damage
- Post-operative complications like infection, loss of correction, pseudoarthrosis or implant related complications

Complications in injuries with neurological deficit:

Acute:

- Pneumonia
- Sepsis
- Autonomic dysreflexia
- Pulmonary embolism

Long term:

- Pulmonary and urologic dysfunction
- Pressure sores
- Scoliosis
- Syringomyelia

Flowchart 29.1

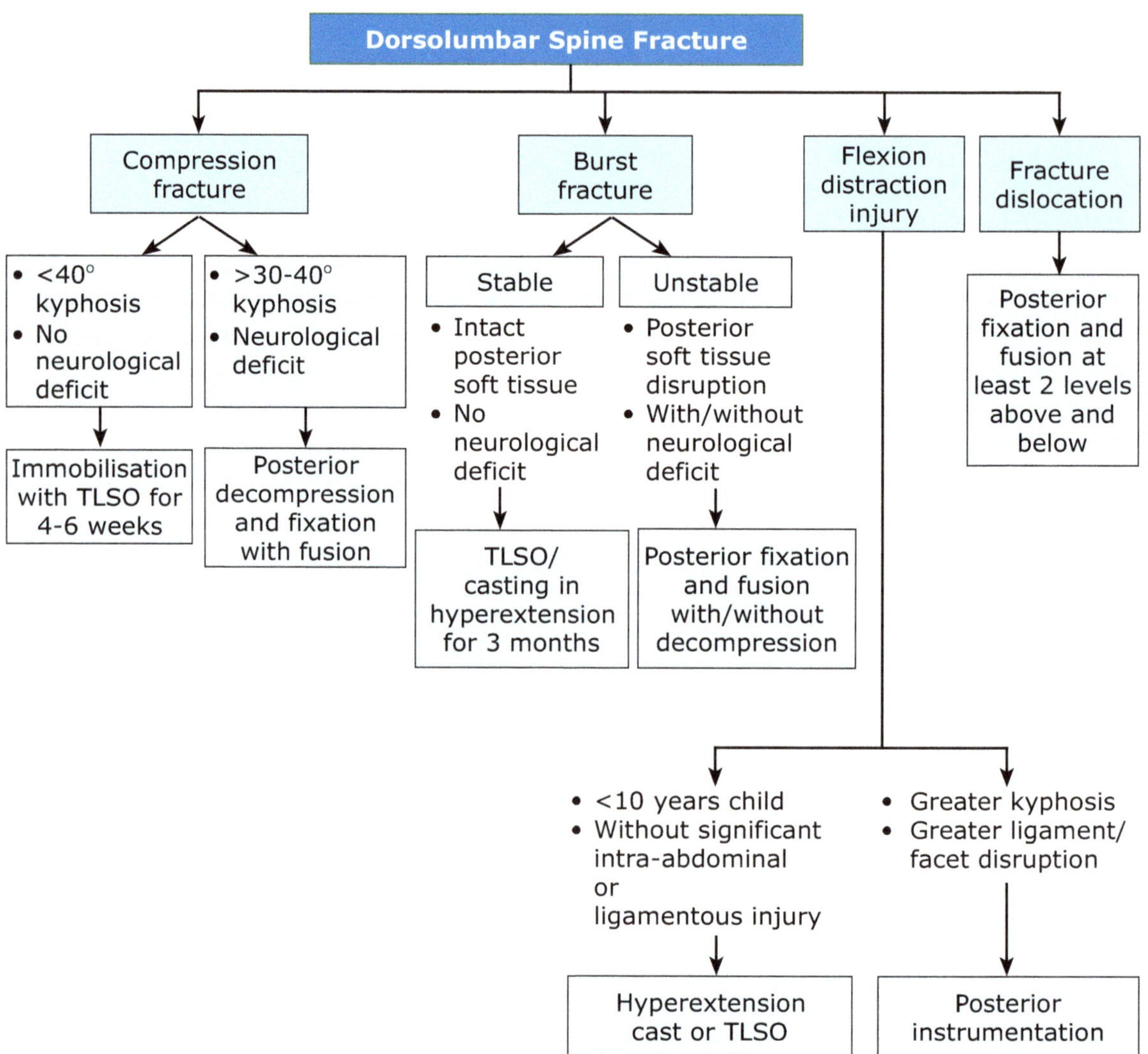

Index

F

G

H

I

J

K

L

M

N

O

P

R

S

www.ingramcontent.com/pod-product-compliance
Ingram Content Group UK Ltd.
Pitfield, Milton Keynes, MK11 3LW, UK
UKHW061952290726
14090UKWH00021B/1186

9 789383 7941